Monitoring in Anesthesia and Perioperative Care

Monitoring in Anesthesia and Perioperative Care is a practical and comprehensive resource documenting the current art and science of perioperative patient monitoring, addressing the systems-based practice issues that drive the highly regulated health care industry of the early 21st century.

Initial chapters cover the history, medicolegal implications, validity of measurement, and education issues relating to monitoring. The core of the book addresses the many monitoring modalities, with the majority of the chapters organized in a systematic fashion to describe technical concepts, parameters monitored, evidence of utility, complications, credentialing and monitoring standards, and practice guidelines.

Describing each device, technique, and principle of clinical monitoring in an accessible style, *Monitoring in Anesthesia and Perioperative Care* is full of valuable advice from the leading experts in the field, making it an essential tool for every anesthesiologist.

David L. Reich, M.D. was named Professor and Chair of Anesthesiology at the Mount Sinai School of Medicine in New York in 2004, where he had been Co-Director of Cardiothoracic Anesthesia since 1990. Dr. Reich's research interests include neurocognitive outcome following thoracic aortic surgery, outcome effects of intraoperative hemodynamics, medical informatics, and hemodynamic monitoring. He has published more than 90 peer-reviewed articles and more than 30 book chapters, and he is an associate editor of the text *Cardiac Anesthesia* and editor-in-chief of *Seminars in Cardiothoracic and Vascular Anesthesia*. He is a member of the International Organization for Terminology in Anesthesia (IOTA) of the Anesthesia Patient Safety Foundation and works with that group, the International Health Terminology Standards Development Organisation (IHTDSO), and High Level Seven International (HL7) to create international standards for anesthesia terminology for electronic patient records.

Ronald A. Kahn, M.D. is Professor of Anesthesiology and Surgery at the Mount Sinai School of Medicine.

Alexander J. C. Mittnacht, M.D. is Associate Professor of Anesthesiology at the Mount Sinai School of Medicine and Director of Pediatric Cardiac Anesthesia at the Mount Sinai Medical Center.

Andrew B. Leibowitz, M.D. is Professor of Anesthesiology and Surgery at the Mount Sinai School of Medicine and Executive Vice Chairman of the Department of Anesthesiology at the Mount Sinai Medical Center.

Marc E. Stone, M.D. is Associate Professor of Anesthesiology at the Mount Sinai School of Medicine and Program Director of the Fellowship in Adult Cardiothoracic Anesthesiology at the Mount Sinai Medical Center.

James B. Eisenkraft, M.D. is Professor of Anesthesiology at the Mount Sinai School of Medicine and Attending Anesthesiologist at the Mount Sinai Medical Center.

Monitoring in Anesthesia and Perioperative Care

Editor

David L. Reich
Mount Sinai School of Medicine

Coeditors

Ronald A. Kahn
Mount Sinai School of Medicine

Alexander J. C. Mittnacht
Mount Sinai School of Medicine

Andrew B. Leibowitz
Mount Sinai School of Medicine

Marc E. Stone
Mount Sinai School of Medicine

James B. Eisenkraft
Mount Sinai School of Medicine

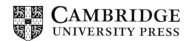

CAMBRIDGE
UNIVERSITY PRESS

CAMBRIDGE UNIVERSITY PRESS
Cambridge, New York, Melbourne, Madrid, Cape Town,
Singapore, São Paulo, Delhi, Tokyo, Mexico City

Cambridge University Press
32 Avenue of the Americas, New York, NY 10013-2473, USA

www.cambridge.org
Information on this title: www.cambridge.org/9780521755986

First published 2011

Printed in the United States of America

A catalog record for this publication is available from the British Library.

Library of Congress Cataloging in Publication data

Monitoring in anesthesia and perioperative care / [edited by] David L.
Reich, Ronald A. Kahn, Alexander J. C. Mittnacht, Andrew B.
Leibowitz, Marc E. Stone, James B. Eisenkraft.
   p.;   cm.
Includes bibliographical references and index.
ISBN 978-0-521-75598-6 (hardback)
1. Anesthesia.   2. Patient monitoring.   I. Reich, David L.
(David Louis), 1960– , editor.   II. Kahn, Ronald A., editor.
III. Mittnacht, Alexander J. C., editor.   IV. Leibowitz, Andrew B.,
editor.   V. Stone, Marc E., editor.   VI. Eisenkraft, James B., editor.
[DNLM: 1. Monitoring, Intraoperative – methods.   2. Anesthesia –
methods.   3. Perioperative Care – methods.   WO 181]
RD82.M68   2011
617.9′6–dc22   2010045695

ISBN 978-0-521-75598-6 Hardback

Contents

Contributors

Eric Adler, M.D.
Assistant Professor
Department of Cardiology
Mount Sinai School of Medicine
New York, NY

Anoushka Afonso, M.D.
Anesthesia Resident
Department of Anesthesiology
Mount Sinai School of Medicine
New York, NY

Dean B. Andropoulos, M.D., M.H.C.M.
Chief of Anesthesiology
Texas Children's Hospital
Professor, Anesthesiology and Pediatrics
Baylor College of Medicine
Houston, TX

Adel Bassily-Marcus, M.D.
Assistant Professor
Department of Surgery
Division of Critical Care Medicine
Mount Sinai School of Medicine
New York, NY

Yaakov Beilin, M.D.
Professor
Department of Anesthesiology
Department of Obstetrics, Gynecology, and Reproductive
   Science
Mount Sinai School of Medicine
New York, NY

Elliott Bennett-Guerrero, M.D.
Professor and Director of Perioperative Clinical Research
Duke Clinical Research Institute
Duke University Medical Center
Durham, NC

Howard H. Bernstein, M.D.
Associate Professor
Department of Anesthesiology
Mount Sinai School of Medicine
New York, NY

Marc J. Bloom, M.D., Ph.D.
Associate Professor of Anesthesiology
New York University School of Medicine
New York, NY

David Bronheim, M.D.
Associate Professor
Department of Anesthesiology
Mount Sinai School of Medicine
New York, NY

Albert T. Cheung, M.D.
Professor
Department of Anesthesiology and Critical
   Care
University of Pennsylvania School of Medicine
Philadelphia, PA

Samuel DeMaria, Jr., M.D.
Instructor in Anesthesiology
Department of Anesthesiology
Mount Sinai School of Medicine
New York, NY

Deborah Dubensky, M.D.
Department of Anesthesiology
University of Rochester Medical Center
Rochester, NY

James B. Eisenkraft, M.D.
Professor
Department of Anesthesiology
Mount Sinai School of Medicine
New York, NY

Jonathan Elmer, M.D.
Clinical Fellow
Department of Emergency Medicine
Brigham and Women's Hospital
Boston, MA

Liza J. Enriquez, M.D.
Fellow
Department of Anesthesiology
Montefiore Medical Center
Bronx, NY

Jonathan Epstein, M.D., M.A.
Attending Anesthesiologist
St. Luke's–Roosevelt Hospital Center
New York, NY

Jeffrey M. Feldman, M.D., M.S.E.
Associate Professor of Clinical Anesthesiology
Department of Anesthesiology and Critical Care
    Medicine
University of Pennsylvania School of Medicine
Division Chief, General Anesthesia
Children's Hospital of Philadelphia
Philadelphia, PA

Gregory W. Fischer, M.D.
Associate Professor of Anesthesiology and Cardiothoracic
    Surgery
Director of Adult Cardiothoracic Anesthesia
Mount Sinai School of Medicine
New York, NY

Brigid Flynn, M.D.
Assistant Professor
Department of Anesthesiology
Mount Sinai School of Medicine
New York, NY

Jennifer A. Frontera, M.D.
Assistant Professor
Departments of Neurology and Neurosurgery
Mount Sinai School of Medicine
New York, NY

Richard S. Gist, M.D.
Professor
Department of Anesthesiology
Mount Sinai School of Medicine
New York, NY

Glenn P. Gravlee, M.D.
Professor
Department of Anesthesiology
University of Colorado Denver
Aurora, CO

Christina L. Jeng, M.D.
Assistant Professor of Anesthesiology and Orthopaedics
Department of Anesthesiology
Mount Sinai School of Medicine
New York, NY

Ronald A. Kahn, M.D.
Professor of Anesthesiology
Department of Anesthesiology
Mount Sinai School of Medicine
New York, NY

Jenny Kam, M.D.
Chief Resident
Department of Anesthesiology

Mukul Kapoor, M.D.
Senior Adviser
Anaethesiology and Cardiothoracic Anaesthesiology
Command Hospital
Lucknkow, India

Jung Kim, M.D.
Department of Anesthesiology
St. Luke's–Roosevelt Hospital Center
New York, NY

Roopa Kohli-Seth, M.D.
Assistant Professor
Department of Surgery
Division of Critical Care Medicine
Mount Sinai School of Medicine
New York, NY

Aaron F. Kopman, M.D.
Professor of Clinical Anesthesiology
Weill Cornell Medical College
New York, NY

Tuula S. O. Kurki, M.D., Ph.D.
Head of the Preoperative Clinic
Department of Anesthesia and Intensive Care
Helsinki University Central Hospital
Helsinki, Finland

Andrew B. Leibowitz, M.D.
Professor of Anesthesiology and Surgery
Department of Anesthesiology
Mount Sinai School of Medicine
New York, NY

Matthew Levin, M.D.
Mount Sinai School of Medicine
New York, NY

Adam I. Levine, M.D.
Associate Professor
Department of Anesthesiology
Mount Sinai School of Medicine
New York, NY

Michael S. Lewis, M.D.
Director of Transfusion Medicine and Histology
Assistant Professor of Pathology
University of Southern California, Keck School of Medicine
Attending Pathologist
West Los Angeles VA Hospital
Mount Sinai School of Medicine
Los Angeles, CA

Justin Lipper, M.D.
Mount Sinai School of Medicine
New York, NY

Martin London, M.D.
Professor of Clinical Anesthesia
University of California, San Francisco
San Francisco, CA

Michael L. McGarvey, M.D.
Assistant Professor
Department of Neurology
University of Pennsylvania
Philadelphia, PA

Alexander J. C. Mittnacht, M.D.
Associate Professor
Department of Anesthesiology
Mount Sinai School of Medicine
New York, NY

Timothy Mooney, MD
Fellow
Duke University Medical Center
Durham, NC

Diana Mungall, B.S.
Department of Anesthesiology
Mount Sinai School of Medicine
New York, NY

Yasuharu Okuda, M.D.
Associate Clinical Professor
Department of Emergency Medicine
Mount Sinai School of Medicine
New York, NY

Peter J. Papadakos, M.D., F.C.C.M.
Professor of Anesthesiology, Surgery, and Neurosurgery
Director, Division of Critical Care Medicine
University of Rochester
Rochester, NY

Jayashree Raikhelkar, M.D.
Assistant Professor
Departments of Anesthesiology and Cardiothoracic Surgery
Mount Sinai School of Medicine
New York, NY

Lakshmi V. Ramanathan, Ph.D.
Assistant Professor
Department of Pathology
Mount Sinai School of Medicine
Director, Chemistry, Endocrinology, Stat Lab, and Point of Care Testing
Mount Sinai Medical Center
New York, NY

David L. Reich, M.D.
Professor and Chair of Anesthesiology

Department of Anesthesiology
Mount Sinai School of Medicine
New York, NY

Meg A. Rosenblatt, M.D.
Professor
Department of Anesthesiology
Mount Sinai School of Medicine
New York, NY

Corey Scurlock
Assistant Professor
Departments of Anesthesiology and Cardiothoracic Surgery
Mount Sinai School of Medicine
New York, NY

Tamas Seres, Ph.D.
Associate Professor
Department of Anesthesiology
University of Colorado Denver
Aurora, CO

Linda Shore-Lesserson, M.D.
Professor of Anesthesiology
Montefiore Medical Center
Bronx, NY

Marc E. Stone, M.D.
Associate Professor
Department of Anesthesiology
Mount Sinai School of Medicine
New York, NY

Daniel M. Thys, M.D.
Chairman Emeritus
Department of Anesthesiology
St. Luke's–Roosevelt Hospital Center
New York, NY

Judit Tolnai, B.S.
Department of Pathology
Mount Sinai School of Medicine
New York, NY

David Wax, M.D.
Assistant Professor
Department of Anesthesiology
Mount Sinai School of Medicine
New York, NY

Nathaen Weitzel, M.D.
Assistant Professor
Department of Anesthesiology
University of Colorado Denver
Aurora, CO

Foreword

Carol L. Lake

Training and practicing the specialty of anesthesiology, and specifically cardiac anesthesia, during the last three decades of the 20th century provides a unique perspective from which to address the state of clinical monitoring for health care. The advent and growth of sophisticated physiologic monitoring clearly advanced the anesthesiology subspecialty of cardiac anesthesia, and vice versa. Likewise, it seems especially prudent that Dr. David L. Reich, a cardiac anesthesiologist, and many of the chapter authors, represent the subspecialty of cardiac anesthesia.

From using a manual blood pressure cuff, precordial stethoscope, and a finger on the pulse to the current American Society of Anesthesiologists standards of monitoring the patient's oxygenation, ventilation, circulation, and temperature continually (usually with pulse oximetry, electrocardiogram, end-tidal carbon dioxide, temperature, inspired/expired anesthetic gases, and automated blood pressure cuff during general anesthesia) was the great leap forward in perioperative monitoring in the 20th century. Similarly, the plethora of devices developed during the past century to allow monitoring of depth of anesthesia, respiratory compliance, ventricular contractility, coagulation, tissue oxygenation, and blood flow, rather than only basic cardiovascular parameters such as heart rate and blood pressure, is truly amazing progress. The past and present of physiologic monitoring are represented in the history chapter and the chapters on equipment, procedures, techniques, and technologies, respectively, in this book. Unfortunately, at the present time, many of the critical incidents during anesthesia still result from inadequate or incomplete monitoring of the patient, the anesthesia machine, or the patient–machine interface.

What is the future for monitoring in health care in general and anesthesiology, critical care, and pain management in particular? With the miraculous advances in clinical monitoring have come associated challenges that are addressed in this book. How can information overload from monitors be minimized? How are trainees educated and trained in multiple monitoring techniques? How can practitioners beyond training maintain their skills with infrequently used, complex monitors? How will future anesthesiologists and intensivists know whether a new device or monitoring technique is useful and reliable? Has a cost–benefit analysis of a specific monitor demonstrated effectiveness? Similar demanding questions need to be answered. Finally, is the ongoing research to develop new devices or techniques to monitor parameters currently judged difficult to assess, such as intraoperative, global cerebral or renal function, being adequately supported? Dr. Reich and his many distinguished contributing authors provide a comprehensive practical review of these questions while preparing the reader to confront these future monitoring challenges.

Information overload occurs when there are many parameters to observe, necessitating the provision of alarm systems, set to indicate when a particular parameter or device is outside set limits. However, these same alarms do not always indicate true life-threatening emergencies. Attending to false alarms adds to the workload and encourages ignoring them, obviously to the detriment of the patient if the alarm is not false. Ways to prioritize and display alarms, and to prevent unnecessary alarms, will continue to be the subject of research until user-friendly, ergonomic, common anesthesia workstations exist.

Reliance on alarms may also encourage inattention by the person providing anesthesia or critical care. Although a recent single-institution study demonstrated that intraoperative reading and nonpatient-related conversation did not adversely affect recognition of a randomly illuminated alarm light (Slagle JM, Weinger MB. Effects of intraoperative reading on vigilance and workload during anesthesia care in an academic medical center. *Anesthesiology* 2009;110:275–283), recognizing an impending disaster *before* the alarm sounds may save precious seconds, and those seconds count if you or your loved one is the anesthetized or critically ill patient.

The training, retraining, and ongoing evaluation of competence of the anesthesia team to use complex and sophisticated monitoring devices remains an educational conundrum. Although textbooks and lectures continue to be the mainstay of health care educational material, interactive computer programs; standardized patients; part-task trainers; human patient simulators mimicking neonates, children, and adults; and realistic simulation laboratories configured to be operating rooms, intensive care units, emergency departments, or patient rooms appear likely to become the major training and examination venues in the 21st century. A simulation laboratory is an ideal environment to learn to use monitoring devices and techniques and is particularly applicable to demonstration of competence with monitoring techniques.

Are there hazards to the extensive use of monitoring? Possibly. Could the increased technology of monitoring occur at the expense of clinical acumen? We have already seen that over-reliance on monitors leads to both amusing and deleterious situations, such as the pronouncement of ventricular fibrillation by a new anesthesiology resident when an electrocardiograph lead falls off the patient or the inability to assess anesthetized patient well-being when electrical power is interrupted in a developing country or following a disaster. Could sophisticated 21st-century perioperative monitoring expose the specialty of anesthesiology to eventual substitution by robots with artificial intelligence? Probably not, because the monitors still lack the completeness, continuousness, and adaptability to human natural variation in perioperative situations.

Despite all the extensive and sophisticated devices and techniques described in this book, there is nothing at present that can replace the vigilance of a professional anesthesia or intensive care team providing the human-to-human interaction essential to patient safety and well-being in operating rooms, intensive care units, or the myriad venues in which patients receive general anesthesia or its equivalents. As Dr. Reich's book aptly illustrates, 21st-century monitoring for anesthesiology, pain management, and critical care must focus on striking the optimal balance among such factors as patient safety, cost, clinical outcomes, innovation, and complexity. However, the patient, not the monitor, must always come first!

Preface

Monitoring in Anesthesia and Perioperative Care follows the tradition of previous texts that document the current art and science of perioperative patient monitoring. Additionally, the text addresses the systems-based practice issues that drive the highly regulated health care industry of the early 21st century. The initial chapters cover the concepts of history, medicolegal implications, validity of measurement, and education. The core of the book addresses the many monitoring modalities. To the extent possible, each chapter is organized in a systematic fashion to describe:

1. **Technical concepts**: How does it work?
2. **Parameters monitored**: What information do you get from it?
3. **Evidence of utility**: Is there evidence that it makes a difference in outcome?
4. **Complications**: What harm can it cause?
5. **Credentialing and monitoring standards**: What is the educational or credentialing process, if any?
6. **Practice guidelines**: When should/must I use it?

Ultrasonic guidance of invasive catheterization and regional anesthesia are included as monitoring concepts. The next group of chapters addresses scales and assessments that are increasingly evidence-based documentation standards. Finally, electronic health records, alarm systems, and automated medication delivery systems complete the body of the text. A table in the appendix is intended to help residents and other anesthesia care providers know the typical monitoring modalities that are chosen for major categories of operations.

The target audience for this text is medical students, anesthesia residents, Fellows, nurse anesthetists, anesthesia assistants, and anesthesia and critical care practitioners who are acquiring or updating their knowledge of patient monitoring during anesthesia and the perioperative period. There is significant overlap with critical care monitoring, and the intensive care physician will find nearly all concepts of critical care monitoring to be covered.

Patient monitoring in anesthesia and perioperative care has changed drastically since the specialty of anesthesiology emerged in the 19th century. The pace of that change has accelerated in recent decades as one sees in the preceding texts on the subject, which are snapshots of the monitoring practices of their eras. The earliest of those texts that I located illustrated an important juncture in the art and science of patient monitoring. In these two quotes from the preface of Dornette and Brechner's *Instrumentation in Anesthesiology* (Philadelphia: Lea & Febiger, 1959), we see the point in anesthesia history at which the emphasis shifted from direct patient observation to reliance on mechanical instrumentation:

> [The anesthesiologist] feels the pulse and rebreathing bag to determine rate, rhythm and volume of the pulse waves and respiratory efforts. He sees the eye signs and thoracic excursions to assess depth of anesthesia. He hears the sound generated by compression of the brachial artery during auscultation of the blood pressure. He smells the anesthetic atmosphere to determine the approximate concentration of ether or cyclopropane. He tastes the fluid dripping from the epidural needle to differentiate bitter procaine from tasteless cerebrospinal fluid.

> [Instrumentation] increases the perceptibility of our senses, and also allows the study of physiologic signals not capable of being detected by these senses.

The monitoring texts in more recent years, including those edited by Lake, Saidman and Smith, Blitt and Hines, Gravenstein and colleagues, and Dorsch and Dorsch, have chronicled these continuing changes in both instrumentation and standards. Their erudition and eloquence set a high standard. The current publication is intended to continue the tradition of anesthesiologists as the leaders in patient monitoring education and standards creation.

David L. Reich, M.D.
Professor and Chair
Department of Anesthesiology
Mount Sinai School of Medicine
New York, NY

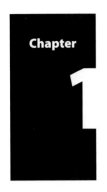

Chapter

1

The history of anesthesia and perioperative monitoring

David L. Reich

Introduction

The discoveries that facilitated patient monitoring in the perioperative period occurred long before the introduction of clinical anesthesia. Respiratory patterns had been described since antiquity. The rise of scientific methods in Renaissance Europe led to the initial experiments in hemodynamics – specifically, animal experiments demonstrating that blood flows under pressure. The earliest source that cited correct observations of arterial and venous flow and pressures was William Harvey's *De Motu Cordis*, published in 1628.[1] In the following century, Stephen Hales offered the first quantification of arterial blood pressure measured in the horse.[2] The first cardiac catheterization was performed by Claude Bernard in 1844.[3]

Soon after the introduction of clinical general anesthesia by W. T. G. Morton in 1846 and John Snow in 1847, the need to monitor patients was recognized by the leaders of the new specialty. The first documented death under chloroform anesthesia (that of fifteen-year-old Hannah Greener in 1848) led the early practitioners to highlight the importance of monitoring simple vital signs – respiration, pulse, and skin color. Since that time, patient safety concerns have invariably driven the development of monitoring modalities and standards in perioperative monitoring practice. This chapter recounts important milestones of perioperative patient monitoring and the historical events and clinical developments that influenced them.

Early advocacy of monitoring the pulse and respiration

As news of the Boston public demonstration reached London late in 1846, John Snow, M.D. personally adopted the technique, publishing his series of eighty anesthetized patients, ranging in age from children to octogenarians, in *Inhalation of the Vapour of Ether in Surgical Operations*. He mentioned the customary monitoring under anesthesia to include respiration depth and frequency, muscle movements, skin color, and stages of excitation or sedation. Although the pulse was continually palpated, its characteristics were not considered worth studying.[4] By 1855, the Edinburgh surgeon James Syme, M.D., lectured on the importance of monitoring respiration

and explained in his surgical lectures that, in his opinion, chloroform was safer than ether anesthesia if it was administered properly. The key, however, to proper administration was monitoring the patient's respiration.[5]

Joseph Lister, M.D., the founder of the principles of antisepsis in surgery, was an eminent surgeon in Scotland and the United Kingdom from the 1850s through the 1890s. He protested against palpation of the pulse as "a most serious mistake. As a general rule, the safety of the patient will be most promoted by disregarding it altogether, so that the attention may be devoted exclusively to the breathing."[6] Dr. Lister's instruction to the senior students who served as his anesthetists was "that they strictly carry out certain simple instructions, among which is that of never touching the pulse, in order that their attention may not be distracted from the respiration." His airway management strategy included "the drawing out of the tongue" and he believed that the services of special anesthetists were unnecessary if simple routines were followed by his assistants while administering chloroform.

Joseph Thomas Clover, M.D., was the leading clinical anesthetist in Victorian England during his professional life, from the beginning of his anesthesia practice in 1846 until his death in 1882. In 1864, the Royal Medico-Chirurgical Society established a committee to investigate chloroform fatalities, and as an expert assistant to that group, Dr. Clover described his innovations in apparatus and animal experimentation with anesthetics. He strongly advised that the pulse be continuously observed during an anesthetic and that irregularities such as a diminution should alert the anesthetist to discontinue the anesthetic. He also advised monitoring the pulse continuously while administering an anesthetic. "If the finger be taken from the pulse to do something else, I would give a little air."[7] James Young Simpson, M.D., also voiced caution during the administration of chloroform when snoring ensued and the pulse became "languid."[8]

With continuing deaths associated with chloroform use, a group led by Edward Lawrie formed a commission in Hyderabad, India to investigate causes. In 1888, the first commission report asserted the safety of chloroform anesthesia.[9] In 1889, the Second Hyderabad Chloroform Commission concluded that chloroform deaths were related to respiratory depression and not a directly injurious effect on the heart. The commission reported that anesthetists should be guided entirely by respiration, as pupil size and pulse were not significant enough to monitor.[10,11]

Auscultation of heart tones

The earliest clinical account of auscultation in the operating room was reported in 1896 by Robert Kirk, M.D., of the Glasgow Western Infirmary. An ordinary binaural stethoscope lengthened by Indian rubber tubing was first used. Later, 200 patients anesthetized with chloroform were auscultated using a "phonendoscope" with timing of heart rate and rhythm by a watch.[12] Dr. Kirk was involved at the time with the Glasgow Committee on Anesthetic Agents and saw the stethoscope as a clinical research tool to assess the effects of chloroform on cardiac physiology.

Charles K. Teter, D.D.S., described the benefits of using a stethoscope during anesthesia, especially in poor-risk patients.[13] He praised the convenience of the flat Kehler stethoscope, which "will usually stay without being held" on the precordium. When necessary, adhesive tape prevented its being dislodged. Dr. Teter praised the stethoscope because "uninterrupted information will be given to any and all change[s] in the heart beat and respiration." He expressed his feeling of confidence when "every variation of heart sound is at once discernable, and what might be serious complications can be averted by the premonitory symptoms thus made manifest."[13]

The strong advocacy of routine, continuous monitoring of cardiac and respiratory sounds under anesthesia by Harvey Cushing, M.D., gave impetus to the widespread clinical use of intraoperative auscultation[14] (see Figure 1.1). An esophageal stethoscope was described in 1893 by Solis-Cohen[15] for diagnostic purposes, but it was not adopted as a routine monitoring technique until nearly seventy-five years later.

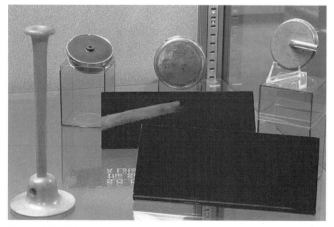

Figure 1.1. Early stethoscopes used for intraoperative monitoring are displayed. (Courtesy of the Wood Library-Museum of Anesthesiology, Park Ridge, IL)

The anesthesia record

Once the idea that monitoring patients under anesthesia was clinically useful and early tools were developed to do so, the anesthetic record could not be far behind. B. Raymond Fink, M.D., credits the first anesthetic record to A. E. Codman, M.D., at the Massachusetts General Hospital in 1894[16] (Figure 1.2). Dr. Codman's chief, F. B. Harrigan, M.D., recommended recording the patient's pulse during an anesthetic. This practice was encouraged by Dr. Cushing, who published a classic paper in 1902 reproducing an actual patient's anesthetic record.[17] Dr. Cushing's initiatives were not accepted easily, and opponents to the newer devices to measure temperature, pulse, blood pressure, and the auscultation of the heart were castigated by an editorial in the *British Medical Journal* claiming that "by such methods we pauperize our senses and weaken clinical acuity."[18]

Indirect measurement of arterial blood pressure

In 1901, during a visit to Italy, Harvey Cushing met Scipione Riva-Rocci, who, a few years earlier, had developed a practical sphygmomanometer for measuring blood pressure indirectly.[19] Subsequently, Cushing recommended the routine use of this sphygmomanometer to determine blood pressure during anesthesia.[20] Because the return-to-flow method was employed by palpation of the radial pulse, only the systolic pressure could be determined. Furthermore, this was inaccurate, as the cuff used was a bicycle inner tube, which gave excessively high values owing to the ratio of the region of compression to arm circumference. At that time, however, normal values for systolic blood pressure were unknown and the instrument provided the first clinical example of following trends of blood pressure change during surgery.

In 1905, Korotkoff described the sounds heard when flow occurs distal to the deflating cuff.[21] This, together with the use of a wider cuff advocated by von Recklinghausen,[22] allowed more accurate determination of blood pressure and is the basis of current auscultatory blood pressure monitoring. Further advances in the indirect measurement of blood pressure largely involved the development of alternative means of "sensing" systolic and diastolic points and automating the process.

In 1931, von Recklinghausen[23] described a semiautomated device for measuring blood pressure, known as an oscillotonometer. A double-cuff system was used, with the proximal cuff occluding the artery and the distal cuff acting as the sensor to detect the onset of arterial pulsations. The introduction of ultrasound into clinical medicine in the 1940s allowed the application of the Doppler principle to detect blood flow[24] and movement of the arterial wall under the distal edge of the sphygmomanometer cuff.[25] The Arteriosonde (Roche) used ultrasound at 3 mHz that reflected off the vibrating arterial wall, which the practitioner heard as an electronically conditioned audible signal. The device was accurate and found its greatest application for measurement of blood pressure in infants.[26] The

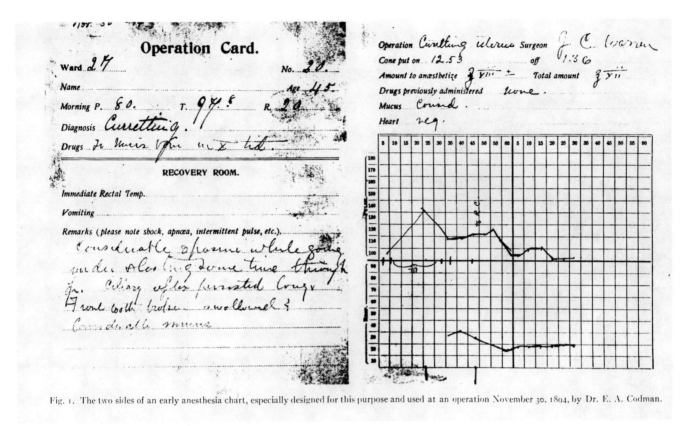

Figure 1.2. One of the first known anesthesia records is reproduced. (Courtesy of the Wood Library-Museum of Anesthesiology, Park Ridge, IL)

desire for more automated and rapid acquisition of noninvasive blood pressure led to the development of automated devices has allowed frequent estimation of indirect blood pressure. The first wide commercial success was the Dinamap (Critikon), which essentially was an automated oscillotonometer. The instrument was simple to use and produced accurate results.[27]

Eye signs of anesthesia depth

Although Snow and other early leaders of the specialty described the monitoring of depth of anesthesia, the individual given greatest credit for standardizing the process was Arthur Guedel, M.D. The eye signs of ether anesthesia were the most significant contribution to his schematic approach to identifying signs of anesthesia.[28] The eye signs included the activity of motor muscles of the eyeball, pupillary dilation, and, later, the eyelid reflex. The eyelid reflex was tested by gently raising the upper eyelid with the finger. If the reflex was present, the eyelid would attempt to close at once or within a few seconds. The corneal and eyelash reflexes known today were not mentioned.[29]

The setting for these contributions was the complete lack of trained anesthesia specialists when the United States entered World War I.[30] Dr. Guedel experienced a crush of casualties from a major battle, where his staff of three physicians and one dentist ran as many as forty operating room tables at a time. He concluded that additional anesthesia care providers would have to be trained quickly to meet this overwhelming need and created a school that trained physicians, nurses, and orderlies in open-drop ether.[29] He prepared a chart of his version of the signs and stages of ether anesthesia, the most common agent in use at the time because of its wide margin of safety (Figure 1.3). Armed with their charts, the trainees went out to nearby hospitals to work on their own, as Dr. Guedel made weekly motorcycle rounds to check on his trainees at the six hospitals for which he was responsible.[30]

Direct measurement of arterial blood pressure

Poiseuille, in 1828, described the mercury manometer.[31] In 1847, Karl Ludwig made use of Poiseuille's device and applied it to his invention of the kymograph.[32] A column of mercury on the kymograph moved, and thus directed a floating needle against a moving drum. This device allowed animal hemodynamic physiology to be recorded continuously for research purposes. The application to humans, however, was limited by problems of vascular access and control of bleeding and infection. Almost one century later, direct recording of arterial blood pressure continued to be difficult, even though problems of sepsis and coagulation were solved.

The discovery of plastic "nonthrombogenic" sterile tubing and its medical applications occurred in 1945–46. In 1949, Lyle Peterson and Robert Dripps described the technique of percutaneous placement of a plastic catheter for continuous measurement of arterial blood pressure during anesthesia and surgery.[33]

3

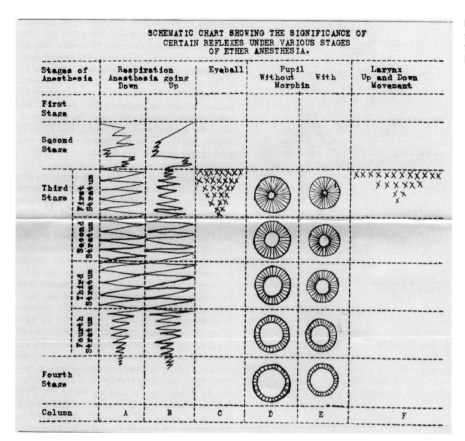

Figure 1.3. One version of Guedel's chart demonstrating stages of ether anesthesia. (Courtesy of the Wood Library-Museum of Anesthesiology, Park Ridge, IL)

The value of this measurement was widely recognized, but the technique remained unpopular. The recording equipment was impractical and too expensive.

The technique of surgical cut-down was used to gain access to peripheral arteries during cardiac surgery in the 1950s. In 1960, the catheter-over-the-needle technique was introduced, and the wide medical application of polytetrafluoroethylene (PTFE; Teflon, Dupont, Inc.) Teflon made possible convenient percutaneous access, leading to easier and smoother percutaneous placement of cannulae for continuous monitoring of arterial blood pressure by surgeons, anesthesiologists, and intensive care specialists. Simultaneous technological advances in pressure transducers, continuous flush systems, and transistor-based display and recording equipment made invasive arterial monitoring commonplace.

The electrocardiogram in the operating room

In 1918, Heard and Strauss[34] reported two cases of atrioventricular rhythm, one of which occurred immediately following ether anesthesia. They reported that "no other cases of nodal rhythm have been observed by us in a series of 21 cases in which electrocardiographic records have been taken during anesthesia." No further details were given. Levine[35] reported two cases of paroxysmal atrial tachycardia under ether anesthesia, documented by electrocardiography.

The first prospective study of the practical use of the electrocardiograph (ECG) for monitoring patients in the operating room was reported in 1922. Lennox, Graves, and Levine[36] studied fifty operations performed on forty-nine patients at the Peter Bent Brigham Hospital in Boston. The monitoring method was onerous. The electrocardiographer was summoned by a buzzer in the operating room at the beginning and end of the operation and during critical moments in the operation. ECG tracings were produced by a string galvanometer, at average intervals of 2.5 minutes. For a permanent record, photographic paper had to be exposed to light. The heart rate calculated from the ECG tracings was much higher than the count of the anesthetist. The most marked discrepancies usually occurred during induction of anesthesia, when the pulse rate was taken by a nurse from the ward. Abnormalities of conduction (displacement of pacemaker) were found in 15 (30%) of the cases and 11 cases developed premature beats, seven of them ventricular in origin. None of these premature beats was noted by the anesthetist. Analysis of the patients' characteristics, type of surgery, and type of anesthesia failed to demonstrate predisposing factors apart from alterations in vagal tone.

The value of the electrocardiogram during surgery was demonstrated by further similar studies.[37-39] The intermittent nature of the recording and the inevitable delay in developing ECG tracings on photographic paper, however, limited the usefulness of these observations for diagnosis and therapy.

Direct-writing ECG recorders eliminated the delay associated with processing films but were impractical for obtaining continuous records.[40]

In 1952, Himmelstein and Scheiner described a cardiotachoscope, which permitted continuous display of the ECG on a cathode ray screen.[41] The heart rate, obtained by measuring the time interval between successive beats, appeared as a moving line on the calibrated screen of a cathode ray tube. A direct writing cardiograph could be attached to the instrument to obtain permanent records.

With the advent of continuous ECG monitoring devices, the routine use of the ECG to detect abnormalities of rhythm and rate became practical, albeit too expensive for routine use. Several reviews and studies[42,43] documented the type and incidence of dysrhythmias that could occur during anesthesia. Lead II was usually monitored because the axis paralleled the normal P wave vector, facilitating easy recognition of dysrhythmias. The application of the ECG to detect myocardial ischemia during anesthesia was first proposed by Kaplan and King.[44] In patients undergoing stress tests, Blackburn[45] had previously found that the majority of ischemic episodes could be detected by precordial lead V_5 of a 12-lead electrocardiogram. Kaplan[46] demonstrated successful use of a modified CM_5 lead in anesthetized patients. This lead was practical with three-lead ECG systems, then in common clinical use in the operating room.

Central venous and pulmonary artery catheterization

Werner Forssmann is credited with being the first person to pass a catheter into the heart of a living person[47], using himself as the subject. He passed a ureteral catheter through one of his left antecubital veins, guiding it by fluoroscopy into his right atrium, and then confirming the position by chest roentgenogram. In 1930, Klein reported eleven catheterizations of the right side of the heart, including catheterization of the right ventricle and measurement of cardiac output in humans, using Fick's principle.[48] In the 1940s, catheterization of the right side of the heart began to be used to investigate problems of cardiovascular physiology by Cournand,[49] who later received the Nobel prize (together with Forssmann) for his pioneering efforts.

In 1947, Dexter[50] and Werko[51] reported on oxygen saturation in the pulmonary artery and demonstrated, for the first time, the value of the pulmonary artery wedge pressure in estimating left atrial pressure. In 1970, a balloon-tipped flow-guided catheter technique was introduced by Swan and Ganz, making possible the use of the catheter outside the catheterization laboratory in intensive care units and operating rooms.[52]

Monitoring of oxygenation, blood gases, and acid–base status

As related by John W. Severinghaus, respiratory physiology became important when World War II pilots trying to fly higher than their enemies became hypoxic (without cabin pressurization), lost consciousness, and crashed. Physicist Glen Millikan (1906–1947) developed oximetry in 1940 as a pilot warning device, but the technology became practical only when pulse oximetry was introduced in approximately 1980. The polio epidemics drove the development of artificial ventilation, with the need for carbon dioxide analysis to guide the ventilation of a paralyzed patient. The mid-20th-century advances in the use of hypothermia and cardiopulmonary bypass necessitated frequent monitoring of oxygenation and acid–base status.[53]

Severinghaus built a cuvette for the carbon dioxide electrode and mounted it in a 37°C water bath. His modifications of Stow's invention cut analysis time from an hour to two minutes. Clark had built a successful bubble-type blood oxygenator to perfuse livers.[54] To measure PO_2 in the oxygenator, he turned to polarography. In 1954, Clark made an electrically insulated polarographic sensor with cathode and reference electrode combined, permitting it to work in either air or liquid.

With Clark's approval, Severinghaus used his electrode and his modification of Stow's carbon dioxide electrodes in a blood gas analyzer. Severinghaus displayed the first blood PO_2 and PCO_2 analyzer at the fall American Society of Anesthesiologists meeting in 1957.[55] The addition of a pH electrode completed the modern arterial blood analysis device.

In the 1960s, with the advent of oxygen therapy and positive pressure ventilation of premature infants, it became apparent that excessive oxygenation was associated with blindness. Transcutaneous blood gas monitoring was developed primarily to avoid oxygen-induced retinopathy of prematurity. A skin surface oxygen electrode heated to 44°C accurately monitored PaO_2.[56] Severinghaus further developed a transcutaneous PCO_2 electrode[57] and combined oxygen and carbon dioxide electrodes under a single membrane.[58]

Neuromuscular monitoring

At the time when d-tubocurarine (1942), alcuronium (1964), and pancuronium (1967) were the staple relaxants, Christie and Churchill-Davidson[59] and Katz[60] first popularized the use of peripheral nerve stimulation in the mid-1960s (the Block-Aid monitor) to evaluate neuromuscular function. This device applied a twitch (every four seconds) or tetanic stimulation (30 Hz on demand). These investigators popularized the observation and recording of adductor responses from the thumb, elicited via the ulnar nerve at the wrist.[60] Shortly thereafter, Ali and others (1971)[61] introduced train-of-four (TOF) stimulation, and Lee (1975)[62] further popularized this technique by quantifying and correlating depth of blockade (percent twitch inhibition) according to the TOF count.

The TOF technique has remained the most useful method of evaluation of neuromuscular function in clinical anesthesia practice for more than thirty years because of its simplicity and ease of evaluation and because the stimulus pattern creates its own internal standard each time the response is evaluated; that is, the strength of the fourth response is simply compared with that of the first without the need for establishment of a baseline prior to the administration of neuromuscular blocking drugs.[63]

Safety-driven monitoring standards

As recounted by Ellison Pierce, the latest historical drivers of improvements in anesthesia monitoring were a combination of media attention to anesthetic deaths and a malpractice insurance rate crisis of the 1970s and 1980s.[64] The field of anesthesia safety research was advanced in 1978 with the publication of Jeffrey Cooper's first paper describing critical incident analysis applied to anesthesia.[65] Cooper stated, "Factors associated with anesthetists and/or factors that may have predisposed anesthetists to err have, with a few exceptions, not been previously analyzed. Furthermore, no study has focused on the process of error – its causes, the circumstances that surround it, or its association with specific procedures, devices, etc. – regardless of final outcome."

Data for this first critical incident technique study were obtained from 47 interviews of staff and resident anesthesiologists. In a follow-up paper published in 1984, the database was enlarged to include 139 practitioners and 1089 descriptions of preventable critical incidents.[66] Cooper proposed corrective strategies to lessen the likelihood of an incident occurring, including using appropriate monitoring instrumentation and vigilance.[67]

Major mortality studies have come from the United Kingdom, where Lunn and associates established a confidential, anonymous system to report anesthesia deaths associated with surgery. Their initial report was published in 1982, and anesthesia was considered partly or totally causative of mortality in one or two cases per 10,000 and to be totally causative in nearly 1 per 10,000. Their monitoring-related findings were that that large numbers of patients did not have blood pressure recorded intraoperatively and did not have intraoperative monitoring with the electrocardiogram.[68]

The Closed Claims Project of the American Society of Anesthesiologists (ASA) found that adverse respiratory events constituted the single largest class of injury, some 35 percent of the total.[69] The first three mechanisms of adverse respiratory events were inadequate ventilation (38%), esophageal intubation (18%), and difficult intubation (17%), and the majority of respiratory claims were lodged before widespread adoption of pulse oximetry and capnography. The reviewers concluded that better monitoring would have prevented adverse outcomes in three-quarters of the respiratory claims, compared with only around 10 percent in the nonrespiratory cases.

There is indirect evidence that the advent of ASA basic monitoring standards has diminished the incidence of adverse respiratory events in anesthesia. Eichhorn reviewed 1 million anesthetics administered to ASA physical status 1 and 2 patients at the various Harvard hospitals between 1976 and 1985, and noted 11 major intraoperative anesthesia accidents (2 cardiac arrests, 4 cases of severe brain damage, and 5 deaths).[70] The most common cause (7 of 11) was an unrecognized lack of ventilation. He concluded that these seven, as well as one other, in which oxygen was discontinued inadvertently, would have been prevented by "safety monitoring." Of the next 300,000 anesthetics after the institution of the Harvard capnography and pulse oximetry monitoring standards in 1985, there were no major preventable intraoperative anesthesia injuries.

The evidence-based monitoring standards and guidelines that emerged in the 1980s and 1990s have changed the practice of anesthesia and evolved over time. The ASA and peer organizations embraced evidence-based standards and practice parameters related to basic monitoring standards, transesophageal echocardiography, and pulmonary artery catheterization (http://www.asahq.org/publicationsAndServices/sgstoc.htm, accessed February 7, 2011).

In conclusion, the history of anesthesia monitoring is a fascinating prelude to the remainder of this text. A remarkable group of perioperative physicians who were dedicated to improving patient outcomes persevered to advance the specialty, despite resistance from peers who did not share their vision. The gradual advance in the quality and sophistication of instrumentation and the regression of clinician observations of physical signs is another theme that is remarked on by every chronicler of anesthesia history. The recent decades have also brought the rise of standards in monitoring practice. The history of anesthesia clearly shows how safer anesthesia practices have arisen through improved patient monitoring. The lesson to be taken from this chapter is that we still have the capacity for further improvements in perioperative patient safety, and that we will remember most clearly those perioperative physicians who advance that goal.

Acknowledgments

The author is indebted to Selma Harrison Calmes, M.D., Lydia A. Conlay, M.D., Ph.D., Doris K. Cope, M.D, James C. Erickson III, M. Ellison C. Pierce, Jr., M.D., John Severinghaus, M.D., and George Silvay, whose writings served as the source material for this chapter. Additionally, the staff of the Wood Library–Museum of Anesthesiology, Park Ridge, IL, were instrumental in providing research and support.

References

1. Harvey W. *De Motu Cordis* (translated by Chauncey Leake), Tercentenary ed. Springfield, IL: Charles C. Thomas, 1928.
2. Hales S. An account of some hydraulic and hydrostatical experiments made on the blood and blood vessels of animals. In Willus FA, Keyes RE, eds. *Cardiac Classics*. St. Louis: Mosby, 1941;I:131–155.
3. Bernard C. *Leçon sur la chaleur animale*. Paris: Libraire J-M. Bailliere et Fils, 1876.
4. Snow J. *On the Inhalation of the Vapour of Ether in Surgical Operations*. London: John Churchill, 1847; reproduced by Lea & Febiger, Philadelphia, 1959.
5. Syme WS. The Scottish chloroform legend – Syme and Simpson as practical anesthetists. In *Essays on the First Hundred Years of Anesthesia*. Huntington, NY: Robert Kreiger, 1972, Chapter 8.

6. Duncum B. *The Development of Inhalation Anaesthesia*. Part 9: The beginnings of modern anaesthesia. Chapter 18: The jubilee of anaesthesia. Geoffrey Cumberlege, London: Oxford University Press. 1947:537–540.

7. Clover JT. On an Apparatus for Administering Nitrous Oxide Gas and Ether, Singly or Combined. Br Med J 1876;2(Issue 811):74–75 (Published 15 July 1876).

8. Simpson WG, ed. *Works of Sir J. J. Simpson*. New York: Appleton & Co., 1872.

9. Sreevastava DK, Mohan CVR. First lady physician anaesthesiologist in the world: an Indian. *Indian J Anaesth* 2006;50:103.

10. Pierce EC, Jr. Does monitoring have an effect on patient safety? Monitoring instruments have significantly reduced anesthetic mishaps. *J Clin Monit* 1988;4(2):111–114.

11. Momin Ali, Asrit Ramachari. About the participants in the Hyderabad Choloform Commissions. In Fink BR, Morris LE, Stephen CR (eds). *The History of Anesthesia: Third International Symposium*. Wood Library Museum of Anaesthesiology, Illinois. 1992; 28–31.

12. Kirk R. On auscultation of the heart during chloroform narcosis. *Br Med J* 1896;2:1704–1706.

13. Teter CK. Thirteen thousand administrations of nitrous oxid with oxygen as an anesthetic. *JAMA* 1909;53:448–454.

14. Cushing H. Technical methods of performing certain cranial operations. *Surg Gynecol Obstet* 1908;VI:227–234.

15. Solis-Cohen S. Exhibition of an oesophageal stethoscope, with remarks on intrathoracic auscultation. *Trans Cell Physicians Philadelphia* 1893;3.5 XV:218–221.

16. Fink, BR. *Times of the Signs, The Origins of Charting, The History of Anesthesia, 3rd International Symposium Proceedings*. B.R. Fink, L.E. Morris, C.R. Stephen, eds. Chicago: Wood Library-Museum, 1992.

17. Cushing HW. On the avoidance of shock in major amputations by cocainization of large nerve trunks preliminary to their diversion, with observations on blood-pressure changes in surgical cases. *Ann Surg* 1902;36:321–343.

18. Major RH. The history of taking the blood pressure. *Ann Medical Hist*. 1930;**2**:47–55.

19. Riva-Rocci S. A new sphygmomanometer. In Faulconer A, Keyes TE, eds. *Foundations of Anesthesiology*. Springfield, IL: Charles C. Thomas, 1965;2:1043–1075.

20. Cushing HW. On routine determinations of arterial tension in operating room and clinic. *Boston Med Surg J* 1903;148: 250–256.

21. Korotkoff NS. On the subject of methods of determining blood pressure. *Bull Imp Mel Med Acad St. Petersburg* 1905; 11:365.

22. von Recklinghausen H. Ueber Blutdruckmessung bein menschen. *Arch F exp Path U Pharmakol* 1901: 46:78.

23. Von Recklinghausen H. *Neue Wege zur Blutdruckmessung*. Berlin: Springer-Verlag, 1931.

24. Kazamias TM, Gander MP, Franklin DL, Ross J Jr. Blood pressure measurement with Doppler unltrasonic flowmeter. *J Appl Physiol* 1971;30:585–588.

25. Kirby RR, Kemmerer WT, Morgan JL. Transcutaneous measurement of blood pressure. *Anesthesiology* 1969;31: 86–89.

26. Zahed B, Sadove MS, Hatano S, Wu HH. Comparison of automated Doppler ultrasound and Korotkoff measurements of blood pressure of children. *Anesth Analg* 1971;50:699–704.

27. Silas JH, Barker AT, Ramsey LE. Clinical evaluation of Dinamap 845 automated blood pressure recorder. *Br Heart J* 1980;43: 202–205.

28. Gillespie NA. The signs of anesthesia. *Anesth Analg*. 1943;22:275–282.

29. Calmes SA. Arthur Guedel, M.D. and the eye signs of anesthesia. *ASA Newsletter*, September 2002. https://www.asahq.org/Newsletters/2002/9_02/feature5.htm (accessed May 25, 2009).

30. Courington FW, Calverley RK. Anesthesia on the western front: the Anglo-American experience of World War I. *Anesthesiology* 1986;65:642–653.

31. Poiseuille JLM. Récherches sur la force du Coeur aortique. *Arch Gen Med* 1828;18:550–555.

32. Ludwig C. Beitrage zur kenntniss des einflussen der respiratiores bewegungen auf den blut auf in aortensysteme. *Muller's Arch Anat* 1847;240–302.

33. Peterson LH, Dripps RD, Risman GC. A method for recording the arterial pressure pulse and blood pressure in man. *Am Heart J* 1949;37:771–782.

34. Heard JD, Strauss AE. A report on the electrocardiographic study of two cases of nodal rhythm exhibiting R-P intervals. *Am J Med Soc* 1918;75:238–251.

35. Levine SA. Acute cardiac upsets occurring during or following surgical operations. *JAMA* 1920;75:795–799.

36. Lennox WG, Graves RC, Levine SA. An electrocardiographic study of fifty patients during operation. *Arch Int Med* 1922;30:57–72.

37. Maher CJ, Crittenden PJ, Shapiro PT. Electrocardiography study of viscerocardiac reflexes during major operations. *Am Heart J* 1934;9:664–676.

38. Kurtz CM, Bennet JH, Shapiro HH. Electrocardiographic studies during surgical anesthesia. *JAMA* 1936;**106**:434–441.

39. Feil H, Rossman PL. Electrocardiographic observations in cardiac surgery. *Ann Intern Med* 1939;13:402–414.

40. Ziegler RF. Cardiac mechanism during anesthesia and operation in patients with congenital heart disease and cyanosis. *Bull Johns Hopkins Hosp* 1948;83:237–71.

41. Himmelstein A, Scheiner M. The cardiotachoscope. *Anesthesiology* 1952;13:62–64.

42. Cannard TH, Dripps RD, Helwig J Jr, Zinsser HF. The electrocardiogram during anesthesia and surgery. *Anesthesiology* 1960; 21:194–202.

43. Russell PH, Coakley CS. Electrocardiographic observation in the operating room. *Anesth Analg* 1969;48:474–488.

44. Kaplan JA, King SB. The precordial electrocardiographic lead V5 in patients who have coronary artery disease. *Anesthesiology* 1976;45:570–574.

45. Blackburn H, Taylor HL, Okamoto N, Rautaharju P, Mitchell PL, Kerkhof AC. Standardization of the exercise electrocardiogram. A systematic comparison of chest lead configuration employed for monitoring during exercise. In Karvaner MJ, Barry AD, eds. *Physical Activity and the Heart*. Springfield, IL: Charles C. Thomas, 1967; 101–133.

46. Kaplan JA. Electrocardiographic monitoring. In Kaplan, JA, ed. *Cardiac Anesthesia*. New York: Grune and Stratton, 1979; 149–151.

47. Forssmann W. *Die Sondierung de rechten Herzens Klin Wochenschr* 1929; 8:2085–2087.

48. Klein O. Zur Bestimmung de zerkulatorischen minutens. Volumen nach dem Fickschen Prinzip. *Munch Med Wochenschr* 1930; 77:1311.

49. Cournand AF. Measurement of cardiac output in man using the technique of catheterization of the right auricle. *J Clin Invest* 1945;24:105–116.

50. Dexter L, Haynes FW, Burwell CS, Eppinger EC, Sagerson RP, Evans JM. Studies of congenital heart disease: II. The pressure and

oxygen content of blood in the right auricle, right ventricle and pulmonary artery in control patients, with observations on the oxygen saturation and source of pulmonary "capillary" blood. *J Clin Invest* 1947;26:554–560.

51. Lagerlof H, Werko L. Studies on the circulation of blood in man. VI. The pulmonary capillary venous pressure pulse in man. *Scand J Clin Lab Invest* 1949;1:147–161.

52. Swan HJC, Ganz W, Forrester J, Marcus H, Daimond G, Chonette D. Catheterization of the heart in man with use of a flow directed balloon-tipped catheter. *N Engl J Med* 1970;283:447–451.

53. Severinghaus JW. Gadgeteering for health care: The John W. Severinghaus Lecture on Translational Science. *Anesthesiology* 2009;110:721–728.

54. Clark LC Jr, Gollan F, Gupta VB. The oxygenation of blood by gas dispersion. *Science* 1950;111:85–87.

55. Severinghaus JW, Bradley AF. Electrodes for blood pO2 and pCO₂ determination. *J Appl Physiol* 1958;13:515–520.

56. Severinghaus JW, Peabody JL, Thunstrom A, Eberhard P, Zappia E, eds. Workshop on methodologic aspects of transcutaneous blood gas analysis. *Acta Anaesthesiol Scand Suppl* 1978;68:1–144.

57. Severinghaus JW. A combined transcutaneous PO_2-PCO_2 electrode with electrochemical HCO_3-stabilization. *J Appl Physiol* 1981;51:1027–32.

58. Palmisano BW, Severinghaus JW. Clinical accuracy of a combined transcutaneous PO_2-PCO_2 electrode. *Crit Care Med* 1984;12:276.

59. Christie TH, Churchill-Davidson HC. The St. Thomas's Hospital nerve stimulator in the diagnosis of prolonged apnoea. *Lancet* 1958;1:776.

60. Katz RL. A nerve stimulator for the continuous monitoring of muscle relaxant action. *Anesthesiology* 1965;26:832.

61. Ali HH, Utting JE, Gray C. Quantitative assessment of residual antidepolarizing block (part II). *Br J Anaesth.* 1971; 3:478.

62. Lee CM. Train-of-4 quantitation of competitive neuromuscular block. *Anesth Analg* 1975;54:649.

63. Savarese JJ. Monitoring of neuromuscular function: past, present and future. *ASA Newsletter*, September 2002. https://www.asahq.org/Newsletters/2002/9_02/feature6.htm (accessed May 25, 2009)

64. Eichhorn JH. Prevention of intraoperative anesthesia accidents and related severe injury through safety monitoring. *Anesthesiology* 1989;70:572–577.

64. Cooper JB, Newbower RS, Long CD, McPeek B. Preventable anesthesia mishaps: a study of human factors. *Anesthesiology* 1978;49:399–406.

66. Cooper JB, Newbower RS, Kitz RJ. An analysis of major errors and equipment failures in anesthesia management: considerations for prevention and detection. *Anesthesiology* 1984;60:34–42.

67. Cooper JB. Toward prevention of anesthetic mishaps. In Pierce EC Jr, Cooper JB, eds. *Analysis of Anesthetic Mishaps*. Boston: Little, Brown, 1984:167–183.

68. Lunn JN, Mushin WW. *Mortality Associated with Anaesthesia*. London: Nuffield Provincial Hospitals Trust, 1982.

69. Caplan RA, Posner KL, Ward RJ, Cheney FW. Adverse respiratory events in anesthesia: A closed claims analysis. *Anesthesiology* 1990;72:828–833.

70. Eichhorn JH. Prevention of intraoperative anesthesia accidents and related severe injury through safety monitoring. *Anesthesiology* 1989;70:572–577.

Medicolegal implications of monitoring

Jeffrey M. Feldman

Introduction

If you have never received a letter with the return address of an unknown law firm, consider yourself lucky. In the case of a malpractice proceeding, you will open the letter and typically find your name in a long list of defendants. Sometimes the letter is anticipated, but often, the precipitating events occurred so long ago that the details are difficult to recall.

Whatever the circumstances, a malpractice suit unleashes a sequence of events with an unpredictable outcome. The trial venue, the quality of the attorneys, the members of the jury, the expert witnesses involved, the ability of the plaintiff to engender sympathy, the perceived credibility of the defendant, and the quality of the documentation all play a role in the ultimate outcome. The plaintiff's attorney will leave no stone unturned in building the case for malpractice. Because physiologic monitoring is essential to safe patient care, the plaintiff's attorney is likely to scrutinize how the patient was monitored in building the case. The intent of this chapter is to explore the ways in which physiologic monitoring and exposure to malpractice liability are related. The intent is not to offer a comprehensive discussion of the nuances of malpractice liability. If you are named in a malpractice suit, there is no better resource than a skilled defense attorney.

In a chapter titled "Medical Liability and the Culture of Technology," Jacobsen argues, "The history of medical liability is a struggle between technological advances and injuries suffered when those advances fail."[1] He goes on to observe that technical advances empower physicians to tackle ever more complex and challenging medical problems with the attendant increased risks. In some cases, the outcome is a return to the previous state of health, but that is not always the case. The public, on the other hand, demands – and has come to expect – perfect outcomes. Although a physician may clearly understand that a less-than-perfect outcome is much better than even more severe disability or death, the patient perceives only the loss of his or her health. Physiologic monitoring has facilitated increasingly complex surgical procedures for sicker patients. Even the most confident clinician would be unlikely to attempt to provide anesthesia for liver transplantation using just a finger on the pulse. The most sophisticated monitoring, however, cannot prevent undesired outcomes in sick patients undergoing complex procedures and the resulting exposure to malpractice suits.

Although the proliferation of technology can increase the potential for malpractice liability, Jacobsen recognizes that the specialty of anesthesiology provides one example in which technology, and patient monitoring in particular, has actually reduced malpractice liability by reducing the risk of serious injury. For a number of years, anesthesiology ranked at the top of the medical specialties in malpractice claims and the severity of patient injury. In 1986, the Harvard Medical School Department of Anesthesia adopted a minimum standard for patient monitoring during anesthesia.[2] This standard included provisions for monitoring ventilation, preferably by capnography. Interestingly, pulse oximetry, which had only recently been introduced, was advocated as a means to monitor the circulation, not oxygenation. The primary goal of the Harvard standard was to improve patient safety by reducing adverse events, with a secondary goal of reducing malpractice claims. Malpractice insurance carriers became convinced of the value of these guidelines to mitigate malpractice exposure and, in an effort to catalyze more widespread adoption, offered to reduce premiums to practices that adhered to the monitoring guidelines. The result was a significant reduction in the number and severity of claims against anesthesiologists.[3] A review of 1175 closed malpractice claims filed between 1974 and 1988 underscores the potential for physiologic monitoring to reduce malpractice claims. The reviewers determined that one-third of the injuries could have been prevented by the use of monitoring devices, most notably pulse oximetry and capnometry.[4]

Establishing monitoring standards was facilitated by the development of monitoring devices that were easy to use and cost-effective. The resulting outcome clearly established the relationship between physiologic monitoring and patient safety. The motivation for these efforts was to reduce the risk of patient injury. The financial realities of the malpractice system created the business case, as avoiding even one wrongful death or hypoxic injury suit would pay for multiple patient monitors.

Risk management strategies typically focus on adherence to the standard of care, the importance of documentation, and the patient–physician relationship. Monitoring patients appropriately reduces the risk of significant injury and is therefore an important part of risk management in anesthesia. As a result of the Harvard experience, the American Society of Anesthesiologists (ASA) established a standard for anesthetic monitoring.

It is notable that the ASA has chosen to include the word "standard" in the title of this document, which establishes the content to indicate the standard of care.* As we will see, this monitoring standard is the most unambiguous evidence that can be presented in court for the standard of care because it does not require the opinion of an expert witness. Furthermore, there is good evidence from the ASA closed-claims database that when adherence to a standard of care can be demonstrated, there is a reduced chance of payment for a malpractice claim.[5] To better understand the importance of the standard of care, consider the elements of proof that are required in a malpractice proceeding.

Burden of proof

Although the outcome of a malpractice suit can sometimes seem capricious, the burden of proof that must be satisfied by the plaintiff's attorney is well defined. Understanding the burden of proof is a useful foundation for evaluating the role of any aspect of care that is used to build a case for malpractice.

In the broad sense, health care malpractice liability arises from five areas of exposure:[6]

- Professional negligence (substandard care delivery)
- Intentional misconduct
- Breach of a therapeutic promise (breach of contract)
- Patient injury from dangerous treatment-related activities, regardless of fault (strict liability)
- Patient injury from dangerous devices (product liability)

Of these areas of exposure, professional negligence is the most common basis for suit against an individual health care provider. Most of the discussion in this chapter focuses on the role of physiologic monitoring in establishing a case for negligence against a health care provider. Physiologic monitors can be involved in a suit related to strict or product liability. In the latter case, the liability suit would typically be directed toward the manufacturer, and debate would ensue about whether it was the device or failure to use it correctly that caused the injury.

Negligence is defined as "conduct which falls below the standard established by law for the protection of others against unreasonable risk of harm."[7] When professional negligence is considered, the "standard" by which the care is measured is considered to be the minimally acceptable practice. Practitioners accused of negligence in a malpractice case are judged not by the standard set by the most skilled practitioner, but by the standard set by an ordinary practitioner under usual circumstances. The role of the expert witness is therefore to articulate not how he or she personally would have treated the patient, but what is generally considered to be the minimal safe practice standard. Different rules can be applied to defining the

minimal safe practice standard. In some cases, the professional is held to the standard in his or her geographic practice area so, for example, a rural physician in a community hospital is not held to the same standard as a physician with the resources of a tertiary-care urban hospital. For individual specialties, the standard could be applied to a reasonably prudent professional in the same specialty.

Negligent acts can be acts of commission or omission. In the former case, the liable party must *do* something that, under similar circumstances, a reasonably prudent professional would have done differently or not at all. An act of omission is the *failure to do* something that a reasonably prudent professional would have done under the same circumstances. An act of commission in patient monitoring, for example, would involve using a monitoring device that exposes a patient to injury when using that device would not be considered standard of care. An act of omission in patient monitoring would involve failing to use a monitoring modality that is considered the minimal safe practice. The terminology "reasonably prudent professional" is an attempt to create an objective standard for evaluating a person's actions. In the case of an anesthesia provider, the "reasonably prudent" definition would indicate an individual who is trained and licensed in accordance with applicable laws and professional standards.

The failure to follow indicated monitoring standards is not in itself sufficient proof of negligence. The plaintiff's attorney has the burden to prove the following four elements:[8]

- The professional had a duty to care for the patient.
- The professional breached the duty to care for the patient by providing substandard care.
- The injury suffered by the patient was caused by the breach of duty.
- The damages to the patient are compensable.

Of these four elements, the second and third can be related to the manner in which a physiologic monitor is used. Using a device that may cause injury when the device is not indicated, or failing to use a device when it is indicated, are examples of substandard care absent a compelling explanation by the provider. Other examples would include pulmonary artery rupture from placing a pulmonary artery catheter that is not indicated, or hypoxic injury when a pulse oximeter is not used.

The burden of proof also requires that the injury suffered by the patient be related to the breach of duty to provide care consistent with the prevailing standard. In the strictest definition, one would need to establish a clear link between the aspect(s) of the care that are substandard and the injury suffered by the plaintiff. Given the uncertainties of medicine, it is not always possible to establish direct causation for a particular injury. The plaintiff's attorney may argue that breach of duty need not be proven based on the principle of *res ipsa loquitur,* or "the thing speaks for itself." This burden of proof is not as rigorous as in the case of strict professional negligence, as a causative link between the care lapse and the injury is not required. To argue

---

* The ASA also issues "Guidelines" and "Statements" that are intended to provide information about practice decisions but are not considered a standard of care. The distinction is important in a malpractice proceeding. For more information, see http://www.asahq.org/publicationsAndServices/sgstoc.htm.

for liability on the basis of *res ipsa loquitur*, the attorney must prove that

- The injuries suffered by the plaintiff would not normally occur in the absence of negligence;
- The defendant(s) had both the ability and the duty to prevent such injuries; and
- The plaintiff did not contribute to causing his or her own injury.

Although the burden of proof for professional negligence is clearly established, differences of opinion between expert witnesses are typical. In a review of 103 closed anesthesia malpractice claims, independent paired reviewers disagreed about the appropriateness of care in 38 percent of the cases using the standard of a reasonable and prudent anesthesia practitioner.[9] These findings underscore the fact that the standard of care is a matter of opinion, and both plaintiffs and defense attorneys are likely to find well-intentioned credible experts to support their views. The ultimate decision of a lay jury can be swayed by many factors. As we will see, failure to monitor can cast a very negative light on the health care practitioner, and if the patient has suffered injury, the jury is likely to provide compensation. Under the principle of *res ipsa loquitur*, linking the injury directly to the failure to monitor may not be needed to convince the jury to find for the defendant.

Monitoring standards

> It is 2 AM. A 24-year-old patient is on the way to the operating room for an emergency appendectomy. You check the anesthesia machine and find that the inspired oxygen monitor cannot be calibrated and does not provide a reading. Do you proceed with the case?

When it comes to defining the standard of care with regard to physiologic monitoring, we are fortunate to have the ASA Standards for Basic Anesthetic Monitoring.[10] As noted previously, that document clearly defines the recognized minimum standard for patient monitoring, inclusive of all regional, general, and monitored-care anesthetics.

The standard guidelines are divided broadly into two categories. The first emphasizes that the anesthesia provider be physically present at all times to ensure adequate patient monitoring. The second category requires, "During all anesthetics, the patient's oxygenation, ventilation, circulation and temperature shall be continually evaluated." For the most part, these standards are self-explanatory. The language in the standard is carefully chosen in an attempt to limit malpractice exposure when adherence to the standard either is impractical or would present a greater risk to the patient. For virtually all the recommended monitoring strategies, there is an opportunity to waive a specific requirement under extenuating circumstances. The standard emphasizes the importance, however, of documenting the reasons for waiving the requirement in the patient's medical record.

One can be certain that in the event of a patient injury that could even remotely be related to physiologic monitoring, adherence to the ASA Standards for Basic Anesthetic Monitoring will be scrutinized by the plaintiff's attorney. Any variation from this standard will be used to identify a cause for the injury and to impugn the quality of care rendered by the anesthesia provider. An interesting example of this scenario has been reported by Vigoda and Lubarsky.[11] The report describes the case of a 58-year-old male who underwent a craniotomy for a brain tumor while in the sitting position and suffered new-onset quadriplegia after the procedure. During the case, the Standards for Basic Anesthesia Monitoring were followed and, in particular, arterial pressure monitoring was performed using an intraarterial catheter for continuous measurement. The case involved the use of an anesthesia information management system (AIMS) to acquire data from the monitors and create the anesthetic record. During the procedure, there was a 93-minute period of time during which the data from the arterial pressure monitor did not appear on the automated anesthesia record.

It turned out that there was a problem with the cable connecting the physiologic monitor to the AIMS, so blood pressure data were not transferred to the recordkeeper. The providers caring for the patient did not notice this problem, as they were able to follow the blood pressure on the display of the physiologic monitor, and the blood pressure data on the AIMS display were covered by an informational window. A malpractice claim was filed and ultimately settled during the trial phase. Although the patient's injury was not clearly linked to substandard monitoring, conformance with the standard of care was not documented by the record, and successful defense became unlikely.

This case report raises another interesting consideration regarding the use of an AIMS and liability exposure related to monitoring standards. In contrast to a paper record, the AIMS provides a continuous electronic record of monitored information. In addition to the paper record printed at the conclusion of a case, all the data are time-stamped and archived to an electronic database. Both the paper record and the electronic database are discoverable and will provide the most authoritative information available to a jury to decide how a patient was monitored. The design of the AIMS used by Vigoda and Lubarsky has been changed, as a consequence of their experience, to alert the provider when a monitoring failure has occurred. Anyone using an AIMS would do well to review the case report and understand how the system will document conformance with minimal monitoring standards.

Given these considerations, in general, one should not render anesthetic care unless conformance with the standards for basic monitoring can be met. Exceptions to this rule involve emergency procedures when delaying the start of care would increase the risk to the patient. If the scenario of the appendectomy was, instead, that of a trauma victim who is rushed from the emergency department to the OR for a lifesaving surgical intervention, it would not be advisable to delay the procedure to troubleshoot an oxygen monitor. It is important, however, to document as soon as possible why the procedure started without that monitoring modality, and to make every effort to institute the ability to monitor that parameter.

Monitoring beyond the standards

The ASA Standards for Basic Anesthesia Monitoring should be followed for every anesthetic, but additional monitoring is often used. Additional monitored parameters include cardiac output, mixed venous oxygen saturation, processed electroencephalography, evoked potentials, and echocardiography. Although these monitoring modalities are not included in the minimum monitoring standard, there is significant potential for the use of these monitors to be scrutinized in the event of a malpractice suit. This is especially true when one considers that these additional devices are typically used for patients and procedures where there is an increased risk of an untoward outcome. Clearly, if the risk of a bad outcome is increased, then the risk of a malpractice suit is increased as well. Unfortunately, both using a monitor and failing to use a monitor can result in liability exposure.

> A 35-year-old healthy male patient is scheduled for an open removal of a renal staghorn calculus and possible nephrectomy. After induction of general anesthesia, a central venous catheter is placed; shortly thereafter, the patient becomes hypotensive, suffers a cardiac arrest, and cannot be resuscitated. The postmortem examination identifies hemopericardium, with resulting cardiac tamponade, as the cause of death.

Complications related to central venous catheter placement are well recognized. In 2004, Domino and coworkers used the ASA closed-claims database to evaluate claims related to central venous catheter placement. They identified 110 claims related to central venous catheters with a greater severity of injury and proportion of death than the other claims in the database. Cardiac tamponade, hemothorax, and pulmonary artery rupture were the common causes of death.[12] In the case example, there is little doubt that central venous catheter placement led to the patient's demise. From a malpractice perspective, one question that will be raised is whether central venous catheter placement was indicated in this case. In the absence of a reference for the standard of care, the professional is in the position of having to justify the risk to the patient based on the potential benefit. Secondarily, plaintiff's attorneys could question the experience of the person placing the catheter and the method of placement. Ultrasound guidance has proven to be useful for central catheter placement (see Chapter 12). Although it is useful for directing needle placement, ultrasound has not been shown to prevent the serious complications that can result from central catheter placement, especially those that can occur after finding the vein. Well-considered differences of opinion on the standard of care will exist when attempting to address the questions raised by this case scenario.

Although a monitor may not be considered a "standard," using that monitor could be considered part of the duty to use reasonable care to protect a patient from harm.[13] Adopting a monitor into clinical practice is an implicit statement that it is useful for patient care. Scientific documentation linking a monitor to improved outcome may not exist, but expert witnesses can use evidence from the literature that these monitors reduce the risk of serious complications and are considered part of the reasonable duty to protect a patient from harm.

> A 60-year-old man with a history of peripheral vascular disease is scheduled for a lower-extremity arterial bypass. General anesthesia is administered, including the use of a muscle relaxant. During the surgical preparation, the patient's arterial blood pressure is 100/50 and the concentration of inhaled anesthetic is minimized. After awakening, the patient reports recall of the surgical preparation and the pain from the incision, including the inability to move or talk.

Existing literature suggests that the incidence of awareness during general anesthesia may be as high as 0.2 percent, or up to 26,000 occurrences per year in the United States alone.[14] Patients who experience awareness may be left with a posttraumatic stress-like disorder and permanent psychologic impairment. There is a high likelihood, therefore, that an incident of awareness will lead to a malpractice suit. The ASA Closed Claims project has documented 56 claims for recall during general anesthesia between 1990 and 2006, although this number likely underrepresents the total number of cases. Interestingly, payment was made in just 52 percent of the claims, suggesting that the burden of proof can be difficult. A large number of awareness claims were not associated with any one single factor, but "there were indications that lower doses of anesthetic agents may be associated with recall."[15]

How would monitoring modalities intended to assess the risk of awareness be viewed in a malpractice proceeding? Could it be considered negligence if one of these monitors was not used and the patient suffered intraoperative recall? Monitoring exhaled anesthetic agent concentration is not considered a monitoring standard but is certainly widely used, and the information is often recorded to a handwritten record or AIMS. A variety of neurophysiologic monitors are available that are designed to help the clinician assess anesthetic depth (see Chapter 18). Neither anesthetic agent monitors nor neurophysiologic monitors are included in the ASA basic monitoring standards. Nevertheless, there is an accumulating body of literature that could be used to argue for the use of these monitors, especially in selected "high-risk" patients. In 2004, the Joint Commission (TJC; formerly known as the Joint Commission on the Accreditation of Healthcare Organizations, abbreviated as JCAHO) issued a sentinel event alert on Preventing and Managing the Impact of Anesthesia Awareness. In this alert, TJC recommended "[the] effective application of available anesthesia monitoring techniques" as a preventive strategy.[16] In that same year, the ASA published a practice advisory on Intraoperative Awareness and Brain Function Monitoring.[17] The report specifically states that the practice advisory is not intended as a standard, guideline, or absolute requirement. With regard to preventing awareness, the advisory states that "brain function monitoring is not routinely indicated for patients undergoing general anesthesia, either to reduce the frequency of intraoperative awareness or to monitor depth of anesthesia," and further stated that "the decision to use a brain function monitor should be made on a case-by-case basis by the individual practitioner for selected patients." The practice advisory does advocate for multimodality monitoring (including anesthetic agent monitoring) to minimize the occurrence of awareness and does state that the use of a muscle relaxant "adds additional importance to the use of monitoring methods that assure the adequate delivery of anesthesia."

Whether a jury would consider an anesthetic agent or depth-of-anesthesia monitor to be consistent with minimally acceptable practice will depend on the arguments of the attorneys and the testimony of expert witnesses. Even though awareness monitoring is not included in the ASA Basic Anesthesia Monitoring Standards, the language in the practice advisory suggests that selected high-risk patients would benefit from monitoring for awareness. Regardless of what monitoring strategy is used, whenever a patient receives general anesthesia there is the potential for awareness, and the anesthesia professional should be able to articulate the strategy that was employed to prevent awareness.

Patient awareness is just one of the events that has a high likelihood of resulting in a malpractice suit when monitoring beyond the basic standard can be involved. Patients with significant hemodynamic compromise (e.g., trauma patients), or patients at risk for intraoperative stroke (e.g., major vascular or neurosurgery) also have a high likelihood of poor outcome and a related increased likelihood of suit. Even though there may not be specific indications for monitoring beyond the standards defined by the ASA, there is enough literature about the potential value of advanced monitoring devices that *not* using these devices may be called into question. It is beyond the scope of this chapter to explore all of these potential sources of liability. Further, the indications for most advanced monitoring techniques are not so well established that one can define when and how monitoring beyond the ASA standard would be considered a community standard. Any attempt to do so would likely create literature that could be exploited by a plaintiff's attorney without any scientific basis.

Importance of training

The evolution of physiologic monitors has led to devices that are both easy to use and reliable. Gone are the days of calibrating pressure transducers against mercury manometers. Today, most physiologic monitors need only be turned on and connected to the patient to obtain monitored information. Nevertheless, misuse of the monitor or the information from

the device can be the basis for malpractice liability related to negligence or strict liability.

> A 32-year-old woman was admitted to the intensive care unit in a coma following closed head trauma. At the change of the nursing shift, the intracranial pressure (ICP) transducer is found to have been affixed 15 centimeters above the zero point. This error occurred several hours earlier during adjustment of the height of the bed as the patient was turned for decubitus ulcer prevention. The zero is reestablished and the ICP measurement of 12 cmH_2O, which had been stable for the last six hours, is now 27 cmH_2O. Measures to reduce ICP are instituted. The patient is left with significant neurologic injury.

Monitors that measure pressure are likely to provide misleading or incorrect information if they are used improperly. Even though modern transducers do not require calibration, they all require establishing a zero reference point for pressure measurement. The anatomical relationship of this reference point to the patient must be carefully established and maintained to prevent erroneous readings that can easily be clinically significant. In the case of an arterial pressure transducer, there is the potential for falsely high or falsely low measurements if the transducer is too low or too high, respectively, relative to the heart or brain.

In the case of central venous pressure or ICP monitors, the location of the zero point is even more critical. Because the absolute values of those pressure measurements are relatively low, small errors in the location of the transducer relative to the zero point can have a significant impact on the monitored information. Given the severity of the injury in patients who require ICP monitoring, undesired outcomes are common, with the corresponding increased risk of a malpractice suit. Providers caring for these patients must understand the principles of pressure measurement, carefully locate the zero reference point for pressure measurement, and be sure to maintain accurate monitoring over time. Mounting transducers to the patient or the patient's bed is useful for preventing the problem of moving the patient relative to the zero reference of the transducer.

Even though many monitors have become easy to use and require little training, some advanced approaches to monitoring require significant training. Perhaps the most notable example relevant to the practice of anesthesiology is transesophageal echocardiography (TEE), which is often employed during high-risk procedures involving high-acuity patients. Proper use of this monitor requires training and experience. The National Board of Echocardiography offers a certification exam for special competence in perioperative transesophageal echocardiography, which is intended to "serve the public by encouraging quality patient care in the practice of echocardiography."[18] Although certification is not required for anesthesia professionals to perform echocardiography exams, significant patient management decisions are often guided by the results of these exams. Should an untoward outcome occur that could be related to the interpretation of the TEE, the credentials of the clinician performing the TEE would almost certainly be questioned in the event of a malpractice proceeding. The existence of the certification process creates a competency standard even though it is not required for practice. Accreditation of skills related to physiologic monitoring is available only for certain devices. Documentation of training and proficiency is currently not employed in a rigorous fashion for most devices but, from a medicolegal/risk management perspective, competency documentation can only be a benefit.

Physiologic alarms – unintended consequences?

The ASA Standards for Basic Anesthesia Monitoring include the recommendation for audible alarms for low inspired oxygen concentration, low arterial oxygen saturation, the absence of end-tidal carbon dioxide, and ventilator disconnection. Audible alarms were not included in the monitoring standard until the most recent revision in 2005, despite the fact that audible alarms have been a standard feature of physiologic monitors for many years. Why were audible alarms not part of the monitoring standard from the outset? Furthermore, physiologic monitors incorporate audible alarms that are tied to virtually all the parameters monitored during anesthesia. Why is the recommendation for using audible alarms during monitoring restricted to the four alarms currently mentioned in the monitoring standard?

The technology for audible physiologic alarms is, for the most part, based on setting high and low thresholds for a monitored parameter, and sounding an audible tone when the actual measured value crosses that threshold (see Chapter 35). This approach is practical from an engineering perspective, but for the most part has not resulted in clinically useful alarms. In fact, this approach to alarms has resulted in a high rate of audible alarms that are clinically meaningless (false-positive alarms), and are either disabled or just add noise and distraction to the clinical environment.[19] Similar to the fable attributed to Aesop, "The Boy Who Cried Wolf," current alarms are so often meaningless that they are either disabled or do not catch the user's attention when an important event occurs. Several strategies have been proposed to standardize and improve on clinical alarms, yet none has been adopted in any widespread fashion.[20] Given the obvious shortcomings of current alarm technology, why has there been so little progress toward improving the alarms?

The inadequacy of the current alarm technology and lack of progress toward improving alarms is an unintended consequence of the medicolegal protections afforded to patients. Failure to notify the user of an important physiologic change that could lead to patient injury can only open the door for product liability. From the perspective of a manufacturer, the goal in designing audible alarms is to incorporate highly sensitive alarms that will not miss any important events. The consequence of a highly sensitive alarm is a high false-alarm rate.

There is little or no incentive for the manufacturer to make the alarms more specific, as the cost is almost certain to be a reduced sensitivity and the potential to miss an important event. Until a manufacturer can create a competitive advantage by improving alarm technology, there is little chance that the basic technology will be improved.

Fortunately, there are efforts under way to improve the clinical utility of audible alarms. Numerous strategies have been investigated that range from simple time delays to suppress alarms from transient artifacts, to multivariate statistical approaches.[21] International standards efforts are focusing on tailoring alarm tones to the specific type of alarm rather than having a nonspecific tone that is related to a certain manufacturer. Given the potential costs to manufacturers of a product liability suit, there is little incentive to take any risk with new alarm algorithms that reduce the sensitivity of the alarms unless the improved specificity is clearly documented. Because new developments are unlikely to come from industry, we will be left with the unintended consequence of audible alarms that are not clinically useful unless research can lead us to improved alarm algorithms.

Conclusions

As a medical specialty, anesthesiology has been a leader in establishing the connection between the appropriate use of physiologic monitors and enhanced patient safety. The ASA Standards for Basic Anesthesia Monitoring provide an unambiguous definition of the minimum standards for monitoring. These standards should be followed for every patient unless the reasons for not following the standard can be clearly documented. As sicker patients present for more complicated procedures, the risks of undesirable outcomes increase, with the consequence of greater liability exposure. When the outcome leads to a malpractice suit, reasonable expert witnesses may argue that monitoring beyond the standard would be indicated to protect a patient from harm. From a risk management perspective, it is important to be able to explain why a device that could be considered useful to protect the patient was not used, or why a device that has inherent risks was chosen.

Experience has demonstrated that keeping patients safe reduces malpractice exposure and is the best risk management strategy one can employ. Proper use of physiologic monitors can help to achieve that goal.

Acknowledgment

Special thanks to Teresa Salamon, CRNA, JD, of Dechert LLP in Philadelphia for her critical review of this chapter.

References

1. Jacobsen PD. Medical liability and the culture of technology. In Sage WM, Kersh R, eds. *Medical Malpractice and the US Health Care System*. New York: Cambridge University Press, 2006, p. 116.

2. Eichhorn JH, Cooper JB, Cullen DJ, Maier WR, Philip JH, Seeman RG. Standards for patient monitoring during anesthesia at Harvard Medical School. *JAMA* 1986;256:1017–1020.

3. Jacobsen PD. Medical liability and the culture of technology, p. 126.

4. Tinker JH, Dull DL, Caplan RA, Ward RJ, Cheney FW: Role of monitoring devices in prevention of anesthetic mishaps: A closed claims analysis. *Anesthesiology* 1989;71:541–546.

5. Cheney FW, Posner K, Caplan RA, Ward RJ. Standard of care and anesthesia liability. *JAMA* 1989;261:1599–1603.

6. Scott RW. *Health Care Malpractice. A Primer on Legal Issues for Professionals*. 2nd Ed. New York: McGraw Hill, 1999, p. 5.

7. Boumil MM, Elias CE. *The Law of Medical Liability*. West Publishing, St Paul, 1995. p. 24.

8. Scott RW. *Health Care Malpractice*, pp. 16–18.

9. Posner KL, Caplan RA, Cheney FW: Variation in expert opinion in medical malpractice review. *Anesthesiology* 1996;85:1049–54.

10. American Society of Anesthesiologists. ASA Basic Monitoring Standards. Amended October 25, 2005. http://www.asahq.org/publicationsAndServices/sgstoc.htm (as of 1/10/2009).

11. Vigoda MM, Lubarsky DA. Failure to recognize loss of incoming data in an anesthesia record-keeping system may have increased medical liability. *Anesth Analg* 2006;102:1798–802.

12. Domino KB, Bowdle TA, Posner KL, Spitellie PH, Lee LA, Cheney FW. Injuries and liability related to central vascular catheters: a closed claims analysis. *Anesthesiology*. 2004;100:1411–1418.

13. Pegalis SE. *American Law of Medical Malpractice*, 3d ed., vol 2. West Eagan, MN: Thomson, 2005;11:7.

14. Sebel PS, Bowdle TA, et al. The incidence of awareness during anesthesia: a multicenter United States study. *Anesth Analg* 2004;99:833–9.

15. Kent CD. Liability associated with awareness during anesthesia. *ASA Newsletter* 2006;70(6): 8–10.

16. JCAHO Sentinel Alert. Preventing, and managing the impact of, anesthesia awareness. Volume 32, October 6, 2004.

17. Practice Advisory for Intraoperative Awareness and Brain Function Monitoring. *Anesthesiology* 2006;104:847–64.

18. National Board of Echocardiography, http://www.echoboards.org/certification/certexpl.html (as of 1/10/2009).

19. Block FE, Nuutinen L, Ballast B. Optimization of alarms: a study on alarm limits, alarm sounds and false alarms intended to reduce annoyance. *J Clin Monit Comput* 1999;15:75–83.

20. IEC 60601-1-8 (2005–08): Medical electrical equipment – Part 1–8: General requirements for safety – Collateral standard: general requirements, tests and guidance for alarm systems in medical electrical equipment and medical electrical systems. Geneva: International Electrotechnical Commission, 2005.

21. Imhoff M, Kuhls S. Alarm algorithms in critical care monitoring. *Anesth Analg* 2006;102:1525–37.

Validity, accuracy, and repeatability of monitoring variables

Daniel M. Thys and Jung Kim

Introduction

Most of the physiologic variables (they are variables, not parameters, because they vary from individual to individual) that we monitor in our daily practice are expressed as numerical values.[1] There are many advantages to the conversion of physiologic activities into numbers. In the digital age, numbers are easy to compute, analyze, display, or convert into graphic format. Additionally, most of us are very comfortable with the use of numbers. From early ages, we are able to estimate numbers in a linear manner.[2] We have an intrinsic understanding of what a "normal" value represents, of how a "range" characterizes the limits of a normal value, and how the magnitude of a change in a numerical value quantitates a deviation from normal physiologic function. We can intervene to correct abnormal values and tailor our response to the magnitude of the numerical change that we intend to achieve.

The purpose of this chapter is to reflect on numbers as representations of physiologic data. Many different variables will be alluded to, but to make the analysis more palatable, one variable, cardiac output (CO), will frequently be used as an example. Cardiac output was selected because it constitutes an important physiologic variable that we are keen to monitor, because it has been studied extensively and because new techniques to monitor CO continue to be introduced. Under no circumstances should this chapter be construed as a detailed review of CO monitoring. Such a review is provided in Chapter 8.

What is the monitored variable?

"My patient's heart rate is 96 beats per minute."

The definition of heart rate is self-explanatory and has been known to us since long before we entered medical school: heart rate is the number of heartbeats per unit of time, usually expressed as beats per minute (bpm). The principal purpose of heart rate monitoring is to detect numerical changes from normal or baseline. A low number draws our attention to various potential physiologic disturbances, whereas a high number suggests other disorders. We know that for the normal adult, the average heart rate is around 70 bpm. We are also well aware that it is more rapid in younger age groups. A heart rate of 96 bpm may be bradycardia in the newborn, but tachycardia in the elderly. In our practice, we interpret a numerical value such as heart rate within the context of its clinical setting. As scientific knowledge expands, however, the context within which a numerical value needs to be interpreted broadens.

Monitoring devices incorporate a variety of smoothing technologies to provide us with a relatively steady heart rate number that is free of artifacts. In our effort to obtain a steady or reliable heart rate number, however, we may be shrinking the clinical context and ignoring information that is of great value. When we observe changes in heart rate, they are usually the result of changes in the tone of the autonomic nervous system or reflex responses triggered by these changes. In a recent editorial, Deschamps and Denault explained how, in the future, the study of heart rate variability by quantitating autonomic tone may help us anticipate changes in heart rate and blood pressure.[3] This knowledge would allow us to apply our therapeutic interventions with greater efficacy. To gauge heart rate variability, time intervals between cardiac contractions are measured, and their variability is analyzed using statistical analysis or other techniques. Absence of, or a decrease in, heart rate variability has been associated with various disease states, poor prognosis, and negative outcomes.[4-9] On the contrary, preservation of, or increase in, heart rate variability has been related to good health and identified as a predictor of survival in critically ill patients.[7,8]

More recently, gender and postural position have been independently associated with heart rate (Figure 3.1).[10] In the supine position, heart rate is higher in women than in men, whereas on standing, heart rate increases significantly in both genders. Additionally, investigators have observed that in middle-aged women, parasympathetic modulation dominates heart rate control, whereas sympathetic tone is dominant in middle-aged men (Figure 3.2).[11] Finally, attention has recently turned to another measure of heart rate, called *intrinsic heart rate* (HR_{int}). HR_{int} is defined as the heart rate seen in the absence of ongoing sympathetic or parasympathetic influences on the heart.[12] We all know that heart rate increases with exercise, yet we also know that the maximal heart rate (HR_{max}) that can be achieved during exercise decreases with age. Christou and colleagues have investigated the mechanisms that underlie these age-related differences.[13] They observed that the lower mean HR_{max} achieved by older men is associated with lower mean levels of HR_{int} and chronotropic responsiveness to β-adrenergic

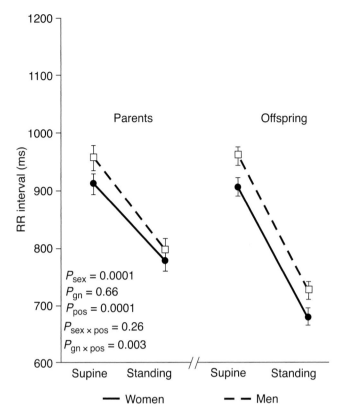

Figure 3.1. Influence of sex, generation, and posture on RR interval (P_{sex}, P_{gn}, P_{pos}, respectively) and two-way interaction terms. RR interval is the inverse of heart rate. Reproduced with permission from reference 10.

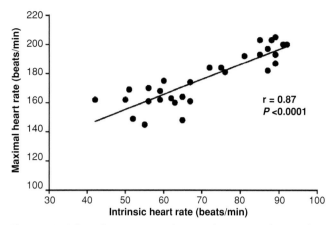

Figure 3.3. Relation between maximal exercise heart rate and intrinsic heart rate. Modified and reproduced with permission from reference 13.

same heart rate may be well below the HR_{max}; it all depends on the patient's HR_{int}.

As scientific knowledge evolves, it will become more and more challenging to provide a suitable context for each numerical value; our example of a heart rate of 96 bpm may need to be qualified for the patient's age, gender, HR_{int}, and heart rate variability, among many variables. It will be interesting to observe how monitoring technology evolves to incorporate some of these qualifiers into the monitoring of standard physiologic variables.

How is the variable measured?

"My patient's blood pressure is 137/81."

We routinely refer to normal arterial pressure as being 120 over 80 mmHg. This is certainly correct when considering average blood pressures measured by cuff inflation in large adult populations. In individual patients, however, the normal blood pressure may vary significantly from these values, depending on the method of measurement. There is a large volume of literature documenting differences in blood pressure measurements depending on whether the variable was measured by sphygmomanometry, oscillometry, or invasive methods.[14–17] Even within each technique, measurements will vary depending on equipment and procedures: aneroid versus mercury

stimulation when compared with young healthy men. They also noted that among individual subjects, HR_{int} shows a particularly strong correlation with HR_{max} (Figure 3.3).

The purpose of this brief discussion is not to review the autonomic determinants of heart rate, but to highlight the complexity of interpreting a single number, such as heart rate. A heart rate of 96 bpm can have widely differing meanings, depending on the clinical context. In a critically ill patient, a heart rate of 96 bpm will carry negative outcome implications if heart rate variability is absent. However, if heart rate variability is preserved, survival may be more likely. Similarly, a heart rate of 96 bpm may constitute one patient's HR_{max}; additional stress or β-adrenergic stimulation is unlikely to result in further increases in heart rate and/or CO. In a different subject, the

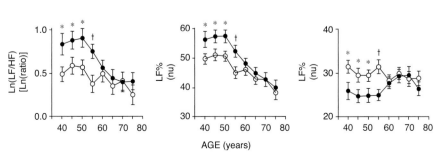

Figure 3.2. Effect of gender and age on all measures of heart rate variability at five-year intervals from 40 to 79 years. (HF: high frequency; LF: low frequency; In: natural logarithm; ● male; ○ female). Values are means ± SE; nu, no units (normalized). * $P < 0.05$; $P < 0.01$ between genders by Student's t-test. Modified and reproduced with permission from reference 11.

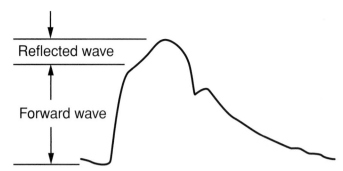

Figure 3.4. Carotid pressure waveform showing the forward and reflected wave pressures. Modified and reproduced with permission from reference 22.

manometer in sphygmomanometry, first-reading effect in oscillometry (the first of several readings obtained within a few minutes of each other tends to be higher, by about 3 to 5 mmHg, than subsequent readings), and location of the intraarterial catheter for invasive measurements.[18,19]

Because invasive blood pressure is often considered to be more reliable than noninvasive blood pressure, it is worth taking a closer look at its measurement. As the arterial pressure wave travels down the aortic tree, it is amplified by reflected waves and its amplitude increases in the periphery (Figures 3.4 and 3.5).[20] The magnitude of the reflected wave will depend on a complex relationship among the patient's age, the elastic properties of the arterial tree, and the location of the pressure measurement.[21] Wave reflection is most pronounced in subjects between the ages of 20 and 40. In a 2004 study, Mitchell and associates have shown that in healthy middle-aged and elderly individuals with no known cardiovascular disease, aortic stiffness increases dramatically with advancing age, whereas the stiffness of second- and third-generation muscular arteries increases minimally with age (Figure 3.6).[22] Therefore, in healthy elderly subjects, changes in central aortic stiffness and forward wave amplitude, rather than wave reflection, are responsible for most of the increase in pulse pressure. These

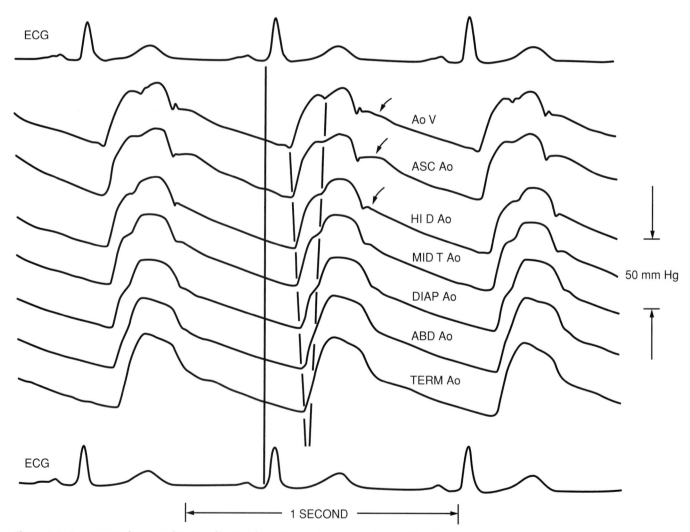

Figure 3.5. Pressure waveforms as a function of location from the ascending aorta to the iliac bifurcation in one patient. Figure constructed from single pulse or pairs of pulses selected from cardiac cycles with equal RR intervals and from similar phases of respiration. Ao V = sensor just above aortic valve; Asc Ao = ascending aorta; Hi D Ao = high descending aorta; Mid T Ao = midthoracic aorta; Diap Ao = diaphragmatic aorta; Abd Ao = abdominal aorta; Term Ao = terminal abdominal aorta just before iliac bifurcation. Reproduced with permission from reference 20.

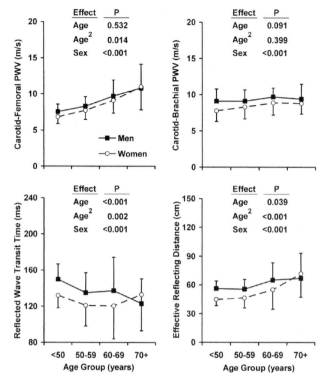

Figure 3.6. Means of regional pulse wave velocities (PWVs) and reflected wave variables by sex and decade of age. Carotid–femoral PWV increased substantially with advancing age (age^2 term), whereas an insignificant increase in carotid–brachial PWV was found in these unadjusted analyses. As a result, carotid–femoral PWV exceeded carotid–brachial PWV in older participants. Aortic stiffening was accompanied by a proportional decrease in reflected wave transit time in younger but not older groups; therefore, distance to the effective reflecting site increased in older individuals. Numbers per group (men/women): <50 years, $n = 43/52$; 50 to 59 years, $n = 74/172$; 60 to 69 years, $n = 57/82$; and 70+ years, $n = 14/27$. Reproduced with permission from reference 22.

observations provide insights into the variable mechanisms of age-related loss of peripheral pressure amplification: In young adults with a reflected pressure wave arriving centrally during diastole, pulse pressure is substantially higher in the periphery as compared with the central aorta. In middle age, increasing pulse wave velocity leads to premature return of the reflected pressure wave to the central aorta during systole, which augments central systolic and pulse pressure and reduces peripheral amplification. Finally, in the elderly, central arterial stiffness exceeds peripheral arterial stiffness. This loss of the normal arterial stiffness gradient reduces amplification and reflection. These changes are more pronounced in women than in men.

In summary, invasive systolic and diastolic blood pressure recordings will vary with the sampling location (central versus peripheral), the age of the patient (young versus middle-aged versus elderly), and the patient's gender. Compared with central aortic pressure, invasive pulse pressure measured in the dorsalis pedis artery will be markedly amplified in the young, moderately amplified in the middle-aged, and equivalent in the elderly. Gender may further accentuate these differences. Normal blood pressure is indeed a complicated concept. In many instances, it will be difficult to interpret a blood pressure value

of 137/81 mmHg if the patient's characteristics and the method of pressure measurement are unknown. Similar limitations are associated with the monitoring of most other variables.

At first glance, the definition of CO is also straightforward: it is the volume of blood pumped in one minute by the heart. In the laboratory, CO can be measured accurately because the blood ejected by the heart in one minute can be collected and measured. In clinical practice, however, such a simple measurement is obviously not available; over the years, a variety of indirect measures of CO have been introduced. The earliest method was described by Adolph Fick in 1870 and was based on the principle that oxygen consumption is equal to the product of blood flow and oxygen consumed by the tissues.[23] The calculation of CO by the Fick principle requires that in addition to oxygen consumption, the oxygen content of arterial and mixed venous blood be measured. Subsequently, different techniques, including indicator dilution, Doppler velocimetry, pulse pressure analysis, impedance cardiography, CO_2 or inert gas rebreathing, and echocardiographic volumetry, have been introduced.[24–27] In each of these techniques, different entities are being measured and different assumptions relied on to derive CO; each method also has its own limitations and intrinsic errors.

The major limitations of the direct Fick technique are well recognized. They are related to errors in sampling and analysis, or to the inability to maintain steady-state hemodynamic and respiratory conditions. To minimize errors in sampling, the venous blood must be truly mixed venous blood and the samples must represent average, rather than instantaneous, samples. The most serious errors in the measurement of CO by the direct Fick technique result from changes in pulmonary volumes. Indeed, the methods used to measure oxygen consumption measure the uptake of oxygen by the lungs, rather than by the blood. Because lung volumes can change, the tissues' oxygen consumption is not necessarily being measured. In addition to these technical exigencies, one must wonder about the clinical usefulness of a CO measurement technique that requires steady-state conditions; indeed, it is during conditions of hemodynamic instability that CO measurements are of the greatest use.

Limitations of other CO measurement techniques are also manifold. In the dilution techniques, errors result from inadequate mixing and recirculation of the dye, as well as from respiratory variability. Doppler measurements are dependent on beam orientation and flow profile assumptions. Thoracic impedance measurements are influenced by lead placement and body habitus assumptions. In brief, none of these techniques is devoid of problems, and therefore establishing their accuracy is challenging.

How accurate is the measurement?

"My patient's cardiac output is 4.76 L/min."

Accuracy is the degree of closeness of a measured or calculated variable to its true value. In the physical sciences, the accuracy of a measurement technique is usually determined by repeatedly measuring a well-defined reference standard. The reference standards are obtained from an organization such as the National Institute of Standards and Technology. This federal organization supplies industry, academia, government, and other users with more than 1300 reference materials that are of the highest quality and have metrologic value. Obviously, there is no equivalent process to characterize the accuracy of clinical monitoring techniques.

When the accuracy of a new CO technique is investigated, it often involves a comparison with thermodilution. But is thermodilution CO truly a valid standard? As mentioned previously, CO can be measured accurately if the heart's output is pumped into a measurement bucket and quantitated over time. Although this approach is not practical in the clinical environment, it is certainly feasible in the laboratory. Interestingly, thermodilution has been studied in vitro, using a variety of mechanical models to produce precisely controlled blood flows.[28–33] Although not all these studies are comparable, there is broad agreement that thermodilution measurements deviate from the calibrated flows by ± 10 percent to 20 percent. Therefore, the concept of thermodilution as a gold standard is mostly fallacious. As a similar absence of true quantity or absolute standards applies to many clinical variables, a different approach is necessary to validate the accuracy of new monitoring techniques.

In their landmark publication, Bland and Altman addressed this issue.[34] The statistical method that they described allows one to compare a new method with an established technique rather than with a true quantity. The purpose of such an analysis is to define by how much the new method is likely to differ from the old technique. If the new method differs little from the old method, the two techniques can be used interchangeably. Ideally, the clinically acceptable difference will be defined *before* conducting the comparison; this facilitates interpretation of the results and the selection of a sample size.

In a comparison of two measurement techniques, a first step consists of building a plot with the difference between the results obtained with each of the two methods on the vertical axis and the mean of the results on the horizontal axis (Figure 3.7). One must then establish that there is no pattern or relationship in the plot of the averages versus the differences; it may be useful to calculate a correlation coefficient for the data and test it against the null hypothesis of $r = 0$. Assuming that there is no obvious relationship between the differences and the mean, one can calculate the bias and the limits of agreement. The bias is equal to the mean of the differences, whereas the 95 percent limits of agreement are the bias plus and minus two standard deviations of the differences (this assumes a normal or Gaussian distribution of the differences). If the bias or mean difference is small, it can be ignored. If the bias is consistent, an adjustment can be applied; one can subtract the bias or mean difference from the new method. The 95 percent limits of agreement are used to determine the clinical validity of the new technique. As stated earlier, ideally the acceptable

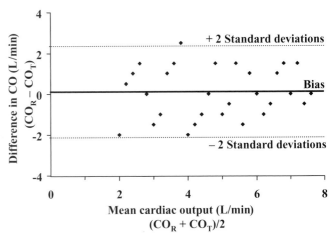

Figure 3.7. Typical Bland–Altman plot for the comparison of two cardiac output techniques (CO_R: cardiac output from reference technique; CO_T: cardiac output from tested technique).

difference between the two techniques would have been defined before the conduct of the comparison. If the differences within the 95 percent limits of agreement are not clinically important, the two measurements methods can be used interchangeably.

Bias analysis has been used extensively in the evaluation of new CO monitoring techniques and examples from the literature will be used to clarify this method of comparison. To assess the validity of a new continuous CO (CCO) device, Bein and associates studied 113 CO measurements in 10 patients and compared them with measurements of CO by pulse contour analysis and ultrasound (Doppler) techniques.[35] The authors plotted the mean of the results on the horizontal axis and the difference between the results on the vertical axis. As indicated previously, the next step in the analysis consists of determining whether an obvious relationship exists between the differences and the mean results. For both comparisons, this certainly was the case ($r = -0.69$ and $r = -0.52$, respectively; Figures 3.8 and 3.9). When compared with pulse contour and ultrasound, the new technique (CCO) appeared to systematically overestimate CO at low values (2 to 4 L/min) and to underestimate CO at high values (> 5 L/min). When such a data distribution occurs, little useful information can be derived from the bias calculation (Bland and Altman suggest that a log transformation of the data may occasionally be helpful). Indeed, the purpose of the bias calculation is to define the systematic adjustment that needs to be made to the measurements by the new technique so they are in agreement with those of the established technique. In the current example, one would need to make a negative adjustment at low CO, no adjustment at normal CO, and a positive adjustment at high CO. Clinically, this is highly impractical.

In a different study, Missant et al. compared CO by pulse contour analysis and Doppler echocardiography with thermodilution CO.[36] The investigators compared 149 pulse contour measurements with 84 Doppler measurements with thermodilution in 20 patients. When the means of the results were plotted on the horizontal axis and the difference between the results

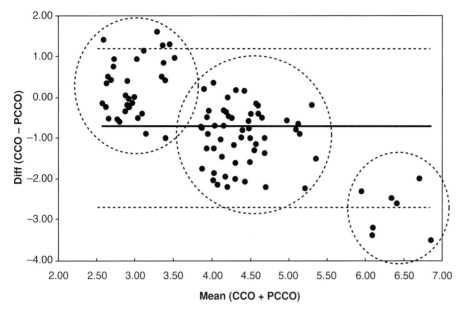

Figure 3.8. Bland–Altman plot between continuous cardiac output (CCO) and pulse-contour cardiac output (PCCO) techniques. The solid line represents the mean difference (bias); the dotted line represents the 2SD limits of agreement. Dotted circles added for emphasis. Modified and reproduced with permission from reference 35.

on the vertical axis, no obvious relationship could be discerned for either comparison (Figures 3.10 and 3.11). For a range of CO values between 2 and 7.5 L/min, the data points distributed randomly around the average difference between the measurements. The bias or average difference between the measurements was –0.03 L/min for the comparison between pulse contour and thermodilution, and +0.45 L/min for the comparison between Doppler and thermodilution. Although a systematic error of –0.03 L/min has little clinical significance and can be ignored, the same most likely cannot be said about an error of 0.45 L/min. Therefore, CO measured by the Doppler technique

that is described in the manuscript would require a systematic adjustment of +0.45 L/min to be comparable with thermodilution CO.

The next step in the analysis of the results requires that the 95 percent limits of agreement be calculated (± 2 standard deviations of the differences). For the comparison between pulse contour and thermodilution, they were found to be +1.26 L/min and –1.33 L/min, whereas they were +2.38 L/min and –1.49 L/min for Doppler and thermodilution. Finally, one must decide whether the 95 percent limits of agreement are clinically acceptable. In the current example, assuming a true CO of

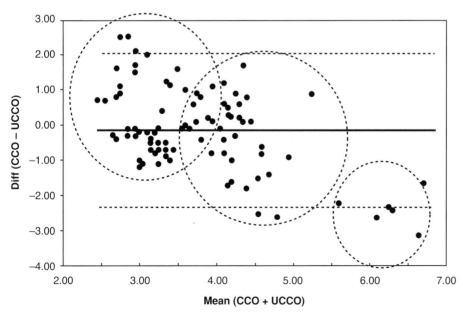

Figure 3.9. Bland–Altman plot between continuous cardiac output (CCO) and ultrasound cardiac output (UCCO) techniques. The solid line represents the mean difference (bias); the dotted line represents the 2SD limits of agreement. Dotted circles added for emphasis. Modified and reproduced with permission from reference 35.

21

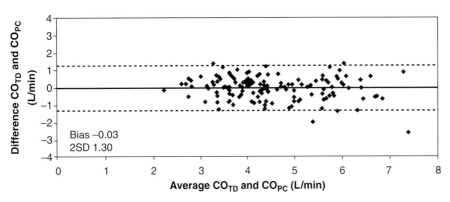

Figure 3.10. Bland–Altman plot of cardiac output measurements by pulmonary artery thermodilution (CO$_{TD}$) and pulse contour analysis (CO$_{PC}$). Reproduced with permission from reference 36.

4.5 L/min, pulse contour analysis will yield CO values between 3.2 L/min and 5.8 L/min in 95 percent of measurements. For Doppler echocardiography, they will fall between 2.57 L/min and 6.43 L/min. Are those values clinically acceptable?

In 1999, Critchley and Critchley published a very elegant study that answered this question.[37] They conducted a meta-analysis of studies that compared methods of CO measurement and used Bland–Altman statistics for analysis. They identified 25 comparative studies and stated that acceptance of a new method of CO measurement needed to be judged against the accuracy of the reference method. In most studies, the reference method is thermodilution, which has an accuracy of ± 20 percent, as stated earlier. They concluded that a new CO measurement technique should be accepted if the percentage error (± 2 standard deviations divided by the mean CO for the study) did not exceed ± 30 percent.

We can now apply these acceptability criteria to the study of Missant et al. Although the authors do not provide the mean CO for the study, one can deduce from the published data that it was 4.5 L/min. Therefore, the percentage error for pulse contour analysis was 29 percent (2 standard deviations = 1.3; mean CO = 4.5 L/min; percentage error = 1.3/4.5). This falls within the acceptable range as defined by Critchley and Critchley, and thus pulse contour analysis can be substituted for thermodilution. For Doppler echocardiography, the percentage error was 43 percent and thus, in these investigators' experience, it is not an acceptable substitute for thermodilution.

One must obviously keep in mind that these findings apply only to this one specific study. Indeed, other studies yield very different findings. When Darmon and colleagues compared CO by Doppler echocardiography and thermodilution, they found a percentage error of 19 percent.[38] Such an error is well within the acceptable range and, in these latter investigators' clinical practice, Doppler echocardiography and thermodilution are interchangeable.

The reasons that studies can yield such divergent findings are myriad and related to differences in patient population, experimental circumstances, and methodological variations. Evidently, a clinician can draw conclusions about the acceptability of a new technique only by consulting the broadest body of evidence available.

Although Bland–Altman analysis is now widely used in the assessment of new monitoring techniques, clinically acceptable 95 percent limits of agreement are seldom defined before the onset of a study. In a review by Mantha and associates of 42 anesthesia reports that used limits of agreement methodology to analyze comparisons between measurement techniques, only three reports included an *a priori* definition of limits of agreement.[39]

Furthermore, the 30 percent acceptability criteria that were defined by Critchley and Critchley for the comparison of new CO techniques with thermodilution cannot be applied to the comparison of measurement techniques for other variables, as they sometimes are.[40] Clearly, for each physiologic variable,

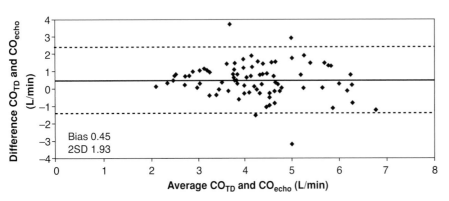

Figure 3.11. Bland–Altman plot of cardiac output measurements by pulmonary artery thermodilution (CO$_{TD}$) and pulse contour analysis (CO$_{echo}$). Reproduced with permission from reference 36.

clinically acceptable limits need to be determined. For example, in a study of transcutaneous PCO_2 monitoring devices, the clinically acceptable limits were set at ± 7.5 mmHg.[41] How such a value was arrived at is unclear, but it is at least a step in the right direction. The European Society of Hypertension recommends that automated sphygmomanometers differ from a mercury standard by a standard deviation of less than 8 mmHg.[42,43] For laboratory analysis of PO_2 and PCO_2, limits of ± 7.5 percent have been recommended.[44]

How reproducible is the measurement?

"My patient's second cardiac output is 4.15 L/min."

When interpreting data from a monitoring or measurement technique, it is important to know not only the technique's accuracy, but also its repeatability or reproducibility. Indeed, from a clinical standpoint, one needs to know whether the second measurement of a variable is significantly different from a prior measurement. Does the new value represent a true decrease in CO (e.g., a real decrease of 13% from 4.76 L/min to 4.15 L/min), or are the two values within the measurement technique's expected range of variability?

To understand the difference between accuracy and reproducibility, it is useful to refer to a target comparison (Figure 3.12). If a number of rounds are fired at a target, *accuracy* will describe the closeness of the hits to the bull's-eye of the target. Rounds that hit close to the center of the target are considered to be accurate. As additional rounds are fired, their location in relation to prior hits will determine *reproducibility*. If all the hits are clustered together, the reproducibility is

considered to be high (Figure 3.12A, C); if they are widely dispersed, the reproducibility is low (Figure 3.12D). A few additional observations are worth considering. (1) As shown in Figure 3.12C, a measurement system can have high reproducibility, but low accuracy. The reverse is not true, however. For a system to be accurate, the hits must be close to the center of the target, and therefore, by necessity, they will also be close together. (2) Average accuracy measurements can be misleading. Indeed. if one were somehow able to calculate an average accuracy for the four hits in Figure 3.12D, one would end up with a high mean accuracy (a hit above the center is counterbalanced by a hit below the center, etc.). However, each individual hit is highly inaccurate and poorly reproducible. Therefore, knowing a measurement system's average accuracy without knowing its reproducibility is of limited use.

When Bland and Altman published their method to test agreement between two methods of clinical measurement, they also referred to *repeatability* as relevant to the assessment of agreement. It is indeed obvious that if there is considerable variability in the results obtained with a certain method, agreement with another method will, by definition, be poor. To gauge reproducibility, they suggest that a coefficient of repeatability be calculated. This can be done in a manner similar to the one used to test the limits of agreement: the mean of repeated measurements are plotted on the horizontal axis, and the differences between measurements are plotted on the vertical axis. Theoretically, the mean of the differences should be zero, as the same measurement method was used. The standard deviation of the differences is calculated, and the value of two standard deviations is considered to be the coefficient of repeatability. The coefficient of repeatability represents the value below which the

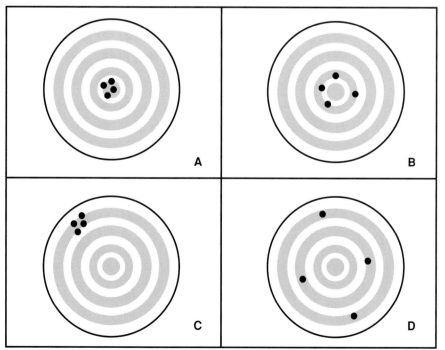

Figure 3.12. Target comparison of accuracy and reproducibility. (A) High accuracy and reproducibility; (B) moderate accuracy and reproducibility; (C) low accuracy and high reproducibility; (D) low accuracy and reproducibility.

absolute difference between two repeated test results is expected to lie, with a probability of 95 percent. If several repeated measurements are obtained per subject, the standard deviations of the measurements are plotted against their mean and analyzed by one-way analysis of variance.

It is worth noting that when Mantha and colleagues analyzed the anesthesia literature, they observed that repeatability was assessed in only 9 of 42 reports (21.4%). In addition, the manner by which repeatability was evaluated varied markedly from study to study. For instance, Seguin and associates used two different approaches to assess reproducibility of semicontinuous thermodilution CO and bolus thermodilution CO.[45] The first approach was the one described by Stetz and colleagues in 1982.[46] The Stetz group reviewed 14 publications on the use of thermodilution in clinical practice and concluded that with the use of commercial thermodilution devices, a minimal difference of 12 percent to 15 percent (average 13%) between determinations was required to be statistically significant, provided that each determination was obtained by averaging three measurements. If each determination was the result of only a single measurement, a minimal difference of 20 percent to 26 percent (average 22%) was required for statistical significance. In practice, a standard error of the mean can be calculated for the measurements. A variation of at least three standard errors of the mean is necessary to establish with confidence that two values of CO differ from each other. With this analysis, Seguin and associates determined that the threshold required to establish that two CO measurements are different was 0.54 L/min for bolus CO and 0.465 L/min for continuous CO. Although they also tested repeatability by the Bland–Altman method, they did not provide a coefficient of repeatability for their measurements, and therefore, the meaning of their analysis is unclear.

Reproducibility will be influenced by myriad factors, some intrinsic to the measurement technique and others determined by technical aspects of the measurement. These technical factors have been well studied for thermodilution CO. Factors such as temperature and volume of injectate, speed and rate of injection, and timing in the respiratory cycle have all been shown to influence the reproducibility of thermodilution CO.[47,48]

Finally, two additional observations related to this discussion of accuracy and reproducibility merit comment. First, in most of the studies that were referenced previously, the number of data points plotted in the Bland–Altman analysis exceeds the number of studied patients – that is, multiple measurements are included for each patient. Therefore, the bias analysis will be influenced not only by the differences between the two measurement techniques but also by the reproducibility of each of the measurement techniques. In most publications, however, this obvious limitation is never mentioned.

Second, it is often suggested that the monitoring of changes in physiologic variables is more important than a focus on specific values. Even though this may be true, interpretation of change is feasible only if the repeatability of the measurement technique is known. As mentioned earlier, most investigations of new measurement techniques fail to include an analysis of reproducibility. In its absence, the meaning of changes cannot be interpreted.

Conclusions

In our daily management of patients, we collect a large quantity of numbers from a variety of physiologic monitors. We interpret these values and tailor our therapeutic interventions to the results of our interpretations. The purpose of this brief discussion was to stimulate thought about the meaning of some of the numbers that we use in our clinical management. The following conclusions can be drawn:

1. An individual value, even one as simple as heart rate, is meaningless if it is not analyzed within its clinical context; as scientific knowledge expands, the importance of the clinical context increases.
2. For each measured variable, the values that one obtains will be influenced by a large number of factors. These include the underlying physiologic process, but also factors related to patient characteristics, the measurement technique, and the manner in which the technique is applied.
3. It is seldom possible to determine the accuracy of a new measurement technique, because reference standards rarely exist in clinical medicine. The best one can hope for is to ascertain whether a new technique is interchangeable with an older, established technique. The Bland–Altman analysis was designed to test such interchangeability.
4. One needs to know the reproducibility of a measurement technique to gauge its value; a technique that yields results that are poorly reproducible is of limited value. In addition, because absolute values are often influenced by a large number of confounding factors, the monitoring of changes is often recommended. However, changes cannot be interpreted if one does not know the measurement technique's reproducibility.

References

1. Altman DG, Bland JM. Variables and parameters. *Br Med J* 1999; 318:1667.
2. Ebersbach M, Luwel K, Frick A, Onghena P, Verschaffel L. The relationship between the shape of the mental number line and familiarity with numbers in 5- to 9-year old children: Evidence for a segmented linear model. *J Exper Child Psychol* 2008;99:1–17.
3. Deschamps A, Denault A. Analysis of heart rate variability: a useful tool to evaluate autonomic tone in the anesthetized patient? *Can J Anaesth* 2008; 55(4):208–13.
4. Carpeggiani C, Emdin M, Raciti M, et al. Heart rate variability and myocardial infarction: acute and sub-acute phase. CNR-PF FATMA Multicenter Study on psycho-neurological risk factors in acute myocardial infarction. *Clin Sci (Lond)* 1996;91 Suppl:28–9.
5. Piepoli M, Coats AJ. Autonomic abnormality in chronic heart failure evaluated by heart rate variability. *Clin Sci (Lond)* 1996;91Suppl:84–6.

6. Voss A, Wessel N, Sander A, Malberg H, Dietz R. Requirements on sampling rate in Holter systems for analysis of heart rate variability. *Clin Sci (Lond)* 1996;91 Suppl:120–1.

7. Maier P, Toepfer M, Dambacher M, Theisen K, Roskamm H, Frey AW. Heart rate variability and its relation to ventricular tachycardia in patients with coronary artery disease. *Clin Sci (Lond)* 1996;91Suppl:67.

8. Schmidt H, Muller-Werdan U, Hoffmann T, et al. Autonomic dysfunction predicts mortality in patients with multiple organ dysfunction syndrome of different age groups. *Crit Care Med* 2005;33:1994–2002.

9. Winchell RJ, Hoyt DB. Analysis of heart-rate variability: a noninvasive predictor of death and poor outcome in patients with severe head injury. *J Trauma* 1997;43:927–33.

10. Stolarz K, Staessen J, Kuznetsova T, et al. Host and environmental determinants of heart rate and heart rate variability in four European populations. *J Hypertens* 2003;21:525–35.

11. Kuo TBJ, Lin T, Yang CCH, Li CL, Chen CF, Chou P. Effect of aging on gender differences in neural control of heart rate. *Am J Physiol Heart Circ Physiol* 1999;277:H2233-H2239.

12. Joyner MJ. Not so fast: intrinsic heart rate vs. beta-adrenergic responsiveness in the aging human heart. *J Appl Physiol* 2008;105(1):3–4.

13. Christou D, Seals D. Decreased maximal heart rate with aging is related to reduced β-adrenergic responsiveness but is largely explained by a reduction in intrinsic heart rate. *J Appl Physiol* 2008;105(1):24–9.

14. Park MK, Menard SW, Yuan C. Comparison of auscultatory and oscillometric blood pressures. *Arch Pediatr Adolesc Med* 2001;155:50–53.

15. Goonasekera CD, Dillon MJ. Random zero sphygmomanometer versus automatic oscillometric blood pressure monitor; is either the instrument of choice? *J Hum Hypertens* 1995;9:885–9.

16. Gillman MW, Cook NR. Blood pressure measurement in childhood epidemiological studies. *Circulation* 1995;92:1049–57.

17. Park MK, Menard SM. Accuracy of blood pressure measurement by the Dinamap monitor in infants and children. *Pediatrics* 1986;79:907–14.

18. Perloff D, Grim C, Flack J, et al. Human blood pressure determination by sphygmomanometry. *Circulation* 1993;88:2460–70.

19. Park MK, Menard SM. Normative oscillometric blood pressure values in the first 5 years in an office setting. *Am J Dis Child* 1989;143:860–4.

20. Murgo JP, Westerhof N, Giolma JP, Altobelli SA. Aortic input impedance in normal man: relationship to pressure wave forms. *Circulation* 1980;62:105–16.

21. Westerhof BE, Guelen I, Westerhof N, Karemaker JM, Avolio A. Quantification of wave reflection in the human aorta from pressure alone: a proof of principle. *Hypertension* 2006;48:595–601.

22. Mitchell GF, Parise H, Benjamin EJ, et al. Changes in arterial stiffness and wave reflection with advancing age in healthy men and women: the Framingham Heart Study. *Hypertension* 2004;43:1239–45.

23. Fick A. Über die Messung des Blutquantums in den Hertzventrikln. *Sitz Physik Med Würzburg* 1870; p. 16.

24. Albert NM, Hail MD, Li J, Young JB. Equivalence of the bioimpedance and thermodilution methods in measuring cardiac output in hospitalized patients with advanced, decompensated chronic heart failure. *Am J Crit Care* 2004;13(6):469–79.

25. Haryadi DG, Orr JA, Kuck K, McJames S, Westenskow DR. Partial CO_2 rebreathing indirect Fick technique for non-invasive measurement of cardiac output. *J Clin Monit Comput* 2000;16(5–6):361–74.

26. Spiess BD, Patel MA, Soltow LO, Wright IH. Comparison of bioimpedance versus thermodilution cardiac output during cardiac surgery: evaluation of a second-generation bioimpedance device. *J Cardiothorac Vasc Anesth* 2001;15(5):567–73.

27. Parra V, Fita G, Rovira I, Matute P, Gomar C, Paré C. Transoesophageal echocardiography accurately detects cardiac output variation: a prospective comparison with thermodilution in cardiac surgery. *Eur J Anaesthesiol* 2008;25(2):135–43.

28. Jebson P, Karkow W. Pulsatile flow simulator for comparison of cardiac output measurements by electromagnetic flow meter and thermodilution. *J Clin Monit* 1986;2:6–14.

29. Bilfinger TV, Lin CY, Anagnostopoulos CE. In vitro determination of accuracy of cardiac output measurements by thermal dilution. *J Surg Res* 1982;33(5):409–14.

30. Norris SL, King EG, Grace M, Weir B. Thermodilution cardiac output – an in vitro model of low flow states. *Crit Care Med* 1986;14(1): 57–9.

31. Runciman WB, Ilsley AH, Roberts JG. An evaluation of thermodilution cardiac output measurement using the Swan-Ganz catheter. *Anaesth Intensive Care* 1981;9(3):208–20.

32. Powner DJ, Snyder JV. In vitro comparison of six commercially available thermodilution cardiac output systems. *Med Instrum* 1978;12(2):122–7.

33. Renner LE, Morton MJ, Sakuma GY. Indicator amount, temperature, and intrinsic cardiac output affect thermodilution cardiac output accuracy and reproducibility. *Crit Care Med* 1993;21(4):586–97.

34. Bland JM, Altman DG. Statistical methods for assessing between two methods of clinical measurement. *Lancet* 1986;1(8476):307–10.

35. Bein B, Worthmann F, Tonner PH, Paris A, Steinfath M, Hedderich J, Scholz J. Comparison of esophageal Doppler, pulse contour analysis, and real-time pulmonary artery thermodilution for the continuous measurement of cardiac output. *J Cardiothorac Vasc Anesth* 2004;18:185–189.

36. Missant C, Rex S, Wouters, PF. Accuracy of cardiac output measurements with pulse contour analysis (PulseCO) and Doppler echocardiography during off-pump coronary artery bypass grafting. *Eur J Anaesthesiol* 2008;25:243–48.

37. Critchley LAH, Critchley JAHJ. A meta-analysis of studies using bias and precision statistics to compare cardiac output measurement techniques. *J Clin Monit Comput* 1999;15:85–91.

38. Darmon PL, Hillel Z, Mogtader A, Mindich B, Thys D. Cardiac output by transesophageal echocardiography using continuous-wave Doppler across the aortic valve. *Anesthesiology* 1994;80(4):796–805.

39. Mantha S, Roizen MF, Fleisher LA, Thisted R, Foss J. Comparing methods of clinical measurement: reporting standards for Bland and Altman analysis. *Anesth Analg* 2000;90(3):593–602.

40. Molnar Z, Umgelter A, Toth I, et al. Continuous monitoring of ScvO(2) by a new fibre-optic technology compared with blood gas oximetry in critically ill patients: a multicentre study. *Intensive Care Med* 2007;33(10):1767–70.

41. Bendjelid K, Schütz N, Stotz M, Gerard I, Suter PM, Romand JA. Transcutaneous PCO_2 monitoring in critically ill adults: clinical

evaluation of a new sensor. *Crit Care Med* 2005;33(10): 2203–6.

42. Association for the Advancement of Medical Instrumentation. American National Standard. Electronic or Automated Sphygmomanometers. ANSI/AAMI SP 10–1992. Arlington, VA: AAMI, 1993:40.

43. O'Brien E, Waeber B, Parati G, Staessen J, Myers MG. Blood pressure measuring devices: recommendations of the European Society of Hypertension. *BMJ* 2001;322:531–6.

44. Zollinger A, Spahn DR, Singer T, et al. Accuracy and clinical performance of a continuous intra-arterial blood-gas monitoring system during thoracoscopic surgery. *Br J Anaesth* 1997;79: 47–52.

45. Seguin P, Colcanap O, Le Rouzo A, Tanguy M, Guillou YM, Malledant Y. Evaluation of a new semi-continuous cardiac output system in the intensive care unit. *Can J Anesth* 1998;45:578–83.

46. Stetz CW, Miller RG, Kelly GE, Raffin TA. Reliability of the thermodilution method in the determination of cardiac output in clinical practice. *Am Rev Respir Dis* 1982;126(6):1001–4.

47. Stevens JH, Raffin TA, Mihm FG, Rosenthal MH, Stetz CW. Thermodilution cardiac output measurement. Effects of the respiratory cycle on its reproducibility. *JAMA* 1985;253(15):2240–2.

48. Pearl RG, Rosenthal MH, Nielson L, Ashton JP, Brown BW Jr. Effect of injectate volume and temperature on thermodilution cardiac output determination. *Anesthesiology* 1986;64(6):798–801.

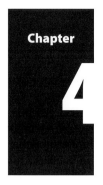

Chapter 4

Teaching monitoring skills

Samuel DeMaria Jr., Adam I. Levine, and Yasuharu Okuda

Introduction

Most medical schools and residency programs do not have a formalized training and assessment program dedicated to the acquisition of skills and knowledge needed for monitoring the perioperative patient. This is understandable, as the current model of medical education was developed during the early 20th century, when the act of monitoring during a procedure meant a very different enterprise from the current state of the art in anesthesiology. Typically, information related to monitor output was first learned piecemeal throughout medical school, and only when it was necessary to demonstrate changes in patient physiology related to a drug or disease process. It was rarely taught as a stand-alone topic, even at the graduate medical education (GME) level. Although the Accreditation Council for Graduate Medical Education (ACGME) defines the scope of practice for anesthesiology to include "monitoring and maintenance of normal physiology during the perioperative period" and mandates that anesthesiology residents have "significant experience with central vein and pulmonary artery catheter placement and the use of transesophageal echocardiography and evoked potentials," a standardized curriculum and a standardized assessment for monitor training do not currently exist.[1] Physicians in training learn monitoring skills in the same way they learn other procedures, by "seeing, doing, and teaching."

Over the past 20 years, there have been significant advances in available monitoring modalities. Although the complexity of monitoring has become daunting, physicians are now able to continuously measure physiologic parameters such as core temperature, end-tidal CO_2, and arterial blood pressure. With each of these advanced capabilities comes a need to learn new skills and knowledge in new ways. As an emphasis on patient safety and error reduction has become paramount, it is increasingly difficult for medical students and residents to "learn on the job" on actual patients. This situation creates an opportunity for innovative educators to develop and implement unique educational modalities using state-of-the-art technologies to teach and evaluate perioperative physiologic monitoring skills.

The traditional method of passive learning through lectures and reading is not ideal for teaching the majority of monitoring skills, given the dynamic nature of these devices and the data they generate. Although some basic concepts can be effectively taught in a lecture format, the development of psychomotor skills needed for invasive monitor placement, as well as the development of cognitive skills needed for data analysis, data synthesis, and data fidelity determination, are best been taught at the bedside. Unfortunately, the bedside teaching of monitoring skills has become challenging in the current medicolegal climate and has put an increased demand on faculty efficiency and productivity.

Unlike passive instruction, adult learning theory emphasizes the need for adults to learn in an environment that promotes experience and self-direction.[2] Based on this learning theory, adult learners need to understand the benefits of knowledge as well as its potential applications for their learning to be successful. This was corroborated by a review by Davis and associates.[3] In an attempt to determine formal continuing medical education (CME) effectiveness, the authors reviewed a wide variety of CME formats, including conferences, refresher courses, seminars, lectures, and workshops, and explored the effect of formal CME on American, Canadian, and French internists, pediatricians, and family practitioners. The authors concluded that "interactive educational sessions that enhance participant activity and provide the opportunity to practice skills can effect change in professional practice and, on occasion, health care outcome." They also concluded that "didactic sessions alone do not appear to be effective in changing physician performance."

Not surprisingly, increased learner participation and interaction between educator and student also increased overall satisfaction with the teaching program.[4] Cantillion and Jones determined that although interactive experience is important, it is much more effective for the adult learner when it is accompanied by feedback.[5] The use of evaluation and feedback was support by Reiter and associates, who determined that adults are not innately self-directed learners who can accurately assess their own strengths and weaknesses.[6] It follows that educational modalities that encourage interactive, hands-on, small-group sessions that include immediate feedback would be the most effective.

With the understanding of adult learning and effective teaching modalities, an innovative model for teaching monitoring skills that takes a logical, chronologic approach is described in this chapter. Implementing new technologies, such as simulation for monitor skill teaching, is also expanded on. Implementing such a program will afford the educator the opportunity to teach monitoring skills in an active and explicit fashion that is more likely to affect a student's knowledge base in an efficient and effective way.

Philosophical framework for teaching monitoring skills in perioperative medicine

The numerous effects of anesthesia on the normal physiologic state mandate that practitioners engaged in the delivery of perioperative care be facile with a number of monitoring skills and modalities. Only through such competence can the mission of the Anesthesia Patient Safety Foundation (APSF), "[t]hat no patient shall be harmed by anesthesia," be realized. Successfully teaching such complex skills to clinicians and students relies on multimodality techniques based firmly in adult learning theory. Because the practitioner is the final common conduit through which all input gleaned from monitors passes, he or she should be optimally trained to process, interpret, and act on such information on the patient's behalf. He or she must also understand that monitoring is a process that is ongoing and does not occur in isolation from other clinical information.

Interpreting and placing physiologic monitors is second nature for the seasoned anesthesiologist. Many do not normally consider all the components involved with successfully monitoring patients in their day-to-day activities. Therefore, deconstructing the skills necessary for safe and effective patient monitoring placement and interpretation is critical in the development of an effective and systematic educational methodology of teaching monitoring skills.

Monitoring skills can be divided into psychomotor and cognitive skills. These skills can be further subdivided into various components. Educators can determine from these lists which specific goals and objectives they hope to accomplish during a particular monitoring skills teaching session (Box 4.1).

In 1999, the ACGME and the American Board of Medical Specialties (ABMS) defined competency in terms of six domains to be used in the evaluation of new practitioners (Table 4.1).[7] In each of these domains, a set of unique knowledge, skills, and attitudes (which include behaviors) must be developed for the competencies to be achieved effectively.

An effective way for educators to approach the teaching of monitoring skills is to consider the ACGME core competencies within a *chronological* framework to identify the attitudes, skills, and knowledge necessary at each step in the monitoring process in the preoperative, intraoperative, and postoperative periods. We have coined this framework the "ASK [attitudes, skills, and knowledge] to achieve" model for developing monitoring skills (Boxes 4.2, 4.3, and 4.4).

Preoperative phase

Monitor selection and the timing of the monitor placement are critical components of monitoring skills. This preplacement stage is crucial to the anesthesia provider and is best approached systematically during the assessment of the patient and the anticipated surgical factors. Educators should emphasize which

---

Box 4.1 Psychomotor and cognitive components of monitoring skills

Psychomotor skills
Landmark identification
Patient positioning
Sterile patient and monitor kit preparation
Development of an ergonomic work environment
Hand–eye coordination
Procedure sequence
Intraprocedure troubleshooting
Proper placement confirmation
Securing monitor site

Cognitive skills
Monitor selection
  Indications
  Contraindications
Monitor site insertion
  Indications
  Contraindications
Timing of placement
  Preanesthetic induction
  Postanesthetic induction
Monitor interpretation
  Data validity
  Data corroboration
  Data analysis
Clinical management
  Development of differential diagnosis
  Therapeutic intervention
  Patient reassessment
  Monitor selection

Table 4.1. The ACGME core competencies

Domain of competency	Description of domain
Patient care	Compassionate and medically appropriate treatment of health problems
Medical knowledge	Understanding of established and evolving medical evidence and the application of such evidence to patient care
Practice-based learning and improvement	Evaluation of one's own patient care and utilization of medical knowledge to improve the delivery of this care to patients
Interpersonal and communication skills	Professional and appropriate interactions with patients and other health care providers to improve patient care
Professionalism	Carrying out professional responsibilities, adherence to ethical tenets, and sensitivity to diversity
Systems-based practice	Appropriate practice within the modern system of health care and the ability to effectively call on system resources to provide optimal care

Adapted from http://www.acgme.org/outcome/comp/compMin.asp.

Box 4.2 Preoperative ASK to achieve

1. **Evaluation of monitor necessity**
   - Gather surgical/patient information that supports/obviates the need for the monitor
   - Consider indications/contraindications
   - Consider invasive versus noninvasive monitors
   - Consider the timing of invasive monitor placement
   - Consider the evidence and cost/benefit ratio (e.g., use of bispectral index monitor for a patient with a low preoperative risk of intraoperative awareness)
   - Discuss the decision to place or forgo the monitor with the surgical team and patient
   - Ensure that the patient understands risks/benefits and has had questions answered

2. **Placement of monitors**
   - Anticipate the logistics/ergonomics of monitor placement and use
   - Master and practice the psychomotor skills necessary to safely place and activate monitor
   - Ensure patient comfort
   - Ensure patient safety (e.g., ultrasound-guided central venous catheter placement and maintenance of sterile technique)

   - Develop and adopt methods to combat error fixation and decreased vigilance (e.g., mandatory breaks and enabling all audible alarms)
   - Develop and implement scanning skills

3 **Intervention**
   - Apply knowledge of normal values and predetermined thresholds to clinical scenario
   - Decide what treatment is appropriate to correct a perceived abnormal monitor value
   - Cross-check and double-check fidelity of data before intervening or failing to intervene
   - Consider all corroborating and conflicting data
   - Recognize that no intervention is without risks and benefits
   - Communicate to appropriate team members that an intervention is being made

4 **Reevaluation**
   - Repeat steps 1–3 above after intervention as necessary
   - Consider expected response to the intervention
   - Communicate problems to team and seek assistance where appropriate
   - Be a patient advocate despite potential conflicting pressures

Box 4.3 Intraoperative ASK to achieve

1 **Interpretation of monitors**
   - Consider the technology and theory behind the monitor of interest
   - Consider the strengths/weaknesses
   - Consider the importance of corroborating/conflicting data as well as interfering factors (e.g., effect of electrocautery on ECG tracing)
   - Consider common pitfalls (e.g., importance of a good waveform in interpretation of the pulse oximeter reading)
   - Understand and anticipate the normal values for the particular patient
   - Master the intricacies of reading monitor changes (e.g., recognition of cannon waves on the arterial line tracing in a patient with AV block)
   - Develop troubleshooting and salvage skills (e.g., fixing a positional monitor)
   - Determine threshold values at which to consider an intervention (e.g., decision to switch to 100% oxygen if pulse oximeter continues to read less than 92%)
   - Develop confidence in physical exam skills to confirm or disprove potentially erroneous data (i.e., appreciate the importance of the practitioner as a monitor)

2 **Vigilance**
   - Recognize and correct barriers to proper vigilance (e.g., fatigue and distraction)

Box 4.4 Postoperative ASK to achieve

1 **Evaluation of monitor necessity**
   - Use a similar approach to monitor necessity as in preoperative phase
   - Determine need for new monitors
   - Consider logistics/ergonomics of the postoperative setting (e.g., will the intensive care unit be able to use monitors already in place?)
   - Communicate effectively the monitoring endpoints used to intervene for the patient intraoperatively and any problems encountered with the monitors

2 **Removal of monitors**
   - Predetermine what defines "stable" and discontinue monitors that are no longer necessary
   - Discontinue invasive monitors as soon as possible to prevent patient discomfort and likelihood of infection

monitors are standard (as defined by the ASA) and which monitor options are indicated and necessary based on the patient's comorbidities and/or the anticipated surgical derangements. After the array of monitors to be used is determined, the timing of monitor placement must also be considered and taught. Should the monitor be placed before the anesthetic induction, or can the monitor be placed safely after the anesthetic induction? Are the indications for a particular monitor based on the patient's comorbidities (e.g., severe coronary artery disease, raised intracranial pressure, decompensated congestive heart failure) or are the indications based on the anticipated surgical physiologic derangements? Will the data provided by the specific monitor be necessary for the administration of a safe anesthetic induction, or will these data be necessary only intraoperatively?

The student or resident physician is obligated to conduct a thorough history, physical exam, and review of available medical records to determine what, if any, patient factors mandate monitoring beyond the ASA standards. In addition, the planned surgical technique, which often is an unknown variable to the novice anesthesia provider, should be discussed with more experienced anesthesia or surgical staff. This helps the novice anticipate important determinants of monitor choice (e.g., expected blood loss) and augments his or her knowledge of accepted indications for the monitor to be placed. This also offers an opportunity for communication with the perioperative team and fosters open dialogue regarding the best interests of the patient. The patient must also be included in the preplacement discussion so he or she can be truly informed and will not be distressed if he or she emerges from anesthesia with additional monitors in place.

The psychomotor skills involved in monitor placement can be mastered at varying speeds, depending on the difficulty of actual placement. Many novice practitioners will place most of their focus on these skills, so effective instruction mandates patience and a consistent, systematic approach to accepted techniques for monitor placement. In fact, deemphasizing the importance of these motor skills and highlighting the indications, risks, and benefits is more important, as most practitioners will become technically proficient with time. Most new anesthesia providers will learn on real patients by trial and error, but other devices exist for practicing the psychomotor skills necessary to achieve competency in a safe and effective environment that does not subject the patient to the practicing student during the early phase of the learning curve (see the section on full environment simulation later in this chapter).

Safely placing invasive monitoring techniques will also require the teaching of anatomy with a consideration of potential placement sites, emphasizing the risks and benefits of the site selection. Sterile technique during invasive monitor placement will also need to be taught and stressed; a standardized approach using mannequins in a nonclinical environment is ideal.

Patient comfort and safety should also be emphasized, as all monitors, whether invasive or noninvasive, carry with them some inherent risks and discomfort. One consideration that is often learned the hard way by novices is the importance of the ergonomics of an operating room. Emphasizing the importance of planning ahead for the particular facets of a surgery (e.g., properly positioning the monitoring cables before turning the head of the bed 180 degrees), or actual work environment (e.g., being able to fit an echocardiography machine next to the patient) helps the operating room run more efficiently and saves

the new practitioner undue embarrassment and conflict in the operating room.

Intraoperative phase

During the intraoperative period, monitors are active and interpretation of data becomes the main focus. Although a working knowledge of normal human physiology underlies all successful monitor interpretation, many other facets of monitoring must be taught "on the job." The technology behind a particular monitor and its inherent strengths, weaknesses, and corroborating, conflicting, or interfering factors are necessary pieces of information for the novice anesthesiologist to understand if he or she is to trust the data seen. An experienced practitioner can help novices develop and target these factors so when data deviate from normal or expected values, technical influences can quickly be ruled out and pathophysiologic sources of abnormal data can be pursued and corrected. Therapeutic interventions based on monitoring data rely on the data being correct; therefore, the gravity of intervening or not intervening must be emphasized.

Teaching new practitioners to be vigilant is a component of monitoring not to be overlooked by educators. The conventional wisdom is that vigilance cannot be taught and will develop over time. Many novices experience information overload when they are first immersed in the operating room. A systematic approach (e.g., scanning the anesthetizing environment periodically by starting at the patient and making one's way back to the machine and monitor) is learned more easily if it is taught explicitly. This gives a framework for vigilance and can then be modified as new practitioners become more experienced. In times of stress, inexperienced practitioners may rely on simple strategies to make disordered situations more manageable. In this way, teaching vigilance may increase patient safety by allowing the novice to make difficult decisions and interpretations in a distracting and demanding environment.

Postoperative phase

Postoperative monitoring depends on similar factors considered in the preoperative phase. One crucial component is the predetermined definition of stability after the procedure is finished. Based on the patient's state after the surgery, monitors are discontinued or new ones are placed and the patient's destination (e.g., intensive care unit versus home) is determined.

Role of simulation in teaching monitoring skills

The use of patient simulation to educate and evaluate providers of anesthesia (traditionally, anesthesiology residents) has become increasingly accepted. Although anesthesiology took the initiative in incorporating simulation into its culture, its use in education and evaluation has been widely embraced during the last two decades by both medical schools and postgraduate training programs. The American Board of Anesthesiology (ABA) now requires simulator-based education to fulfill maintenance of certification in anesthesia (MOCA) requirements,[8] and the ACGME has recognized simulation as a useful assessment tool.[9] The Israeli Board of Anesthesiology Examination Committee has given some primacy to simulation as an element in credentialing and certifying anesthesiologists.[10] Indeed, the role of simulation appears to be evolving from that of an educational adjunct to an additionally useful tool in the assurance of clinical competence. Because monitoring skills are most important in dynamic perioperative settings, it follows that being trained in similar fashion would be beneficial. Hence, simulator-based education and evaluation are uniquely suited to this scope of anesthesia-based practice.

History and classification of medical simulation

Although an exhaustive review of the history of medical simulation is beyond the scope of this chapter, a brief overview is in order. Cooper and Taqueti give a comprehensive survey of simulation and note that because the field is arguably in its infancy, few accepted conventions exist.[11] Some basic terms with which the reader should be familiar are listed in Table 4.2.

These definitions provide a broad framework with which to describe the various types of simulators available in medical education today and encompass a wide array of human (e.g., standardized patients) and manufactured (e.g., mannequins) simulation techniques. A more extensive system of classification has been described by Cumin and Merry.[12]

Inspired by the aviation industry, the first mannequin-based medical simulators were introduced in the early 1960s. Resusci-Anne, designed by Asmund Laerdal, was developed during this time to teach mouth-to-mouth resuscitation. The concept of basic life support training using a mannequin-based simulator would grow out of this simple design as Laerdal partnered with Peter Safar, a Baltimore anesthesiologist, to enhance his simulator's capabilities and realism.[13] The model did not undergo significant improvement until the 1990s, when more anatomically correct airway features were added and the model was renamed SimMan, which is still commercially available.[14]

Table 4.2. Common definitions in simulation

Term	Definition
Simulator	Any object or representation of the full or part task to be replicated
Simulation	Application of simulator to training and/or assessment
Immersive simulation	Recreation of actual environment in which tasks are to be performed (e.g., OR, ICU)
Part-task simulation	Technologies that replicate only a portion of a process or system
Fidelity	The nearness to "true life" achieved by simulation

Adapted from reference 4.

Table 4.3. Features of the HPS by METI

1. Pupils that automatically dilate and constrict in response to light
2. Thumb twitch in response to a peripheral nerve stimulator
3. Automatic recognition and response to administered intravenous and inhaled drugs and drug dosages
4. Variable lung compliance and airway resistance
5. Real-time oxygen consumption and carbon dioxide production
6. Automatic response to cardiovascular conditions, including ischemia needle decompression of a tension pneumothorax, chest tube drainage, and pericardiocentesis
7. Automatic control of urine output

Adapted from www.meti.com.

Computer-driven simulators were first developed in the mid-1960s with SimOne, a full-scale mannequin with a chest capable of rise-and-fall action during respiration, blinking eyes, and a jaw that could open and close.[15] A single SimOne was manufactured and was eventually lost to obscurity largely because it was ahead of its time, despite the fact that residents trained on the simulator acquired airway management skills more quickly than their colleagues. The Harvey cardiology mannequin was also developed in the 1960s but, unlike the Sim One, it has had sustainable use to the present day. This simulator is capable of a wide array of cardiac disease scenarios, has been researched and validated extensively and has evolved over time to include multimedia programs that enhance its fidelity.[16–18]

The development of mathematical modeling programs for human physiology and drug pharmacodynamics and pharmacokinetics led to the development of modern mannequin and screen-based simulators. Various evolutions of these mathematically driven simulators have been developed at Stanford and University of Florida Gainesville and are described elsewhere.[4,19] Today the Human Patient Simulator (HPS), based on the Gainesville simulator and now manufactured by Medical Education Technologies Inc. (METI), is the prototypical full-scale, mathematical–model-driven product. This simulator can be used to stage full-scale simulations whereby realistic monitoring, physiologic response to drugs, and high-fidelity pathologic conditions can be encountered by participants. Key features of the HPS are listed in Table 4.3.[20]

A simple classification system of simulator types uses three categories: part-task trainers, computer-driven mannequins, and virtual reality simulators, on a continuum from low to high fidelity.[21] Part-task trainers usually represent anatomical parts for teaching and/or evaluating skills (e.g., central line placement trainers for practicing sterile technique, landmark identification, and monitor placement and suturing) and are generally passive, noncomputerized models. However, part-task does not imply less sophisticated technology; more advanced part-task trainers have been designed, such as the various transesophageal echocardiography simulators. These simulators also include cursory responses to noxious stimuli, including audible sounds of discomfort from the "patient," increased heart rate, and blood pressure, along with the ability to administer medications commonly used for sedation.

Computer-driven mannequins, or realistic patient simulators (RPSs), possess anatomic features and process advanced pharmacologic and physiologic models to respond to stimuli and medication administration. Such mannequins are ideally suited for immersive and full environment simulation (FES), in which individuals or entire teams of health care providers can perform tasks, manage potentially deadly scenarios, and improve skills, including leadership, communication, delegation, and prioritization.[22-25] Virtual reality (VR) simulations are the newest types of simulator, in which a computer-driven scenario is created and the user can interact with all the elements of the scenario. Visual, auditory, and haptic (touch and pressure) feedback are all available in VR simulations, but much work needs to be done to incorporate VR technology into the field of medical simulation.

General uses and benefits of simulated patients

The growing interest in medical simulation for education and assessment of physicians has been fueled by many of the same factors that led to the use of simulation in the aviation and nuclear industries.[26] The importance of simulation is evident in aviation, in which commercial pilots take their first flight only after a rigorous simulation program. The extensive use of simulation in the aviation industry has been driven not purely by evidence, but also by intuition and common sense. To date there is a lack of convincing evidence that simulator training improves health care education, practice, and patient safety, but, Gaba argues, "no industry in which human lives depend on skilled performance has waited for unequivocal proof of the benefits of simulation before embracing it."[27] Certainly, adopting simulation for the training in monitoring skills seems logical.

An educational imperative is one obvious utility of simulation. Simulation is learner-centered in that the participant's education receives highest priority. There exist no competing patient needs; therefore, the participant is afforded a unique opportunity to perform tasks without the looming stress of medical error. Medical clerkships and residency training rely on apprentice-based, chance encounters in which learning time is limited and not standardized. Simulation eliminates these limitations and, in doing so, benefits teachers by allowing for an optimal learning environment and a predesigned curriculum that emphasizes points deemed germane by the teacher. Also, presentation of uncommon but critical situations in which a rapid intervention is required is possible. This offers the learner the benefit of experience with a particular disease state in a safe environment rather than a purely "textbook" knowledge of the subject.

Full environment simulation, in particular, allows for assessment and education that extends beyond simple cognitive measures. A participant or team of participants can be evaluated and trained in domains of clinical knowledge, communication, and teamwork and procedural and technical skills in one environment and in one simulation session. An expert

for the domain(s) of interest can then debrief the participant(s).[28] Debriefings are vital, as one can learn from mishaps that occurred during a scenario and also speak openly about perceived and actual errors and limitations without fear of liability, blame, or guilt. Errors are deliberately allowed to occur and reach their end, whereas in real life, a more capable clinician would necessarily be called. In this way, participants can see the results of their choices. Patient safety and medical errors have come to the forefront of health care since the Institute of Medicine released *To Err is Human: Building a Safer Health System* in 2000.[29] The effective integration of simulation into medical education and assessment can address this modern health care challenge.

In addition to the more obvious and intended benefits of simulation, the ethical benefits are also pronounced. Patients entrust health care providers with their well-being and enter into a relationship in which they believe their providers to be expertly trained. It follows that being trained in simulated scenarios before a real patient encounter reduces a patient's exposure to less-seasoned professionals. Thus, patients theoretically receive a higher quality of care than they might otherwise get from those trained in apprentice-based systems, in which the adage of "see one, do one, teach one" may in fact overestimate the experience the provider has attained. As alluded to previously, other high-risk fields, such as aviation and the nuclear power industry, have adopted simulation in training personnel to acquire skills and knowledge and prove competency.[30,31]

Utility of simulation for monitoring skills development

A formalized teaching philosophy with regard to monitor skills is lacking in many, if not most, medical education curricula. An understanding of human physiology is essential if one is to be adept at the science of monitoring, which is, in fact, a form of applied physiology. In the most traditional sense, physiology has been, and still is, taught to students throughout the world in the classroom. The emphasis on linear thinking (i.e., teaching a single concept at a time) helps learners digest complex information. However, complex human processes do not function in linear fashion and, although this setting has served numerous clinicians well since the advent of modern medical education, the past 20 years have seen the rise of new educational techniques to replace or augment this approach.

Simulation provides an ideal format for teaching the attitudes, skills, and knowledge needed in monitoring. As defined by Gaba, "simulation is a technique—not a technology—to replace or amplify real experiences with guided experiences that evoke or replicate substantial aspects of the real world in a fully interactive manner."[32] Simulation enables both teacher and learner to engage in bedside teaching outside of the clinical setting with no patient risk, and creates an ideal environment for adult learning.

One reason simulation has become more prominent in medical education is that modern medicine requires the move from theory to practice to occur faster than in the past. The health care industry has changed markedly and, in turn, medical education has had to evolve.[33] Shorter hospital stays, a generally sicker hospitalized patient population, and greater legal concerns have decreased the number of patients a medical student is likely to encounter during his or her training.[34] Simulation permits students and residents to function in an environment in which no actual patients can be harmed.

At many medical schools, the traditional subject-based basic sciences are being replaced by system-based teaching. Lectures are often replaced or augmented by problem-based learning and small-group discussions regarding hypothetical, simulated case scenarios.[35] In essence, simulation of patients is superseding the traditional teaching of pathophysiology. Building on the history of simulation in the aviation and defense industries, computer-based simulations and full-body human patient simulators now augment traditional medical education. In similar fashion, simulation techniques are necessarily assuming important roles in teaching more advanced concepts, such as monitoring skills.

In a simulated environment, monitor skills can be taught as "pieces of a puzzle" that can be mastered individually. Monitor selection, monitor placement, monitor interpretation, data corroboration, monitor failure, data analysis, and medical management can each be taught in a standardized, digestible fashion without the time pressure or variability of the actual clinical environment. Only after mastery of each "piece" can the student then synthesize the "pieces" to formulate the entire "puzzle" of a simulated full-scale clinical environment.

The chronological model outlined in the beginning of this chapter can be applied using FES and allows new anesthesia providers to practice the important components of the monitoring process. Using FES, an instructor can recreate an operating room setting using real patient monitors attached to a high-fidelity mannequin simulator patient. An important benefit of FES is that the scenario can be tailored to the type and level of the learner. This is the key advantage of simulation education over traditional medical education that relies on chance encounters with relatively rare clinical situations for monitoring skills to be observed, learned, or practiced. The preoperative phase can be simulated with a standardized patient or actor playing the patient. This allows the participant in the FES to elicit a history and physical and review any lab data. Monitor placement can even be practiced at this point, using task-trainers set up in the FES. The learner can practice the psychomotor tasks needed in monitor skills, be exposed to rare events related to monitor malfunction or adverse medication reactions, and understand difficult-to-conceptualize topics such as monitor ergonomics. At each phase in the simulation, the learner can be asked about his or her rationale in choosing a particular monitor, as well as any other important points the educator seeks to review, such as theory behind the monitor, technology, and the like. Simulation also allows the teacher to assess learner performance and knowledge using reproducible clinical encounters rather than through standardized exams, which often require only the memorization of facts.

As the scenario moves to the intraoperative phase, data can be manipulated to teach proper interpretation, corroboration, and intervention based on different deviations from normal values. The use of FES acknowledges that monitoring data are not interpreted in a quiet or isolated environment, but in a stressful and often dizzying workplace. This adds an element of difficulty in the interpretation of data; FES provides an opportunity to practice vigilance, as well as cognitive and social skills, allowing learners to "think on their feet" in an environment fraught with demands and distractions. This makes good sense, considering that adult learners thrive in environments that are participative and interactive. This kind of contextual learning also allows the practitioner to experience the demands of monitor interpretation within an environment similar to what he or she will be experiencing in the actual operating room.

The postoperative phase provides another opportunity to review the rationale behind any plans to continue or discontinue the monitors chosen at the start of the scenario. At the end of the simulation, a videotape of the learner's performance can be reviewed and a debriefing with experienced practitioners can take place, something that is virtually impossible to do in actual practice and that is crucial for adult learners (i.e., immediate feedback). This opportunity to assess a learner's monitoring skills using FES is superior to that offered in an operating room setting, where distractions and important patient care duties abound. Although the resources required to run a successful simulation program are possibly prohibitive at many centers, the potential benefits are apparent. The opportunity to teach nuances of monitoring skills is unparalleled and takes reliance on chance encounters with rare clinical situations out of the equation. The numerous advantages and disadvantages of simulation are listed in Table 4.4.[36]

Simulation need not occur on a grand scale such as FES, but may use simple screen-based simulators with continuous feeds

Table 4.4. Advantages/disadvantages of simulation as an educational technique[36]

Advantages
No actual patient is threatened
Standardized educational experience for each student
Learner-centered, instructor-controlled
Can be paused for reflection and correction
Complex environment with multiple problems can be presented
Rare situations can be reliably reproduced and practiced
Interactive
Immediate feedback
Leadership and communication skills can be practiced
Psychomotor skills can be taught and practiced
Sessions can be recorded and reviewed after completion
Disadvantages
Expensive to start, house, and maintain simulation curriculum
Only small groups of learners can be accommodated
Performance anxiety may hinder learning
Time required for preparing scenarios
Learner may anticipate problems and be hypervigilant

Source: From reference 36.

of monitoring data. Such simulations may be best suited to less-advanced practitioners acquiring a foundation of skills. However, for the high-stakes interpretation of monitors involved in anesthesiology, FES seems best suited to practicing true-to-life skills.

Simulation not only should be thought of as a tool to educate new trainees, but can also serve practicing anesthesiologists and their educational needs. Of particular interest is the use of full-scale simulators to allow practicing health care providers the opportunity to learn and perfect clinical skills and techniques not available or mastered during training. Medical technology has expanded, and is anticipated to continue to expand, exponentially. It is likely that new and novel monitoring technologies will be introduced into the practice of anesthesiology. The full-scale simulated environment is ideal for anesthesiologists to practice and familiarize themselves with new technology without sacrificing operating room efficiency or patient safety.

As patient care environments become increasingly complex, it becomes necessary for practitioners to use equally complex modalities of monitoring to optimize patient care. The rapid pace of monitor development often supersedes the time available to trainees and practitioners that is necessary to learn new monitor skills or refresh facility with extant ones. Complexity, increased demand to practice efficiently, and the demand to reduce patient errors have made the actual clinical environment less conducive for education. Gone are the days when the educational dictum of "see one, do one, teach one" was law. Modern educational programs will need to promote the use of multimodality formats to enhance learning, protect patients during the learning process, and create sustained skill acquisition in practicing anesthesiologists. The availability of new educational technology, such as computers, virtual reality, and mannequin-based simulators, will support such endeavors. Here we describe one possible teaching module that fosters the use of multimodality formats and simulation-based technology that addresses the needs of students in an efficient, learner-centered way that protects patients now and in the future.

References

1. http://www.acgme.org/acWebsite/RRC_040/040_prIndex.asp.
2. Bryan R, Kreuter M, Brownson R. Integrating adult learning principles into training for public health practice. *Health Promotion Practice*. 2008;10(4):557–563.
3. Davis, D et al. Impact of formal continuing medical education: do conferences, workshops, rounds and other traditional continuing education activities change physician behavior or health care outcome? *JAMA* 1999;282(9):867–874.
4. Gercenshtein L, Fogelman Y, Yaphe J. Increasing the satisfaction of general practitioners with continuing medical education programs: A method for quality improvement through increasing teacher-learner interaction. *BMC Family Prac* 2002;3:15–19.
5. Cantillion P, Jones R. Does continuing medical education in general practice make a difference? *Br Med J* 1999;318:1276–1279.
6. Reiter HI, Eva KW, Hatala RM, Norman GR. Self and peer assessment in tutorials: application of a relative-ranking model. *Acad Med* 2002;77:1134–1139.
7. 6 http://www.acgme.org/outcome/comp/compMin.asp.
8. American Board of Anesthesiology: http://www.theaba.org/anes-moc.asp.
9. *Toolbox of Assessment Methods* 2000. Accreditation Council for Graduate Medical Education (ACGME), and American Board of Medical Specialties (ABMS). Version 1.1.
10. Ziv A, Rubin O, Sidi A, Berkenstadt H. Credentialing and certifying with simulation. *Anesthesiol Clin* 2007;25:261–269.
11. Cooper JB, Taqueti VR. A brief history of the development of mannequin simulators for clinical education and training. *Qual Saf Health Care* 2004;13(Suppl1):i11–i18.
12. Cumin D, Merry AF. Simulators for use in anaesthesia. *Anaesthesia* 2007;62:151–162.
13. Grevnik A, Schaefer JJ. From Resusci-Anne to Sim Man: The evolution of simulators in medicine. *Crit Care Med* 2004;32:556–557.
14. Schaefer J, Gonzalez R. Dynamic simulation: a new tool for difficult airway training of professional healthcare providers. *Am J Clin Anesth* 2000;27:232–242.
15. Denson J, Abrahamson S. A computer-controlled patient simulator. *JAMA* 1969;208:504–508.
16. Gordon MS. Cardiology patient simulator: development of an automated manikin to teach cardiovascular disease. *Am J Cardiol* 1974;34:350–355.
17. Issenberg SB, Gordon MS, Gordon DL, et al. Simulation and new learning technologies. *Med Teach* 2001;23:16–23.
18. Sajid AW, Ewy GA, Felner JM, et al. Cardiology patient simulator and computer-assisted instruction technologies in bedside teaching. *Med Educ* 1990;24:512–517.
19. Gaba DM, DeAnda A. A comprehensive anesthesia simulation environment: recreating the operating room for research and training. *Anesthesiology* 1988;69:387–394.
20. METI: http://www.meti.com.
21. Scalese RJ, Obeso VT, Issenberg SB. Simulation technology for skills training and competency assessment in medical education. *J Gen Intern Med* 2007;23(Suppl 1):46–49.
22. Howard SK, Gaba DM, Fish KJ, et al. Anesthesia crisis resource management training: Teaching anesthesiologists to handle critical incidents. *Aviat Space Environ Med* 1992;63: 763–770.
23. Gaba DM, Fish KJ, Howard SK. *Crisis Management in Anesthesiology*. New York: Churchill Livingstone, 1994.
24. Holzman RS, Cooper JB, Gaba DM, et al. Anesthesia crisis resource management: Real-life simulation training in operating room crises. *J Clin Anesth* 1995;7:675–687.
25. Gaba DM, Howard SK, Fish KJ, et al. Simulation-based training in anesthesia crisis resource management (ACRM): A decade of experience. *Simul Gaming* 2001;32:175–193.
26. Ziv A, Small SD, Wolpe PR. Patient safety and simulation-based medical education. *Med Teach* 2000;22(5):489–495.
27. Gaba DM. Improving anesthesiologists' performance by simulating reality. *Anesthesiology* 1992;76:491–494.
28. Issenberg SB, McGaghie WC, Petrusa ER, et al. Features and uses of high-fidelity medical simulations that lead to effective learning: a BEME systematic review. *Med Teach* 2005;27(1):10–28.
29. Institute of Medicine. *To Err is Human: Building a Safer Healthcare System*. Washington DC: National Academy Press, 2000.
30. Goodman W. The world of civil simulators. *Flight Intl* 1978;18:435.
31. Wachtel J. The future of nuclear power plant simulation in the United States. In: *Simulation for Nuclear Reactor Technology*.

Walton DG (ed.). Cambridge: Cambridge University Press, 1985:339–349.

32. Gaba DM. The future vision of simulation in health care. *Qual Saf Health Care.* 2004;13 Suppl 1:i2–i10.

33. Richardson WC, et al. *Crossing the Quality Chasm: A New Health System for the 21st Century.* Washington, DC: National Academy Press, 2000.

34. Mardis R, Brownson K. Length of stay at an all time low. *Health Care Manager* 2003;22:122–127.

35. Shokar G, Shokar N, Romero C. Self-directed learning: looking at outcomes with medical students. *Fam Med* 2002;34:197–200.

36. Rauen CA. Simulation as a teaching strategy for nursing education and orientation in cardiac surgery. *Crit Care Nurse* 2004;24(3):46–51.

Electrocardiography

Alexander J. C. Mittnacht and Martin London

Introduction

Electrocardiography (ECG) monitoring and interpretation are considered part of the basic or minimal monitoring requirements in all patients undergoing diagnostic and/or therapeutic procedures, regardless of the anesthesia technique administered. The American Society of Anesthesiologists (ASA) guidelines for basic anesthesia monitoring, available online at http://www.asahq.org/publicationsAndServices/standards/02. pdf (last amended October 2005), mandate continuous ECG monitoring for the evaluation of a patient's circulation during all anesthetics from the beginning of anesthesia until preparing to leave the anesthetizing location. The ASA guidelines also state that under extenuating circumstances, the responsible anesthesiologist may waive ECG monitoring, but recommends that when this is done, the anesthesiologist should leave a note in the patient's medical record, excluding the reason for not excluding ECG monitoring. Consequently, all practitioners involved in perioperative patient care should have at least a basic understanding of ECG monitoring.

With advances in computer technology, the diagnostic and monitoring capabilities of the ECG for the detection of arrhythmias and myocardial ischemia and infarction continue to develop and expand, and the distinction between diagnostic ECG carts and bedside ECG monitoring units is narrowing. The universal availability of affordable digital storage allows for almost continuous recording of large amounts of perioperative data, including information derived from ECG monitoring. The ability to retrieve such ECG data can serve as invaluable information in analyzing perioperative cardiac events.

Although it seems obvious that patients should benefit from continuous ECG monitoring, evidence-based medicine would require proof of improved patient outcome, preferably including data from several large randomized prospective studies. However, given the stated ASA recommendations, randomizing patients to ECG monitoring would be nearly impossible. The American Heart Association (AHA) has published practice standards for ECG monitoring in hospital settings. Based mostly on expert opinion, recommendations are given regarding cardiac arrhythmia, ischemia, and QT interval ECG monitoring.[1] Furthermore, the most recent American College of Cardiology/AHA Task Force on Practice Guidelines in patients undergoing noncardiac surgery include recommendations on pre- and postoperative 12-lead ECG monitoring.[2]

The following text is intended not to be a substitute for extensive cardiology textbooks written on ECG monitoring, but rather to provide the practitioner involved in patient anesthesia care with a basic understanding of ECG monitoring requirements and ECG interpretation, as well as an overview of recent developments and available data on ECG monitoring and patient outcome.

Technical concepts
Historical perspective

Willem Einthoven is universally considered the father of electrocardiography (for which he won the 1924 Nobel Prize). However, Augustus Waller actually recorded the first human ECG in 1887, using a glass capillary electrometer. This early device used changes in surface tension between mercury and sulfuric acid in a glass column induced by a varying electric potential. The level of the meniscus was magnified and recorded on moving photographic paper, describing what were initially termed "A–B–C–D waves." In 1895, Einthoven published his observations using this crude device. Frustration with its low-frequency resolution led him to develop the string galvanometer, using a silver-coated quartz fiber suspended between the poles of a magnet. Changes induced by the electrical potentials conducted through the quartz string resulted in its movement at right angles to the magnetic field. The shadow of the string, backlit from a light source, was transmitted through a microscope (the string was only 2.1 mm in diameter) and was recorded on a moving photographic plate. He renamed the signal the P–QRS–T complex (based on standard geometric convention for describing points on curved lines).

Many of the basic clinical abnormalities (i.e. bundle-branch block, delta waves, ST-T changes with angina) in electrocardiography were first described using the string galvanometer. It was used until the 1930s, when it was replaced by a system using vacuum tube amplifiers and a cathode ray oscilloscope. A portable direct-writing ECG cart was not introduced until the early 1950s (facilitated at first by transistor technology and subsequently by integrated circuits), which allowed widespread use of the ECG in clinical practice. The first analog-to-digital (A/D) conversion systems for the ECG were introduced in the early 1960s, but their clinical use was restricted until the late 1970s. Today, with advances in microcomputer technology, most ECG machines convert the analog ECG signal to digital form before further processing.

Power spectrum of the ECG

The ECG signal must be considered in terms of its amplitude (or voltage) and its frequency components (generally termed its *phase*). The power spectrum of the ECG is derived by Fourier transformation, in which a periodic waveform is mathematically decomposed to its harmonic components (sine waves of varying amplitude and frequency). The frequency of each of these components can be equated to the slope of the component signal. The R wave, with its steep slope, is a high-frequency component, whereas the P and T waves have lesser slopes and are lower in frequency. The ST segment has the lowest frequency, not much different from the underlying electrical (i.e. isoelectric) baseline of the ECG.

Prior to the introduction of digital signal processing (DSP), accurately displaying the ST segment presented significant technical problems, particularly in operating room (OR) and ICU bedside monitoring units (discussed later). Although the overall frequency spectrum of the QRS complex in Figure 5.1 does not appear to exceed 40 Hz, many components of the QRS complex, particularly the R wave, exceed 100 Hz. Thus, reducing the ECG signal to a bandwidth between 0.5 Hz and 40 Hz (monitoring mode) reduces artifacts but is unacceptable for diagnostic purposes (diagnostic mode 0.05–150 Hz; also see discussion later). Very high-frequency signals of particular clinical significance are pacemaker spikes. Their short duration and

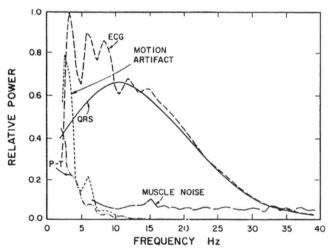

Figure 5.1. The typical power spectrum of the electrocardiography (ECG) signal, including its subcomponents and common artifacts (motion and muscle noise). The power of the P and T waves (P–T) is low-frequency, and the QRS complex is concentrated in the mid-frequency range, although residual power extends up to 100 Hz. From Thakor NV et al. Estimation of QRS complex power spectra for design of a QRS filter. *IEEE Trans Biomed Eng* 1984;31(11):702–6 (Figure 4), with permission.

high amplitude present technical challenges for proper recognition and rejection to allow accurate determination of the heart rate (HR). Spectra representing some of the major sources of artifact must be eliminated during processing and amplification of the QRS complex.

Frequency response of ECG monitors: monitoring and diagnostic modes

Given the importance of the ECG in diagnosing myocardial ischemia, it is important to realize that significant ST segment depression or elevation can occur solely as a result of improper ECG signal filtering.[3] This was a particular problem prior to the introduction of DSP. The AHA Electrocardiography and Arrhythmias Committee released specific recommendations regarding ECG signal sampling, filtering, and further processing.[4,5] To reproduce the various frequencies components accurately, they all must be amplified equally. Thus, the monitor must have a flat amplitude response over the wide range of frequencies present. Similarly, because the slight delay in a signal as it passes through a filter or amplifier may vary in duration with different frequencies, all frequencies must be delayed equally. This is termed *linear phase response*. If the response is nonlinear, various components may appear temporally distorted (termed *phase shift*). The AHA recommends a bandwidth from 0.05 Hz to 150 Hz (250 Hz for children) for all 12-lead diagnostic ECGs. A low-frequency cutoff of 0.5 Hz and a high-frequency cutoff of 40 Hz is commonly referred to as a *monitoring mode*. This produces a more stable signal with less baseline noise and fewer high-frequency artifacts. According to the most recent AHA recommendations, ECG machines should alert the user when used in the monitoring mode. Because most newer monitors use signal-averaging techniques that effectively eliminate most artifacts even in the diagnostic mode, the clinician can usually (and should) avoid using the monitoring mode whenever possible.

Intrinsic and extrinsic artifacts

ECG artifacts and baseline wander may result from several causes.[6–11] Even though the development of DSP techniques has helped to minimize these artifacts, new sources of electrical interference have emerged. Implantable, miniaturized devices such as neurostimulators, pacemaker/defibrillators, and infusion pumps are almost unrecognizable, and artifacts resulting from such devices must be carefully evaluated and correctly interpreted. Table 5.1 lists more common causes of such artifacts.

To avoid or minimize such artifacts, signal acquisition should be optimized. Proper electrode application and positioning are simple methods in improving ECG quality. Monitoring electrodes should preferentially be placed directly over bony prominences of the torso (i.e. clavicular heads and iliac prominences) to minimize excursion of the electrode during respiration, which could cause baseline wander. Electrode impedance must be optimized to avoid loss and alteration of the signal.

Table 5.1. Common causes of ECG artifacts

- Skin impedance
- ECG electrodes, cables
- Electromyographic (EMG) noise (motor activity)
- Electrical power line interference, line isolation monitor (LIM)
- Electrocautery
- Evoked potential monitoring
- Mechanical ventilation
- Magnetic resonance imaging (MRI)
- Extracorporeal shock wave lithotripsy (ESWL)
- Neurostimulators, implantable infusion pumps
- Infusion pumps, blood warmers
- Extracorporeal blood circulation devices, such as cardiopulmonary bypass devices and renal replacement therapy

By removing a portion of the stratum corneum (gentle abrasion with a dry gauze pad, resulting in a minor amount of surface erythema, works well), skin impedance can be reduced by a factor of 10 to 100. Optimal impedance is 5000 ohms or less. The electrode may be covered with a watertight dressing to prevent surgical scrub solutions from undermining electrode contact. To minimize electrocautery artifact, the right leg reference electrode should be placed as close as possible to the grounding pad, and the ECG monitor should be plugged into a different power outlet than the electrosurgical unit. Devices with which the patient is in physical contact, particularly via plastic tubing, may at times cause clinically significant ECG artifacts. Although the exact mechanism is uncertain, two leading explanations are either a piezoelectric effect caused by mechanical deformation of the plastic, or buildup of static electricity between two dissimilar materials, especially those in motion. This effect has been noted with the use of cardiopulmonary bypass, renal replacement therapy, and the like and usually mimics atrial arrhythmias (also see Figure 5.2). A grounding lead on the external device usually eliminates this.

Lead systems

Where and how ECG electrodes are placed on the body is a critical determinant of the morphology of the ECG signal. Lead systems have been developed based on theoretical considerations (i.e. the orthogonal arrangement of the Frank XYZ leads) and/or references to anatomic landmarks that facilitate consistency between individuals (i.e. standard 12-lead system).

History and description of the 12-lead system

Einthoven established electrocardiography using three extremities as references: the left arm (LA), right arm (RA), and left leg (LL). He recorded the difference in potential between the LA and RA (lead I), LL and RA (lead II), and LL and LA (lead III). Because the signals recorded were differences between two electrodes, these leads were termed *bipolar*. The right leg (RL) served only as a reference electrode. Einthoven postulated that the three limbs defined an imaginary equilateral triangle with the heart at its center. Because Kirchoff's loop equation states that the sum of the three voltage differential pairs must equal zero, the sum of leads I and III must equal lead II (which is therefore redundant). Given the influence of Einthoven's vector analyses of frontal plane forces, others eventually incorporated the other two orthogonal planes (transverse and sagittal).

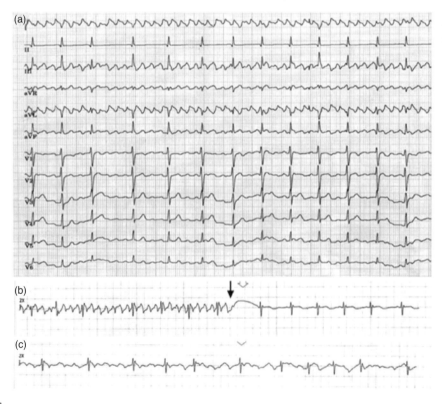

Figure 5.2. Artifactual atrial flutter during continuous venovenous hemofiltration. (a) Initial 12-lead electrocardiogram during hemofiltration; (b) rhythm strip at time hemofiltration was turned off (black arrow); (c) rhythm strip with flow rate of filtration system decreased by half. Kaltman JR, Shah MJ. Artefactual atrial flutter. *Cardiol Young* 2006;16:195–196 (Figure 1), with permission.

Wilson refined and introduced the unipolar precordial leads into clinical practice. To implement these leads, he postulated a mechanism whereby the absolute level of electrical potential could be measured at the site of the exploring precordial electrode (the positive electrode). A negative pole with zero potential was formed by joining the three limb electrodes in a resistive network in which equally weighted signals cancel each other out. He termed this the *central terminal*, and in a fashion similar to Einthoven's vector concepts, he postulated that it was located at the electrical center of the heart, representing the mean electrical potential of the body throughout the cardiac cycle. He described three additional limb leads (VL, VR, and VF). These leads measured new vectors of activation; thus, the hexaxial reference system for determination of electrical axis was established. Wilson subsequently introduced the six unipolar precordial V leads in 1935.[12]

Clinical application of the unipolar limb leads was limited because of their significantly smaller amplitude relative to the bipolar limb leads from which they were derived. They were not clinically applied until Goldberger augmented their amplitude (by a factor of 1.5) by severing the connection between the central terminal and the lead extremity being studied (which he termed *augmented limb leads*) in 1942.

The three limb leads (I, II, and III), the three augmented limb leads (aVR, aVL, and aVF), and the six precordial leads (V1 through V6) have been universally accepted as the conventional 12-lead ECG system. However, in the AHA's most recent recommendations for the standardization and interpretation of the ECG, the use of the terms "unipolar" and "bipolar" is discouraged and should be avoided, as all leads are effectively bipolar.[13]

Additional lead systems, and other expanded and derived lead systems, have been developed for specific clinical applications. The EASI-derived 12-lead ECG system is a based on vectorcardiography,[14] and uses fewer electrodes (four chest electrodes and one reference electrode) and well-defined convenient landmarks (see Figure 5.3). The EASI system has been shown to compare favorably with the standard 12-lead ECG system for ischemia and arrhythmia detection and offers advantages in long-term continuous patient monitoring (e.g., fewer electrodes, increased patient comfort, less interference with patient care).[15–19]

At this point, the AHA does not recommend derived lead systems as a substitute for standard 12-lead (10 electrodes) ECGs.[13]

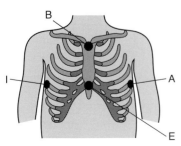

Figure 5.3. Location of the four EASI electrodes. A ground electrode can be placed anywhere on the body. From reference 17 (Figure 1), with permission.

Detection of myocardial ischemia
Pathophysiology of ST segment responses

The ST segment is the most important portion of the QRS complex for evaluating ischemia. The origin of this segment at the point where the QRS complex joins the ST segment (junction between QRS complex and ST segment or J point) may deviate from baseline in myocardial ischemia and is easy to locate. Its end, which is generally accepted as the beginning of any change of slope of the T wave, is more difficult to determine. In normal individuals, there may be no discernible ST segment, as the T wave starts with a steady slope from the J point, especially at rapid heart rates. The T–P segment has been used as the isoelectric baseline from which changes in the ST segment are evaluated, but, with tachycardia, this segment is eliminated and, during exercise testing, the P–R segment is used. The P–R segment is used in all ST segment analyzers as well. Repolarization of the ventricle proceeds from the epicardium to the endocardium, opposite to the vector of depolarization. The ST segment reflects the midportion, or phase 2, of repolarization, during which there is little change in electrical potential. Thus, it is usually isoelectric.

Ischemia causes a loss of intracellular potassium, resulting in a current of injury. The electrophysiologic mechanism accounting for ST segment shifts (either elevation or depression) remains controversial. The two major theories are based on either a loss of resting potential as current flows from the uninjured to the injured area (diastolic current), or a true change in phase 2 potential as current flows from the injured to the uninjured area (systolic current). With subendocardial injury, the ST segment is depressed in the surface leads. With epicardial or transmural injury, the ST segment is elevated. When a lead is placed directly on the endocardium, opposite patterns are recorded.

ECG manifestations of ischemia

With myocardial ischemia, repolarization is affected, resulting in downsloping or horizontal ST segment depression. Varying local effects and differences in vectors during repolarization result in different ST morphologies that are recorded by the different leads. It is generally accepted that ST changes in multiple leads are associated with more severe degrees of coronary artery disease (CAD).

The classic criterion for ischemia is a 0.1 mV (1 mm) depression measured 60 to 80 msec after the J point. The slope of the segment must be horizontal or downsloping. Downsloping depression may be associated with a greater number of diseased vessels and a worse prognosis than horizontal depression. Slowly upsloping depression with a slope of 1 mV/sec or less is also used but is considered less sensitive and specific (and difficult to assess clinically). Nonspecific ST segment depression can be related to the use of drugs, particularly digoxin.[20,21] Interpretation of ST segment changes in patients with left ventricular hypertrophy (LVH) is particularly controversial, given the tall

R wave baseline, J point depression, and steep slope of the ST segment.

The criteria for ischemia with ST segment elevation (≥ 0.1 mV in ≥ 2 contiguous leads) are used in conjunction with clinical symptoms or elevation of biochemical markers to diagnose acute coronary syndromes. ST segment elevation is usually caused by transmural ischemia, but may potentially represent a reciprocal change in a lead oriented opposite the primary vector with subendocardial ischemia (as may be seen in the reverse situation).[22,23] Perioperative ambulatory monitoring studies have also included > 0.2 mV in any single lead as a criterion, but ST elevation is rarely reported in the setting of noncardiac surgery. It is commonly observed, however, during weaning from cardiopulmonary bypass (CPB) in cardiac surgery with relative frequency, and during coronary artery bypass graft (CABG) surgery (both on and off pump) with interruption of coronary flow in a native or graft vessel. ST elevation in a Q wave lead should not be analyzed for acute ischemia, although it may indicate the presence of a ventricular aneurysm.

Despite the clinical focus on the ST segment for monitoring, the earliest ECG change at the onset of transmural ischemia is the almost immediate onset of tall and peaked (hyperacute) T waves, a so-called primary change. This phase is often transient. A significant increase in R wave amplitude may also occur at this time. T wave inversions (symmetrical inversion) commonly accompany transmural ST segment elevation changes, although the vast majority of T wave inversions and/or flattening observed perioperatively are nonspecific, resulting from transient alterations of repolarization caused by changes in electrolytes, sympathetic tone, and other noncardiac factors.

Although repolarization changes (e.g. ST–T wave) have long been the focus of ischemia detection, it has been well documented that changes in the high-frequency (150–250 Hz) recordings of the QRS complex may be a more sensitive marker for ischemia.[24] This effect is likely the result of slowing of conduction velocity in the ischemic region.[25] Such changes are not visible on the standard ECG, and large intra- and interindividual variations in the high-frequency recordings of the QRS complex are present even in healthy individuals (also see Figure 5.4).[26] Absolute changes in the root mean square (RMS) of measured QRS amplitudes > 0.6 μV or relative changes >20 percent are considered clinically significant.[27]

Pettersson and colleagues documented a higher sensitivity of this approach compared with 12-lead ST segment analysis in the detection of acute coronary occlusion during percutaneous transluminal coronary angioplasty (PTCA).[28] The overall sensitivity was 88 percent, compared with 71 percent using ST-segment elevation criteria, or 79 percent by combining ST-segment elevation and depression. Its greatest value was in the detection of circumflex and right coronary occlusions. Anesthesia induction also seems to change high-frequency ECG parameters; however, a small study found these changes to be within the described normal limits.[29] Although intriguing, further studies are clearly required, and it is unlikely that high-frequency ECG analysis will be used commonly in the

(a)

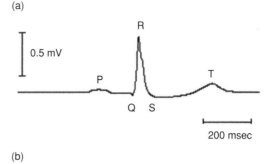

(b)

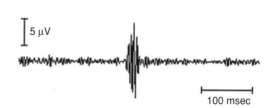

(c)

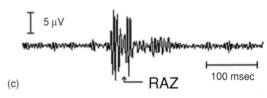

Figure 5.4. Twelve-lead high-frequency QRS electrocardiograms. (a) A conventional surface electrocardiogram signal from a healthy subject. (b) High-frequency QRS signal in a healthy individual in whom ECG signals were analyzed at a sampling rate of >1000/s, signal-averaged, and then passed through a filter excluding frequencies outside a range of 150–250 Hz. Note the reduced voltage scale compared with trace (a). (c) High-frequency QRS signal from a patient with myocardial ischemia. There are two peaks in the envelope of the high-frequency QRS signal, rather than the single peak in trace (b). The dip in the envelope (arrow) is denoted as a reduced-amplitude zone (RAZ). From reference 29 (Figures 1–3), with permission.

near future, given the expense of replacing or upgrading existing equipment.

Perioperative ECG ischemia monitoring

Detection of perioperative myocardial ischemia has received considerable attention over the past several decades and, more recently, with publication of several studies of clinical monitoring and therapy (e.g. perioperative beta blockade).[30] Many of these studies demonstrated associations of perioperative ischemia with adverse cardiac outcomes in adults undergoing a variety of cardiac and noncardiac surgical procedures, particularly major vascular surgery.[31–33]

With regard to ECG devices, advances in ECG technology now allow for automated ST segment trend monitoring in almost all perioperative clinical settings. However, applying this technology routinely, even in low-risk surgical patients, may yield false-positive responses (although these are uncommon). Perhaps the bigger challenge is interpreting minor ST segment changes in the context of the overall risk profile of the patient. Recent studies document that transient myocardial ischemia occurs in the absence of significant CAD in unexpected patients, such as parturients, particularly with significant hemodynamic stress and/or hemorrhage.[34] Although the precise etiology of such changes is uncertain, significant troponin release has been recently documented in these patients, confirming the suspicion that these ECG changes are true ischemic responses (likely related to subendocardial ischemia owing to global hypoperfusion).

The recommended leads for perioperative ECG monitoring, based on several clinical studies, do not differ substantially from those used during exercise testing, although considerable controversy as to the optimal lead(s) persists in both clinical settings. Early clinical reports of intraoperative monitoring using the V_5 lead in high-risk patients were based on observations during exercise testing, in which bipolar configurations of V_5 demonstrated high sensitivity for myocardial ischemia detection (up to 90%). Subsequent studies using 12-lead monitoring (torso-mounted for stability during exercise) confirmed the sensitivity of the lateral precordial leads.[35,36] Some studies, however, reported higher sensitivity for leads V_4 or V_6 compared with V_5, followed by the inferior leads (in which most false-positive responses were reported).[37–44]

With the widespread growth of percutaneous coronary intervention (PCI) for acute myocardial infraction and unstable angina in the 1990s, a number of investigators have reported on the use of continuous ECG monitoring (3 or 12 leads) in this setting. The controlled occlusion of specific coronary artery branches during PCI has extended our knowledge regarding vessel-specific ECG responses to acute myocardial ischemia. Horacek and Wagner found ST segment elevation in leads V_2 and V_3 to be most sensitive for occlusion of the left anterior descending artery, and leads III and aVF most sensitive for the right coronary artery.[45] In contrast, circumflex occlusion results in variable responses, with primary elevation in the posterior precordial leads V_7 through V_9 (which are rarely monitored clinically), and reciprocal ST segment depression in the standard precordial leads (V_2 or V_3).[46,47] For transmural ischemia, sensitivity is highest in the anterior rather than in the lateral precordial leads. The most widely quoted clinical study using continuous, computerized 12-lead ECG analysis in a mixed cohort (vascular and other noncardiac procedures) by London and coworkers reported that nearly 90 percent of responses involved ST segment depression alone (75% in V_5 and 61% in V_4).[48] In approximately 70 percent of patients, significant changes were noted in multiple leads. When considered in combination (as would be done clinically), the use of both leads V_4 and V_5 increased sensitivity to 90 percent, whereas the standard clinical combination, leads II and V_5, was only 80 percent sensitive. Use of leads V_2 through V_5 and lead II captured all episodes (see Table 5.2).

A larger clinical study by Landesberg and associates of patients undergoing vascular surgery using a longer period of monitoring (up to 72 hours) with more specific criteria for ischemia (>10 minute duration of episode) extended these observations. They reported that V_3 was most sensitive for

Table 5.2. Sensitivity for different ECG lead combinations for intraoperative ischemia detection

Lead Combination		Sensitivity (%)
1 lead	II	33
	V_4	61
V_5		75
2 leads	II/V_5	80
	II/V_4	82
	V_4/V_5	90
3 leads	V_3/V_4/V_5	94
	II/V_4/V_5	96
4 leads	II/V_2–V_5	100

Based on data presented in reference 48.

ischemia (87%) followed by V_4 (79%), while V_5 alone was only 66 percent sensitive (also see Figure 5.5).[49] In the subgroup of patients for whom prolonged ischemic episodes ultimately culminated in infarction, however, V_4 was most sensitive (83%). In this study, all myocardial infarctions were non–Q-wave events detected by troponin elevation. Use of two precordial leads detected 97 percent to 100 percent of changes. Based on analysis of the resting isoelectric levels of each of the 12 leads (a unique component of this study), it was recommended that V_4 was the best single choice for monitoring of a single precordial lead, as it was most likely to be isoelectric relative to the resting 12-lead preoperative ECG. In contrast, the baseline ST segment was more likely above isoelectric in V_1–V_3 and below isoelectric in V_5–V_6. Surprisingly, no episodes of ST elevation were noted in this study, as opposed to 12 percent in the earlier study of London and colleagues, in which such changes were noted in inferior and anteroseptal precordial leads. A multidisciplinary working group specifically recommends continuous monitoring of leads III, V_3, and V_5 for all acute coronary syndrome patients.[50]

The coronary care unit's use of continuous ECG monitoring has received increasing attention recently as well.[51] Martinez et al. evaluated a cohort of vascular patients monitored in the ICU for the first postoperative day using continuous 12-lead monitoring using a threshold of 20 minutes for an ischemic episode.[52] Eleven percent of patients (of 149 patients) met the criteria, with ST depression in 71 percent and ST elevation alone in 18 percent (12% with both). The majority of changes were detected in V_2 (53%) and V_3 (65%). Using the standard two-lead system (II and V_5), only 41 percent of episodes would have been detected.

Although these studies clearly support the value of precordial monitoring in patients at risk for subendocardial ischemia, one must be vigilant for the rare patient with acute Q-wave infarction (most commonly in the inferior leads). The use of multiple precordial leads, although appealing, is not likely to become common clinical practice, owing to the limitations of existing monitors (and cables). Even if such equipment were available, it is likely that considerable resistance would occur from practitioners because of the extra effort associated with this approach. Perhaps, in the future, when lower-cost wireless

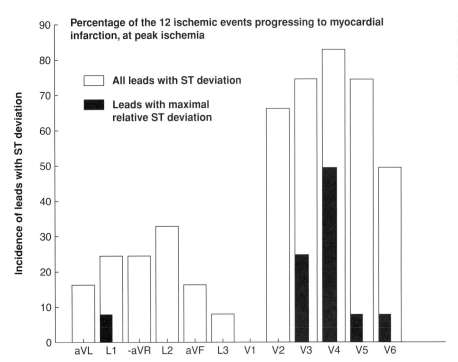

Figure 5.5. Histogram showing the incidence of all electrocardiographic leads, demonstrating greater than 1 mm relative ST deviation during peak ischemia and the electrocardiographic lead with the maximal ST deviation in 12 patients with myocardial infarction. From reference 49 (Figure 5), with permission.

technologies are perfected, this approach may become a clinical reality.

Perioperative arrhythmia monitoring

Heart rhythm diagnosis is one of the main features of perioperative ECG monitoring. Consequently, there has been considerable interest in the refinement of arrhythmia detection algorithms and their validation.[53] Most modern ECG machines feature real-time automated computerized arrhythmia detection algorithms, allowing for the detection, audiovisual signaling, and recording of clinical relevant arrhythmias, including asystole, ventricular tachycardia/fibrillation, bradycardia, R on T, and irregular rhythm recognition. As expected, the devices' accuracy for detecting ventricular arrhythmias is high but is much lower for detecting atrial arrhythmias. Typically, inferior ECG leads are preferred in rhythm diagnosis, allowing superior discrimination of the P wave morphology. Particularly in the OR setting, a variety of artifacts – for example, those caused by electrocautery – are common causes of false-positive responses.

Aside from rhythm diagnosis, an increasing number of patients are presenting for surgery with a pacemaker or an automated implantable defibrillator (which also has a pacemaker function) implanted. The anesthesiologist should not only be familiar with the latest recommendations regarding perioperative management of patients presenting with such devices but should also be aware of possible interference with normal ECG monitoring. The detection of pacemaker spikes may be complicated by very-low-amplitude signals related to bipolar pacing leads, varying amplitude with respiration, and total body fluid accumulation.[53] Most critical care and ambulatory monitors incorporate pacemaker spike enhancement for small high-frequency signals (typically 5–500 mV with 0.5–2 ms pulse duration) to facilitate recognition. However, this can lead to artifacts if there is high-frequency noise within the lead system.

Summary

ECG monitoring has been used for perioperative hemodynamic monitoring for more than four decades. Most of its basic features remain unchanged, although improvements in automated ischemia and arrhythmia detection have increased its clinical utility. It is relatively inexpensive, completely noninvasive, and can easily be used for continuous monitoring in every patient, extending into the postoperative setting. Unlike newer modalities, such as transesophageal echocardiography, that may have a higher sensitivity for ischemia detection, only basic training is necessary for most ECG monitoring purposes.

References

1. Drew BJ, Califf RM, Funk M, et al. Practice standards for electrocardiographic monitoring in hospital settings. An American Heart Association Scientific Statement from the councils on cardiovascular nursing, clinical cardiology, and cardiovascular disease in the young. *Circulation* 2004;110: 2721–46.
2. Fleisher LA, Beckman JA, Brown KA, et al. ACC/AHA 2007 guidelines on perioperative cardiovascular evaluation and care for noncardiac surgery: executive summary: a report of the American College of Cardiology/American Heart Association Task Force on Practice Guidelines (Writing Committee to Revise the 2002 Guidelines on Perioperative Cardiovascular Evaluation for Noncardiac Surgery). *Anesth Analg* 2008;106:685–712.
3. Kligfield P, Okin PM. Prevalence and clinical implications of improper filter settings in routine electrocardiography. *Am J Cardiol* 2007;99:711–3.

4. Kligfield P, Gettes LS, Bailey JJ, et al. Recommendations for the standardization and interpretation of the electrocardiogram. Part I: the electrocardiogram and its technology, a scientific statement from the American Heart Association Electrocardiography and Arrhythmias Committee, Council on Clinical Cardiology; the American College of Cardiology Foundation; and the Heart Rhythm Society endorsed by the International Society for Computerized Electrocardiology. *J Am Coll Cardiol* 2007;49:1109–27.

5. Mason JW, Hancock EW, Gettes LS. Recommendations for the standardization and interpretation of the electrocardiogram. Part II: electrocardiography diagnostic statement list, a scientific statement from the American Heart Association Electrocardiography and Arrhythmias Committee, Council on Clinical Cardiology; the American College of Cardiology Foundation; and the Heart Rhythm Society Endorsed by the International Society for Computerized Electrocardiology. *J Am Coll Cardiol* 2007;49:1128–35.

6. Patel SI, Souter MJ. Equipment-related electrocardiographic artifacts: causes, characteristics, consequences, and correction. *Anesthesiology* 2008;109:138–48.

7. McGrath B, Columb M. Renal replacement therapy causing ECG artefact mimicking atrial flutter. *Br J Intensive Care* 2004;14:49–52.

8. Marples IL. Transcutaneous electrical nerve stimulation (TENS): An unusual source of electrocardiogram artefact. *Anaesthesia* 2000;55:719–20.

9. Khambatta HJ, Stone JG, Wald A, Mongero LB. Electrocardiographic artifacts during cardiopulmonary bypass. *Anesth Analg* 1990;71:88–91.

10. Toyoyama H, Kariya N, Toyoda Y. Electrocardiographic artifacts during shoulder arthroscopy using a pressure-controlled irrigation pump. *Anesth Analg* 2000;90:856–7.

11. Marsh R. ECG artifact in the OR. *Health Devices* 1991;20:140–141.

12. Kossman CE. Unipolar electrocardiography of Wilson: a half century later. *Am Heart J* 1985;110:901–4.

13. Kligfield P, Gettes LS, Bailey JJ, et al. Recommendations for the standardization and interpretation of the electrocardiogram. Part II: the electrocardiogram and its technology, a scientific statement from the American Heart Association Electrocardiography and Arrhythmias Committee, Council on Clinical Cardiology; the American College of Cardiology Foundation; and the Heart Rhythm Society endorsed by the International Society for Computerized Electrocardiology. *J Am Coll Cardiol* 2007;49:1109–27.

14. Frank E. Theoretic analysis of the influence of heart-dipole eccentricity on limb leads, Wilson central-terminal voltage and the frontal-plane vectocardiogram. *Circ Res* 1953;1:380–8.

15. Wehr G, Peters RJ, Khalife K, et al. A vector-based, 5-electrode, 12-lead monitoring ECG (EASI) is equivalent to conventional 12-lead ECG for diagnosis of acute coronary syndromes. *J Electrocardiol* 2006;39:22–28.

16. Chantad D, Krittayaphong R, Komoltri C. Derived 12-lead electrocardiogram in the assessment of ST-segment deviation and cardiac rhythm. *J Electrocardiol* 2006;39:7–12.

17. Sejersten M, Wagner GS, Pahlm O, et al. Detection of acute ischemia from the EASI-derived 12-lead electrocardiogram and from the 12-lead electrocardiogram acquired in clinical practice. *J Electrocardiol* 2007;40:120–6.

18. Welinder A, Field DQ, Liebman J, et al. Diagnostic conclusions from the EASI-derived 12-lead electrocardiogram as compared with the standard 12-lead electrocardiogram in children. *Am Heart J* 2006;151:1059–64.

19. Dower GE, Yakush A, Nazzal SB, et al. Deriving the 12-lead electrocardiogram from four (EASI) electrodes. *J Electrocardiol* 1988:21 Suppl:S182–7.

20. Sundqvist K, Jogestrand T, Nowak J. The effect of digoxin on the electrocardiogram of healthy middle-aged and elderly patients at rest and during exercise–a comparison with the ECG reaction induced by myocardial ischemia. *J Electrocardiol* 2002;35:213–21.

21. Mooss AN, Prevedel JA, Mohiuddin SM, et al. Effect of digoxin on ST-segment changes detected by ambulatory electrocardiographic monitotring in healthy subjects. *Am J Cardiol* 1991;68:1503–6.

22. Croft CH, Woodward W, Nicod P, et al. Clinical implications of anterior S–T segment depression in patients with acute myocardial infarction. *Am J Cardiol* 1982;50:428–36.

23. Mirvis DM. Physiologic bases for anterior ST segment depression in patients with acute inferior wall myocardial infarction. *Am Heart J* 1988;116:1308–22.

24. Rahman MA, Gedevanishvili A, Birnbaum Y, et al. High-frequency QRS electrocardiogram predicts perfusion defects during myocardial perfusion imaging. *J Electrocardiol* 2006;39:73–81.

25. Abboud S, Berenfeld O, Sadeh D. Simulation of high-resolution QRS complex using a ventricular model with a fractal conduction system. Effects of ischemia on high-frequency QRS potentials. *Circ Res* 1991;68:1751–60.

26. Pettersson J, Carro E, Edenbrandt L, et al. Spatial, individual, and temporal variation of the high-frequency QRS amplitudes in the 12-lead standard electrocardiographic leads. *Am Heart J* 2000;139:352–8.

27. Aversano T, Rudicoff B, Washington A, et al. High-frequency QRS electrocardiography in the detection of reperfusion following thrombolytic therapy. *Clin Cardiol* 1994;17:175–82.

28. Pettersson J, Pahlm O, Carro E, et al. Changes in high-frequency QRS components are more sensitive than ST-segment deviation for detecting acute coronary artery occlusion. *J Am Coll Cardiol* 2000;36:1827–34.

29. Spackman TN, Abel MD, Schlegel TT. Twelve-lead high frequency QRS electrocardiography during anesthesia in healthy subjects. *Anesth Analg* 2005;100:1043–7.

30. Lindenauer PK, Pekow P, Wang K, et al. Perioperative beta-blocker therapy and mortality after major noncardiac surgery. *N Engl J Med* 2005;353:349–361.

31. Mangano DT, Browner WS, Hollenberg M, et al. Association of perioperative myocardial ischemia with cardiac morbidity and mortality in men undergoing noncardiac surgery. The Study of Perioperative Ischemia Research Group. *N Engl J Med* 1990;323:1781–8.

32. London MJ. Perioperative myocardial ischemia in patients undergoing myocardial revascularization. *Curr Opin Anesthesiol* 1993;6:98–105.

33. McFalls EO, Ward HB, Moritz TE, et al. Predictors and outcomes of a perioperative myocardial infarction following elective vascular surgery in patients with documented coronary artery disease: results of the CARP trial. *Eur Heart J* 2008;29:394–401.

34. Karpati PC, Rossignol M, Pirot M, et al. High incidence of myocardial ischemia during postpartum hemorrhage. *Anesthesiology* 2004;100:30–36.

35. Blackburn H, Katigbak R. What electrocardiographic leads to take after exercise? *Am Heart J* 1964;67:184–5.

36. Mason RE, Likar I. A new system of multiple-lead exercise electrocardiography. *Am Heart J* 1966;71:196–205.

37. Mason RE, Likar I, Biern RO, et al. Multiple-lead exercise electrocardiography: Experience in 107 normal subjects and 67 patients with angina pectoris, and comparison with coronary cinearteriography in 84 patients. *Circulation* 1967;36:517–25.

38. Tubau JF, Chaitman BR, Bourassa MG, et al. Detection of multivessel coronary disease after myocardial infarction using exercise stress testing and multiple ECG lead systems. *Circulation* 1980;61:44–52.

39. Koppes G, McKiernan T, Bassan M, et al. Treadmill exercise testing (part I). *Curr Prob Cardiol* 1977;7:1–44.

40. Chaitman BR, Bourassa MG, Wagniart P, et al. Improved efficiency of treadmill exercise testing using a multiple-lead ECG system and basic hemodynamic exercise response. *Circulation* 1978;57:71–79.

41. Miller TD, Desser KB, Lawson M. How many electrocardiographic leads are required for exercise treadmill tests? *J Electrocardiol* 1987;20:131–7.

42. Lam J, Chaitman BR. Exercise lead systems and newer electrocardiographic parameters. *J Cardiac Rehabil* 1984;4:507–16.

43. Chaitman BR. The changing role of the exercise electrocardiogram as a diagnostic and prognostic test for chronic ischemic heart disease. *J Am Coll Cardiol* 1986;8:1195–1210.

44. Chaitman BR, Hanson JS. Comparative sensitivity and specificity of exercise electrocardiographic lead systems. *Am J Cardiol* 1981;47:1335–49.

45. Horacek BM, Wagner GS. Electrocardiographic ST-segment changes during acute myocardial ischemia. *Card Electrophysiol Rev* 2002;6:196–203.

46. Carley SD. Beyond the 12 lead: review of the use of additional leads for the early electrocardiographic diagnosis of acute myocardial infarction. *Emerg Med (Fremantle)* 2003;15:143–54.

47. Drew BJ, Krucoff MW. Multilead ST-segment monitoring in patients with acute coronary syndromes: a consensus statement for healthcare professionals. ST- Segment Monitoring Practice Guideline International Working Group. *Am J Crit Care* 1999;8:372–86.

48. London MJ, Hollenberg M, Wong MG, et al. Intraoperative myocardial ischemia: localization by continuous 12-lead electrocardiography. *Anesthesiology* 1988;69:232–41.

49. Landesberg G, Mosseri M, Wolf Y, et al. Perioperative myocardial ischemia and infarction: identification by continuous 12-lead electrocardiogram with online ST-segment monitoring. *Anesthesiology* 2002;96:264–70.

50. Drew BJ, Krucoff MW. Multilead ST-segment monitoring in patients with acute coronary syndromes: a consensus statement for healthcare professionals. ST- Segment Monitoring Practice Guideline International Working Group. *Am J Crit Care* 1999;8:372–86.

51. London MJ. Multilead precordial ST-segment monitoring: "the next generation"? *Anesthesiology* 2002;96:259–61.

52. Martinez EA, Kim LJ, Faraday N, et al. Sensitivity of routine intensive care unit surveillance for detecting myocardial ischemia. *Crit Care Med* 2003;31:2302–8.

53. Balaji S, Ellenby M, McNames J, et al. Update on intensive care ECG and cardiac event monitoring. *Card Electrophysiol Rev* 2002;6:190–5.

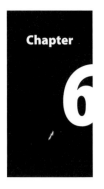

Arterial pressure monitoring

Alexander J. C. Mittnacht and Tuula S. O. Kurki

Introduction

Blood pressure (BP) is the one of the most commonly measured parameters of the cardiovascular system. The American Society of Anesthesiologists (ASA) guidelines for basic anesthesia monitoring, available online at http://www.asahq.org/publicationsAndServices/standards/02.pdf (last amended October 2005), mandate that arterial blood pressure be determined and evaluated at least every five minutes. Numerous methods of noninvasive BP measurement, next to the invasive assessment via an indwelling catheter, are clinically available.[1,2] Technical concepts, evidence of utility, indications, contraindications, and complications of blood pressure monitoring are discussed in this chapter.

Technical concept
General principles

Arterial BP, typically recorded as a systolic, diastolic, and mean arterial pressure (MAP) in millimeters of mercury, is derived from the complex interaction of the heart and the vascular system and varies not only at different sites in the body, but also when individual components of this system are changed. Stroke volume, systemic vascular resistance, the velocity of left ventricular ejection, the distensibility of the aorta and arterial walls, and the viscosity of blood all are components of this complex interaction that ultimately results in a pressure reading.

The arterial BP can also be seen as the force exerted by the blood per unit area on the arterial wall, with kinetic, hydrostatic, and hemodynamic individual pressure components contributing. After an arterial catheter has been placed, the typical arterial waveform can be displayed and recorded. However, this waveform actually represents the summation of a series of mechanical pressure signals or waves (multiple harmonics). The sine wave occurring at the rate of the pulse is called the *fundamental frequency*; each subsequent harmonic is a multiple of this first harmonic. Six to ten of those subsequent harmonics are required to reconstruct and to display the arterial pressure waveform (see Figure 6.1).[3,4] The components of the monitoring system – the cannula, tubing, connectors, and pressure transducer – all have their own natural resonant frequencies. Accurate pressure readings can be obtained only if the natural frequency of the monitoring system does not overlap with harmonic frequencies of the recorded pressure waveforms (also see invasive BP monitoring, discussed later).

Noninvasive BP measurement

Numerous methods of noninvasive BP measurement are clinically available. The American Heart Association (AHA) has published updated recommendations for noninvasive blood pressure measurements in humans.[5,6] The traditional auscultatory method is still considered the gold standard against which all other devices and methods must be compared. Using a stethoscope and a sphygmomanometer with an inflatable cuff placed around the upper arm, one can determine the systolic and diastolic BP. The height of a mercury (Hg) column in millimeters at the auscultatory determined systolic and diastolic points is reported. The systolic BP is the pressure at which the first sound is heard; the exact diastolic BP is more difficult to determine. The use of the fifth Korotkoff sound for diastolic BP measurement is typically used; however, the fourth Korotkoff sound has been recommended in certain clinical situations.[6] Appropriate cuff size is mandatory, as too small a cuff will yield false high, and too large a cuff false low, BP values. Even though a mercury sphygmomanometer does not need repeated calibration, accurate results are operator-dependent (observer error), and limitations of this method in various clinical settings must be recognized.[6]

Automated BP devices have replaced the auscultatory method in most anesthesia practice settings. Most of these devices use a cuff that is inflated by an electrically operated pump. A pressure release valve regulates the pressure in the cuff, with different manufacturers using various algorithms and intervals. All devices display systolic, diastolic, and mean arterial blood pressure and a pulse rate. However, it is important to recognize that typically only the mean arterial BP is determined or measured by oscillatory BP devices; the values of systolic and diastolic BP are computed, not actually measured, from the raw data. Similar to the auscultatory method, the appropriate cuff size is important for determining exact BP values. Available devices and the various methods used vary widely in accuracy; devices should be checked and, if necessary, recalibrated by qualified personal at specified intervals. The US Association for the Advancement of Medical Instrumentation (AAMI) and the British Hypertension Society (BHS) have set standards and

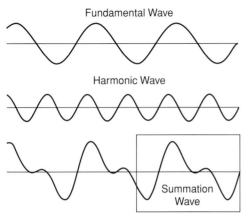

Fundamental Wave

Harmonic Wave

Summation Wave

Figure 6.1. The arterial pressure waveform as a sum of sine waves by Fourier analysis. Summation of the top and middle sine waves produces a waveform with the morphologic characteristics of an arterial blood pressure trace. From Pittman JAL, Ping JS, Mark JB. Arterial and central venous pressure monitoring. *Anesthesiol Clin* 2006;24:717–35 (Figure 1), with permission.

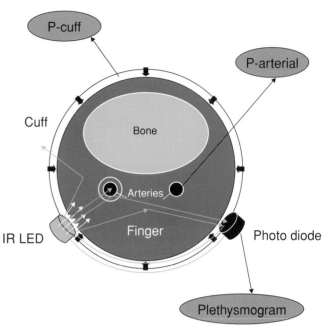

Figure 6.2. Cross-section of a finger at the middle phalanx level with a finger cuff wrapped around on it with built-in infrared (IR) plethysmograph. Source: Nexfin device, BMEYE, Amsterdam, The Netherlands.

protocols for the evaluation of blood pressure device accuracy.[7–9] The Working Group on Blood Pressure Monitoring of the European Society of Hypertension reviews blood pressure measuring devices to guide consumers. There are many sources of inaccurate pressure measurements with automated oscillatory methods, such as irregular heart rate seen with arrhythmias, low flow states, arm movement during BP measurement, and inappropriate positioning of the measurement site or cuff in relation to the heart.

Continuous beat-to-beat BP monitoring with noninvasive devices has been reported.[10,11] The volume-clamp method, tonometry, and photoplethysmographic methods have been described. The volume-clamp method was first described by Jan Peñáz in 1973.[12] The criterion to determine the correct unloaded volume by applying a physiologic calibration (Physiocal) was developed by Wesseling and colleagues.[13] The combination of these methods allows the continuous beat-to-beat BP measurement with a finger cuff placed on a patient's finger (FINAP). Commercially available devices consist of a finger cuff that contains the transducer of an infrared transmission plethysmograph (also see Figures 6.2 and 6.3). Infrared light is absorbed by the blood, and the pulsation of arterial diameter during a heartbeat causes a pulsation in the light detector signal. The cuff is wrapped around the middle phalanx of a finger (index or middle finger is recommended) and is connected to a pressure control valve. This proportional valve modulates the air pressure generated by the air compressor, thus causing changes in the finger cuff pressure in parallel with intraarterial pressure in the finger to dynamically unload the arterial walls in the finger. The cuff pressure thus provides an indirect measure of intraarterial pressure. In addition to continuous arterial BP monitoring, further developments of this technique allow computation of stroke volume, cardiac output, pulse rate variability, baroreflex sensitivity, total peripheral resistance, and systolic pressure variability.[14] The accuracy of the FINAP has been tested in several clinical trials against oscillometric blood

pressure measurement, or noninvasive blood pressure (NIBP), and against invasive intraarterial pressure measurement.[15] The FINAP seems to underestimate the invasive systolic blood pressure (SBP). Raynaud syndrome, anatomical variations in palmar arch arterial circulation, and the use of vasoconstricting agents are some of the factors that, if present, may yield inaccurate BP readings using the FINAP method.[16,17] The under- or overestimation of systolic pressure by changes in vasomotor tone has been mostly corrected for by reconstructing the brachial blood pressure waveform from the measured finger arterial pressure.[18,19] This brachial reconstruction has been validated in a new device based on the integration of these technologies.[20]

Invasive arterial blood pressure monitoring

Pressure waves in the arterial (or venous) tree represent the transmission of forces generated in the cardiac chambers. Measurement of these forces requires their transmission to a device that converts mechanical energy into electronic signals. The components of a system for intravascular pressure measurement include an intravascular catheter, fluid-filled tubing and connections, an electromechanical transducer, an electronic analyzer, and electronic storage and display systems.

Arterial cannulation

For arterial pressure measurements, short, narrow catheters (20-gauge or smaller) are recommended, because they have favorable dynamic response characteristics and are less thrombogenic than larger catheters. An artifact associated with intraarterial catheters has been labeled *end-pressure artifact*.[21] When flowing blood comes to a sudden halt at the tip of the

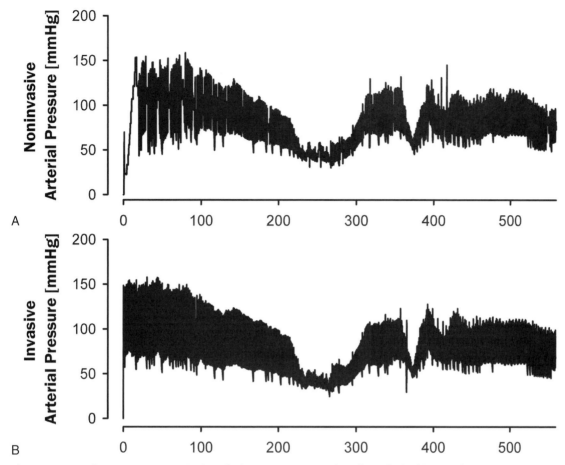

Figure 6.3. Arterial pressure registration (with Nexfin device; BMEYE, Amsterdam, The Netherlands) – nitroglycerin response Top (A): noninvasive–brachial arterial pressure [0-200 mmHG; (B) invasive–radial A-line pressure 0-200 mmHg. Horizontal = time [sec], time in measurement. Patient – female, 62 yrs, supine CABG surgery, anesthetized. Source: JJ Settels, BMEYE, Amsterdam, The Netherlands

catheter, it is estimated that an added pressure of 2 to 10 mmHg results. Conversely, clot formation on the catheter tip will over-damp the system (as discussed later).

Proper technique is helpful in obtaining a high degree of success in arterial catheterization. The wrist should be placed in a slightly dorsiflexed position, preferably over an armboard and over a pack of gauze in a supinated position. Caution should be exercised not to keep the wrist in extreme dorsiflexion, which can lead to median nerve damage by stretching of the nerve over the wrist. The angle between the needle and the skin should be shallow (30 degrees or less), and the needle should be advanced parallel to the course of the artery. When the artery is entered, the angle between the needle and skin is reduced to 10 degrees, the needle is advanced another 1 to 2 mm to ensure that the tip of the catheter also lies within the lumen of the vessel, and the outer catheter is then threaded off the needle whilewatching that blood continues to flow out of the needle hub. If blood ceases flowing while the needle is being advanced, the needle has penetrated the back wall of the vessel. In this technique, the artery has been transfixed by passage of the catheter-over-needle assembly "through-and-through" the artery. The needle is then completely withdrawn. As the catheter is slowly

withdrawn, pulsatile blood flow emerges from the catheter when its tip is within the lumen of the artery. The catheter is then slowly advanced into the artery. A guidewire may be helpful at this point if the catheter does not advance easily into the artery. When using the Seldinger technique, the artery is localized with a needle, and a guidewire is passed through the needle into the artery. A catheter is then passed over the guidewire into the artery.

Doppler-assisted localization of arteries has been used when palpation of the artery is difficult. However, Doppler-assisted techniques have been largely supplanted in clinical practice by two-dimensional ultrasonic methods. In the case of arterial catheterization, especially radial artery cannulation, a high-frequency (e.g. 9 MHz) ultrasonic transducer is required to visualize small structures in the near field. The artery is visualized in transverse section and the catheter-over-needle assembly is advanced at a 30- to 60-degree angle, starting a few millimeters distal to the ultrasonic transducer. With experience, the artery and the catheter are seen to intersect within the ultrasonic imaging plane using a triangulation technique. Alternatively, viewing the artery in a longitudinal imaging plane during needle insertion has been described. Using a two-dimensional ultrasound imaging technique for radial artery cannulation has been shown to increase the success rate at first attempt.[22] Nevertheless, there seems to be a significant learning curve involved.

Following the introduction of two-dimensional ultrasonic vascular access devices, a surgical cutdown as the last resort is typically performed less frequently. For a surgical cutdown technique, an incision is made in the skin overlying the artery, and the surrounding tissues are dissected away from the arterial wall. Proximal and distal ligatures are passed around the artery to control blood loss, but are not tied down. Under direct vision, the artery is cannulated with a catheter-over-needle assembly. Alternatively, a small incision is made in the arterial wall to facilitate passage of the catheter.

Arterial cannulation sites

Factors that influence the site of arterial cannulation include the location of surgery, the possible compromise of arterial flow owing to patient positioning or surgical manipulations, and any history of ischemia of or prior surgery on the limb to be cannulated. Sites for arterial cannulation include the radial, ulnar, brachial, axillary, femoral, and dorsalis pedis or posterior tibial arteries.

The radial artery is the most commonly used artery for continuous invasive BP monitoring. It is usually easy to cannulate with a short (20-gauge) catheter and is readily accessible during surgery. The predictive value of testing adequate palmar collateral circulation with the Allen test has been questioned. The Allen test is performed by compressing both the radial and ulnar arteries and exercising the hand until it is pale. The ulnar artery is then released (with the hand open loosely), and the time until the hand regains its normal color is noted.[23] With normal collateral circulation, the color returns to the hand in about five seconds. If, however, the hand takes longer than 15 seconds to return to its normal color, cannulation of the radial artery on that side is controversial. In a large series of children in whom radial arterial catheterization was performed without preliminary Allen tests, there was an absence of complications.[24] Slogoff and coworkers cannulated the radial artery in 16 adult patients with poor ulnar collateral circulation (assessed using the Allen test) without any complications.[25] An incidence of zero in a study sample of only 16 patients, however, does not guarantee that the true incidence of the complication is negligible. In contrast, Mangano and Hickey reported a case of hand ischemia requiring amputation in a patient with a normal preoperative Allen test.[26] Alternatively, pulse oximetry or plethysmography can be used to assess patency of the hand collateral arteries. Barbeau and associates compared the modified Allen test with pulse oximetry and plethysmography in 1010 consecutive patients undergoing percutaneous radial cannulation for cardiac catheterization.[27] Pulse oximetry and plethysmography were more sensitive than the Allen test for detecting inadequate collateral blood supply, and only 1.5 percent of patients were not suitable for radial artery cannulation.

Brachial artery cannulation is routinely performed at many institutions, although others question the safety of this technique, given the fact that there is little, if any, collateral flow to the hand should brachial artery occlusion occur. Brachial artery pressure tracings resemble those in the femoral artery, with less systolic augmentation than radial artery tracings.[28] Brachial arterial pressures were found to more accurately reflect central aortic pressures than radial arterial pressures, both before and after cardiopulmonary bypass.[29]

The axillary artery is normally cannulated using the Seldinger technique near the junction of the deltoid and pectoral muscles. This approach has been recommended for long-term catheterization in the intensive care unit and in patients with peripheral vascular disease.[30] Because the tip of the 15- to 20-cm catheter may lie within the aortic arch, the use of the left axillary artery is recommended to minimize the theoretical risk of cerebral embolization during flushing. Lateral decubitus positioning or adduction of the arm occasionally results in kinking of axillary catheters with damping of the pressure waveform.

The femoral artery may be cannulated for monitoring purposes but is usually reserved for situations when other sites are unable to be cannulated or it is specifically indicated (e.g. descending thoracic aortic aneurysm surgery for distal pressure monitoring). The use of this site remains controversial because of the risk of ischemic complications and pseudo-aneurysm formation following diagnostic angiographic and cardiac catheterization procedures. However, these data do not pertain to the clinical situation when the femoral artery is used for monitoring purposes, because the size of catheters for BP monitoring is considerably smaller than the size of diagnostic catheters. A literature review on peripheral artery cannulation placed for hemodynamic monitoring purposes (including 3899 femoral artery cannulations) found temporary occlusion in 10 patients (1.45%), whereas serious ischemic complications requiring extremity amputation were reported in only three patients (0.18%).[31] Other complications that were summarized from the published data were pseudoaneurysm formation in six patients (0.3%), sepsis in 13 patients (0.44%), local infection (0.78%), bleeding (1.58%), and hematoma (6.1%). The researchers concluded that, based on the reviewed literature, using the femoral artery for hemodynamic monitoring purposes was safer than radial artery cannulation. Older literature stated that the femoral area was intrinsically dirty, and that catheter sepsis and mortality were significantly increased at this site compared with other monitoring sites. This could also not be confirmed by more recently published literature.[32]

The two main arteries to the foot are the dorsalis pedis artery and the posterior tibial artery, which form an arterial arch on the foot that is similar to the one formed by the radial and ulnar arteries in the hand. The dorsalis pedis or posterior tibial arteries are reasonable alternatives to radial arterial catheterization. The systolic pressure is usually 10 to 20 mmHg higher in the dorsalis pedis artery than in the radial or brachial arteries, whereas the diastolic pressure is 15 to 20 mmHg lower.[33]

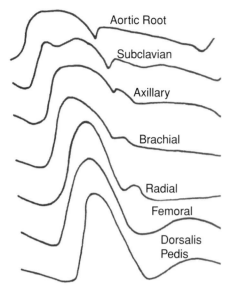

Figure 6.4. The waveform of the arterial pressure changes markedly according to the site of the intraarterial catheter. This illustration demonstrates these changes as a progression from central monitoring (top) through peripheral monitoring (bottom). These changes are believed to be caused by forward wave propagation and wave reflection. In the periphery, systolic pressure is higher, diastolic pressure is lower, and mean pressure is minimally lower. Modified from Bedford RF. Invasive blood pressure monitoring. In Blitt CD (ed.). *Monitoring in Anesthesia and Critical Care*. New York: Churchill Livingstone, 1985, p. 505.

The incidence of failed cannulation is up to 20 percent, and the incidence of thrombotic occlusion is around 8 percent, because of the small size of the artery.[34] In a recently published prospective observational study, dorsalis pedis artery cannulation was found to be a safe and easily available alternative when radial arteries are not accessible.[35] However, these vessels should not be used in patients with severe peripheral vascular disease from diabetes mellitus or other causes.

Arterial pressure waveform

The arterial pressure waveform is ideally measured in the ascending aorta. The pressure measured in the more peripheral arteries is different from the central aortic pressure because the arterial waveform becomes progressively more distorted as the signal is transmitted down the arterial system. The high-frequency components, such as the dicrotic notch, disappear; the systolic peak increases; the diastolic trough decreases; and there is a transmission delay (distal pulse amplification; see Figure 6.4). These changes are caused by decreased arterial compliance in the periphery, and reflection and resonance of pressure waves in the arterial tree.[36] This effect is most pronounced in the dorsalis pedis artery, in which the SBP may be 10 to 20 mmHg higher, and the diastolic blood pressure (DBP) 10 to 20 mmHg lower than in the central aorta. Despite this distortion, the MAP measured in the peripheral arteries should be similar to the central aortic pressure under normal circumstances. Thus, the cannulation of large more central arterial

vessels, such as the femoral and axillary arteries, can be avoided in most clinical settings.[37]

MAP is probably the most useful parameter to measure in assessing organ perfusion, except for the heart, in which the DBP is the most important. MAP is measured directly by integrating the arterial waveform tracing over time, or using the formula: $MAP = (SBP + [2 \times DBP])/3$. The pulse pressure is the difference between SBP and DBP.

Arterial waveform analysis – and, in particular, the influence of positive pressure ventilation on the cyclic variation of the arterial pressure – has been studied.[38–40] The interactions among intrathoracic pressure, lung volume, and left- and right-sided loading conditions are complex, and cannot be easily interpreted. Typically, increased variation in arterial pressure is seen in hypovolemic patients, and its response to fluid administration has been studied in animals and humans. Systolic pressure variation (SPV) is typically described as the increase (Δ up) and decrease (Δ down) from end-expiratory baseline during positive pressure ventilation (see Figure 6.5). In particular, Δ down has been shown to be a sensitive marker for hypovolemia. However, tidal volume, airway pressures, lung and chest wall compliance, positive end-expiratory pressure, and arrhythmias all have been shown to interfere with the magnitude of SPV and its components.

Coupling system and pressure transducers

The coupling system usually consists of pressure tubing, stopcocks, and a continuous flushing device. This fluid-filled system, once attached to the arterial cannula, oscillates in its own inherent frequency. This is called *resonance* and is the major source of distortion of arterial pressure tracings.

The function of transducers is to convert mechanical forces into electrical current or voltage. Modern disposable transducers have eliminated many of the difficulties that formerly required frequent recalibration owing to zero-point drift. Before accurate pressure values can be obtained, transducers must be zeroed against ambient atmospheric pressure and horizontally aligned (leveled) with the right atrium. In fluid-filled catheter systems, incorrect positioning of the transducer can be a major source of inaccurate pressure readings. This is of particular concern in the low-pressure venous system, because small changes in transducer height will have a proportionally large effect on the pressure readings. If cerebral perfusion is of interest – for example, during intracranial procedures in the sitting position – the pressure transducer should be placed at the level of the circle of Willis rather than the right atrium. Calibration of modern transducers is done by the manufacturer and is thus not required in the clinical setting.

Most modern equipment designed to analyze and display pressure information consists of a computerized system that handles several tasks, including the acquisition and display of pressure signals; the derivation of numerical values for systolic, diastolic, and mean pressures; alarm functions; data storage; trend displays; and printing functions. When connected to an

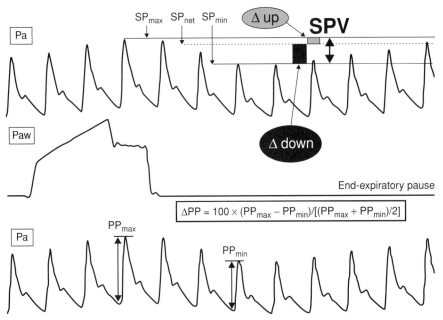

Figure 6.5. Analytic description of respiratory changes in arterial pressure during mechanical ventilation. The systolic pressure and the pulse pressure (systolic minus diastolic pressure) are maximum (SP_{max} and PP_{max}, respectively) during inspiration and minimum (SP_{min} and PP_{min}, respectively) a few heartbeats later – i.e. during the expiratory period. The systolic pressure variation (SPV) is the difference between SP_{max} and SP_{min}. The assessment of a reference systolic pressure (SP_{ref}) during an end-expiratory pause allows the discrimination between the inspiratory increase (Δ up) and the expiratory decrease (Δ down) in systolic pressure. Pa = arterial pressure; Paw = airway pressure. From reference 40.

$$\Delta PP = 100 \times (PP_{max} - PP_{min})/[(PP_{max} + PP_{min})/2]$$

automated anesthesia recordkeeping system, BP readings can be recorded automatically and linked to various perioperative measured parameters and events.

Characteristics of a pressure measurement system

The dynamic response of a pressure measurement system is characterized by its natural frequency and its damping.[41] These concepts are best understood by snapping the end of a transducer–tubing assembly with one's finger. The waveform on the monitor demonstrates rapid oscillations above and below

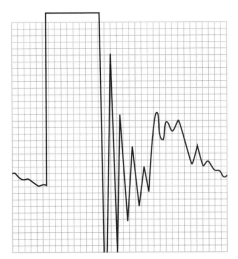

Figure 6.6. The arterial pressure artifact resulting from a fast flush test allows calculation of the natural resonant frequency and the damping coefficient of the monitoring system. The time between adjacent pressure peaks determines the natural frequency and the height or amplitude ratio of adjacent peaks allows determination of the damping coefficient. From reference 27.

the baseline, which is equal to the natural frequency, and then quickly decays to a straight line because of friction in the system (damping; also see Figures 6.6 and 6.7). The peaks and troughs of an arterial pressure waveform will be amplified, resulting in inaccurate pressure readings if the natural frequency of the transducer–tubing–catheter assembly is too low. The natural frequency of the measurement system needs to be at least six to 10 times higher than the fundamental frequency of the pressure wave (heart rate). Consequently, with a heart rate of 120 beats per minute (2 cycles per second or 2 Hz), a natural frequency > 20 Hz of the monitoring system is required to accurately display the arterial pressure.[42] Boutros and Albert demonstrated that by changing the length of low-compliance (rigid) tubing from 6 inches to 5 feet, the natural frequency decreased from 34 to 7 Hz.[43] As a result of the reduced natural frequency, the SBPs measured with the longer tubing exceeded reference pressures by 17.3 percent. Generally, longer transducer tubing lowers the natural frequency of the system and tends to amplify the height of the systolic (peak) and the depth of the diastolic (trough) values of the BP measurement.[44,45]

Damping is the tendency of factors such as friction, compliant (soft) tubing, and air bubbles to absorb energy and decrease the amplitude of peaks and troughs in the waveform. The optimal degree of damping is that which counterbalances the distorting effects of transducer–tubing systems with lower natural frequencies. This is very difficult to achieve. The damping of a clinical pressure measurement system can be assessed by observing the response to a rapid high-pressure flush of the transducer–tubing–catheter system (also see Figures 6.6 and 6.7). In a system with a low damping coefficient, a fast flush test will result in several oscillations above and below the baseline before the pressure becomes constant. In an adequately damped system, the baseline will be reached after one

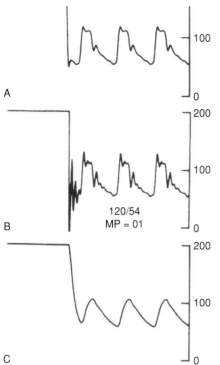

Figure 6.7. The fast flush test demonstrates the harmonic characteristics of a pressure monitoring system (transducer, fluid-filled tubing, and intraarterial catheter). In an optimally damped system (A), the pressure waveform returns to baseline after only one oscillation. In an underdamped system (B), the pressure waveform oscillates above and below the baseline several times. In an overdamped system (C), the pressure waveform returns to the baseline slowly with no oscillations. Modified from reference 49.

oscillation, whereas in an overdamped system, the baseline will be reached after a delay and without oscillations.[46–49]

The formulas for calculating the natural frequency and damping coefficient are as follows:

$$\text{Natural frequency}: f_n = \frac{d}{8}\sqrt{\frac{3}{\pi L \rho V_d}}$$

$$\text{Damping coefficient}: \zeta = \frac{16n}{d^3}\sqrt{\frac{3LV_d}{\pi\rho}},$$

where d = tubing diameter;
L = tubing length;
ρ = density of the fluid;
V_d = transducer fluid volume displacement; and
n = viscosity of the fluid.

Evidence of utility (clinical outcome)

Multiple well-designed prospective studies have established the correlation between elevated BP and cardiovascular events. These data are well presented in the literature and are beyond the scope of this text.[50] Intraoperative measurement of BP is required by the ASA (as mentioned earlier), and outcome studies comparing the use of this parameter to a nonmonitored group are not feasible.

However, there is increasing evidence that an increase in perioperative BP, as well as pulse pressure (PP), are associated with adverse events and outcome measures in cardiac as well as noncardiac surgical settings.[51] Fontes and colleagues recently published on the association between an increased PP and

adverse cerebral and cardiac events.[52] A total of 4801 patients scheduled for elective coronary bypass surgery met the inclusion criteria. Nine hundred seventeen patients (19.1%) had fatal and nonfatal vascular complications, including 146 patients (3.0%) with cerebral events and 715 patients (14.9%) with cardiac events. The incidence of a cerebral event and/or death from neurologic complications nearly doubled for patients with PP >80 mmHg versus PP ≤ 80 mmHg (5.5% vs. 2.8%; $P = 0.004$). PP more than 80 mmHg was also found to be associated with cardiac complications, increasing the incidence of congestive heart failure by 52 percent, and death from cardiac causes by nearly 100 percent ($P = 0.003$ and 0.006, respectively). The same group reported in an earlier study that isolated systolic hypertension is associated with increased cardiovascular morbidity in coronary artery surgery patients.[53] In another large prospective observational study, 7740 noncardiac surgery cases (general, vascular, and urological surgery) were included in the analysis. Intraoperative arterial hypertension was an independent predictor of cardiac adverse events within 30 days of surgery (83 patients, 1.1%).[54]

Complications

The complications of percutaneous arterial cannulation are summarized in Table 6.1. Despite the great advantages of intraarterial monitoring, it does not always give accurate BP values. Equipment misuse and misinterpretation have been reported as the most frequent complications associated with invasive pressure monitoring.[55] The monitoring system may be incorrectly zeroed and calibrated, or the transducers may not be at the appropriate level. The waveform will be dampened if the catheter is kinked or partially thrombosed. In vasoconstricted patients, in patients in hypovolemic shock, and during the post-CPB period, the brachial and radial artery pressures may be significantly lower than the true central aortic pressure. With modern transducers, baseline drift has become less frequent; however, fluid contamination of transducer cable connectors or faulty transducer cables can give inaccurate readings. Another possible etiology for inaccurate measurements is unsuspected arterial stenosis proximal to the monitored artery, as occurs with thoracic outlet syndrome and subclavian stenosis.

One potential complication that is common to all forms of invasive monitoring is infection. Indwelling percutaneous catheters can become infected because of insertion through an

Table 6.1. Complications of invasive arterial pressure monitoring

- False pressure readings (equipment misuse)
- Infection
- Bleeding, hematoma formation
- Thrombosis
- Ischemia
- Cerebral emboli
- Nerve damage
- Pseudoaneurysm

infected skin site, poor aseptic technique during insertion or maintenance, sepsis with seeding of the catheter, and prolonged duration of cannulation with colonization by skin flora.[56] Historically, factors that were associated with catheter infection included nondisposable transducer domes, dextrose flush solutions, contaminated blood gas syringes, and duration of insertion.[57-60] Recently published data suggest that the incidence of arterial catheter infection is similar to infection rates published with the insertion of central venous catheters.[61,62] However, in contrast with central venous catheterization, full sterile barriers during arterial line placement were not found to reduce the risk of arterial catheter infections.[63,64] Nevertheless, these data do not exempt the practitioner from using strict aseptic techniques. Guidelines for the prevention of intravascular catheter related infections have been published by the Hospital Infection Control Practices Advisory Committee and the Centers for Disease Control and Prevention.[65]

The use of an intraarterial catheter carries the potential risk of exsanguination if the catheter or tubing assembly becomes disconnected. The use of Luer-Lok (instead of tapered) connections and monitors with low-pressure alarms should decrease the risk of this complication. Stopcocks are an additional source of occult hemorrhage because of the potential for loose connections or inadvertent changes in the position of the control lever that would open the system to the atmosphere.

Thrombosis of the radial artery following cannulation has been studied extensively. Temporary arterial occlusion is the most common reported complication after radial artery cannulation.[66] Factors that correlate with an increased incidence of thrombosis include prolonged duration of cannulation,[67] larger catheters,[68] and smaller radial artery size (i.e. a greater proportion of the artery is occupied by the catheter).[69] The association between radial artery thrombosis and ischemia of the hand is less certain. As noted above, an abnormal Allen test was not associated with hand complications following radial artery cannulation.[25] Despite the widespread use of radial artery cannulation, hand complications are very rarely reported. Temporary occlusion after arterial cannulation is usually benign. Nevertheless, serious ischemic complications are reported that may require the amputation of a digit or extremity.[70-72] Slogoff and associates stated that, in their experience, most ischemic complications occurred in patients who had had multiple embolic phenomena from other sources or were on high-dose vasopressor therapy, with resultant ischemia in multiple extremities.[25]

The hand should be examined closely at regular intervals in patients with axillary, brachial, radial, or ulnar arterial catheters. Because thrombosis may appear several days after the catheter has been removed,[67] the examinations should be continued through the postoperative period. Although recanalization of the thrombosed artery can be expected in an average of 13 days,[73] the collateral blood flow may be inadequate during this period. The treatment plan should involve consultation with a vascular, hand, or plastic surgeon. Traditionally, treatment for arterial occlusion or thrombosis with adequate collateral flow has been conservative. However, fibrinolytic agents, such as streptokinase, stellate ganglion blockade, and/or surgical intervention are modalities that should be considered. Overall, the evidence of permanent hand ischemia is low.

Particulate matter or air that is flushed forcefully into an arterial catheter can move proximally as well as distally within the artery. Cerebral embolization is most likely from axillary or temporal sites, but is also possible with brachial and radial catheters.[74] Emboli from the right arm are more likely to reach the cerebral circulation than those from the left arm because of the anatomy and direction of blood flow in the aortic arch. Other factors that influence the likelihood of cerebral embolization include the volume of flush solution, the rapidity of the injection, and the proximity of the intraluminal end of the catheter to the central circulation.[75]

Hematoma formation may occur at any arterial puncture or cannulation site, and is particularly common with a coagulopathy. Hematoma formation should be prevented by the application of direct pressure following arterial punctures and, if possible, the correction of any underlying coagulopathy. Posterior puncture or tear of the femoral or iliac arteries can produce massive bleeding into the retroperitoneal area.[76] Surgical consultation should be obtained if massive hematoma formation develops.

Nerve damage is possible if the nerve and artery lie in a fibrous sheath (such as the brachial plexus) or in a limited tissue compartment (such as the forearm).[77] Direct nerve injuries may also occur from needle trauma during attempts at arterial cannulation. The median nerve is in close proximity to the brachial artery, and the axillary artery lies within the brachial plexus sheath.

Incomplete disruption of the wall of an artery may eventually result in pseudoaneurysm formation.[78] The wall of the pseudoaneurysm is composed of fibrous tissue that continues to expand. If the pseudoaneurysm ruptures into a vein, or if both a vein and an artery are injured simultaneously, an arteriovenous fistula may result. Nonsurgical treatment options for the repair of pseudoaneurysms after arterial cannulation have been described recently and may replace surgery that is usually performed to treat this complication.[79]

Credentialing

The AHA recommendations for blood pressure measurements in humans, available online at http://circ.ahajournals.org/cgi/content/full/111/5/697 (last amended 2005), list recommendations for observer training. The training should be the same for health care professionals in ambulatory and community settings, as well as lay observers. Required competencies such as adequate vision, hearing, and eye–hand–ear coordination should be assessed prior to training. Actual training

Table 6.2. Indications for invasive arterial pressure monitoring

- Major surgical procedures involving large fluid shifts and/or blood loss
- Surgery requiring cardiopulmonary bypass
- Surgery of the aorta
- Patients with pulmonary disease requiring frequent arterial blood gases
- Patients with recent myocardial infarctions, unstable angina, or severe coronary artery disease
- Patients with decreased left ventricular function (congestive heart failure) or significant valvular heart disease
- Patients in hypovolemic, cardiogenic, or septic shock, or with multiple organ failure
- Procedures involving the use of deliberate hypotension
- Massive trauma cases
- Patients with right heart failure, chronic obstructive pulmonary disease, pulmonary hypertension, or pulmonary embolism
- Hemodynamic instable patients requiring vasoconstrictive or inotropic pharmacological support
- Patients with electrolyte or metabolic disturbances requiring frequent blood samples
- Inability to measure arterial pressure noninvasively (e.g. morbid obesity)

can be provided in various settings; for clinical trials, however, standardized programs are recommended. For federally funded clinical trials of hypertension care and control, retraining is required every six months. Because the use of automated BP devices does not eliminate all sources of human error, training of observers is also recommended when automated devices are used.

Practice parameters (indications for arterial BP monitoring)

The ASA guidelines for basic anesthesia monitoring mandate that arterial blood pressure be determined and evaluated at least every five minutes during all anesthetic procedures.

There are no specific recommendations as to what procedures or clinical settings require invasive arterial blood pressure monitoring. Some of the typical indications for invasive arterial monitoring are listed in Table 6.2. Intraarterial monitoring provides a continuous, beat-to-beat indication of the arterial pressure and waveform, and having an indwelling arterial catheter enables frequent sampling of arterial blood for laboratory analyses. Thus, even with the ability to measure beat-to-beat BP noninvasively, direct intraarterial monitoring remains the gold standard for cases in which hemodynamic changes occur frequently and large fluid shifts are anticipated. Additionally, the arterial waveform tracing can provide information beyond timely BP measurements. For example, the slope of the arterial upstroke correlates with the derivative of pressure over time, dP/dt, and thus gives an indirect estimate of myocardial contractility. This is not specific information, because an increase in SVR alone will also result in an increase in the slope of the upstroke. The arterial waveform can also present a visual estimate of the hemodynamic consequences of arrhythmias, and the arterial pulse contour can be used to estimate stroke volume and cardiac output. Additionally, hypovolemia is suggested

when the arterial pressure shows large SBP variation during the respiratory cycle in the mechanically ventilated patient (also see previous discussion).[80,81]

Contraindications

Some of the contraindications for noninvasive BP monitoring include prior ipsilateral mastectomy with lymphadenectomy, burns, and cutaneous infections. Contraindications to arterial cannulation include local infection, proximal obstruction, vasoocclusive disorders, and surgical considerations. Coagulopathic patients frequently require invasive BP monitoring, and more central arterial cannulation may result in significant hematoma formation. Thus, in anticoagulated and coagulopathic patients, it is recommended that more peripheral arterial cannulation sites be used when this form of monitoring is required.

Anatomic factors may lead to intraarterial pressure readings that markedly underestimate the central aortic pressure. The thoracic outlet syndrome and congenital anomalies of the aortic arch vessels will obstruct flow to the upper extremities. Aortic coarctation will diminish flow to the lower extremities. Arterial pressure distal to a previous arterial cutdown site may be lower than the central aortic pressure owing to arterial stenosis at the cutdown site. Patients with a prior classic Blalock-Taussig shunt typically have lower BP readings on the upper extremity distal to the shunt. The opposite site should be chosen for arterial BP monitoring.

Radial and brachial arterial cannulation is contraindicated in patients with a history of Raynaud syndrome or Buerger disease (thromboangiitis obliterans). This is especially important in the perioperative setting, because hypothermia of the hand is the main trigger for vasospastic attacks in Raynaud syndrome.[82] It is recommended that large arteries, such as the femoral or axillary arteries, be used for intraarterial monitoring if indicated in patients with either of these diseases.

Several surgical maneuvers may interfere with intraarterial monitoring. During mediastinoscopy, the scope intermittently compresses the innominate artery against the manubrium. In this situation, it is advantageous to monitor radial artery pressure on one side, while a pulse oximeter probe may be placed on the opposite extremity. Invasive BP monitoring on the right extremity allows immediate recognition of innominate artery compression. Alternatively, the pulse oximeter waveform displayed by most modern pulse oximeter devices allows the recognition of innominate artery compression. The invasive BP can then continuously be measured on the opposite side.

References

1. O'Brien E, Waeber B, Parati G, et al. Blood pressure measuring devices: recommendations of the European Society of Hypertension. *BMJ* 2001;322:531–6.

2. Young C, Mark J, White W, et al. Clinical evaluation of continuous noninvasive blood pressure monitoring: Accuracy and tracking capabilities. *J Clin Monit* 1995;11:245–52.

3. Pittman JA, Ping JS, Mark JB. Arterial and central venous pressure monitoring. *Int Anesthesiol Clin* 2004;42:13–30.

4. Kleinman B. Understanding natural frequency and damping and how they relate to the measurement of blood pressure. *J Clin Monit* 1989;5:137–47.

5. Pickering TG, Hall JE, Appel LJ, et al. Recommendations for blood pressure measurements in humans and experimental animals. Part 1: Blood pressure measurement in humans: a statement for professionals from the Subcommittee of Professional and Public Education of the American Heart Association Council on High Blood Pressure Research. *Circulation* 2005;111:697–716.

6. Pickering TG, Hall JE, Appel LJ, et al. Recommendations for blood pressure measurements in humans: an AHA Scientific Statement from the Council on High Blood Pressure Research Professional and Public Education Subcommittee. *J Clin Hypertension* 2005;7:102–107.

7. O'Brien E, Petrie J, Littler WA, et al. The British Hypertension Society Protocol for the evaluation of blood pressure measuring devices. *J Hypertens* 1993;11:S43–63.

8. American National Standard. Electronic or automated sphygmomanometers. ANSI/AAMI SP10–1992. Arlington, VA: Association for the Advancement of Medical Instrumentation, 1993, p. 40.

9. Friedman BA, Alpert BS, Osborn D, et al. Assessment of the validation of blood pressure monitors: a statistical reappraisal. *Blood Press Monit* 2008;13:187–91.

10. Parati G, Ongaro G, Bilo G, Glavina F. Non-invasive beat-to-beat blood pressure monitoring: new developments. *Blood Press Monit* 2003;8:31–6.

11. Belani K, Ozaki M, Hynson J, et al. A new noninvasive method to measure blood pressure: results of a multicenter trial. *Anesthesiology* 1999;91:686–92.

12. Peñáz J. Photoelectric measurement of blood pressure volume and flow in the finger. In *Digest of the 10th International Conference on Medical and Biological Engineering*, Dresden, 1973, p. 104.

13. Wesseling KH, De Wit B, Van Der Hoeven GMA, van Goudoever J, Settels JJ. Physiocal, calibrating finger physiology for Finapres. *Homeostasis* 1995;36:67–82.

14. Wesseling KH, Jansen JR, Settels JJ, Schreuder JJ. Computation of aortic flow from pressure in humans using a nonlinear, three-element model. *J Appl Physiol* 1993;74:2566–73.

15. Kurki TS, Sanford TJ, Smith NT, Dec-Silver H, Head N. Effects of radial artery cannulation on the function of finger blood pressure and pulse oximeter monitors. *Anesthesiology* 1988;69:778–82.

16. Kurki TS, Piirainen HI, Kurki PT. Non-invasive monitoring of finger arterial pressure in patients with Raynaud's phenomenon: effects of exposure to cold. *Br J Anaesth* 1990;65:558–63.

17. Kurki T. Continuous noninvasive monitoring of arterial blood pressure in the emergency department. *Am J Noninv Cardiology* 1991;5:103–5.

18. Bos WJW, Van Den Meiracker AH, Wesseling KH, Schalekamp MAH. Effect of regional and systemic changes in vasomotor tone on finger pressure amplification. *Hypertension* 1995;26:315–20.

19. Bos WJW, van Goeoever J, van Montfrans GA, Van Den Meiracker AH, Wesseling KH. Reconstruction of brachial artery pressure from noninvasive finger pressure measurements. *Circulation* 1996;94:1870–5.

20. Eeftick Schattenkerk DW, van Lieshout JJ, Van Den Meiracker AH, et al. Nexfin noninvasive continuous blood pressure validated against Riva-Rocci/Korotkoff. *Am J Hypertens* 2009;22:378–83.

21. Grossman W, Baim DS. *Cardiac Catheterization, Angiography, and Intervention*. 6th ed. Baltimore: Lippincott Williams & Wilkins, 2000.

22. Levin PD, Sheinin O, Gozal Y. Use of ultrasound guidance in the insertion of radial artery catheters. *Crit Care Med* 2003;31:481–4.

23. Allen EV. Thromboangiitis obliterans: methods of diagnosis of chronic occlusive arterial lesions distal to the wrist with illustrated cases. *Am J Med Sci* 1929;178:237–44.

24. Marshall AG, Erwin DC, Wyse RKH, Hatch DJ. Percutaneous arterial cannulation in children. *Anaesthesia* 1984;39:27–31.

25. Slogoff S, Keats AS, Arlund C. On the safety of radial artery cannulation. *Anesthesiology* 1983;59:42–47.

26. Mangano DT, Hickey RF. Ischemic injury following uncomplicated radial artery catheterization. *Anesth Analg* 1979;58:55–57.

27. Barbeau GR, Arsenault F, Dugas L, et al. Evaluation of the ulnopalmar arterial arches with pulse oximetry and plethysmography: comparison with the Allen's test in 1010 patients. *Am Heart J* 2004;147:489–93.

28. Pascarelli EF, Bertrand CA. Comparison of blood pressures in the arms and legs. *N Engl J Med* 1964;270:693–8.

29. Bazaral MG, Welch M, Golding LAR, Badhwar K. Comparison of brachial and radial arterial pressure monitoring in patients undergoing coronary artery bypass surgery. *Anesthesiology* 1990;73:38–45.

30. Gurman GM, Kriemerman S. Cannulation of big arteries in critically ill patients. *Crit Care Med* 1985;13:217–20.

31. Scheer B, Perel A, Pfeiffer UJ. Clinical review: complications and risk factors of peripheral arterial catheters used for haemodynamic monitoring in anaesthesia and intensive care medicine. *Crit Care* 2002;6:199–204.

32. Frezza EE, Mezghebe H. Indications and complications of arterial catheter use in surgical or medical intensive care units: analysis of 4932 patients. *Am Surg* 1998;64:127–31.

33. Johnstone RE, Greenhow DE. Catheterization of the dorsalis pedis artery. *Anesthesiology* 1973;39:654–655.

34. Youngberg JA, Miller ED. Evaluation of percutaneous cannulations of the dorsalis pedis artery. *Anesthesiology* 1976;44:80–83.

35. Martin C, Saux P, Papazian L, Gouin F. Long-term arterial cannulation in ICU patients using the radial artery or dorsalis pedis artery. *Chest* 2001;119:901–6.

36. Remington JW. Contour changes of the aortic pulse during propagation. *Am J Physiol* 1960;199:331–4.

37. Mignini MA, Piacentini E, Dubin A. Peripheral arterial blood pressure monitoring adequately tracks central arterial blood pressure in critically ill patients: an observational study. *Crit Care* 2006;10:R43.

38. Marx G, Cope T, McCrossan L, et al. Assessing fluid responsiveness by stroke volume variation in mechanically ventilated patients with severe sepsis. *Eur J Anaesthesiol* 2004;21:132–8.

39. Reuter DA, Kirchner A, Felbinger BE, et al. Usefulness of left ventricular stroke volume variation to assess fluid responsiveness

in patients with reduced cardiac function. *Crit Care Med* 2003;31:1399–404.

40. Michard F. Changes in arterial pressure during mechanical ventilation. *Anesthesiology* 2005;103:419–28.

41. Kleinman B. Understanding natural frequency and damping and how they relate to the measurement of blood pressure. *J Clin Monit* 1989;5:137–47.

42. Barbeito A, Mark JB. Arterial and central venous pressure monitoring. *Anesthesiol Clin* 2006;24:717–35.

43. Boutros A, Albert S. Effect of the dynamic response of transducer–tubing system on accuracy of direct blood pressure measurement in patients. *Crit Care Med* 1983;11:124–7.

44. Todorovic M, Jensen EW, Thogersen C. Evaluation of dynamic performance in liquid-filled catheter systems for measuring invasive blood pressure. *Int J Clin Monit Comput* 1996;13:173–8.

45. Heimann PA, Murray WB. Construction and use of catheter-manometer systems. *J Clin Monit* 1993;9:45–53.

46. Kleinman B, Frey K, Stevens R. The fast flush test – is the clinical comparison equivalent to its in vitro simulation? *J Clin Monit Comput* 1998;14:485–9.

47. Kleinman B, Powell S, Kumar P, et al. The fast flush test measures the dynamic response of the entire blood pressure monitoring system. *Anesth* 1992;77:1215–20.

48. Schwid HA. Frequency response evaluation of radial artery catheter–manometer systems: sinusoidal frequency analysis versus flush method. *J Clin Monit* 1988;4:181–5.

49. Gibbs NC, Gardner RM. Dynamics of invasive pressure monitoring systems: clinical and laboratory evaluation. *Heart Lung* 1988;17:43–51.

50. Staessen JA, Asmar R, De Buyzere M, et al. Task Force II: Blood pressure measurement and cardiovascular outcome. *Blood Press Monit* 2001;6:355–70.

51. Aronson S, Fontes ML. Hypertension: a new look at an old problem. *Curr Opin Anaesthesiol* 2006;19:59–64.

52. Fontes ML, Aronson S, Mathew JP, et al. Pulse pressure and risk of adverse outcome in coronary bypass surgery. *Anesth Analg* 2008;107:1103–6.

53. Aronson S, Boisvert D, Lapp W. Isolated systolic hypertension is associated with adverse outcomes from coronary artery bypass grafting surgery. *Anesth Analg.* 2002;94:1079–84.

54. Kheterpal S, O'Reilly M, Englesbe MJ, et al. Preoperative and intraoperative predictors of cardiac adverse events after general, vascular, and urological surgery. *Anesthesiology* 2009;110:58–66.

55. Singleton K, Brady G, Lai S, et al. The Australian Incident Monitoring Study. Problems associated with vascular access: an analysis of 2000 incident reports. *Anaesth Intensive Care* 1993;21:664–669.

56. Khalifa R, Dahyot-Fizelier C, Laksiri L, et al. Indwelling time and risk of colonization of peripheral arterial catheters in critically ill patients. *Intensive Care Med* 2008;34:1820–6.

57. Band JD, Maki DG. Infection caused by arterial catheters used for hemodynamic monitoring. *Am J Med* 1979;67:735–41.

58. Shinozaki T, Deane R, Mazuzan JE, et al. Bacterial contamination of arterial lines: A prospective study. *JAMA* 1983;249:223–5.

59. Weinstein RA, Stamm WE, Kramer L. Pressure monitoring devices: overlooked sources of nosocomial infection. *JAMA* 1976;236:936–8.

60. Stamm WE, Colella JJ, Anderson RL, et al. Indwelling arterial catheters as a source of nosocomial bacteremia. *N Engl J Med* 1975;292:1099–1102.

61. Koh DB, Gowardman JR, Rickard CW, et al. Prospective study of peripheral arterial catheter infection and comparison with concurrently sited central venous catheters. *Crit Care Med* 2008;36:397–402.

62. Traore O, Liotier J, Souweine B. Prospective study of arterial and central venous catheter colonization and of arterial- and central venous catheter-related bacteremia in intensive care units. *Crit Care Med* 2005;33:1276–80.

63. Rijnders BJ, Van Wijngaerden E, Wilmer A, Peetermans WE. Use of full sterile barrier precautions during insertion of arterial catheters: a randomized trial. *Clin Infect Dis* 2003;36:743–8.

64. Sherertz RJ. Update on vascular catheter infections. *Curr Opin Infect Dis* 2004;17:303–7.

65. O'Grady NP, Alexander M, Dellinger EP, et al. Guidelines for the prevention of intravascular catheter-related infections. The Hospital Infection Control Practices Advisory Committee, Center for Disease Control and Prevention. *Pediatrics* 2002;110:e51.

66. Scheer B, Perel A, Pfeiffer UJ. Clinical review: complications and risk factors of peripheral arterial catheters used for haemodynamic monitoring in anaesthesia and intensive care medicine. *Crit Care* 2002;6:199–204.

67. Bedford RF, Wollman H. Complications of percutaneous radial artery cannulation: An objective prospective study in man. *Anesthesiology* 1973;38:228–36.

68. Bedford RF. Radial arterial function following percutaneous cannulation with 18- and 20-gauge catheters. *Anesthesiology* 1977;47:37–39.

69. Bedford RF. Wrist circumference predicts the risk of radial arterial occlusion after cannulation. *Anesthesiology* 1978;48:377–8.

70. Wong AY, O'Regan AM. Gangrene of digits associated with radial artery cannulation. *Anaesthesia* 2003;58:1034–5.

71. Green JA, Tonkin MA. Ischaemia of the hand in infants following radial or ulnar artery catheterisation. *Hand Surg* 1999;4:151–7.

72. Bright E, Baines DB, French BG, et al. Upper limb amputation following radial artery cannulation. *Anaesth Intensive Care* 1993;21:351–3.

73. Kim JM, Arakawa K, Bliss J. Arterial cannulation: Factors in the development of occlusion. *Anesth Analg* 1975;54:836–41.

74. Chang C, Dughi J, Shitabata P, et al. Air embolism and the radial arterial line. *Crit Care Med* 1988;16:141–3.

75. Lowenstein E, Little JW, Lo HH. Prevention of cerebral embolization from flushing radial artery cannulae. *N Engl J Med* 1971;285:1414–5.

76. Zavela NG, Gravlee GP, Bewckart DH, et al. Unusual cause of hypotension after cardiopulmonary bypass. *J Cardiothorac Vasc Anesth* 1996;10:553–6.

77. Qvist J, Peterfreund R, Perlmutter G. Transient compartment syndrome of the forearm after attempted radial artery cannulation. *Anesth Analg* 1996;83:183–5.

78. Edwards DP, Clarke MD, Barker P. Acute presentation of bilateral radial artery pseudoaneurysms following arterial cannulation. *Eur J Vasc Endovasc Surg* 1999;17:456–7.

79. Knight CG, Healy DA, Thomas RL. Femoral artery pseudoaneurysms: risk factors, prevalence, and treatment options. *Ann Vasc Surg* 2003;17:503–8.

80. Rooke GA, Schwid HA, Shapira Y. The effect of graded hemorrhage and intravascular volume replacement on systolic pressure variation in humans during mechanical and spontaneous ventilation. *Anesth Analg* 1995;80: 925–32.

81. Gunn SR, Pinsky MR. Implications of arterial pressure variation in patients in the intensive care unit. *Curr Opin Crit Care* 2001;7:212–7.

82. Porter JM. Raynaud's syndrome. In Sabiston DC, ed. *Textbook of Surgery*. Philadelphia: W. B. Saunders, 1985, pp. 1925–32.

Central venous and pulmonary artery catheterization

Deborah Dubensky and Alexander J. C. Mittnacht

Introduction

Currently, percutaneous central venous cannulation is performed in more than five million patients in the United States annually.[1] Pulmonary artery catheter (PAC) use, after its clinical introduction in the early 1970s, has decreased significantly in the past decade and has been reported in 2 percent of all medical admissions in the United States.[2] The incidence of right heart (PAC) catheterization varies significantly between institutions and hospital settings; even national and international differences have been reported without any apparent difference in patient outcome. This chapter provides an overview of central venous cannulation and right heart catheterization with a critical review of current standards and recommendations.

Technical concept
Techniques and insertion sites

Central venous cannulation may be accomplished by catheter-through-needle, catheter-over-needle, or catheter-over-wire (Seldinger) techniques, the last being used most frequently outside the catheterization laboratory. The considerations for selecting the site of cannulation include the experience of the operator, ease of access, anatomic anomalies, and the ability of the patient to tolerate the position required for catheter insertion.

The most frequently used sites of insertion are the internal jugular vein, subclavian vein, femoral vein, external jugular vein, and large antecubital peripheral veins. Even though the internal jugular approach to central venous cannulation is the most popular, for reasons to be described, other sites may be preferable, considering individual patient characteristics or the particular indication for central venous cannulation.

Cannulation of the internal jugular vein (IJV) was first described by English and colleagues in 1969.[3] Advantages of this technique include (1) the high success rate as a result of the relatively predictable relationship of the anatomic structures; (2) a short, straight course to the right atrium (RA) that almost always ensures positioning of the catheter tip in the RA or superior vena cava (SVC); (3) easy access from the head of the oper-

ating room table; and (4) fewer complications than with subclavian vein catheterization.

The IJV is located under the medial border of the lateral head of the sternocleidomastoid (SCM) muscle. The carotid artery is typically located deeper and more medial to the IJV; however, the use of ultrasound-guided central cannulation has revealed a much less consistent relationship between the two vessels. The right IJV is preferred, because this vein takes the straightest course into the SVC, the right cupola of the lung may be lower than the left, and the thoracic duct is located on the left side.[4]

There are several approaches to right IJV cannulation described in the literature. The close relationship of the IJV to structures such as the carotid artery mandates a technique that poses the lowest risk to the patient. The use of a small-caliber "finder" needle may prevent puncture of the carotid artery with large-bore needles. The use of ultrasound-guided cannulation of large central veins has been advocated and has shown to increase success rate and decrease the incidence of certain complications (as discussed later). The needle should be placed at the apex of the triangle formed by the two heads of the SCM muscle at a 45-degree angle to the skin, and directed toward the ipsilateral nipple. If venous blood return is not obtained, the needle is withdrawn to the subcutaneous tissue and then passed in a more lateral or medial direction until the vein is located.

After the catheter is advanced into the vein, the needle is removed, and the proper intravenous position must be determined. To confirm that an artery has not been inadvertently cannulated, comparison of the color of the blood sample to an arterial sample drawn simultaneously has been described.[5] However, manometry is the preferred method of confirmation. Intravenous tubing attached to the catheter passively fills with blood when lowered below the heart and subsequently recedes to typical central venous pressure (CVP) levels with respiratory variation when held above the heart. Transduction of the pressure waveform is another technique that has been recommended.[6,7] In specific settings such as the cardiac operating room, the placement of a transesophageal echocardiography probe prior to IJV cannulation can help confirm intravenous positioning of the guidewire in the right atrium before a large-bore cannula is advanced.

Ultrasonic guidance of IJV cannulation

Ultrasound has been increasingly used to define the anatomic variations of the IJV.[8] Even though most commonly used for IJV cannulation, it can be useful in cannulating veins at other sites, as well as for arterial cannulation. Recently, a review and meta-analysis of randomized controlled trials looking at ultrasound-guided central venous cannulation found that real-time two-dimensional ultrasound for IJV cannulation in adults had a significantly higher success rate overall and on the first attempt, compared with the landmark method.[9] In 2005, Leyvi and associates[10] showed a higher success rate in IJV cannulation in children with the use of ultrasound compared with the traditional landmark technique, without any difference in complications. Even though most publications including prospective studies advocate the use of ultrasound for IJV cannulation in infants and children,[11–14] a few studies have shown no difference or even an increased risk of complications with ultrasound use compared with the landmark technique.[15,16] Overall, most studies have demonstrated that two-dimensional ultrasonic guidance of IJV cannulation is helpful in locating the vein, permits more rapid cannulation, and decreases the incidence of arterial puncture.[17–24] Circumstances under which ultrasonic guidance of IJV cannulation can be advantageous include patients with difficult neck anatomy (e.g. short neck, obesity), hypovolemia, prior neck surgery or radiation treatment; anticoagulated patients; and infants.[25]

Additionally, ultrasound has provided more precise data regarding the structural relationship between the IJV and the carotid artery. Troianos and coworkers found that in more than 54 percent of patients, more than 75 percent of the IJV overlies the carotid artery.[26] Patients who were over the age of 60 were more likely to have this type of anatomy. In pediatric patients, Alderson and associates found that the carotid artery coursed directly posterior to the IJV in 10 percent of patients.[27] Sulek and colleagues observed that there was greater overlap of the IJV and the carotid artery when the head is rotated 80 degrees toward the contralateral side compared with head rotation of only 0 to 40 degrees.[28] The percentage overlap was larger on the left side of the neck compared with the right. Therefore, excessive rotation of the head of the patient toward the contralateral side may distort the normal anatomy in a manner that increases the risk of inadvertent carotid artery puncture.

Doppler/ultrasound has also been used to demonstrate that the Valsalva maneuver increases IJV cross-sectional area by approximately 25 percent,[29] and that the Trendelenburg position increases it by approximately 37 percent.[30] Suarez and colleagues concluded that the lateral access approach to the internal jugular vein yielded the largest target area.[31] Parry recently published a study showing that maximal right IJV diameter can be achieved by placing the patient in 15 degrees Trendelenburg position, slightly elevating the head with a small pillow, keeping the head close to midline, and releasing the pressure administered to palpate the carotid artery prior to IJV cannulation.[32]

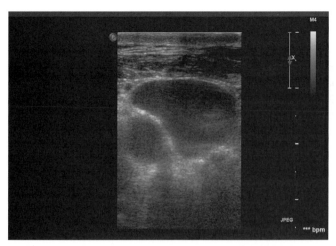

Figure 7.1. Typical relationship between right IJV and carotid artery in the transverse imaging approach. Note that part of the IJV is located above the carotid artery. Slight pressure with the transducer head compresses the IJV compared with the carotid artery. It is important to always demonstrate both IJV and carotid artery to clearly identify the IJV.

At the time of this writing, ultrasonic guidance is not yet the standard of care for IJV cannulation. However, many institutions have departmental policies in place that require ultrasound-guided IJV cannulation, particularly in anticoagulated patients and/or patients with difficult anatomy. The accumulating evidence cited here should be sufficient to justify the cost and effort related to acquiring the equipment and training anesthesiologists in its use. As with most emerging techniques, the practitioner must gain experience in a number of normal IJV cannulations to gain most benefit from the technology in the more complicated patient. Figure 7.1 shows the typical image obtained during two-dimensional ultrasound-guided IJV cannulation.

External jugular vein

Although the external jugular vein (EJV) is another means of reaching the central circulation, the success rate with this approach is lower because of the tortuous path followed by the vein. In addition, a valve is usually present at the point at which the EJV perforates the fascia to join the subclavian vein (SCV). One study, however, reported a success rate of 90 percent using a J-wire to manipulate past obstructions into the central circulation.[33] The main advantage of this technique is that there is no need to advance a needle into the deeper structures of the neck. Manipulation of the shoulder and rotation of the guidewire between the operator's fingers may be useful maneuvers when difficulty is encountered in passing the wire into the SVC.

Subclavian vein

The subclavian vein is readily accessible from supraclavicular or infraclavicular approaches and has long been used for central venous access.[34] The success rate is higher than the EJV approach, but lower than the right IJV approach. Cannulation of the subclavian vein is associated with a higher incidence of complications, especially the risk of a pneumothorax, compared with the IJV approach. Other complications associated with SCV cannulation are arterial punctures, misplacement of the catheter tip, aortic injury, cardiac tamponade, mediastinal hematoma, and hemothorax.[35–38] The SCV may be the cannulation site of choice, however, when CVP monitoring is indicated in patients who have contraindications to IJV cannulation. It is also useful for parenteral nutrition or for prolonged central venous access because the site is easier to maintain and is well tolerated by patients.

The infraclavicular approach is performed with the patient supine or in the Trendelenburg position with a folded sheet between the scapulae to increase the distance between the clavicle and the first rib. The head is turned to the contralateral side. A thin-walled needle or intravenous catheter is inserted 1 cm below the midpoint of the clavicle, the needle is "walked" along the anterior border of the clavicle, and, once the inferior aspect of the clavicle has been reached, the needle is directed toward the suprasternal notch under the posterior surface of the clavicle. When free-flowing venous blood is obtained, the guidewire is passed into the SCV and is exchanged for a CVP catheter. Kinking of the catheter because of the course underneath the clavicle occurs more frequently compared with RIJ cannulation.

The supraclavicular approach is performed with the patient in the Trendelenburg position with the head turned away from the side of the insertion. The finder needle is inserted at the lateral border of the SCM at the point of insertion into the clavicle. The needle is directed to bisect the angle between the SCM and the clavicle, about 15 to 20 degrees posteriorly. The vessel is very superficial (about 1 to 2 cm) and lies very close to the innominate artery and the pleura. There is an increased risk of an injury to the thoracic duct during the left-sided approach.

Antecubital veins

Another route for central venous monitoring is via the basilic or cephalic veins. The advantages of this approach are the low likelihood of complications and the ease of access intraoperatively if the arm is exposed. The major disadvantage is that it is often difficult to ensure placement of the catheter in a central vein. Studies have indicated that blind advancement will result in central venous cannulation in 59 percent to 75 percent of attempts.[39,40] Chest radiographs are usually necessary to confirm that the tip of the catheter has been placed appropriately; this involves some time delay. Alternatively, the guidewire can be attached to a specially designed ECG adapter; a change of the ECG waveform confirms proper positioning. Exact positioning of the catheter tip is crucial, as movement of the arm will result in significant catheter migration and could cause cardiac tamponade.[41–43] Unsuccessful attempts result most frequently from failure to pass the catheter past the shoulder, or retrograde cannulation of the ipsilateral IJV. Turning the head toward the ipsilateral side may help prevent IJV placement of the catheter.[44] These catheters are positioned at the SVC–RA

junction and are used for the aspiration of air emboli in neurosurgical patients. Because of problems inherent with intravascular electrocardiography, Mongan and colleagues described a method for transducing the pressure waveform and identifying the point at which the catheter tip entered the right ventricle.[45] They then calculated the distance required to withdraw the catheters to the SVC–RA junction (for three different types of air-embolism–aspirating catheters). Others have used transesophageal echocardiography (TEE) to assist in the correct placement of these types of catheters.[46] Even though peripherally placed central venous catheters avoid the placement of needles into deep venous structures, there are still significant risks associated with their use.[47–50]

Femoral vein

The femoral vein is less frequently cannulated in the adult patient for intraoperative monitoring purposes. However, cannulation of this vein is technically simple, and the success rate is high. Cannulation of the vessel should be done about 1 to 2 cm below the inguinal ligament. The vein typically lies medial to the artery. Although older literature reported a high rate of catheter sepsis and thrombophlebitis with this approach, this may no longer be valid with increasing awareness of using a full sterile technique, disposable catheter kits, and improved catheter technology.[51,52] Subcutaneous tunneling of femoral central venous catheters has been suggested to reduce the incidence of catheter-related infections.[53,54] In patients with SVC obstruction, or other contraindications to IJV or SCV cannulation, the femoral vein is necessary for intravenous access and to obtain a true CVP measurement. The catheter should be long enough so that the tip lies within the mediastinal portion of the inferior vena cava.

Pulmonary artery catheterization

The considerations for the insertion site of a PAC are the same as for CVP catheters. The right IJV approach remains the technique of choice because of the direct path between this vessel and the RA. In patients undergoing cardiac surgery, the placement of a large-bore introducer sheath and PAC via the SCV may be complicated by kinking of the catheter when the sternum is retracted.[55]

Passage of the PAC from the percutaneous insertion site to the PA can be accomplished by monitoring the pressure waveform from the distal port of the catheter, or under fluoroscopic guidance. Waveform monitoring is the more common technique for perioperative right heart catheterization. First, the catheter must be advanced through the vessel introducer (15–20 cm) before inflating the balloon. The inflation of the balloon facilitates further advancement of the catheter through the RA and right ventricle (RV) into the pulmonary artery. Normal intracardiac pressures are shown in Table 7.1. The pressure waveforms seen during advancement of the PAC are illustrated in Figure 7.2.

Table 7.1. Normal intracardiac pressures (mmHg)

Location	Mean	Range
Right atrium	5	1–10
Right ventricle	25/5	15–30/0–8
Pulmonary arterial systolic/diastolic	23/9	15–30/5–15
Mean pulmonary arterial	15	10–20
Pulmonary capillary wedge pressure	10	5–15
Left atrial pressure	8	4–12
Left ventricular end-diastolic pressure	8	4–12
Left ventricular systolic pressure	130	90–140

The RA waveform is seen until the catheter tip crosses the tricuspid valve and enters the RV. In patients with prior tricuspid valve ring annuloplasty, significant tricuspid regurgitation, or tricuspid stenosis, advancing the catheter past the tricuspid valve (TV) can become cumbersome and, in rare cases, even impossible. Trendelenburg positioning places the RV superior to the RA and, thus, may aid in advancing the PAC past the TV. TEE guidance can prove invaluable in these cases. The experienced echocardiographer can position the catheter tip just proximal to the TV orifice. Further attempts to get past the TV require much less catheter manipulation.

Once the catheter is advanced into the RV, there is a sudden increase in systolic pressure, but little change in diastolic pressure compared with the RA tracing. Arrhythmias, particularly premature ventricular complexes, usually occur at this point, but almost always resolve without treatment once the catheter tip has crossed the pulmonary valve. The catheter is rapidly advanced through the RV toward the PA. Slight reverse Trendelenburg and right lateral decubitus position brings the right ventricular outflow tract anteriorly and superior to the RV and, thus, aids in advancing the catheter into the PA.[56]

As the catheter crosses the pulmonary valve, a dicrotic notch appears in the pressure waveform, and there is a sudden increase in diastolic pressure. The pulmonary capillary wedge pressure (PCWP) – or, more accurately, pulmonary artery occlusion pressure (PAOP) – tracing is obtained by advancing the catheter approximately 3 to 5 cm farther until there is a change in the waveform associated with a drop in the measured

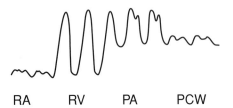

RA   RV   PA   PCW

Figure 7.2. The waveforms encountered during the flotation of a pulmonary artery catheter from the venous circulation to the pulmonary capillary wedge (PCW) position. Note the sudden increase in systolic pressure as the catheter enters the right ventricle (RV), the sudden increase in diastolic pressure as the catheter enters the pulmonary artery (PA), and the decrease in mean pressure as the catheter reaches the PCW position. RA = right atrium. With permission from Reich DL, Mittnacht A, London M, Kaplan JA. Monitoring of the heart and vascular system. In Kaplan JA, Reich DL, Lake CL, Konstadt SL, eds. *Kaplan's Cardiac Anesthesia*, 5th ed. Philadelphia: Saunders Elsevier; 2006, pp. 385–436 (figure 14-13).

mean pressure. Deflation of the balloon results in reappearance of the PA waveform and an increase in the mean pressure value. Benumof and coworkers found that most catheters pass into the right middle or lower lobes.[57]

Using the right IJV approach, the RA is entered at 25 to 35 cm, the RV at 35 to 45 cm, the PA at 45 to 55 cm, and the PCWP at 50 to 60 cm in the vast majority of patients. If the catheter does not enter the PA by 60 cm, the balloon should be deflated and it should be withdrawn into the RA, and another attempt should be made to advance the catheter into proper position. Excessive coiling of the catheter in the RV should be avoided to prevent catheter knotting. The balloon should be inflated for only short periods of time to measure the PCWP. The PA waveform should be monitored continually to be certain that the catheter does not float out into a constant wedge position, because this may lead to pulmonary artery rupture and/or pulmonary infarction.

The PAC is covered by a sterile sheath that must be secured at both ends to prevent contamination of the external portion of the catheter. Not infrequently, the PAC must be withdrawn a short distance as extra catheter in the RV floats out more peripherally into the PA over a period of time as the catheter softens, and during cardiac surgery when manipulation of the heart and cardiopulmonary bypass typically lead to spontaneous wedging of the catheter tip.

The time for the entire PAC insertion procedure is less than 10 minutes in experienced hands. Whether the PAC should be placed prior to anesthesia induction or after the patient has been anesthetized is a matter of personal and institutional preference. However, because the vast majority of outcome studies failed to show any benefit from PAC placement, insertion of a PAC in an awake patient should be considered carefully. Unless the position of the PAC can be confirmed with TEE, a chest radiograph should be obtained postoperatively in all patients to check the position of the PAC.

Parameters monitored
Central venous pressure

CVP catheters are used to measure the filling pressure of the RV, give an estimate of the intravascular volume status, and assess right ventricular function. For accurate pressure measurement, the distal end of the catheter must lie within one of the large intrathoracic veins or the RA. In any pressure monitoring system, it is necessary to have a reproducible landmark (such as the midaxillary line) as a zero reference. This is especially important in monitoring venous pressures, because small changes in the height of the zero reference point produce proportionately larger errors on the venous pressure scale compared with ... in arterial pressure monitoring.

The normal CVP waveform consists of three upward deflections (A, C, and V waves) and two downward deflections (X and Y descents) (see Figure 7.3).

The A wave is produced by right atrial contraction and occurs just after the P wave on the ECG. The C wave occurs as a

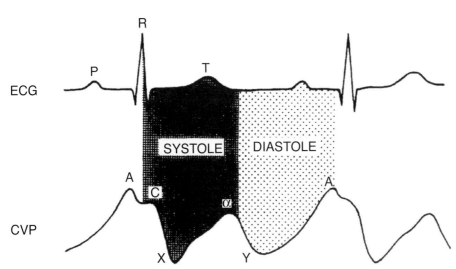

Figure 7.3. The relationship of the central venous pressure (CVP) tracing to the electrocardiogram (ECG) in normal sinus rhythm. The normal CVP waveform consists of three upward deflections (A, C, and V waves) and two downward deflections (X and Y descents). Adapted with permission from reference. 78, figure 2.

result of isovolumic ventricular contraction forcing the tricuspid valve to bulge upward into the right atrium. The pressure within the RA then decreases as the tricuspid valve is pulled away from the atrium during right ventricular ejection, forming the X descent. The RA continues to fill during late ventricular systole, forming the V wave. The Y descent occurs when the tricuspid valve opens and blood from the RA empties rapidly into the RV during early diastole. It is important to remember that many peaks and troughs in the CVP waveform are created artifactually from the transducer–tubing monitoring system. In tachycardic patients, the A and C waves can blend and may not be easily distinguishable.

The CVP waveform may be useful in the diagnosis of pathologic cardiac conditions. For example, onset of an irregular rhythm and loss of the A wave suggest atrial flutter or fibrillation. Cannon A waves occur as the RA contracts against a closed tricuspid valve as in junctional (atrioventricular [AV] nodal) rhythm, complete heart block, and ventricular arrhythmias (see Figure 7.4).

This is clinically relevant because nodal rhythms are frequently seen during anesthesia and may produce hypotension owing to a decrease in stroke volume. Cannon A waves may also be present when there is increased resistance to RA emptying, as in tricuspid stenosis, right ventricular hypertrophy, pulmonary stenosis, or pulmonary hypertension. Early systolic or holosystolic cannon V waves (or CV waves) occur if there is a significant degree of tricuspid regurgitation (see Figure 7.4). Large V waves may also appear later in systole if the ventricle becomes noncompliant as a result of ischemia or right ventricular failure.[58]

Pericardial constriction produces characteristic waveforms in the CVP tracing (see Figure 7.5). There is a decrease in venous return owing to the inability of the heart chambers to dilate because of the constriction. This causes prominent A and V waves and steep X and Y descents (creating an "M" configuration) resembling that seen with diseases that cause decreased right ventricular compliance. Egress of blood from the RA to

the RV is initially rapid during early diastolic filling of the RV (creating a steep Y descent), but is short-lived and abruptly halted by the restrictive, noncompliant RV. The RA pressure then increases rapidly and reaches a plateau until the end of the A wave, at the end of diastole. With pericardial tamponade, the X descent is steep but the Y descent is not present, because early diastolic runoff is impaired by the pericardial fluid collection.

PAC

The PCWP waveform is analogous to the CVP waveform described previously. The A, C, and V waves are similarly timed in the cardiac cycle. Large V waves have been described during mitral regurgitation, LV diastolic noncompliance, and episodes of myocardial ischemia.[59] They are seen on the PCWP tracing as large (or "giant") V waves that occur slightly later than the upstroke on the PA tracing.[60] They can also be identified on the PA waveform tracing, causing the PA waveform to become wider, and the dicrotic notch may be lost. The occurrence of V waves in patients with severe mitral regurgitation has been studied in detail by Grose and colleagues.[61] They found that in some patients severe mitral regurgitation causes reversal of semilunar valve closure. Early pulmonic valve closure with the dicrotic notch in the pulmonary artery V wave preceding the aortic dictrotic notch could be demonstrated in patients with low pulmonary vascular resistance (also see Figures 7.6 and 7.7). The etiology of large V waves during myocardial ischemia is probably caused by a decrease in diastolic ventricular compliance. Alternatively, they may be caused by mitral regurgitation induced by ischemic papillary muscle dysfunction. In this instance, the V waves may occur earlier during the onset of the C wave (CV wave). Large V waves, however, have not been shown to correlate well with other determinants of myocardial ischemia.[62,63]

Specific information that can be gathered from the PAC and the quantitative measurements of cardiovascular and pulmonary function that can be derived from this information are listed in Tables 7.2 and 7.3.

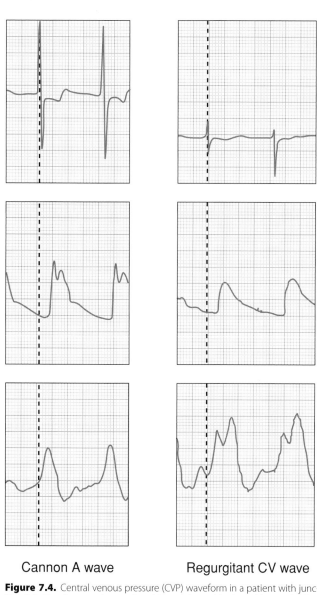

Cannon A wave   Regurgitant CV wave

Figure 7.4. Central venous pressure (CVP) waveform in a patient with junctional rhythm (cannon A waves) and in a patient with tricuspid regurgitation (CV wave). The electrocardiogram (top), arterial blood pressure (middle), and CVP (bottom) traces are shown. Adapted with permission from Pittman JAL, Ping JS, Mark JB. Arterial and central venous pressure monitoring. *Int Anesthesiol Clin* 2004;42:13–30, figure 9.

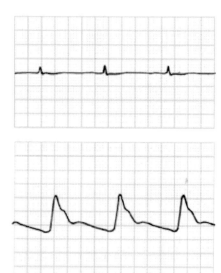

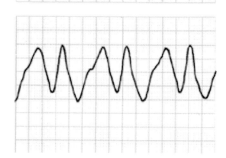

Figure 7.5. Pericardial constriction produces a central venous pressure trace (bottom) that displays tall A and V waves and steep systolic X and diastolic Y descents. The electrocardiogram (top) and arterial blood pressure (middle) traces are also shown. Adapted with permission from Pittman JAL, Ping JS, Mark JB. Arterial and central venous pressure monitoring. *Int Anesthesiol Clin* 2004;42:13–30, figure 10.

One of the main reasons that clinicians measure PCWP and pulmonary artery diastolic pressure (PAD) is that these parameters are estimates of left atrial pressure (LAP), which, in turn, is an estimate of left ventricular end-diastolic pressure (LVEDP). Left ventricular end-diastolic pressure is an index of left ventricular end-diastolic volume (LVEDV), which correlates well with left ventricular preload.[64] The relationship between LVEDP and LVEDV is described by the left ventricular compliance curve. This nonlinear curve is affected by many factors, such as ventricular hypertrophy and myocardial ischemia.[65,66] Thus, the PCWP and PAD do not directly measure left ventricular preload. The relationship of these parameters is diagrammed in Figure 7.8.

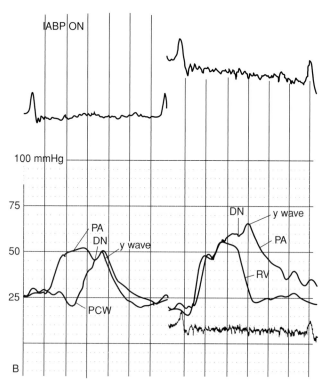

Figure 7.6. V waves can be seen on the PCWP tracing (left) and pulmonary artery pressure tracing in patients with severe mitral regurgitation. PA = pulmonary artery, PCW = pulmonary capillary wedge, RV = right ventricular, DN = dicrotic notch. With permission from reference 61, figure 1B.

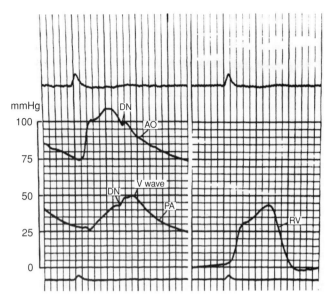

Figure 7.7. Micromanometer pressure tracings from a patient with severe mitral regurgitation. In the main pulmonary artery, a V wave of 50 mmHg is present, which exceeds peak right ventricular or pulmonary artery systolic pressure by 7 mmHg. The incisura of the pulmonary artery dictrotic notch precedes aortic dictrotic notch by 15 msec. With permission from Reference 61, Figure 2.

Table 7.2. Hemodynamic parameters

Formula	Normal Values
Cardiac index CI = CO/BSA	2.8–4.2 l/min/m2
Stroke volume SV = CO *1000/HR	50–110 mL (per beat)
Stroke index SI = SV/BSA	30–65 mL/m2
Left ventricular stroke work index LVSWI = 1.36 * (MAP – PCWP) * SI/100	45–60 gram-meters/m2
Right ventricular stroke work index RVSWI = 1.36 * (MPAP – CVP) * SI/100	5–10 gram-meters/m2
Systemic vascular resistance SVR = (MAP – CVP) * 80/CO	900–1400 dynes-sec/cm5
Systemic vascular resistance index SVRI = (MAP – CVP) * 80/CI	1500–2400 dynes-sec*m2/cm5
Pulmonary vascular resistance PVR = (MPAP – PCWP) * 80/CO	150–250 dynes-sec/cm5
Pulmonary vascular resistance index PVRI = (MPAP – PCWP) * 80/CI	250–400 dynes-sec*m2/cm5

CI = cardiac index; CO = cardiac output; BSA = body surface area; SV = stroke volume; HR = heart rate; MAP = mean arterial pressure; PCWP = pulmonary capillary wedge pressure; PAP = pulmonary arterial pressure; CVP = central venous pressure; SVR = systemic vascular resistance; PVR = pulmonary vascular resistance; SI = stroke index; LVSWI = left ventricular stroke work index; RVSWI = right ventricular stroke work index; SVRI = systemic vascular resistance index; PVRI = pulmonary vascular resistance index. With permission from Reich DL, Mittnacht A, London M, Kaplan JA. Monitoring of the heart and vascular system. In Kaplan JA, Reich DL, Lake CL, Konstadt SL (eds.) *Kaplan's Cardiac Anesthesia* 5th ed. Philadelphia: Saunders Elsevier, 2006, pp. 385–436 (table 14-2).

Table 7.3. Oxygenation parameters

Formula	Normal Values
Arterial O2 content $CaO2 = (1.39 * Hb * SaO2) + (0.0031 * PaO2)$	18–20 mL/dL
Mixed venous O2 content $CvO2 = 1.39 * Hb * SvO2 + 0.0031 * PvO2$	13–16 mL/dL
Arteriovenous O2 content difference $avDO2 = CaO2 – CvO2$	4–5.5 mL/dL
Pulmonary capillary O2 content $CcO2 = 1.39 * Hb * ScO2 + 0.0031 * PcO2$	19–21 mL/dL
Pulmonary shunt fraction $Qs/Qt = 100 * (CcO2 – CaO2)/(CcO2 – CvO2)$	2–8 percent
O2 delivery $DO2 = 10 * CO * CaO2$	800–1100 mL/min
O2 consumption $VO2 = 10 * CO * (CaO2 – CvO2)$	150–300 mL/min

Hb = Hemoglobin; SvO_2 = venous oxygen saturation; PvO_2 venous oxygen tension; ScO_2 = pulmonary capillary oxygen saturation; PcO_2 = pulmonary capillary oxygen tension.
From McGrath R. Invasive bedside hemodynamic monitoring. *Prog Cardiovasc Dis* 1986;29:129. With permission from Reich DL, Mittnacht A, London M, Kaplan JA. Monitoring of the heart and vascular system. In Kaplan JA, Reich DL, Lake CL, Konstadt SL (eds.) *Kaplan's Cardiac Anesthesia* 5th ed. Philadelphia: Saunders Elsevier, 2006, pp. 385–436 (table 14-3).

The PCWP and PAD pressures will not accurately reflect LVEDP in the presence of incorrect positioning of the PAC catheter tip, pulmonary vascular disease, high levels of positive end expiratory pressure (PEEP), or mitral valvular disease. The patency of vascular channels between the distal port of the PAC and the left atrium (LA) is necessary to ensure a close relationship between the PCWP and LAP. This condition is met only in the dependent portions of the lung (West zone III), in which pulmonary venous pressure exceeds alveolar pressure; otherwise, PCWP reflects alveolar pressure, not the LAP. Because PEEP decreases the size of West zone III, it has been shown to adversely affect the correlation between the PCWP and LAP, especially in the hypovolemic patient.[67–71] Interestingly, acute respiratory distress syndrome (ARDS) seems to prevent the transmission of increased alveolar pressure to the pulmonary interstitium. This preserves the relationship between

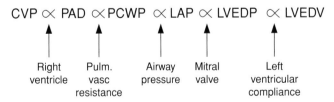

Figure 7.8. The relationship between the various intracardiac pressure measurements and left ventricular preload. The left ventricular end-diastolic volume (LVEDV) is related to left ventricular end-diastolic pressure (LVEDP) by the left ventricular compliance. The LVEDP is related to the left atrial pressure (LAP) by the diastolic pressure gradient across the mitral valve. The pulmonary capillary wedge pressure (PCWP) is related to the LAP by the pulmonary capillary resistance. The pulmonary artery diastolic pressure (PAD) is an estimate of the PCWP. The central venous pressure (CVP) reflects the PAD if right ventricular function is normal. With permission from Reich DL, Mittnacht A, London M, Kaplan JA. Monitoring of the heart and vascular system. In Kaplan JA, Reich DL, Lake CL, Konstadt SL,eds. *Kaplan's Cardiac Anesthesia*, 5th ed. Philadelphia: Saunders Elsevier, 2006, pp. 385–436 (figure 14–11).

Table 7.4. Abnormal central venous and pulmonary artery pressure waveforms

Cannon A wave (central venous waveform)
Right atrium contracts against closed tricuspid valve

- Junctional rhythm
- Complete heart block
- Ventricular arrhythmias
- Ventricular pacing
- Tricuspid stenosis

Increased resistance to right atrial emptying

- Tricuspid stenosis
- Right ventricular hypertrophy
- Pulmonary stenosis
- Pulmonary hypertension

V wave (central venous waveform)

- Tricuspid regurgitation (early systolic or holosystolic)
- Noncompliant right ventricle (late systole)

V wave (pulmonary capillary wedge tracing)

- Mitral regurgitation
- Acute myocardial ischemia
- Noncompliant left ventricle

Table 7.5. Conditions resulting in discrepancies between pulmonary capillary wedge pressure and left ventricular end-diastolic pressure

PCWP > LVEDP

- Positive-pressure ventilation
- PEEP
- Increased intrathoracic pressure
- Non-West lung zone III PAC placement
- Chronic obstructive pulmonary disease
- Increased pulmonary vascular resistance
- Left atrial myxoma
- Mitral valve disease (stenosis, regurgitation)

PCWP LVEDP

- Noncompliant LV (ischemia, hypertrophied LV)
- Aortic regurgitation (premature closure of the mitral valve)
- LVEDP > 25 mmHg

LVEDP = left ventricular end–diastolic pressure; PCWP = pulmonary capillary wedge pressure; PEEP = positive end–expiratory pressure; PAC = pulmonary artery catheter; LV = left ventricle.
Modified from Tuman KJ, Carrol CC, Ivankovich AD. Pitfalls in interpretation of pulmonary artery catheter data. *Cardiothorac Vasc Anesth Update* 1991;2: 1–24.
With permission from: Reich DL, Mittnacht A, London M, Kaplan JA. Monitoring of the heart and vascular system. In Kaplan JA, Reich DL, Lake CL, Konstadt SL, eds. *Kaplan's Cardiac Anesthesia*, 5th ed. Philadelphia: Saunders Elsevier, 2006, pp. 385–436 (box 14–6).

the PCWP and LAP during the application of PEEP.[72] In any case, it is not considered prudent to temporarily disconnect patients from PEEP to measure preload.[73] The presence of large V waves in the PCWP tracing of patients with mitral regurgitation leads to an overestimation of the LVEDP.[74] Table 7.4 lists typical conditions under which cannon A and V waves during central venous and pulmonary artery pressure monitoring are seen.

In patients with mitral stenosis, using the PCWP does not provide an accurate estimate of left ventricular filling pressures and may overestimate true preload conditions. Additionally, it has been demonstrated that there is a significant positive gradient between the PCWP and the LAP in the initial hour following CPB.[75] Table 7.5 is a summary of conditions that may alter the relationship between the PCWP and the LVEDP.

Evidence of utility
CVP monitoring

The CVP is a useful monitor if the factors affecting it are recognized and its limitations are understood. The CVP is influenced by the patient's blood volume, venous tone, and right ventricular performance. However, the complexity of the venous system and right ventricular preload cannot be easily measured or described by measuring right-sided pressures. A true correlation between CVP and left-sided preload is even more difficult to obtain. Mangano showed a good correlation between the CVP and left-sided filling pressures during a change in volume status in patients with coronary artery disease (CAD) and left ventricular ejection fraction (LVEF) greater than 0.4.[76] Other studies, however, have not replicated these results, demonstrating weak relationships between the CVP and measures of left ventricular preload.[77–80] In general, for clinical purposes, following serial measurements (trends) is more useful than

looking at individual numbers. Gelman recently published an extensive review of the venous function and central venous pressure.[81]

PAC monitoring

After its introduction in the 1970s, the PAC instantly increased the amount of diagnostic information that could be obtained at the bedside in critically ill patients.[82] Information about hemodynamic parameters previously obtainable only in the cardiac catheterization laboratory became readily available to physicians taking care of critically ill patients in various settings. It became obvious that the PAC-derived data provided a more accurate assessment of hemodynamic status and oxygenation when compared with clinical evaluation alone. For example, Connors and coworkers prospectively analyzed 62 consecutive pulmonary artery catheterizations.[83] They found that less than half of a group of clinicians correctly predicted the PCWP or cardiac output (CO), and more than 50 percent made at least one change in therapy based on data from the PAC. Waller and associates demonstrated that a group of experienced cardiac anesthesiologists and surgeons who were blinded to the information from the PAC during coronary artery bypass graft (CABG) surgery were unaware of any problem during 65 percent of severe hemodynamic abnormalities.[84] Similarly, Iberti and Fisher showed that ICU physicians were unable to accurately predict hemodynamic data on clinical grounds. Sixty percent made at least one change in therapy and 33 percent changed their diagnosis based on PAC data.[85] As many as 47 percent of physicians could not correctly determine the PCWP to within 5 mmHg in that study.[86]

However, in the late 1990s, the ability of PACs to positively influence patient outcome came under question. In 1996, Connors and associates[87] published the results of a large prospective cohort study. Data were collected from five US teaching hospitals between 1989 and 1994. The researchers enrolled 5735 critically ill adult patients in intensive care settings and surprisingly found that right heart catheterization was associated with an increased mortality in this patient population. The results of this study were instantly criticized and ignited a large number of well-designed studies in the hope of rejecting Connors' findings. However, the more studies emerged, the more convincing was the evidence that PACs have little impact on patients' outcome and may actually cause harm.[88–93] Various hypotheses are being investigated to explain these findings.

Placing a PAC is a highly invasive procedure. Vascular structures are accessed with large-bore introducer sheaths with all possible complications listed below. But most important, even in the best of circumstances, with uncomplicated PAC placement and correct data collection and interpretation, a PAC is a monitoring tool only. As such, we cannot expect a change in patient outcome unless the treatment that is initiated based on our PAC measurements is proven to change patient outcome. In some of the most critically ill patients, such as those with sepsis, ARDS, massive trauma, and so forth, mortality remains high in spite of efforts to find new treatment strategies. Furthermore, diagnoses often can be made on clinical grounds only, and treatment strategies once thought to improve patient outcomes may actually be harmful.

The following paragraphs list some of the landmark studies available today regarding PAC use and patient outcomes in various clinical settings. However, major problems with these studies include flaws in study design, and many lack sufficient statistical power. The most common design flaws were a lack of therapeutic protocols or treatment algorithms based on PAC data and inadequate randomization, which introduces observer bias.

Patients undergoing cardiac surgery

Nearly all studies looking at patient outcome in cardiac surgery are flawed by lack of adequate randomization and control groups. Furthermore, many retrospective analyses investigate patient populations that underwent cardiac surgery in times when other monitoring tools such as TEE were not as widely used. In spite of this, to date, there are no convincing data showing improved outcome in patients undergoing cardiac surgery with PAC placement compared with central venous pressure monitoring only, and few studies actually suggest that PAC use in patients undergoing low-risk cardiac surgery may even cause harm.[94]

Schwann and colleagues[95] retrospectively assessed the outcome of 2685 patients undergoing coronary artery bypass grafting in whom the decision to place a PAC was based on patient characteristics and risk factors. Using a highly selective strategy, no PAC was used in the majority of cases (91%), and the

outcomes were comparable. In another retrospective trial, Ramsey and associates[96] found that pulmonary artery catheterization in elective coronary artery bypass graft surgery was associated with increased in-hospital mortality, longer lengths of stay, and higher total costs. This effect was more pronounced in hospital settings with low overall PAC use. Resano and colleagues looked at PAC use in patients undergoing off-pump coronary artery bypass graft surgery compared with central venous pressure monitoring only and found no difference in outcome.[97]

In a prospective observational study, Djaiani and coworkers[98] looked at 200 consecutive patients undergoing coronary artery bypass surgery when PACs were placed, but the numerical data other than CVP were blinded to the surgeon and anesthesiologist. Patients were managed according to routine, and data could be unblinded if required clinically. Twenty-three percent of patients required unbinding of data; of this 23 percent, preliminary diagnosis was confirmed in 14 percent, and treatment was modified in 9 percent. The patients in the unblinded group went on to experience further morbidity. The researchers thus concluded that placement of a PAC can be safely delayed until the clinical need arises either intraoperatively or in the ICU.

Although patients undergoing low-risk cardiac surgery can probably be managed without PAC placement, many clinicians still consider high-risk cardiac surgery and, in particular, patients with right heart failure or pulmonary hypertension as indications for PAC placement. In a prospective, randomized trial, Pölönen and colleagues applied goal-directed PAC-guided therapy aimed to maintain a mixed venous saturation = 70 percent and blood lactate < 2 mmol/L in patients following cardiac surgery. Using this strategy, they found that increasing oxygen delivery in the immediate postoperative period shortened hospital stay and decreased morbidity.[99]

Patients undergoing major noncardiac surgery

Major noncardiac surgery is composed of a very diverse group of surgeries, including cases in which hemodynamic instability is often anticipated. Examples are trauma, major vascular, abdominal, and thoracic surgeries, including liver resections and transplantations. The differential diagnosis of sudden perioperative hemodynamic decompensation is complicated by numerous comorbidities that are often present in these patient populations. Nevertheless, there are no conclusive data that any patient population undergoing major noncardiac surgery may benefit from PAC monitoring. Some studies even suggest adverse outcomes related to PAC use.

In 2001, Polanczyk and coworkers[100] published the results of an observational study on 4059 patients undergoing major elective noncardiac procedures, looking at the relationship between pulmonary artery catheterization and postoperative cardiac complications. The use of a PAC was associated with an increased incidence of major postoperative cardiac events. Sandham and associates[101] reported a prospective, randomized, controlled outcome study of 1994 high-risk patients (ASA III or IV) scheduled for major noncardiac surgery followed by ICU stay, who were managed with or without the use of a PAC. No benefit in goal-directed therapy with the use of PAC data as compared with standard care (without the use of PAC) was found. Furthermore, they found a higher risk of pulmonary embolism in the PAC group.

Critically ill patients in ICU settings

The trend toward decreasing the use of the PACs continues and includes patients admitted to an ICU setting. The most significant decrease in PAC use has been documented in patients with acute myocardial infarction, whereas patients diagnosed with septicemia show the least decline in PAC use.[102]

Admissions to an ICU typically represent a diverse group of critically ill, multimorbid, and/or high-risk patients prone to adverse events. Nevertheless, to date, there are no data from any large, well-designed, prospective studies showing that PAC placement improves outcome in any of the major clinical ICU diagnoses. Yu and associates[103] performed a prospective cohort study of the relationship between PAC use and outcome in 1010 patients with severe sepsis. PAC monitoring did not improve outcome in this patient population. Sakr and colleagues looked at outcome related to PAC use in 3147 adult patients admitted to an ICU, a subanalysis of a large multicenter prospective observational study designed to evaluate the epidemiology of sepsis in European countries.[104] After propensity score matching, there was no significant difference in outcome with or without PAC placement. Interestingly, significant differences in PAC use were reported between the various participating countries. A prospective randomized study by Rhodes and coworkers[105] found no significant difference in mortality in critically ill patients treated with or without the use of a PAC. Adjusting for the severity of illness, Murdoch and colleagues[106] found that the use of the PAC in patients in the ICU is safe, but no benefit was demonstrated.

Chittock and associates[107] demonstrated that severity of illness may play an important role in defining subgroups of patients who may benefit from PAC monitoring. Of 7310 critically ill adult patients admitted to the ICU, those with APACHE II scores >31 showed decreased mortality with PAC monitoring, whereas patients with lower APACHE II scores had increased mortality. The PAC-Man study, a randomized controlled trial, enrolled 1041 patients from 65 ICUs throughout the United Kingdom. Patients were randomly assigned to management with or without PAC placement. Treatment in both arms of the study was at the discretion of the treating clinician. Neither benefit nor harm related to PAC use was found. This study has been criticized for lack of a standardized treatment protocol based on PAC data, which is a major design flaw in many otherwise well-randomized prospective studies.

The ESCAPE trial (Evaluation Study of Congestive Heart Failure and **P**AC **E**ffectiveness) looked at patients with symptoms of severe heart failure. This multicenter, randomized,

controlled trial enrolled 433 patients at 26 sites. Again, there was no specific treatment protocol to follow. However, the use of inotropes was discouraged, and investigators were asked to follow national guidelines for treatment of heart failure, which promote the use of diuretics and vasodilators. The target in both groups was improvement of clinical symptoms of heart failure. In the PAC group there was an additional target of a pulmonary capillary occlusion pressure of 15 mmHg and a right atrial pressure of 8 mmHg. Overall mortality did not differ between the two groups; however, more adverse events were recorded in the PAC group. Exercise and quality-of-life measures improved in both groups, and the investigators reported a trend toward greater improvement with PAC use.

These findings have been reproduced similarly in patients with ARDS. Two randomized controlled studies could not show improved patient outcome with PAC use.[108,109] Randomized trials including patients with acute myocardial infarction seemed to also confirm these data.[110,111] Cohen and colleagues[112] retrospectively studied 26,437 patients with acute coronary syndromes. A PAC catheter was inserted in 2.8 percent of patients. Patients in the United States were 3.8 times more likely to have a PAC placed than were non-US patients. After adjustment for confounding factors, PAC use was associated with a 2.6-fold increase in hospital mortality. The subset of patients who developed cardiogenic shock had similar outcomes both with and without PAC use. Haupt and coworkers suggested that patients in the ICU might have disease too far advanced to make invasive hemodynamic monitoring useful.[113] Some of the earlier studies that had reported improved outcome used invasive hemodynamic monitoring to optimize oxygen delivery in the perioperative period.[114-117] In a meta-analysis, Heyland and associates argued similarly that "maximizing oxygen delivery" in the perioperative setting (i.e. prior to the onset of irreversible organ damage) is more effective in comparison with doing so in the chronic ICU setting.[118]

The previous discussion illustrated examples of the broad spectrum of critically ill patient populations, and the clinical settings in which PACs have been frequently deployed. The findings regarding patient outcome discussed previously and available in the literature have led to a dramatic decrease in PAC use in many clinical settings. In the 1990s, as TEE began to gain popularity and concern grew as to the risks of PA catheters, there was a significant drop in the use of PACs. A time trend analysis looked at PAC use over 10 years, from 1993 to 2004, and showed a 63 percent decrease in use, which was evident in both cardiac and noncardiac surgical admissions.[119] Wiener and colleagues point out that the decline began in 1994, likely owing to the fact that preliminary data from the Connors group were presented at the American Thoracic Society conference and that early adopters may have stopped placing PACs. However, the largest step-off in use occurred in 1996, likely correlating with the actual publication of the Connors study. Ranucci looked at the PAC and its relationship with TEE.[120] He purported that the information sets gained from each technology are not interchangeable but rather complementary to one another. This may explain why, although TEE is becoming more readily available, PAC has not fallen completely out of favor.

Most practitioners taking care of critically ill patients still value PAC as an important monitoring tool. There are some data showing that small subgroups of patients may benefit from PAC use, and there is enough evidence to prove that if deployed carefully, there is minimal risk with PAC use. It is the opinion of the authors of this text that the PAC still has a role in modern evidence-driven medicine. The risks associated with perioperative PAC monitoring may outweigh the benefits in low-to-moderate–risk patients, whereas high-risk patients undergoing major surgery probably benefit from right heart catheterization. Specific situations in which PAC use may be useful are discussed later in this chapter.

Complications

CVP

The complications of central venous cannulation can be divided roughly into three categories: complications of vascular access, complications of catheter insertion, or complications of catheter presence. These are summarized in Table 7.6.

Specific information regarding several of the complications is detailed below. Inadvertent arterial puncture during central venous cannulation is not uncommon.[121] The two main reasons that this phenomenon occurs are that all veins commonly used for cannulation lie in close proximity to arteries (except the EJV and cephalic vein), and that the venous anatomy is quite variable. Localized hematoma formation is the usual consequence. This may be minimized if a small-gauge needle is initially used to localize the vein[122] or ultrasonic guidance is employed (see previous discussion).

If arterial puncture occurs with a large-gauge needle or catheter, direct pressure may be difficult to apply owing to the location of the artery. If the patient has a coagulopathy, a massive hematoma may form. In the neck, this may lead to airway obstruction, requiring urgent tracheal intubation. In the arm or leg, venous obstruction may occur. If the artery is cannulated with a large-bore catheter, a surgical consultation may be required before its removal. Reports about successful

---

Table 7.6. Complications of central venous cannulation

- Arterial puncture with hematoma
- Arteriovenous fistula
- Hemothorax
- Chylothorax
- Pneumothorax
- Nerve injuries (e.g. brachial plexus)
- Stellate ganglion injury (Horner syndrome)
- Air embolization
- Catheter or wire shearing
- Right atrial or right ventricular perforation
- Thrombosis, thromboembolism
- Infection, sepsis, endocarditis
- Arrhythmias
- Hydrothorax

---

percutaneous repair of inadvertent arterial injuries following central venous cannulation have been published.[123,124]

Arteriovenous fistula from the carotid artery to the IJV has also been reported following central venous cannulation.[125,126] Hemothorax may occur if the subclavian artery is lacerated during cannulation attempts. Symptoms of hypovolemia may predominate because of the large capacity of the pleural cavity.[127]

Injury to the thoracic duct resulting in chylothorax has been reported following left IJV and left subclavian vein cannulation.[128,129] This is a serious complication that may require surgical treatment.[130] Fear of this complication is one of the main reasons for selecting right-sided IJV and subclavian approaches for central venous cannulation.

If the pleural cavity is entered and lung tissue is punctured during an attempt at cannulation, a pneumothorax may result. Tension pneumothorax is possible if air continues to accumulate in the pleural space as a result of a "ball-valve" effect. Pneumothorax is most common with subclavian punctures and occurs only rarely with IJV cannulation.[131,132]

The brachial plexus, stellate ganglion, and phrenic nerve all lie in close proximity to the IJV. These structures may be injured during cannulation attempts. Paresthesias of the brachial plexus are not uncommon during attempts to localize the IJV. Direct needle trauma is the most likely cause of paresthesias or motor deficits; this risk is somewhat increased by the long-beveled needles used for vascular access.[133,134] Transient deficits may result from the deposition of local anesthetic in the brachial plexus, stellate ganglion, or cervical plexus. A large hematoma or pseudoaneurysm could result in nerve injury after an inadvertent arterial puncture.[135,136] Horner's syndrome has also been reported following IJV cannulation.[137]

Venous air embolism is a potentially fatal complication that can occur in situations in which there is negative pressure in the venous system. There is a risk of paradoxical embolization in patients with a patent foramen ovale or other intracardiac defects, such as an atrial or ventricular septal defect. During central venous cannulation, air embolism can usually be prevented with positional maneuvers, such as the Trendelenburg position, which increases the venous pressure in the vessel. After the CVP catheter has been placed, it is important to ensure that the catheter is firmly attached to its connecting tubing. Air embolism may occur even after the catheter has been removed if the subcutaneous tract persists.[138]

The diagnosis of venous air embolism is likely when there is a sudden onset of tachycardia associated with pulmonary hypertension and systemic hypotension. A new murmur may be heard owing to turbulent flow in the RV outflow tract. Two-dimensional echocardiography (transesophageal or transthoracic) and precordial Doppler probe monitoring are highly sensitive methods of detecting air embolism. Venous air embolism is most effectively treated by aspirating the air via a catheter positioned at the SVC–RA junction.

Catheter or guidewire fragments may be sheared off by the inserting needle and may embolize to the right heart and pulmonary circulation when either catheter-through-needle or

Seldinger-type cannulation kits are used. It is also possible to lose a guidewire within the patient by not withdrawing a sufficient length of the wire to grasp it at the external end prior to inserting the catheter.[139] The catheter fragment position within the right-sided circulation will determine whether surgery or percutaneous transvenous techniques are necessary for its removal.[140]

These complications can almost always be avoided by using proper technique. A catheter must never be withdrawn through the inserting needle. Reinsertion of needles into standard (catheter-over-needle) intravenous cannulae is not recommended but should certainly never be performed if the cannula is kinked or resistance is encountered. Similarly, guidewires should not be inserted through cannulae if blood return is not present, or forcefully inserted if resistance is encountered. Additionally, guidewires should not be withdrawn through inserting needles. During unsuccessful catheterization, the needle and catheter, or needle and guidewire, must be withdrawn simultaneously.

If the RA or RV is perforated during central venous cannulation, pericardial effusion or tamponade may result and the patient may require surgical treatment.[141] The likelihood of this complication is increased with the use of inflexible guidewires, long dilators, or long catheters. This complication has also been reported with the use of an indwelling polyethylene catheter.[142] Oropello and colleagues suggested that the dilators used in many of the central catheters kits may be a major cause of vessel perforation.[143] They believe that the dilator may bend the guidewire, creating its own path, thus causing it to perforate a vessel wall. In addition, it was noted that a number of kits have dilators that are much longer than the catheters and present a further risk factor for possible perforation of the heart or vessels. Kinking of the guidewire in large-bore introducer kits can be prevented by guidance of the introducer or catheter distally close to the patient's skin.

If the catheter tip is placed extravascularly in the pleural cavity or erodes into this position, the fluid that is infused into the catheter will accumulate in the pleural cavity, causing hemo- or hydrothorax. A pleurocentesis or thoracostomy (chest) tube might be necessary and surgical consultation may be required.

Transient atrial and/or ventricular arrhythmias commonly occur as the guidewire is passed into the RA or RV during central venous cannulation using the Seldinger technique. This most likely results from the relatively inflexible guidewire causing extrasystoles as it contacts the endocardium. Ventricular fibrillation during guidewire insertion has been reported.[144]

There are also reports of complete heart block from guidewire insertion during central venous cannulation.[145] These cases can be managed successfully using a temporary transvenous or external pacemaker. The problem most likely results from excessive insertion of the guidewire, with irritation of the right bundle branch. It is recommended that, to prevent these complications, the length of guidewire insertion be limited to the length necessary to reach the SVC–RA junction. It is also imperative to monitor the patient appropriately (i.e.

ECG and/or pulse monitoring) and to have resuscitative drugs and equipment immediately available when performing central venous catheterization.

Strict aseptic technique is required to minimize catheter-related bloodstream infections. Full-barrier precautions during insertion of central venous catheters have been shown to decrease the incidence of catheter-related infections.[146,147] Subcutaneous tunneling of catheters inserted into the internal jugular and femoral veins,[148,149] antiseptic-barrier–protected catheter hubs,[150] and antiseptic/antibiotic-impregnated short-term catheters[151,152] have also been shown to reduce catheter-related infections.[153] There is accumulating evidence that 2% chlorhexidine preparation for skin antisepsis is associated with a reduced risk of catheter-related infections.[154–156] Hospital policies differ with respect to the permissible duration of catheterization at particular sites, but routine replacement of central venous catheters to prevent catheter-related infections is not recommended.[157,158]

PAC

The complications associated with PAC placement inherently include almost all those detailed in the section on CVP placement (see previous section). Additional complications that are unique to the PAC are detailed here (also see Table 7.7)

The ASA Task Force on Pulmonary Artery Catheterization concluded that serious complications resulting from PAC catheterization occur in 0.1 percent to 0.5 percent of patients monitored with a PAC.[199] Higher estimates are found in the literature and probably represent different patient populations, hospital settings, level of experience with PAC management, and other factors.[159]

The most common complications associated with PAC insertion are transient arrhythmias, especially premature ventricular contractions (PVCs).[160] However, fatal arrhythmias have rarely been reported.[161,162] Positioning the patient in slight reverse Trendelenburg position and right lateral tilt can help prevent arrhythmias during PAC insertion (compared with the Trendelenburg position).

Complete heart block may develop during PA catheterization in patients with preexisting left bundle-branch block (LBBB).[163–165] This potentially fatal complication is most likely the result of electrical irritability from the PAC tip, causing a transient right bundle-branch block (RBBB) as it passes through the right ventricular outflow tract. The incidence of

Table 7.7. Pulmonary artery specific complications

- Transient dysrhythmias
- Right bundle-branch block
- Complete heart block (in patients with existing left-bundle branch block)
- Pulmonary artery rupture
- Pulmonary infarction
- Pulmonary artery knotting
- Tricuspid valve and subvalvular damage

developing RBBB was 3 percent in a prospective series of patients undergoing PA catheterization.[166] However, none of the patients with preexisting LBBB developed complete heart block in that series. In another study of 47 patients with LBBB, there were two cases of complete heart block, but only in patients with recent onset of LBBB.[167] It is imperative to have an external pacemaker immediately available or to use a pacing PAC when placing a PAC in patients with LBBB.

Hannan and associates reported a 46 percent mortality rate in a review of 28 cases of PAC-induced endobronchial hemorrhage, but the mortality rate was 75 percent in anticoagulated patients.[168] From these reports, several risk factors have emerged: advanced age, female sex, pulmonary hypertension, mitral stenosis, coagulopathy, distal placement of the catheter tip, and balloon hyperinflation. Balloon inflation in distal PAs is probably accountable for most episodes of PA rupture, owing to the high pressures generated by the balloon.[169] Hypothermic cardiopulmonary bypass (CPB) may also increase risk because of the distal migration of the catheter tip with movement of the heart and hardening of the PAC.[170,171] It is common practice to pull the PAC back approximately 3 to 5 cm when CPB is instituted.

It is important to consider the etiology of the hemorrhage when formulating a therapeutic plan. If the hemorrhage is minimal, and a coagulopathy coexists, correction of the coagulopathy may be the only necessary therapy. Protection of the uninvolved lung is of prime importance. Tilting the patient toward the affected side, and isolation of the lungs by placement of a double-lumen endotracheal tube or bronchial blocker, should protect the contralateral lung.[172] Strategies proposed to stop the hemorrhage include the application of PEEP, placement of bronchial blockers, and pulmonary resection.[173,174] The clinician is obviously at a disadvantage unless the site of hemorrhage is known. A chest radiograph will usually indicate the general location of the lesion. Although the etiology of endobronchial hemorrhage may be unclear, the bleeding site must be unequivocally located before surgical treatment is attempted. Using fluoroscopy and a small amount of radiographic contrast dye may help pinpoint the lesion if active hemorrhage is present. In severe hemorrhage and with recurrent bleeding, transcatheter coil embolization has been used. This may emerge as the preferred treatment method.[175,176]

Pulmonary infarction is a rare complication of PAC monitoring. An early report suggested that there was a 7.2 percent incidence of pulmonary infarction with PAC use.[177] However, continuously monitoring the PA waveform and keeping the balloon deflated when not determining the PCWP (to prevent inadvertent wedging of the catheter) were not standard practice at that time. Distal migration of PACs may also occur intraoperatively because of the action of the RV, uncoiling of the catheter, and softening of the catheter over time. Inadvertent catheter wedging occurs during CPB because of the diminished RV chamber size and retraction of the heart to perform the operation. Embolization of thrombus formed on a PAC could also result in pulmonary infarction.

Knotting of a PAC usually occurs as a result of coiling of the catheter within the right ventricle.[178] Insertion of an appropriately sized guidewire under fluoroscopic guidance may aid in unknotting the catheter.[179] Alternatively, the knot may be tightened and withdrawn percutaneously along with the introducer if no intracardiac structures are entangled.[180,181] If cardiac structures, such as the papillary muscles, are entangled in the knotted catheter, or if the knot appears too large, then surgical intervention may be required.[182–184] Sutures placed in the heart may inadvertently entrap the PAC. A report of such a case and the details of the percutaneous removal have been described.[185]

Placement of a PAC may cause or increase tricuspid regurgitation just by its physical presence in the right heart.[186] Additionally, withdrawal of the catheter with the balloon inflated may result in injury to the tricuspid[187] or pulmonary valves.[188] Placement of the PAC with the balloon deflated may increase the risk of passing the catheter between the chordae tendinae.[189] Septic endocarditis has also resulted from an indwelling PAC.[190,191]

The PAC is a foreign body that may serve as a nidus for thrombus formation. Mild thrombocytopenia has been reported in dogs and humans with indwelling PACs.[192] This probably results from increased platelet consumption. Heparin-bonded PACs reduce thrombogenicity for up to 72 hours.[193,194] However, heparin-coated PACs might trigger heparin-induced thrombocytopenia (HIT).[195]

The catheter may pass through an interatrial or interventricular communication into the left side of the heart. It is then possible for the catheter to enter the aorta through the left ventricular outflow tract. This complication should be recognized by the similarity between the presumed PA and systemic arterial waveforms.

Placement of the PAC in the liver has also been described, and the wedged hepatic venous pressures may mimic the PA pressure waveform.[196] Again, if available, TEE has proved invaluable for real-time confirmation of the proper placement of PACs. In many case reports, TEE detected incorrect placement and complications resulting from PACs. Balloon rupture is not uncommon when the PAC has been left in place for several days or when the balloon is inflated with more than 1.5 mL of air. Small volumes of air injected into the PA are of little consequence, and balloon rupture is apparent if the injected air cannot be withdrawn. Right ventricular perforation is an especially rare complication with a balloon-tipped catheter but has been reported in the literature.[197]

Malfunctions of the catheter and balloon can lead to inaccurate PCWP waveforms and data leading to incorrect treatment of the patient. Shin and coworkers reported a problem of eccentric balloon inflation, causing the catheter tip to impinge on the PA wall.[198]

Catheter whip is an artifact that is associated with long catheters, such as PACs. Because the tip moves within the bloodstream of the cardiac chambers and great vessels, the fluid contained within the catheter is accelerated. This can produce superimposed pressure waves of 10 mmHg in either direction.

Credentialing

Currently there are no recommendations for training and credentialing processes regarding PAC monitoring. However, the 2003 ASA guidelines for pulmonary artery catheterization emphasize that patient, surgery, and practice setting must be considered.[199] The ASA Task Force concluded that the practice setting, among other factors, is important, as there is evidence that inadequate training or experience may increase the risk of perioperative complications associated with the use of PACs. Thus, it is recommended that the routine use of PACs should be confined to centers with adequate training and experience in the perioperative management of patients with PACs.

Residents enrolled in an Accreditation Council for Graduate Medical Education (ACGME)–accredited residency program are required to have experience with "patients who require specialized techniques for their perioperative care … [and] significant experience with central vein and pulmonary artery catheter placement." Interestingly, there are no specific requirements for ACGME-accredited cardiothoracic anesthesiology fellowship programs with regard to PACs.

As previously discussed, the use of PACs has been declining significantly as data have emerged questioning their benefit in patient outcome. This then leads to less training and experience in the use PACs. The impact of decreased exposure to PACs may lead to increasing complications secondary to inexperience and operator error.

Practice parameters (indications)

Indications for CVP monitoring

CVP monitoring is often performed to obtain an indication of intravascular volume status. However, the accuracy and reliability of CVP monitoring depend on many factors, including the functional status of the RV and LV, the presence of pulmonary disease, and ventilatory factors, such as PEEP. The CVP may reflect left heart filling pressures, but only in patients with good LV function. Patients undergoing cardiac surgery with CPB should have the CVP monitored. When the catheter tip is positioned in the SVC, it indicates both RA pressure and cerebral venous pressure. Significant increases in CVP can produce critical decreases in cerebral perfusion pressure. During CPB, this is occasionally caused by a malpositioned SVC cannula, resulting in decreased venous drainage to the CPB machine. The surgeon must correct it immediately to prevent cerebral edema and poor cerebral perfusion.

Aside from patient- and surgery-related factors, indications for CVP monitoring may also depend on practice setting and on the preferences of the surgeon and anesthesiologist. If a central venous catheter is used only for volume access, it should be kept in mind that shorter large-bore peripheral lines allow higher flow rates than the longer central line catheters. Table 7.8 summarizes some of the indications for the perioperative use of a central venous catheter.

Table 7.8. Indications and contarindications for central venous catheter placement

Indications

- Major operative procedures involving large fluid shifts and/or blood loss
- Inadequate peripheral venous access
- Frequent venous blood sampling
- Rapid infusion of intravenous fluids (e.g. major trauma, liver transplantation)
- Venous access for vasoactive or irritating drugs
- Chronic drug administration (e.g. antibiotics, chemotherapy)
- Total parenteral nutrition
- Surgical procedures with a high risk of air embolism
- Intravascular volume assessment when urine output is not reliable or unavailable (e.g. renal failure)

Contraindications

- SVC syndrome
- Skin infection at insertion site

Contraindications for CVP monitoring

There are few absolute contraindications for CVP monitoring. In patients with true SVC syndrome, placement of a CVP in the neck, subclavian area, or the upper extremities is contraindicated. Venous pressures in the head and upper extremities are elevated by the SVC obstruction, and therefore do not reflect RA pressure. Medications that are administered into the obstructed venous circulation reach the central circulation via collateral vessels in a delayed fashion. Furthermore, rapid fluid administration into the obstructed venous circulation may exacerbate the elevated venous pressures and cause more pronounced edema. The mild SVC obstruction seen with some ascending aortic aneurysms, however, does not represent a contraindication to central venous cannulation of the upper body. An infection at the side of insertion is another absolute contraindication. In coagulopathic patients, ultrasound-guided central line placement is preferred to reduce the risk of arterial puncture and subsequent hematoma formation in the neck.

Indications for PAC placement

The ability of PACs to positively influence patient outcome has never been conclusively proved in large-scale prospective studies (see previous discussion). To the contrary, enough evidence has been collected to seriously question the indiscriminate use of PA catheters. In general, the risk–benefit ratio of PAC placement should be evaluated for each individual case, rather than based on broad recommendations.[200,201] In 2003, the ASA Task Force on Pulmonary Artery Catheterization published updated practice guidelines for pulmonary artery catheterization (http://www.asahq.org/publicationsAndServices/pulm_artery.pdf). These guidelines emphasized that the combination of patient, surgery, and practice setting had to be considered. Generally, the routine use of PACs is indicated in high-risk patients (e.g. ASA 4 or 5) and high-risk procedures (e.g. where large fluid changes or hemodynamic disturbances are

Table 7.9. ASA practice guidelines for pulmonary artery catheter use

Opinions

- PA catheterization provides new information that may change therapy with poor clinical evidence of its effect on clinical outcome or mortality.
- There is no evidence from large controlled studies to date that *preoperative* PA catheterization improves outcome regarding hemodynamic optimization.
- Perioperative PAC monitoring of hemodynamic parameters leading to goal-directed therapy has produced inconsistent data in multiple studies as well as clinical scenarios.
- Having immediate access to PA catheter data allows important preemptive measures for selected subgroups of patients who encounter hemodynamic disturbances that require immediate and precise decisions about fluid management and drug treatment.
- Experience and understanding are the major determinants of PA catheter effectiveness.
- PA catheterization is inappropriate as a routine practice in surgical patients and should be limited to cases in which the anticipated benefits of catheterization outweighs the potential risks.
- PA catheterization can be harmful.

Recommendations

- The appropriateness of routine PA catheterization depends on a combination of patient-, surgery-, and practice setting-related factors.
- Perioperative PA catheterization should be considered in patients who present with significant organ dysfunction or major comorbidity that poses an increased risk for hemodynamic disturbances or instability (e.g. ASA 4 or 5 patients).
- Perioperative PA catheterization in surgical settings should be considered based on the hemodynamic risk of the individual case rather than generalized surgical setting related recommendations. High-risk surgical procedures are those where large fluid changes or hemodynamic disturbances can be anticipated and procedures that are associated with a high risk of morbidity and mortality.
- Because of the risk of complication from PA catheterization, the procedure should not be performed by clinicians, nursing staff, or in practice settings where competency in safe insertion, accurate interpretation of results, and appropriate catheter maintenance cannot be guaranteed.
- Routine PA catheterization is not recommended when the patient, procedure, and practice setting each pose a low- or moderate- risk for hemodynamic changes.

ASA = American Society of Anesthesiologists; PA = pulmonary artery. American Society of Anesthesiologists: Practice guidelines for pulmonary artery catheterization: http://www.asahq.org/publicationsAndServices/pulm_artery.pdf.

Table 7.10. Contraindications for pulmonary artery catheterization

Absolute contraindications

- Right atrial or right ventricular mass
- Tricuspid or pulmonary stenosis
- Mechanical tricuspid or pulmonary valve prosthesis

Relative contraindications

- Recently placed pacemaker or defibrillator wires
- Patients with left bundle-branch block

very few, if any, clearly defined indications for PAC monitoring left in today's practice. Even though there are no evidence-based data to support this, it is our opinion that patients with known or suspected pulmonary hypertension can benefit from PAC placement.

Significant expertise and training are required for PAC placement as well as for interpretation of PAC-derived data. Many anesthesiology residency training programs, as well as cardiothoracic surgery and intensive care fellowship programs, place PACs more frequently, to provide adequate training. Lack of exposure to PACs could otherwise lead to inadequate expertise among these physicians and potentially increase the risk of complications related to PAC placement.

Contraindications to PAC placement

A list of contraindications to PAC placement is provided in Table 7.10. A right atrial or right ventricular mass (tumor or thrombus) is considered an absolute contraindication to PAC placement. The catheter may dislodge a portion of the mass, causing pulmonary or paradoxical embolization. In patients with tricuspid or pulmonic valvular stenosis, PAC placement should be considered carefully, as it may be difficult or impossible to pass a PAC across a severely stenotic valve and, in fact, it may worsen the obstruction to flow. Patients with certain valvular diseases, such as significant mitral and aortic stenosis, are sensitive to even brief periods of arrhythmias. Brief periods of atrial and ventricular arrhythmias can be seen during PAC placement in the majority of cases and could potentially cause acute hemodynamic instability. Appropriate preparations must be made to enable rapid administration of antiarrhythmic drugs and cardiopulmonary resuscitation, and electrical cardioversion, defibrillation, or pacing if required. In coagulopathic patients PAC is not generally contraindicated; however, increased precautions should be taken to prevent hematoma formation, as mentioned previously. Additionally, the risk of inducing endobronchial hemorrhage may be increased. Newly inserted pacemaker wires may be displaced by the catheter during insertion or withdrawal. After approximately four to six weeks, pacemaker wires become firmly embedded in the endocardium, and wire displacement becomes less likely. Newer generation pacemaker and defibrillator wires are now anchored into the endocardium more securely during placement and are less likely to become dislodged.

expected). The practice setting is important, as there is evidence that inadequate training or experience may increase the risk of perioperative complications associated with the use of PAC. Thus, it is recommended that the routine use of PAC should be confined to centers with adequate training and experience in the perioperative management of patients with PACs. The ASA guidelines specifically do not provide the practitioner with a list of procedures or diagnoses for which PAC placement is indicated (also see Table 7.9). Considering the bulk of literature showing no benefit, or even worse outcome, if PAC was deployed, even in patients with severely compromised cardiac function, the authors of this text also conclude that there are

Specialty catheters

Pacing catheters

Electrode PACs, as well as pacing wire catheters, are available. Electrode PACs (Swan-Ganz Pacing PAC, originally produced by Baxter Edwards) contain five electrodes for bipolar atrial, ventricular, or AV sequential pacing. With appropriate filtering, the catheter may also be used for the recording of an intracardiac ECG. The intraoperative success rates for atrial, ventricular, and AV sequential capture have been reported as 80 percent, 93 percent, and 73 percent, respectively.[202] The Paceport and A-V Paceport catheters (Baxter Edwards) have lumina for the introduction of a ventricular wire (Paceport), or both atrial and ventricular wires (A-V Paceport) for temporary transvenous pacing. The success rate for ventricular pacing capture was 96 percent for the Paceport.[203] The success rates for atrial and ventricular pacing capture prior to CPB were 98 percent and 100 percent, respectively, in a study of the A-V Paceport.[204] The actual use and indications for placement of pacing PAC in a series of cardiac surgery patients has been published.[205] The possible indications for placement of a pacing PAC are shown in Table 7.11.

Right ventricular ejection fraction catheters

The rapid-response thermistor PAC (Baxter Edwards) incorporates three modifications from a standard PAC: a multiorifice injectate port; a rapid-response thermistor; and ECG electrodes. The catheter is positioned so the injectate port is 2 cm cephalad to the tricuspid valve in the RA.[206,207] With each injection, the computer determines the right ventricular ejection fraction (RVEF) from the exponential decay of the thermodilution curve. End-diastolic temperature points in the thermodilution curve are identified using the R-wave signal. The computer also measures heart rate (HR) from the catheter ECG electrodes. From these data, stroke volume (SV), right ventricular end-diastolic volume, and right ventricular end-systolic volume are calculated. Assumptions that are essential to the accuracy of the technique include a regular RR interval, instantaneous mixing of the injectate with the RV blood, and absence of tricuspid regurgitation. The timing of injection with respect to the respiratory cycle also affects the reproducibility of the measurements.[208] The use of this type of monitoring could be justified in patients with severe RV dysfunction caused by myocardial infarction, right-sided CAD, pulmonary hypertension, left-sided failure, or intrinsic pulmonary disease. However, RVEF catheters are rarely used, especially with TEE becoming more readily available in the OR setting.

Mixed venous oxygen saturation catheters

The addition of fiberoptic bundles to PACs has enabled the continuous monitoring of venous oxygen saturation (SvO_2) using reflectance spectrophotometry. The catheter is connected to a device that includes a light-emitting diode and a sensor to detect the light returning from the PA. SvO_2 is calculated from the differential absorption of various wavelengths of light by the saturated and unsaturated hemoglobin.[209]

Monitoring the SvO_2 is a means of providing a global estimation of the adequacy of oxygen delivery relative to oxygen extraction rate. The formula for SvO_2 calculation can be derived by modifying the Fick equation and assuming that the effect of dissolved oxygen in the blood is negligible:

$$SvO_2 = SaO_2 - \frac{\dot{V}O_2}{CO \bullet 1.34 \bullet Hb}$$

A decrease in the SvO_2 can indicate one of the following situations: (1) decreased CO; (2) increased oxygen consumption; (3) decreased arterial oxygen saturation; or (4) decreased hemoglobin concentration (also see the following chapter). If it is assumed that oxygen consumption and arterial oxygen content are constant, then changes in SvO_2 should reflect changes in CO. The values obtained with various fiberoptic catheter systems showed good agreement with in vitro (co-oximetry) SvO_2 measurements.[210–213]

References

1. McGee DC, Gould MK. Preventing complications of central venous catheterization. *N Engl J Med* 2003;348:1123–33.
2. Wiener RS, Welch HG. Trends in use of the pulmonary artery catheter in the United States, 1993–2004. *JAMA* 2007;298:423–9.
3. English IC, Frew RM, Pigott JF, et al. Percutaneous catheterization of the internal jugular vein. *Anesthesia* 1969;24:521–31.
4. Muralidhar K. Left internal versus right internal jugular vein access to central venous circulation using the Seldinger technique. *J Cardiothorac Anesth* 1995;9:115–116.
5. Neustein S, Narang J, Bronheim D. Use of the color test for safer internal jugular vein cannulation. *Anesthesiology* 1992;76:1062.
6. Jobes DR, Schwartz AJ, Greenhow DE, et al. Safer jugular vein cannulation: Recognition of arterial puncture. *Anesthesiology* 1983;59:353–5.
7. Fabian JA, Jesudian MC. A simple method for improving the safety of percutaneous cannulation of the internal jugular vein. *Anesth Analg* 1985;64:1032–3.
8. Denys BG, Uretsky BF. Anatomical variations of internal jugular vein location: Impact on central venous access. *Crit Care Med* 1991;19:1516–9.

Table 7.11. Potential indications for the perioperative placement of pacing pulmonary artery catheters

- Sinus node dysfunction/bradycardia
- Second-degree (Mobitz II) atrioventricular block
- Complete (third-degree) atrioventricular block
- Digitalis toxicity
- Need for AV sequential pacing
- Aortic stenosis (need to maintain sinus rhythm)
- Severe left ventricular hypertrophy or noncompliant left ventricle
- HCM (obstructive type)
- Need for an intracardiac electrogram

HCM = hypertrophic cardiomyopathy

9. Hind D, Calvert N, McWilliams R, et al. Ultrasonic locating devices for central venous cannulation: meta-analysis. *BMJ* 2003;327:361.

10. Leyvi G, Taylor D, Reith E, Wasnick J. Utility of ultrasound guided central venous cannulation in pediatric surgical patients: a clinical series. *Pediatric Anesthesia* 2005;15:953–8.

11. Asheim P, Mostad U, Aadahl P. Ultrasound-guided central venous cannulation in infants and children. *Acta Anaesthesiol Scand* 2002;46:390–2.

12. Liberman L, Hordof AJ, Hsu DT, et al. Ultrasound-assisted cannulation of the right internal jugular vein during electrophysiologic studies in children. *J Interv Card Electrophysiol* 2001;5:177–9.

13. Verghese ST, McGill WA, Patel RI, et al. Ultrasound-guided internal jugular venous cannulation in infants: a prospective comparison with the traditional palpation method. *Anesthesiology* 1999;91:71–7.

14. Verghese ST, McGill WA, Patel RI, et al. Comparison of three techniques for internal jugular vein cannulation in infants. *Paediatr Anaesth* 2000;10:505–11.

15. Hind D, Calvert N, McWilliams R, et al. Ultrasonic locating devices for central venous cannulation: meta-analysis. *BMJ* 2003;327:361.

16. Grebenik CR, Boyce A, Sinclair ME, et al. NICE guidelines for central venous catheterization in children. Is the evidence base sufficient? *Br J Anaesth* 2004;92:827–30.

17. Randolph AG, Cook DJ, Gonzales CA, Pribble CG. Ultrasound guidance for placement of central venous catheters: a meta-analysis of the literature. *Crit Care Med* 1996;24:2053–8.

18. Gratz I, Ashar M, Kidwell P, et al. Doppler-guided cannulation of the internal jugular vein: A prospective, randomized trial. *J Clin Monit* 1994;10(3):185–8.

19. Troianos CA, Jobes DR, Ellison N. Ultrasound-guided cannulation of the internal jugular vein: A prospective, randomized study. *Anesth Analg* 1991;72:823–6.

20. Mallory DL, McGee WT, Shawker TH, et al. Ultrasound guidance improves the success rate of internal jugular vein cannulation. *Chest* 1990;98:157–60.

21. Denys BG, Uretsky BF, Reddy PS. Ultrasound-assisted cannulation of the internal jugular vein. A prospective comparison to the external landmark-guided technique. *Circulation* 1993;87:1557–62.

22. Augoustides J, Horak J, Ochroch A, et al. A randomized controlled clinical trial of real-time needle-guided ultrasound for internal jugular venous cannulation in a large university anesthesia department. *J Cardiothorac Anesth* 2005;19:310–5.

23. Leung J, Duffy M, Finckh A. Real-time ultrasonographically-guided internal jugular vein catheterization in the emergency department increases success rates and reduces complications: a randomized, prospective study. *Ann Emerg Med* 2006;48:540–7.

24. Milling T, Rose J, Briggs W, et al. Randomized, controlled clinical trial of point-of-care limited ultrasonography assistance of central venous cannulation: The Third Sonography Outcomes Assessment Program (SOAP-3) Trial. *Crit Care Med* 2005;33:1764–9.

25. Hayashi H, Amano M. Does ultrasound imaging before puncture facilitate internal jugular vein cannulation? Prospective randomized comparison with landmark-guided puncture in ventilated patients. *J Cardiothorac Anesth* 2002;16:572–5.

26. Troianos CA, Kuwik R, Pasqual J, et al. Internal jugular vein and carotid artery anatomic relation as determined by ultrasonography. *Anesthesiology* 1996;85:43–48.

27. Alderson PJ, Burrows FA, Stemp LI, et al. Use of ultrasound to evaluate internal jugular vein anatomy and to facilitate central venous cannulation of paediatric patients. *Br J Anaesth* 1993;70:145–8.

28. Sulek CA, Gravenstein N, Blackshear RH, Weiss L. Head rotation during internal jugular vein cannulation and the risk of carotid artery puncture. *Anesth Analg* 1996; 82:125–8.

29. van de Griendt EW, Muhiudeen I, Cassoria L, et al. The effects of Trendelenburg position and Valsalva maneuver on the cross-sectional area of the internal jugular vein. *Anesthesiology* 1991;75:A423.

30. Mallory DL, Showker T, Evans G, et al. Effects of clinical maneuvers on sonographically determined internal jugular vein size during venous cannulation. *Crit Care Med* 1990;18:1269–73.

31. Suarez T, Baerwald J, Kraus C. Central venous access: the effects of approach, position, and head rotation on internal jugular vein crosssectional area. *Anesth Analg* 2002;95:1519–24.

32. Parry G. Trendelenburg position, head elevation and a midline position optimize right internal jugular vein diameter. *Can J Anaesth* 2004;51:379–81.

33. Blitt CD, Wright WA, Petty WC, et al. Cardiovascular catheterization via the external jugular vein: A technique employing the J-wire. *JAMA* 1974;229:817–8.

34. Defalque RJ. Subclavian venapuncture: a review. *Anesth Analg* 1968;47:677–82.

35. Ruesch S, Walder B, Tramer M. Complications of central venous catheters: internal jugular versus subclavian access – a systematic review. *Crit Care Med* 2002;30:486–7.

36. Lefrant JY, Muller L, De La Coussaye JE, et al. Risk factors of failure and immediate complication of subclavian vein catheterization in critically ill patients. *Intensive Care Med* 2002;28:1036–41.

37. Fangio P, Mourgeon E, Romelaer A, et al. Aortic injury and cardiac tamponade as a complication of subclavian venous catheterization. *Anesthesiology* 2002;96:1520–2.

38. Mansfield PF, Hohn DC, Fornage BD, et al. Complications and failures of subclavian-vein catheterization. *N Engl J Med* 1994;331:1735–8.

39. Kellner GA, Smart JF. Percutaneous placement of catheters to monitor "central venous pressure." *Anesthesiology* 1972;36:515–6.

40. Webre DR, Arens JF. Use of cephalic and basilic veins for introduction of cardiovascular catheters. *Anesthesiology* 1973;38:389–92.

41. Nadroo AM, Lin J, Green RS, et al. Death as a complication of peripherally inserted central catheters in neonates. *J Pediatr* 2001;138:599–601.

42. Nadroo AM, Glass RB, Lin J, et al. Changes in upper extremity position cause migration of peripherally inserted central catheters in neonates. *Pediatrics* 2002;110:131–6.

43. Loewenthal MR, Dobson PM, Starkey RE, et al. The peripherally inserted central catheter (PICC): a prospective study of its natural history after cubital fossa insertion. *Anaesth Intensive Care* 2002;30:21–4.

44. Burgess GE, Marino RJ, Peuler MJ. Effect of head position on the location of venous catheters inserted via the basilic vein. *Anesthesiology* 1977;46:212–3.

45. Mongan P, Peterson R, Culling R. Pressure monitoring can accurately position catheters for air embolism aspiration. *J Clin Monit* 1992;8:121–5.

46. Roth S, Aronson S. Placement of a right atrial air aspiration catheter guided by transesophageal echocardiography. *Anesthesiology* 1995;83:1359–60.

47. Kumar M, Amin M. The peripherally inserted central venous catheter; friend or foe? *Int J Oral Maxillofac Surg* 2004;33:201–4.

48. Parikh S, Narayanan V. Misplaced peripherally inserted central catheter: an unusual cause of stroke. *Pediatr Neurol* 2004;30:210–2.

49. Pettit J. Assessment of infants with peripherally inserted central catheters: Part 1. Detecting the most frequently occurring complications. *Adv Neonatal Care* 2002;2:304–15.

50. Smith JR, Friedell ML, Cheatham ML, et al. Peripherally inserted central catheters revisited. *Am J Surg* 1998;176:208–11.

51. Durbec O, Viviand X, Potie F, et al. A prospective evaluation of the use of femoral venous catheters in critically ill adults. *Crit Care Med* 1997;25:1986–9.

52. Pawar M, Mehta Y, Kapoor P, et al. Central venous catheter-related bloodstream infections: incidence, risk factors, outcome, and associated pathogens. *J Cardiothorac Vasc Anesth* 2004;18:304–8.

53. Timsit JF, Bruneel F, Cheval C, et al. Use of tunneled femoral catheters to prevent catheter-related infection. A randomized, controlled trial. *Ann Intern Med* 1999;130:729–35.

54. Nahum E, Levy I, Katz J, et al. Efficacy of subcutaneous tunneling for prevention of bacterial colonization of femoral central venous catheters in critically ill children. *Pediatr Infect Dis J* 2002;21:1000–4.

55. Mantia AM, Robinson JN, Lolley DM, et al. Sternal retraction and pulmonary artery catheter compromise. *J Cardiothorac Anesth* 1988;2:430–9.

56. Keusch DJ, Winters S, Thys DM. The patient's position influences the incidence of dysrhythmias during pulmonary artery catheterization. *Anesthesiology* 1989;70:582–4.

57. Benumof JL, Saidman IJ, Arkin DB, et al. Where pulmonary artery catheters go: Intrathoracic distribution. *Anesthesiology* 1977;46:336–8.

58. Mark JB. Central venous pressure monitoring: clinical insights beyond the numbers. *J Cardiothorac Vasc Anesth* 1991;5:163–73.

59. Schmitt EA, Brantigan CO. Common artifacts of pulmonary artery pressures: recognition and interpretation. *J Clin Monit* 1986;2:44–53.

60. Moore RA, Neary MJ, Gallagher HD, Clark DL. Determination of the pulmonary capillary wedge position in patients with giant left atrial V waves. *J Cardiothorac Anesth* 1987;1:108–113.

61. Grose R, Strain J, Cohen MV. Pulmonary arterial V waves in mitral regurgitation: clinical and experimental observations. *Circulation* 1984;69:214–22.

62. Haggmark S, Hohner P, Ostman M, et al. Comparison of hemodynamic, electrocardiographic, mechanical, and metabolic indicators of intraoperative myocardial ischemia in vascular surgical patients with coronary artery disease. *Anesthesiology* 1989;70:19–25.

63. van Daele ME, Sutherland GR, Mitchell MM, et al. Do changes in pulmonary capillary wedge pressure adequately reflect myocardial ischemia during anesthesia? *Circulation* 1990;81:865–71.

64. Lappas D, Lell WA, Gabel JC, et al. Indirect measurement of left atrial pressure in surgical patients – pulmonary capillary wedge and pulmonary artery diastolic pressures compared with left atrial pressure. *Anesthesiology* 1973;38:394–7.

65. Nadeau S, Noble WH. Misinterpretation of pressure measurements from the pulmonary artery catheter. *Can Anaesth Soc J* 1986;33:352–63.

66. Tuman KJ, Carroll G, Ivankovich AD. Pitfalls in interpretation of pulmonary artery catheter data. *J Cardiothorac Anesth* 1989;3:625–41.

67. Shasby DM, Dauber IM, Pfister S, et al. Swan-Ganz catheter location and left atrial pressure determine the accuracy of the wedge pressure when positive end-expiratory pressure is used. *Chest* 1980;80:666–70.

68. Lorzman J, Powers SR, Older T, et al. Correlation of pulmonary wedge and left atrial pressure: A study in the patient receiving positive end-expiratory pressure ventilation. *Arch Surg* 1974;109:270–7.

69. Kane PB, Askanazi J, Neville JF Jr, et al. Artifacts in the measurement of pulmonary artery wedge pressure. *Crit Care Med* 1978;6:36–8.

70. Rajacich N, Burchard KW, Hasan FM, Singh AK. Central venous pressure and pulmonary capillary wedge pressure as estimates of left atrial pressure: effects of positive end-expiratory pressure and catheter tip malposition. *Crit Care Med* 1989;17:7–11.

71. Shasby DM, Dauber IM, Pfister S, et al. Swan-Ganz catheter location and left atrial pressure determine the accuracy of the wedge pressure when positive end-expiratory pressure is used. *Chest* 1981;80:666–70.

72. Teboul J–L, Zapol WM, Brun-Buisson C, et al. A comparison of pulmonary artery occlusion pressure and left ventricular end-diastolic pressure during mechanical ventilation with PEEP in patients with severe ARDS. *Anesthesiology* 1989;70:261–266.

73. Pinsky M, Vincent JL, DeSmet JM. Estimating the left ventricular filling pressure during positive end-expiratory pressure. *Am Rev Respir Dis* 1991;25:143.

74. Haskell RJ, French WJ. Accuracy of left atrial and pulmonary artery wedge pressure in pure mitral regurgitation in predicting left ventricular end-diastolic pressure. *Am J Cardiol* 1988;61:136–41.

75. Entress JJ, Dhamee S, Olund T, et al. Pulmonary artery occlusion pressure is not accurate immediately after CPB. *J Cardiothorac Anesth* 1990;4:558–63.

76. Mangano DT. Monitoring pulmonary arterial pressure in coronary artery disease. *Anesthesiology* 1980;53:364–70.

77. Kumar A, Anel R, Bunnell E, et al. Pulmonary artery occlusion pressure and central venous pressure fail to predict ventricular filling volume, cardiac performance, or the response to volume infusion in normal subjects. *Crit Care Med* 2004;32:691–9.

78. Buhre W, Weyland A, Schorn B, et al. Changes in central venous pressure and pulmonary capillary wedge pressure do not indicate changes in right and left heart volume in patients undergoing coronary artery bypass surgery. *Eur J Anaesthesiol* 1999;16:11–17.

79. Godje O, Peyerl M, Seebauer T, et al. Central venous pressure, pulmonary capillary wedge pressure and intrathoracic blood volumes as preload indicators in cardiac surgery patients. *Eur J Cardiothorac Surg* 1998;13:533–9.

80. Lichtwarck-Aschoff M, Beale R, Pfeiffer UJ. Central venous pressure, pulmonary artery occlusion pressure, intrathoracic blood volume, and right ventricular end-diastolic volume as indicators of cardiac preload. *J Crit Care* 1996;11:180–8.

81. Gelman S. Venous function and central venous pressure. *Anesthesiology* 2008;108:735–48.

82. Swan HJC, Ganz W, Forrester JS, et al. Catheterization of the heart in man with the use of a flow-directed balloon-tipped catheter. *N Engl J Med* 1970;283:447–51.

83. Connors AF, McCaffree DR, Gray BA. Evaluation of right heart catheterization in the critically ill patient. *N Engl J Med* 1983;308:263–7.

84. Waller JL, Johnson SP, Kaplan JA. Usefulness of pulmonary artery catheters during aortocoronary bypass surgery. *Anesth Analg* 1982;61:221–2.

85. Iberti T, Fisher CJ. A prospective study on the use of the pulmonary artery catheter in a medical intensive care unit – its effect on diagnosis and therapy. *Crit Care Med* 1983;11: 238.

86. Iberti TJ, Fischer EP, Leibowitz AB, et al. A multicenter study of physicians' knowledge of the pulmonary artery catheter. *JAMA* 1990;264:2928–32.

87. Connors AF, Speroff T, Dawson NV, et al. The effectiveness of right heart catheterization in the initial care of critically ill patients. *JAMA* 1996;276:889–97.

88. Barone JE, Tucker JB, Rassias D, Corvo PR. Routine perioperative pulmonary artery catheterization has no effect on rate of complications in vascular surgery: a meta-analysis. *Am Surg* 2001;67(7):674–9.

89. Shah MR, Hasselblad V, Stevenson LW et al. Impact of the pulmonary artery catheter in critically ill patients. *JAMA* 2005;294:1664–70.

90. Afessa B, Spencer S, Khan W, et al. Association of pulmonary artery catheter use with in-hospital mortality. *Crit Care Med* 2001;29:1145–8.

91. Gattinoni L, Brazzi L, Pelosi P, et al. A trial of goal-oriented hemodynamic therapy in critically ill patients. *N Engl J Med* 1995;333:1025–32.

92. Tuman KJ, McCarthy RJ, Spiess BD, et al. Effect of pulmonary artery catheterization on outcome in patients undergoing coronary artery surgery. *Anesthesiology* 1989;70:199–206.

93. Taylor RW. Controversies in pulmonary artery catheterization. *New Horizons* 1997;5:173–296.

94. Steward RD, Psyhojos T, Lahey SJ, et al. Central venous catheter use in low-risk coronary artery bypass grafting. *Ann Thorac Surg* 1998;66:1306–11.

95. Schwann TA, Zacharias A, Riordan CJ, et al. Safe, highly selective use of pulmonary artery catheters in coronary artery bypass grafting: an objective patient selection method. *Ann Thorac Surg* 2002;73:1394–401.

96. Ramsey SD, Saint S, Sullivan SD, et al. Clinical and economic effects of pulmonary artery catheterization in nonemergent coronary artery bypass graft surgery. *J Cardiothorac Vasc Anesth* 2000;14:113–8.

97. Resano FG, Kapetanakis EI, Hill PC, et al. Clinical outcomes of low-risk patients undergoing beating-heart surgery with or without pulmonary artery catheterization. *JCVA* 2006;20: 300–6.

98. Djaiani G, Karski J, Yudin M et al. Clinical outcomes in patients undergoing elective coronary artery bypass graft surgery with and without utilization of pulmonary artery catheter-generated data. *J Cardiothorac Vasc Anesth* 2006;20:307–10.

99. Pölönen P, Ruokonen E, Hippeläinen M, et al. A prospective, randomized study of goal-oriented hemodynamic therapy in cardiac surgical patients. *Anesth Analg* 2000;90: 1052–9.

100. Polanczyk CA, Rohde LE, Goldman L, et al. Right heart catheterization and cardiac complications in patients undergoing noncardiac surgery: an observational study. *JAMA* 2001;286:309–14.

101. Sandham JD, Hull RD, Brant RF, et al. A randomized, controlled trial of the use of pulmonary-artery catheters in high-risk surgical patients. *N Engl J Med* 2003;348:5–14.

102. Wiener RS, Welch HG. Trends in use of the pulmonary artery catheter in the United States, 1993–2004. *JAMA* 2007;298:423–429.

103. Yu DT, Platt R, Lanken PN, Black E, et al. Relationship of pulmonary artery catheter use to mortality and resource utilization in patients with severe sepsis. *Crit Care Med* 2003;31:2734–41.

104. Sakr Y, Vincent JL, Reinhard K, et al. Use of the pulmonary artery catheter is not associated with worse outcome in the ICU. *Chest* 2005;128:2722–31.

105. Rhodes A, Cusack RJ, Newman PJ, et al. A randomised, controlled trial of the pulmonary artery catheter in critically ill patients. *Intensive Care Med* 2002;28:256–64.

106. Murdoch SD, Cohen AT, Bellamy MC. Pulmonary artery catheterization and mortality in critically ill patients. *Br J Anaesth* 2000;85:611–5.

107. Chittock DR, Dhingra VK, Ronco JJ, et al. Severity of illness and risk of death associated with pulmonary artery catheter use. *Crit Care Med* 2004;32:911–5.

108. Richard C, Warszawski J, Anguel N, Deye N, et al. Early use of the pulmonary artery catheter and outcomes in patients with shock and acute respiratory distress syndrome: a randomized controlled trial. *JAMA* 2003;290:2713–20.

109. Wheeler AP, Bernard GR, Thompson BT, et al. Pulmonary-artery versus central venous catheter to guide treatment of acute lung injury. National Heart, Lung, and Blood Institute Acute Respiratory Distress Syndrome (ARDS) Clinical Trials Network. *N Engl J Med* 2006;354:2213–24.

110. Guyatt G, Ontario Intensive Care Group. A randomised control trial of right heart catheterization in critically ill patients. *J Intensive Care Med* 1991;6:91–5.

111. Gore JM, Goldberg RJ, Spodick DH, et al. A community-wide assessment of the use of pulmonary artery catheters in patients with acute myocardial infarctions. *Chest* 1987;92:721–7.

112. Cohen MG, Kelly RV, Kong DF, et al. Pulmonary artery catheterization in acute coronary syndromes: Insights from the GUSTO IIb and GUSTO III trials. *Am J Med* 2005;118: 482–8.

113. Haupt M, Shoemaker W, Haddy F, et al. Correspondence: Goal-oriented hemodynamic therapy. *N Engl J Med* 1996;334:799–800.

114. Shoemaker WC, Appel PL, Kram HB, et al. Prospective trial of supranormal values of survivors as therapeutic goals in high-risk surgical patients. *Chest* 1988;94:1176–86.

115. Boyd O, Grounds RM, Bennett ED. The beneficial effect of supranormalization of oxygen delivery with dopamine hydrochloride on perioperative mortality. *JAMA* 1993;270:2699–707.

116. Rao TLK, Jacobs KH, El-Etr AA. Reinfarction following anesthesia in patients with myocardial infarction. *Anesthesiology* 1983;59:499–505.

117. Moore CH, Lombardo TR, Allums JA, Gordon FT. Left main coronary artery stenosis: Hemodynamic monitoring to reduce mortality. *Ann Thorac Surg* 1978;26:445–51.

118. Heyland DK, Cook DL, King D, et al. Maximizing oxygen delivery in critically ill patients: A methodologic appraisal of the evidence. *Crit Care Med* 1996;24:517–24.

119. Wiener RS, Welch HG. Trends in use of the pulmonary artery catheter in the United States, 1993–2004. *JAMA* 2007;298:423–9.

120. Ranucci M. Which cardiac surgical patients can benefit from placement of a pulmonary artery catheter? *Crit Care* 2006;10(Suppl3):S6.

121. Applebaum RM, Adelman MA, Kanschuger MS, et al. Transesophageal echocardiographic identification of a retrograde dissection of the ascending aorta caused by inadvertent cannulation of the common carotid artery. *J Am Soc Echocardiogr* 1997;10:749–51.

122. Eckhardt W, Iaconetti D, Kwon J, et al. Inadvertent carotid artery cannulation during pulmonary artery catheter insertion. *J Cardiothorac Vasc Anesth* 1996;10:283–90.

123. Fraizer MC, Chu WW, Gudjonsson T, Wolff MR. Use of a percutaneous vascular suture device for closure of an inadvertent subclavian artery puncture. *Catheter Cardiovasc Interv* 2003;59:369–71.

124. Berlet MH, Steffen D, Shaughness G, Hanner J. Closure using a surgical closure device of inadvertent subclavian artery punctures during central venous catheter placement. *Cardiovasc Intervent Radiol* 2001;24:122–4.

125. Gobiel F, Couture P, Girard D, et al. Carotid artery-internal jugular fistula: Another complication following pulmonary artery catheterization via the internal jugular venous route. *Anesthesiology* 1994;80:230–1.

126. Robinson R, Errett L. Arteriovenous fistula following percutaneous internal jugular vein cannulation: A report of carotid artery-to-internal jugular vein fistula. *J Cardiothorac Anesth* 1988;2:488–91.

127. Kim J, Ahn W, Bahk JH. Hemomediastinum resulting from subclavian artery laceration during internal jugular catheterization. *Anesth Analg* 2003;97:1257–9.

128. Kwon SS, Falk A, Mitty HA. Thoracic duct injury associated with left internal jugular vein catheterization: anatomic considerations. *J Vasc Interv Radiol* 2002; 13:337–9.

129. Khalil DG, Parker FB, Mukherjee N, Webb WR. Thoracic duct injury: a complication of jugular vein catheterization. *JAMA* 1972;221:908–9.

130. Teba L, Dedhia HV, Bowen R, Alexander JC. Chylothorax review. *Crit Care Med* 1985;13:49–52.

131. Cook TL, Deuker CW. Tension pneumothorax following internal jugular cannulation and general anesthesia. *Anesthesiology* 1976;45:554–5.

132. Plewa MC, Ledrick D, Sferra JJ. Delayed tension pneumothorax complicating central venous catheterization and positive-pressure ventilation. *Am J Emerg* 1995;Med 13:532–5.

133. Porzionato A, Montisci M, Manani G. Brachial plexus injury following subclavian vein catheterization: a case report. *J Clin Anesth* 2003;15:582–6.

134. Selander D, Dhuner K-G, Lundborg G. Peripheral nerve injury due to injection needles used for regional anesthesia. An experimental study of the acute effects of needle point trauma. *Acta Anaesth Scand* 1977;21:182.

135. Karakaya d, Baris S, Guldogus F, et al. Brachial plexus injury during subclavian vein catheterization for hemodialysis. *J Clin Anesth* 2000;12:220–3.

136. Nakayama M, Fulita S, Kawamata M, et al. Traumatic aneurysm of the internal jugular vein causing vagal nerve palsy: a rare complication of percutaneous catheterization. *Anesth Analg* 1994;78:598–600.

137. Parikh RD. Horner's syndrome: a complication of percutaneous catheterization of the internal jugular vein. *Anaesthesia* 1972;27:327–9.

138. Turnage WS, Harper JV. Venous air embolism occurring after removal of a central venous catheter. *Anesth Analg* 1991;72:559–60.

139. Akazawa S, Nakaigawa Y, Hotta K. Unrecognized migration of an entire guidewire on insertion of a central venous catheter into the cardiovascular system. *Anesthesiology* 1996;84:241–2.

140. Smyth NPD, Rogers JB. Transvenous removal of catheter emboli from the heart and great veins by endoscopic forceps. *Ann Thorac Surg* 1971;11:403–8.

141. Bossert T, Gummert J, Bittner H, et al. Swan-Ganz catheter-induced severe complications in cardiac surgery: right ventricular perforation, knotting, and rupture of a pulmonary artery. *J Card Surg* 2006;21:292–5.

142. Friedman BA, Jergeleit HC. Perforation of atrium by polyethylene central venous catheter. *JAMA* 1968;203:1141–2.

143. Oropello J, Leibowitz A, Manasia A, et al. Dilator-associated complications of central venous catheter insertion: Possible mechanisms of injury and suggestions. *J Cardiothorac Vasc Anesth* 1996;10:634–7.

144. Royster RL, Johnston WE, Gravlee GP, et al. Arrhythmias during venous cannulation prior to pulmonary artery catheter insertion. *Anesth Analg* 1985;64:1214–6.

145. Eissa NT, Kvetan V. Guide wire as a cause of complete heart block in patients with preexisting left bundle-branch block. *Anesthesiology* 1990;73:772–4.

146. O'Grady NP, Alexander M, Dellinger EP, et al. Guidelines for the prevention of intravascular catheter-related infections. *Infect Control Hosp Epidemiol* 2002;23:759–69.

147. Hu KK, Lipsky BA, Veenstra DL, Saint S. Using maximal sterile barriers to prevent central venous catheter-related infection: a systematic evidence-based review. *Am J Infect Control* 2004;32:142–6.

148. Timsit JF, Sebille V, Farkas JC, et al. Effect of subcutaneous tunneling on internal jugular catheter-related sepsis in critically ill patients: a prospective randomized multicenter study. *JAMA* 1996;276:1416–20.

149. Timsit JF, Bruneel F, Cheval C, et al. Use of tunneled femoral catheters to prevent catheter-related infection. A randomized, controlled trial. *Ann Intern Med* 1999;130:729–35.

150. Leon C, Alvarez-Lerma F, Ruiz-Santana S, et al. Antiseptic chamber-containing hub reduces central venous catheter-related infection: a prospective, randomized study. *Crit Care Med* 2003;31:1318–24.

151. Veenstra DL, Saint S, Saha S, et al. Efficacy of antiseptic-impregnated central venous catheters in preventing catheter-related bloodstream infection: a meta-analysis. *JAMA* 1999;281:261–7.

152. Kamal GD, Pfaller MA, Rempe LE, Jebson PJR. Reduced intravascular catheter infection by antibiotic bonding: a prospective, randomized, controlled trial. *JAMA* 1991;265:2364–8.

153. Cicalini S, Palmieri F, Petrosillo N. Clinical review: new technologies for prevention of intravascular catheter-related infections. *Crit Care* 2004;8:157–62.

154. Maki DG, Ringer M, Alvarado CJ. Prospective randomised trial of povidone-iodine, alcohol, and chlorhexidine for prevention of infection associated with central venous and arterial catheters. *Lancet* 1991;338:339–43.

155. Mimoz O, Pieroni L, Lawrence C, et al. Prospective, randomized trial of two antiseptic solutions for prevention of central venous or arterial catheter colonization and infection in intensive care unit patients. *Crit Care Med* 1996;24:1818–23.

156. Chaiyakunapruk N, Veenstra DL, Lipsky BA, Saint S. Chlorhexidine compared with povidone-iodine solution for vascular catheter-site care: a meta-analysis. *Ann Intern Med* 2002;136:792–801.

157. Mermel LA. Prevention of intravascular catheter-related infections. *Ann Intern Med* 2000;132:391–402.

158. Polderman KH, Girbes AR. Central venous catheter use. Part 2: infectious complications. *Intensive Care Med* 2002;28:18–28.

159. Poses RM, McClish DK, Smith WR, et al. Physicians' judgments of the risks of cardiac procedures. Differences between cardiologists and other internists. *Med Care* 1997;35:603–17.

160. Shah KB, Rao TLK, Laughlin S, El-Etr AA. A review of pulmonary artery catheterization in 6245 patients. *Anesthesiology* 1984;61:271–5.

161. Lopez-Sendon J, Lopez de Sa E, Gonzalez Maqueda I, et al. Right ventricular infarction as a risk factor for ventricular fibrillation during pulmonary artery catheterization using Swan-Ganz catheters. *Am Heart J* 1990;119:207–9.

162. Spring CL, Pozen RG, Rozanski JJ, et al. Advanced ventricular arrhythmias during bedside pulmonary artery catheterization. *Am J Med* 1982;72:203–8.

163. Patil AR. Risk of right bundle-branch block and complete heart block during pulmonary artery catheterization. *Crit Care Med* 1990;18:122–3.

164. Abernathy WS. Complete heart block caused by a Swan-Ganz catheter. *Chest* 1974;65:349.

165. Thomson IR, Dalton BC, Lappas DG, et al. Right bundle-branch block and complete heart block caused by the Swan-Ganz catheter. *Anesthesiology* 1979;51:359–62.

166. Sprung CL, Elser B, Schein RMH, et al. Risk of right bundle-branch block and complete heart block during pulmonary artery catheterization. *Crit Care Med* 1989;17:1–3.

167. Morris D, Mulvihill D, Lew WYW. Risk of developing complete heart block during bedside pulmonary artery catheterization in patients with left bundle-branch block. *Arch Intern Med* 1987;147:2005–10.

168. Hannan AT, Brown M, Bigman O. Pulmonary artery catheter-induced hemorrhage. *Chest* 1984;85:128–31.

169. Durbin CG. The range of pulmonary artery catheter balloon inflation pressures. *J Cardiothorac Anesth* 1990;4:39–42.

170. Dhamee MS, Pattison CZ. Pulmonary artery rupture during cardiopulmonary bypass. *J Cardiothorac Anesth* 1987;1:51–56.

171. Cohen JA, Blackshear RH, Gravenstein N, Woeste J. Increased pulmonary artery perforating potential of pulmonary artery catheters during hypothermia. *J Cardiothorac Vasc Anesth* 1991;5:234–6.

172. Stein JM, Lisbon A. Pulmonary hemorrhage from pulmonary artery catheterization treated with endobronchial intubation. *Anesthesiology* 1981;55:698–9.

173. Sirivella S, Gielchinsky I, Parsonnet V. Management of catheter-induced pulmonary artery perforation: a rare complication in cardiovascular operations. *Ann Thorac Surg* 2001;72:2056–9.

174. Purut CM, Scott SM, Parham JV, Smith PK. Intraoperative management of severe endobronchial hemorrhage. *Ann Thorac Surg* 1991;51:304–7.

175. Laureys M, Golzarian J, Antoine M, Desmet JM. Coil embolization treatment for perioperative pulmonary artery rupture related to Swan-Ganz catheter placement. *Cardiovasc Intervent Radiol* 2004;27:407–9.

176. Abreu AR, Campos MA, Krieger BP. Pulmonary artery rupture induced by a pulmonary artery catheter: a case report and review of the literature. *J Intensive Care Med* 2004;19:291–6.

177. Foote GA, Schabel SI, Hodges M. Pulmonary complications of the flow-directed balloon-tipped catheter. *N Engl J Med* 1974;290:927–31.

178. Ahmed H, Kaufman D, Zenilman M. A knot in the heart. *Am Surg* 2008;74:235–6.

179. Mond HG, Clark DW, Nesbitt SJ, Schlant RC. A technique for unknotting an intracardiac flow-directed balloon catheter. *Chest* 1975;67:731–733.

180. England MR, Murphy MC. A knotty problem. *J Cardiothorac Vasc Anesth* 1997;11:682–3.

181. Eshkevari L, Baker B. Occurrence and removal of a knotted pulmonary artery catheter: a case report. *AANA Journal* 2007;75:423–8.

182. Georghiou GP, Vidne BA, Raanani E. Knotting of a pulmonary artery catheter in the superior vena cava: surgical removal and a word of caution. *Heart* 2004;90:e28.

183. Arnaout S, Diab K, Al-Kutoubi A, Jamaleddine G. Rupture of the chordae of the tricuspid valve after knotting of the pulmonary artery catheter. *Chest* 2001;120:1742–4.

184. Bagul N, Menon N, Pathak R, et al. Knot in the cava – an unusual complication of Swan-Ganz catheters. *Eur J Vasc Endovasc Surg* 2005;29:651–3.

185. Lazzam C, Sanborn TA, Christian F. Ventricular entrapment of a Swan-Ganz catheter: A technique for nonsurgical removal. *J Am Coll Cardiol* 1989;13:1422–4.

186. Sherman S, Wall M, Kennedy D et al. Do pulmonary artery catheters cause or increase tricuspid or pulmonic valvular regurgitation? *Anesth Analg* 2001:92:1117–22.

187. Boscoe MJ, deLange S. Damage to the tricuspid valve with a Swan-Ganz catheter. *BMJ* 1981;283:346–7.

188. O'Toole JD, Wurtzbacher JJ, Wearner NE, Jain AC. Pulmonary valve injury and insufficiency during pulmonary-artery catheterization. *N Engl J Med* 1979;301:1167–8.

189. Kainuma M, Yamada M, Miyake T. Pulmonary artery catheter passing between the chordae tendineae of the tricuspid valve [correspondence]. *Anesthesiology* 1995;83:1130.

190. Rowley KM, Clubb KS, Smith GJ, Cabin HS.: Right-sided infective endocarditis as a consequence of flow-directed pulmonary-artery catheterization. A clinicopathological study of 55 autopsied patients. *N Engl J Med* 1984;311:1152–6.

191. Greene JF Jr, Fitzwater JE, Clemmer TP. Septic endocarditis and indwelling pulmonary artery catheters. *JAMA* 1975;233:891–2.

192. Kim YL, Richman KA, Marshall BE. Thrombocytopenia associated with Swan-Ganz catheterization in patients. *Anesthesiology* 1980;53:261–2.

193. Hofbauer R, Moser D, Kaye AD, et al. Thrombus formation on the balloon of heparin-bonded pulmonary artery catheters: an ultrastructural scanning electron microscope study. *Crit Care Med* 2000;28:727–35.

194. Mangano DT. Heparin bonding and long-term protection against thrombogenesis. *N Engl J Med* 1982;307:894–5.

195. Moberg PQ, Geary VM, Sheikh FM. Heparin-induced thrombocytopenia: A possible complication of heparin-coated pulmonary artery catheters. *J Cardiothorac Anesth* 1990;4:226–8.

196. Tewari P, Kumar M, Kaushik S. Pulmonary artery catheter misplaced in liver. *J Cardiothorac Vasc Anesth* 1995;9:482–4.

197. Karakaya D, Baris S, Tur A. Pulmonary artery catheter-induced right ventricular perforation during coronary artery bypass surgery. *Br J Anaesth* 1999;82:953.

198. Shin B, McAslan TC, Ayella RJ. Problems with measurements using the Swan-Ganz catheter. *Anesthesiology* 1975;43:474–6.

199. American Society of Anesthesiologists Task Force on Pulmonary Artery Catheterization. Practice guidelines for pulmonary artery catheterization: an updated report by the American Society of Anesthesiologists Task Force on Pulmonary Artery Catheterization. *Anesthesiology* 2003;99:988–1014.

200. Robin ED. Defenders of the pulmonary artery catheter. *Chest* 1988;93:1059–66.

201. Dalen JE, Bone RC. Is it time to pull the pulmonary artery catheter? *JAMA* 1996;276:916–8.

202. Zaidan J, Freniere S. Use of a pacing pulmonary artery catheter during cardiac surgery. *Ann Thorac Surg* 1983;35:633–6.

203. Mora CT, Seltzer JL, McNulty SE. Evaluation of a new design pulmonary artery catheter for intraoperative ventricular pacing. *J Cardiothorac Anesth* 1988;2:303–8.

204. Trankina MF, White RD. Perioperative cardiac pacing using an atrioventricular pacing pulmonary artery catheter. *J Cardiothorac Anesth* 1989;3:154–62.

205. Risk SC, Brandon D, D'Ambra MN, et al. Indications for the use of pacing pulmonary artery catheters in cardiac surgery. *J Cardiothorac Vasc Anesth* 1992;6:275–80.

206. Kay HR, Afshari M, Barash P, et al. Measurement of ejection fraction by thermal dilution techniques. *J Surg Res* 1983;34:337–46.

207. Spinale FG, Zellner JL, Mukherjee R, Crawford FA. Placement considerations for measuring thermodilution right ventricular ejection fraction. *Crit Care Med* 1991;19:417–21.

208. Assmann R, Heidelmeyer CF, Trampisch HJ, et al. Right ventricular function assessed by thermodilution technique during apnea and mechanical ventilation. *Crit Care Med* 1991;19:810–7.

209. Krouskop RW, Cabatu EE, Chelliah BP, et al. Accuracy and clinical utility of an oxygen saturation catheter. *Crit Care Med* 1983;11:744–9.

210. Reinhart K, Kuhn HJ, Hartog C, Bredle DL. Continuous central venous and pulmonary artery oxygen saturation monitoring in the critically ill. *Intensive Care Med* 2004;30:1572–8.

211. Scuderi P, MacGregor D, Bowton D, et al. A laboratory comparison of three pulmonary artery oximetry catheters. *Anesthesiology* 1994;81(1):245–53.

212. Pond CG, Blessios G, Bowlin J, et al. Perioperative evaluation of a new mixed venous oxygen saturation catheter in cardiac surgical patients. *J Cardiothorac Vasc* 1992;6:280–2.

213. Armaganidis A, Dhainaut JF, Billard JL, et al. Accuracy assessment for three fiberoptic pulmonary artery catheters for SvO2 monitoring. *Intensive Care Med* 1994;20:484–8.

Chapter

8

Cardiac output and intravascular volume

Mukul Kapoor and Marc Stone

It is absolutely necessary to conclude that the blood in the animal body is impelled in a circle, and is in a state of ceaseless motion; that this is the act or function which the heart performs by means of its pulse; and that it is the sole and only end of the motion and contraction of the heart.

William Harvey (1578–1657)

Introduction

The management of a hemodynamically unstable patient is one of the most challenging experiences for the acute care physician; incorrect treatment or delay in appropriate treatment can result in morbidity and mortality. Anesthesia- and sepsis-induced changes in arterial or venous tone, intravascular volume, ventricular performance, peripheral vascular reactivity, core temperature, and blood rheology sum to make the moment-to-moment assessment of cardiovascular status difficult. Monitoring the heart rate and blood pressure may be adequate for many patients, but in a milieu of cardiovascular abnormality, more detailed measurements are needed, as the cardiovascular system is too complex for assessment with something as ingenuous as heart rate and systemic blood pressure.[1]

Hypovolemia, systemic vasodilation, and myocardial dysfunction are frequently responsible for hemodynamic instability during the perioperative period and in the intensive care unit. An accurate assessment of cardiac preload is of paramount importance in critically ill patients with true/relative hypovolemia to direct therapy and optimize the cardiac output. Although the majority of patients with hemodynamic compromise are preload-responsive, excessive fluid administration will provoke fluid overload in the remaining ones.[2] Cardiac filling pressures, measured using a pulmonary artery catheter (PAC), are still widely used to guide fluid therapy in major surgery and critical care, but critical analysis of clinical studies has shown that cardiac filling pressures are of little value to predict ventricular filling volume, or the hemodynamic effects of intravascular volume expansion.[3,4]

The first method to measure cardiac output (CO) in humans was described by Adolf Fick in 1870.[5] In 1954, Fegler introduced CO measurement by thermodilution, but it was the development of the balloon-tipped PAC by Swan and Ganz in the 1970s that made the technique more practicable.[6] The PAC was initially used to measure intracardiac pressures, but CO measurement later became its primary function. At the time of this writing, the PAC remains the gold-standard device for determination of CO, although it is hardly ideal, for a variety of reasons (discussed subsequently).

An ideal device to measure CO would be continuous, automated, self-calibrating, easy to use, and noninvasive. It would rapidly provide an accurate and comprehensive measure of cardiac performance (contractility, preload, and afterload) in an operator-independent, cost-effective, and reproducible manner, without increasing morbidity and mortality.[7,8] A number of devices to estimate CO have since been introduced, but the search for an ideal CO monitor continues.

This chapter discusses the basic and essential principles underlying determination of CO by various methodologies. Specific devices that employ the different methodologies are discussed, including PAC, NICO, CCCombo, OptiQ CCO/Q-vue, truCATH, PiCCO, LiDCO, Finometer, FloTrac/Vigileo, endotracheal CAO monitor (ECOM), and ultrasonic CO monitor (USCOM). The chapter concludes with discussions of complications, accreditation, and practice parameters.

Technical aspects of the measurement of cardiac output

Systems based on Fick's principle

Fick's principle is based on the conservation of mass. Fick postulated that all oxygen taken up by the lungs is completely transferred to the blood, and the oxygen consumption per unit time is the product of blood flow through the lungs and the arteriovenous oxygen content difference. The application of the principle provides an accurate and reproducible measure of CO. The arterial–mixed venous oxygen content difference is calculated by analysis of arterial and mixed venous blood samples, drawn from an arterial line and the distal port of a PAC, respectively, whereas the oxygen consumption is calculated by inspired/expired gas analysis and minute ventilation. CO is calculated by relating oxygen consumption to arterial and mixed venous oxygen content using the equation

$$Q = [VO_2/(CaCo_2 - CvCO_2)] \times 100,$$

where Q is the cardiac output, VO_2 is the oxygen consumption (content difference between inspired and exhaled gas), CaO_2 is oxygen content of arterial blood, and CvO_2 is oxygen content of mixed venous blood.

This estimation is accurate when the hemodynamic status is sufficiently stable to allow constant gas diffusion during transit of blood through the lungs. However, the estimation may not be valid in critically ill patients with unstable hemodynamics and who require high fractional inspired oxygen. In theory, Fick's technique is the gold standard for cardiac output measurement, but it is invasive, complex in methodology, and difficult to perform.

Differential carbon dioxide Fick partial rebreathing technique

A modification of the Fick principle is used in the differential carbon dioxide partial rebreathing method used by the NOVA NICO monitor (Novametrix Medical Systems; Wallingford, CT). Changes in CO_2 elimination and partial pressure of end-tidal CO_2 following a brief period of partial rebreathing are used to estimate pulmonary capillary blood flow, instead of oxygen consumption, as CO_2 elimination is easier to measure. The rebreathing maneuver is used to estimate mixed venous partial pressure of CO_2, which, combined with concurrent measurements of end-tidal CO_2 and CO_2 production, gives a non-invasive estimate of CO.[9] The monitor offers the advantage of also measuring CO_2 production, continuous tidal volumes and flows, and compliance assessment on a breath-by-breath basis, and provides a continuous estimate of metabolic demand. The NOVA NICO rebreathing circuit can be incorporated into both the anesthesia machine breathing circuit and the ventilator circuit (Figure 8.1).

Rebreathing CO_2 reduces the blood–alveolar gradient and thereby reduces the CO_2 flux. This elevates arterial CO_2 content, which restabilizes during the next baseline phase. CO_2 data

measured during the rebreathing and the nonrebreathing periods is used to calculate the ratio of the change in CO_2 elimination and computation of CO[10] using the formula

$$Q = VCO_2/(CvCO_2 - CaCO_2),$$

where Q is the cardiac output, VCO_2 is the carbon dioxide output (content difference between exhaled and inspired gas), $CaCO_2$ is the carbon dioxide content of arterial blood, and CvO_2 is the carbon dioxide content of mixed venous blood.

Clinical trials with NICO have shown reasonably good correlation with CO measured by thermodilution CO (TDCO).[11,12] However, the monitor requires stable CO_2 elimination for reliable CO measurements and has been reported to be unreliable at low-volume minute ventilation and in spontaneous breathing;[13] during rapid changes in pulmonary shunts and dead-space, as in thoracic surgery;[14] and after cardiopulmonary bypass and aortic clamping/unclamping.[15] In intensive care, as the majority of patients are ventilated with modes that allow some spontaneous breathing, the use of the device is limited to patients who are deeply sedated or anesthetized and/or paralyzed.[16] Although the technology was introduced nearly two decades ago, its use remains limited.

Systems based on indicator dilution

The principle of indicator dilution for measuring CO was first described by Stewart.[17] These methods make use of the time taken by flowing blood to dilute an indicator substance introduced to the circulatory system at a given point until it reaches a point downstream to obtain a time dilution curve. Usually these methods require a PAC because the indicator substance must be introduced at a point at which uniform mixing will occur within the total blood flow, prior to the measurement of a dilution curve. The average volume flow is inversely proportional to the integrated area under the dilution curve. The CO, being inversely proportional to the concentration of the indicator sampled downstream, is estimated using the Stewart–Hamilton principle, wherein CO is estimated from the quantity of indicator injected divided by the area under the dilution curve measured downstream.

Dye dilution

A known quantity of dye (normally indocyanine green) is injected into the pulmonary artery, and timed arterial samples are analyzed using a photoelectric spectrometer. Plotting the concentration of dye against time on a semilogarithmic plot (with extrapolation of the straight line created to correct for dye recirculation) allows calculation of cardiac output by the mass of injectate used and the area under the extrapolated curve.

Lithium indicator dilution

A bolus of isotonic lithium chloride solution is injected via a central or peripheral vein. The lithium concentration–time curve is recorded by withdrawing arterial blood past a lithium sensor attached to the arterial line. CO is calculated from the

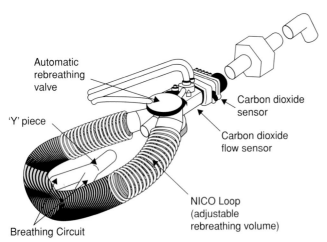

Figure 8.1. NOVA NICO breathing circuit. A pneumatically controlled rebreathing valve is sited within a large-bore tubing loop and a CO_2/flow sensor in the ventilator circuit between the patient and the Y-connector. The rebreathing valve cycles through two phases. During the first phase, the rebreathing valve directs the flow straight through the valve, whereas during the second phase, positive pressure activates the valve to direct the end-expired gas into the expandable large-bore tubing loop. This end-exhaled gas is accumulated for inspiration during the patient's next breath. (Modified from ref. 8, *permission granted*).

lithium dose and the area under the concentration–time curve prior to recirculation. Blood flows into the sensor assembly at a rate controlled by a peristaltic pump. A bolus dose of 0.15 to 0.30 mmol of lithium chloride is needed for an average adult.

Thermodilution cardiac output

Pulmonary artery thermodilution methods use change of temperature of blood flowing in the right-sided circulation for the measurement of blood flow. The thermodilution principle is based on the injection of a quantified cold charge and registration of its dilution (i.e. the subsequent change in temperature of the blood at a point downstream in the direction of the blood flow). As heat, unlike a dye, will mix well irrespective of laminar flow in the blood vessels, the thermoindicator can be injected into the right atrium and the temperature registered in the pulmonary artery.

The TDCO method uses a cold solution to create a thermal deficit as a variant of the indicator–dilution method.

A known bolus of a cold sterile solution is injected, as a thermal indicator, into the right atrium through the proximal port of a PAC. A thermistor located at the distal end of the PAC detects the change in temperature of the blood downstream. The distance between the injection and detection sites should be as short as possible to reduce extravascular loss of the thermal indicator owing to heat exchange in the pulmonary vascular bed. This can be attained by injecting into the right atrium and detection in the PA.

The normal thermodilution curve peaks rapidly and then follows an exponential decay, until there is recirculation or delayed cooling from the residual indicator in the PA catheter (Figure 8.2). CO is inversely proportional to the area under the curve (temperature change over time). A small area under the curve indicates a high CO. The faster blood flows through the heart, the earlier the peak and sharper the drop, because the catheter senses temperature change over a short period.

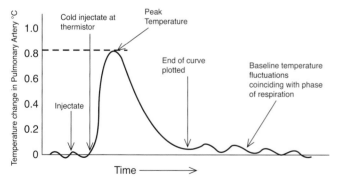

Figure 8.2. Typical thermodilution curve. CO is determined using the Stewart–Hamilton equation: $Q = K_1 \times K_2 \times V_I \times (T_B - T_I)/\int T_b(t)\,dt$, where Q is the cardiac output; K_1 is a density factor defined as the specific heat multiplied by the specific gravity of the injectate divided by the product of the specific heat and gravity of blood; K_2 is a computation constant taking into account the catheter dead space, the heat exchange in transit, and injection rate; V_I is the volume of injectate; T_B and T_I the initial temperature of the blood and injectate respectively; and $\int Tb(t)\,dt$ is the change of blood temperature as a function of time and corresponds to the area under the thermodilution curve.

A low cardiac output results in a larger area under the curve. When blood flows slowly (low cardiac output), the area under the curve is greater because the catheter senses changes in temperature over a longer period.

The change in temperature of blood in the PA causes a change in the thermistor (Wheatstone bridge) resistance, which allows calculation of the area under the thermodilution curve. A correction factor is introduced for the loss of indicator by transit of the cold solution through the catheter into the right atrium. From the Stewart–Hamilton equation, the cardiac output is calculated by a computer, and a thermodilution curve also can be recorded. As there are limits to the numerical values the computer can handle, the computation factor must be altered for very low and for very high outputs.

Even under ideal circumstances, TDCO measurements have a 10 percent error rate.[18,19] The accuracy of the thermodilution technique can be influenced by various factors:

1. Presence of a cardiac shunt: right and left ventricular output may differ.
2. Tricuspid or pulmonary valve regurgitation: backflow of blood and indicator causes underestimation of CO.
3. Variations in blood temperature affecting measurements: after cardiopulmonary bypass, intravenous fluid administration.
4. Speed of the bolus injection and its timing relative to the phase of the respiratory cycle: positive pressure ventilation produces beat-to-beat variations in right ventricular stroke volume during the cycle.
5. Positive end-expiratory pressure.
6. Catheter dysfunction and position of the PAC.
7. Volume and temperature of the injectate.
8. Patient's body position.

To ensure the validity and reliability of the measurement, the following should be checked meticulously:

- Position of the pulmonary artery catheter
- Computation constant of the pulmonary artery catheter (PAC)
- Catheter size
- Temperature of the injectate
- Volume of injectate, 10 mL at room temperature (5 mL if iced)

The difference between the temperature of the injectate and the temperature of the patient's blood should be 10°C.[20] Ten mL of iced injectate produces a greater signal-to-noise ratio than does ten mL of room-temperature injectate or smaller volumes of either iced. Pearl and colleagues recommended the use of 10 mL iced or room-temperature injectate for CO determinations, because 10-mL injectates produced less variability than 3 or 5 mL of injectate.[21] Most reports show no difference in the accuracy or reproducibility whether iced or room-temperature injectate was used.[21,22]

To accurately measure CO, inject cold saline at a constant rate (10 mL within 4 seconds; 5 mL within 2 seconds) during end expiration, using a closed injectate delivery system. Obtain three measurements and assess the cardiac output curve. The average value computed should be within 10 percent of the median value.

Continuous CO monitoring

Advances in technology have allowed for the development of continuous CO monitoring by the use of a random sequence of temperature changes generated by a heating coil within the PAC, which is located in the right ventricle (CCOmbo/Vigilance, Edwards Lifesciences LLC, Irvine, CA; Opti Q CCO/Q-vue, Abbott Critical Care Systems, Mountain View, CA). A monitor computes the CO in real time from the fractional changes in temperature detected distally. The heat impulses are generated in a stochastic pattern, and subsequent processing allows for automated updating of CO within minutes.[23] The heating filament is cycled on and off in a pseudorandom sequence, and CO is calculated using a cross-correlation algorithm that combines the measured pulmonary artery temperature and the pseudorandom sequence of filament activation.[24] A faulty thermal filament, blood temperature ≤31°C or ≥41°C, electrical interference from electrocautery, and large blood temperature variations can affect calculations.

Other specialized pulmonary artery catheters are available that also use the principle of mass heat transfer. The truCATH (BD Medical Systems) obtains data from the measured amount of energy required to maintain a thermistor, located in the right atrium, at 1°C above the measured blood temperature in the pulmonary artery. Delays in data acquisition prevent these systems from being truly real-time, as there is an inherent delay in response to sudden flow changes. However, there is a reduced need for bolus injections and they provide a better average CO over time compared with intermittent bolus techniques. These systems offer the advantages of possibly being more accurate, convenient, and user-independent; reducing demands on the time of carers; and providing an early signal of hemodynamic alterations.[23,25]

The passage of the PAC catheter into the right-sided circulation has the added advantage of measuring the right atrial, pulmonary artery, and the pulmonary artery occlusion pressure.

Estimation of the preload of the cardiac chambers – and, indirectly, the intravascular volume – is thus possible. Advances in computation techniques have also resulted in development of algorithms to calculate the global end-diastolic volume and the right ventricular end-diastolic and end-systolic volumes, facilitating better estimation of the intravascular blood volume.[26] With advances in technology, the continuous CO catheters have also been incorporated with oximetry sensors to continuously measure mixed venous oxygen saturation online.

Systems based on pulse contour analysis

Arterial pulse contour analysis was first described in the early 1940s. It is a technique to measure and monitor stroke volume on a beat-to-beat basis from the arterial pulse pressure waveform and is based on the principle that the magnitude of the arterial pulse pressure and the pressure decay profile describe a unique stroke volume for given arterial input impedance (Figure 8.3). A number of devices are commercially available that provide CO data following calibration by an independent CO measurement. Some of them require central venous access to perform a TDCO measurement for calibration (analyzed by a thermistor present in the arterial catheter tip), but cannulation of the right heart or pulmonary artery is not required.

Based on models representing the systemic circulation, several methods are used to analyze the pressure waveform, which include the Windkessel model, its modification, and new advanced models. The basic Windkessel model (two-element model – aortic impedance, arterial and peripheral vascular resistance) assumes that the time constant of the monoexponential pressure decay is determined by the product of systemic vascular resistance and aortic compliance, whereas the modified Windkessel model (three-element model- aortic impedance, arterial compliance, and peripheral vascular resistance), assumes that compliance of the arterial system can be partitioned into central and distal compartments, in which central compliance is distinct from distal compliance.[27,28]

Mechanical ventilation induces cyclic variations in cardiac preload that are reflected in changes in aortic blood flow and arterial pulse pressure within a period of a few pulses.[29]

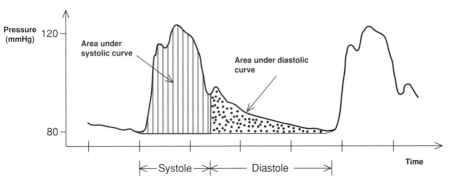

Figure 8.3. Pulse contour analysis waveform. The area under the measured waveform is analyzed to derive ejection systolic area by identifying ventricular ejection and the appearance of the dicrotic notch (closure of the aortic valve). The pulsatile systolic area under the pressure curve above a horizontal line drawn from the diastolic point and bounded by a vertical line through the lowest point of incisura (area under the pressure curve from the start of the upstroke to the incisura) and stroke volume are related by means of characteristic impedance of the aorta.

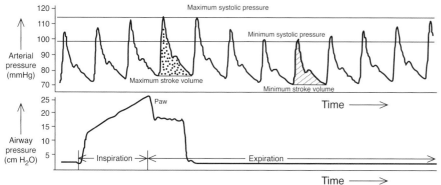

Figure 8.4. Pulse pressure and stroke volume variations, as functional hemodynamic variables, are based on the heart–lung interactions during mechanical ventilation. Respiration-induced changes in left ventricular preload result in cyclic changes in left ventricular stroke volume and in arterial pressure. The left ventricular stroke volume increases during inspiration because left ventricular preload increases, whereas left ventricular afterload decreases. In hypo-volemic patients, the respiratory variations in stroke volume and arterial pressure are of greater magnitude because the venous system is more collapsible. The pulse contour analysis, based on the computation of the area under the systolic portion of the arterial pressure curve, allows a beat-to-beat measurement of left ventricular stroke volume and the quantification of its variation during a short period of a few seconds.

The arterial pulse pressure variation and stroke volume variation, induced by mechanical ventilation, have been shown to be useful in identifying patients likely to respond to volume therapy.[2,30–32] Arterial pulse contour analysis allows the use of arterial pressure waveforms to calculate stroke volume and its change during ventilation, and thus helps determine pulse pressure variation and stroke volume variation (Figure 8.4). The technique helps calculates CO changes and assess global cardiovascular responsiveness to therapies such as fluid and inotropes.

The ratio of pulse pressure variation to stroke volume variation reflects the central capacitor tone, whereas the ratio of mean arterial blood pressure changes to stroke volume variation reflects the arterial tone. The technique thus helps monitor both the arterial and venous tone, which are major determinants of cardiovascular performance.

Concerns have been raised about issues that affect the accuracy of pulse contour analysis-based systems.[33] The major issues raised are

- Nonlinearity of the waveform will affect the algorithm-based calculations, as the compliance of the aorta varies at different arterial pressures. Properties of the aorta also vary with age, gender, distending pressure, and atherosclerosis. Aortic valve pathology, aortic aneurysms, and sympathetic outflow status also influence aortic characteristics.
- The aortic pulse waveform reflects the stroke volume. However, the peripheral arterial pressure waveform (which has higher resonance) is used for monitoring, and thus there is a need for accurate compensation with antiresonance. In addition, continuous flush devices need to be used because damped waveforms may result in an inaccurate assessment of CO.
- Supine/prone position and increased abdominal pressure in obesity may affect aortic distending properties.

The available devices use varied patented algorithms but essentially provide a continuous estimate of CO through analysis of the shape of the pulse wave from a peripherally placed arterial catheter. The stroke volume is estimated from the systolic, diastolic, or both components of the pressure waveform. However, these algorithm-based estimations fail to remain accurate in aortic regurgitation, with use of high-dose vasodilators or vasoconstrictors, and with the use of intraaortic balloon pumps.[34]

Diastolic pulse contour analysis

Diastolic pulse contour analysis is based on the basic Windkessel model and assumes that the arterial blood pressure should decay exponentially during diastolic time intervals with a time constant. By fitting the diastolic decay portion of an individual's arterial waveform to a first-order model (basic Windkessel) or third-order model (modified Windkessel), compliance variables can theoretically be derived. In this model, because the arterial compliance is assumed to be constant, the derived stroke volume values do not reflect the true stroke volume. For accurate values, calibration against a standard method is carried out.

Systolic pulse contour analysis

Wesseling and coworkers developed a pulse contour analysis technique based on a transmission line model of the arterial tree. The Wesseling algorithm involves measuring the systolic portion of the ejection phase divided by aortic impedance to provide a measure of stroke volume.[35] The algorithm uses the three major properties of the aorta and the arterial system (aortic impedance, Windkessel compliance of the arterial system, and peripheral vascular resistance) to compute a flow pulse from an arterial pressure pulsation.[36] According to the Wesseling model, total systemic vascular resistance is a time-varying property of the vascular bed.[37] CO determined by an independent alternative method is used to calibrate the device.

The PiCCO system (Pulsion Medical System; Munich, Germany) is a commercially available continuous CO monitor with a working principle based on the preceding model. However, it differs from this model in that no age-related corrections for pressure-dependent nonlinear changes in aortic cross-sectional area are incorporated. In the newer version of the equipment, the algorithm analyzes the actual shape of the waveform, in addition to computing the pulsatile systolic area.[38] With improvement in computation technology, the device can measure vascular volumes from advanced analysis of the thermodilution curve.

In the PiCCO system, a 20-cm–long arterial catheter with a thermistor embedded in its wall is inserted in the femoral artery. The arterial catheter is connected to the pulse contour analysis computer for monitoring of arterial blood pressure, heart rate, temperature, and measurements derived from the arterial pressure wave. The device is initially calibrated by TDCO measurements, randomized within the respiratory cycle, by injection of saline solution at a temperature lower than 7°C via a central venous catheter, and the subsequent detection of the cold saline injection by the thermistor in the arterial catheter. Beat-to-beat calculations are averaged over 30-second cycles and displayed as a numerical value.

Continuous CO assessed by PICCO and by TDCO have been found to be comparable by a number of studies; however, the monitor needs to be recalibrated if the systemic vascular resistance changes markedly.[37,39–41]

Modelflow pulse contour analysis

The Modelflow method computes an aortic flow waveform from the arterial pressure waveform using the three-element model developed by Wesseling and associates.[36] It computes the arterial flow waveform from the pressure waveform with continuous nonlinear corrections for variations in aortic diameter, impedance, and compliance during the arterial pulsation. The patient's gender, age, height, and weight are entered into the Modelflow computer to determine pressure–volume, pressure–compliance, and pressure–characteristic impedance relationships using Langewouters' equations, which are based on population averages. This model is simulated digitally in real time and supplied with the sampled arterial pressure waveform.[42]

The aortic impedance is a function of aortic cross-sectional area, the instantaneous flow, and compliance. Postmortem studies have shown that aortic cross-sectional area is a function of pressure by an arctangent relation and also of the patient's age, gender, height, and weight.[43,44] The aortic impedance and arterial compliance are computed making use of a built-in database of arctangent area–pressure relationships derived from these studies. Both compliance and impedance are nonlinear and are functions of the elasticity of the aorta. This nonlinear property is taken into account to calculate stroke volume and is presented in terms of the aortic pressure area relation and its derivative. The subject's gender and age are also input. The instantaneous impedance and compliance values obtained are used in a model simulation to compute an aortic flow waveform. The peripheral vascular resistance is calculated for each beat and updated. Integration of flow waveform per beat gives stroke volume.

The Finometer (Finapres Medical Systems BV; Amsterdam, The Netherlands) is a noninvasive blood pressure measurement monitor that uses proprietary Modelflow methodology to provide beat-to-beat CO monitoring. The system can operate noninvasively by using the volume–clamp method of obtaining finger arterial pressure tracings with the Physiocal algorithm to periodically correct the system for changes such as hematocrit, physiologic stress, or smooth muscle tone. The system includes a servo-controlled pressure device for applying the rapidly changing pressures to the finger-pressure cuff as well as a photoplethysmography light source and a detector for application of the volume–clamp method. The front-end unit is connected to the Finometer for finger arterial tracing determination, brachial pressure derivations, and CO determinations. The system has the ability to trend changes in CO. However, if absolute CO values are desired, a calibration with another CO determination is necessary.[38]

The Modelflow and Finometer have been reported as inaccurate when evaluated against TDCO.[45,46] However, when the devices are calibrated by an independent mode of CO determination, the CO values are reliable and accurate.[47,48]

Pulse power analysis

The arterial blood pressure waveform measured in a peripheral artery arises from the interaction between the arterial system and the heart (i.e. an incident pressure wave ejected from the heart and a reflected wave from the peripheral arterial system). At any point in the arterial system, a measured waveform may be decomposed into its forward and backward components. Theoretically, if wave reflection were absent, then the pressure and flow contours in the aorta would be identical, their magnitudes being related by the aortic characteristic impedance. Differences between the pressure and flow contours in the aorta occur because backward waves result in augmentation of the pressure but retardation of the flow. Depending on the distance of the sampling site from the heart and the patient's age, the reflected wave characteristics change. To calculate stroke volume, the two waves need to be analyzed individually.[49]

The algorithm used is based on the assumption that the net power change in a cardiac cycle is stroke volume, less the blood lost to the periphery during the beat, and that the net power and net flow relate to each other. The algorithm used thus caters to this aspect. The method is independent of the position of the sampling site, as the whole beat is analyzed. The pressure wave is transformed to a volume wave and the net power and beat period are derived from the volume waveform, using autocorrelation. Net power is proportional to net flow. Changes in stroke volume, rather than absolute values, are calculated using this method.[49]

Popular commercial equipment that make use of pulse power analysis include the LiDCO *plus* (LiDCO Ltd; Cambridge, UK) and the Flo Trac/Vigileo (Edwards Lifesciences LLC; Irvine, CA). Both the devices use proprietary algorithms to derive CO and other derived parameters. Similar to the PiCCO system, both these devices also display the pulse pressure variation and the stroke volume variation, which are indicative of the patient's intravascular volume status.

The LiDCO system needs to be calibrated using the lithium dilution technique, by placing 0.3 mmol of lithium chloride in an indwelling central venous line and then flushing this line rapidly with 20 mL of 0.9% saline, ensuring a rapid bolus of lithium chloride entering into the circulation. A lithium-specific sensor connected to the arterial line detects the change in lithium ion concentration in blood coming in contact with it and generating a lithium indicator dilution curve to derive the CO. Although this dose has no known pharmacological effect, the technique is contraindicated in patients receiving therapeutic lithium. High doses of neuromuscular blocking agents, with quaternary ammonium ions, can interfere with the sensing electrode; hence, lithium calibration should be performed prior to the administration of these agents.[38]

The Flo Trac/Vigileo system can derive CO from the arterial waveform without the need for an independent method of calibration. It bases its calculations on arterial waveform characteristics in conjunction with patient demographic data. CO can be measured directly from a conventional arterial line attached to the sensor of the monitor, making CO monitoring appear "deceptively simple."[34]

The performance of LiDCO and the Flo Trac has been evaluated vis-à-vis PAC and found to be comparable in patients.[50] CO value measures were found to be interchangeable with TDCO in 80 percent of uncomplicated cardiac surgical patients.[51] However, CO measurements by the devices have been reported as inaccurate in hyperdynamic circulations;[52] in the presence of altered arterial pressure waveform, as in aortic regurgitation and aortic counter-pulsation;[53] and in the presence of alterations of vascular tone.[54]

Pressure-recording analytical method

The pressure-recording analytic method (PRAM) determines continuous CO changes from the arterial pressure wave via mathematic analysis of the arterial pressure profile changes. It is a technique based on the mathematical analysis of pulse profile changes based on the theory of perturbations, by which any physical system under the effect of a perturbation tends to react to achieve its own state of minimum energy. The basic principle is that in any given vessel, volume changes occur mainly because of radial expansion of the artery in response to variations in pressure. The method analyzes the arterial pressure wave from a standard peripheral or centrally inserted arterial catheter, without need for independent CO calibration.

The algorithm does not use retrospectively collected aortic impedance and compliance data obtained. PRAM analyzes the entire waveform, including the systolic ejection, compliance, and impedance, as well as the diastolic portion of flow related to peripheral vascular resistance. The technique recognizes that volume changes in the arterial system are related primarily to the radial expansion of the system in response to blood pressure changes. Involved in this process are the force of cardiac ejection, aortic impedance to inflow into the aorta, arterial compliance that elastically stores energy of the cardiac ejection, and the vascular resistance providing retrograde reflections.[38] In an animal study, the PRAM device was reported to measure CO comparable with TDCO, during various hemodynamic states.[55]

Systems based on electrical impedance cardiography

William Kubicek and National Aeronautical and Space Administration (NASA) researchers developed thoracic electrical bioimpedance to study cardiovascular hemodynamics of astronauts in absence of gravity – that is, under conditions mimicking space.[56] Kubicek described the thorax as a cylinder evenly perfused with blood of specific resistivity, but Sramek later showed that the thorax behaves electrically more like a truncated cone.[57] Aortic blood volume varies during systole and diastole, which results in a phasic change in electrical resistance through the thorax during the cardiac cycle. The technique involves continuous measurement of this change in impedance, caused by a fluctuation of blood volume, to measure and calculate stroke volume, CO, myocardial contractility, and total thoracic fluid status.

The electrodes define the upper and lower limits of the thorax, and the distance between them is measured to obtain the thoracic length (Figure 8.5). A high-frequency, low-amplitude alternating current is introduced through the transmitting thoracic electrodes; the sensing thoracic electrodes measure impedance associated with the blood flow in the aorta during the cardiac cycle. By measuring the impedance changes during the pulse flow and the time intervals between these changes, stroke volume can be calculated. Increased blood volume, flow velocity, and alignment of red blood cells reduce impedance during systole, whereas the opposite effects during diastole increase impedance (Figure 8.6).

Stroke volume can be determined from the impedance curve by extrapolating to the impedance change that would result if no blood were to flow out of the thorax during systole. Impedance change is approximated by drawing a tangent to the impedance

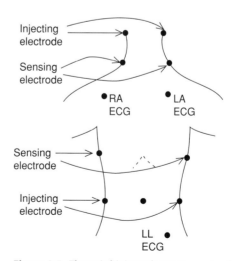

Figure 8.5. Thoracic bioimpedance. Four pairs of electrodes and a set of ECG leads are used to measure the impedance changes and, thereby, the hemodynamic parameters. Each pair of electrodes consists of a transmitting and a sensing electrode. Two pairs are applied to the base of the neck on directly opposite sides, and two pairs are placed at the level of the sterno–xiphoid junction, directly opposite from each other.

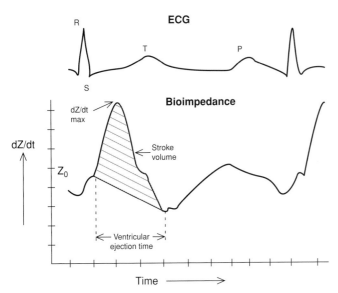

Figure 8.6. Bioimpedance. The change in impedance is measured from the baseline impedance (Z_0), which reflects total thoracic fluid volume. The change in impedance related to time (dZ/dt) generates a waveform similar to the aortic flow curve and is a reflection of left ventricular contractility. Simultaneous ECG recording helps calculation of ventricular ejection time of each cardiac cycle.

curve at the point of its maximum rate of change. The stroke volume is calculated using the formula

$$Stroke\ Volume = \rho \times L^2 / Z_0^2 x(dZ/dt)_{max} \times VET$$

where ρ is the resistivity of blood, L is the mean distance between the inner electrodes, VET is the ventricular ejection time, $(dZ/dt)_{max}$ is the maximum value of change in impedance relative to time, and Z_0 is the basal thoracic impedance. VET is obtained from the dZ/dt versus time curve and ECG.

Electrocautery, mechanical ventilation, and surgical manipulations distort the impedance signal, leading to inaccurate readings. Alterations in cardiac performance resulting from anesthetics, myocardial ischemia, and alterations in loading conditions may cause errors in measurements, limiting the usefulness of bioimpedance cardiac output measurement in patients with coronary artery disease and impaired ventricular function. Changes in lead placement or changes in tissue water content, as seen in fluid shifts and pulmonary edema, may interfere with the signal. Bioimpedance systems have little control over the percentage of current passing through the vascular structures as the electrical impedance of the lungs changes with respiration, thus varying the total current passing through blood-containing structures. Bioimpedance systems are not reliable in patients after cardiopulmonary bypass, kidney transplants, congestive heart failure, pulmonary edema, sepsis, pregnancy, abdominal surgery, or critical illness.[58–64]

A novel system for the measurement of CO based on bioimpedance, called the *endotracheal cardiac output monitor* (ECOM), has also been assessed. It provides a continuous measurement of CO derived from impedance measurements from electrodes on the balloon and on the shaft of an endotracheal

tube. The shaft electrode serves as a ground. The field current is produced between the balloon electrode and the ground electrode on the tube. Orthogonal pairs of sensing electrodes on the balloon are used to measure the impedance signals.[65]

Thoracic electrical bioimpedance has been evaluated and compared with TDCO. CO values measured were reported equivalent to TDCO-derived values.[66,67]

Systems based on Doppler ultrasound

High-frequency sound waves easily penetrate skin and other body tissues. On encountering tissues of different acoustic density, a fraction of an emitted ultrasound signal is reflected.[68] When a sound beam is directed to a moving object, such as blood, the reflected sound wave changes its frequency (Doppler shift). The magnitude of this shift is directly proportional to the velocity of blood flow. Mathematically it is expressed as

$$Fd = 2fo/C \times V \times cos\theta,$$

where Fd represents the Doppler shift, fo is the transmitted frequency, C is the velocity of ultrasound in blood (constant), V is the velocity of the moving blood, and $cos\theta$ is the cosine of the angle between the direction of the moving blood and the transmitted ultrasound beam.[69] Stroke volume can be calculated by multiplying the average blood velocity during a systolic cycle by the ejection time (stroke distance) and by the cross-sectional area through which blood flows.[70] Doppler signals can be obtained with an ultrasound probe placed externally at the suprasternal notch directed at the ascending aorta, at the tip of an endotracheal tube, or at the tip of an esophageal probe directed at the descending thoracic aorta.

To measure peak velocity blood flow in the ascending aortic or pulmonary artery with surface ultrasound, the transducer is positioned either in the left parasternal position to measure transpulmonary blood flow or the suprasternal position to measure transaortic blood flow. The ultrasound beam should be transmitted parallel to the direction of blood flow; only angles up to 20° are clinically acceptable for measurements of blood velocity and, consequently, of CO. The cross-sectional area of the aorta can be determined by two-dimensional or M-mode echocardiography but more commonly is derived from a nomogram stored in the computer based on age, sex, height, and weight. There is 5 percent to 17 percent variation in the cross-sectional area of the aorta between systole and diastole; this can introduce error in calculations. Although nomograms may correlate well in large population studies, they may be invalid for an individual patient.[71]

The USCOM ultrasonic cardiac output monitor (USCOM Pty Ltd; Coffs Harbour, NSW, Australia) is a commercially available device that measures cardiac output transcutaneously using such a transducer, based on continuous-wave Doppler ultrasound. It is more accurate than pulsed Doppler at higher velocities and does not need to obtain a two-dimensional image of the heart/outflow tract and accurate selection of a sample area.[72]

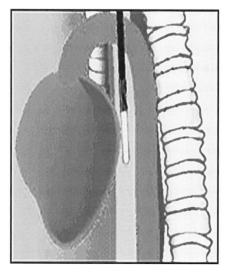

Figure 8.7. Esophageal Doppler. The esophageal Doppler probe remains stable in the esophageal lumen and is positioned to maximize descending aortic flow signals.

Esophageal Doppler monitoring offers the advantages of the probe being in close proximity of the descending aorta, thus providing an excellent window for obtaining Doppler signals (Figure 8.7). A correction factor (K-factor) is incorporated in the equation to account for blood flow distributed to the head and upper extremities, but this itself may introduce a source of error in the measurement of CO, as it can fluctuate during surgery as a response to changes in sympathetic tone, arterial blood pressure, and alterations in anesthetic depth.[73,74] Esophageal probes are available that allow near-simultaneous measurement of the velocity of the descending aortic flow and the descending aortic diameter.

Transtracheal Doppler monitoring uses a pulsed Doppler probe transducer mounted on the tip of a standard endotracheal tube to obtain the aortic diameter and measure the Doppler shift of the ultrasound beam reflected by the blood in the ascending aorta. The patient's trachea is intubated with a Doppler Tube (Applied Biometrics; Minetonka, MN); Doppler flow signals and visual representation of forward and reverse flow are used for optimum positioning of the transducer. The angle between the vector of the ultrasound signal and the direction of blood flow is used to calculate both the aortic diameter and blood velocity; this angle is assumed to be constant. Similarly, the aortic diameter is assumed to be constant throughout the cardiac cycle.[75]

Transesophageal echocardiography (TEE) is an essential perioperative diagnostic and monitoring tool; it is widely used to assess cardiac anatomy, left ventricular function, preload, myocardial ischemia, and cardiac valve function and repair. With TEE, CO can be derived by measurement of flow through a cardiac valve (most commonly, the mitral or aortic valve), left ventricular outflow tract, or main pulmonary artery. Perrino and colleagues have described a single transducer probe position to monitor left ventricular regional/global wall motion and also measure CO, with minimal positioning adjustments.[76]

The TEE probe is positioned to obtain a transverse plane, transgastric short-axis view of the left ventricle at the midpapillary level. By rotating the imaging array to approximately 120°, the left ventricular outflow tract and ascending aorta can be imaged lying parallel to the ultrasound beam, and aortic blood flow velocities measured by a continuous-wave Doppler beam focused at the level of the aortic valve. The aortic valve area is measured by planimetry. The CO may also be calculated by calculating the stroke volume, from the end-diastolic and end-systolic volume, and multiplying it by the heart rate.

The USCOM device has been found to be reliable, on evaluation in animal experiments and clinical trials.[72,77,78] Clinical trials using esophageal Doppler devices have given inconsistent results, probably because the techniques are operator-dependent and need frequent manipulation of the probe.[74,79]

A comparison of various modalities available to measure CO are presented in Table 8.1.

Parameters monitored

The parameters monitored by the different CO monitoring modalities are tabulated in Table 8.2.

The TDCO-based systems (the most practical dye dilution-based systems) are capable of measuring and deriving, with help of specialized PAC catheters and monitoring computers, the following parameters or indices continuously or intermittently: CO; central venous pressure; pulmonary artery pressure; pulmonary artery occlusion pressure; systemic vascular resistance and index; pulmonary vascular resistance and index; left/right ventricular stroke work index; right ventricular stroke volume and index; right ventricular end-diastolic volume and index; right ventricular end-systolic volume and index; right ventricular stroke volume and index; and right ventricular ejection fraction.

In addition, the computer can derive the global end-diastolic volume, intrathoracic volume, and extravascular lung water from the collected data. The thermoindicator injectate disperses volumetrically and thermally within the pulmonary and cardiac volumes. The volume of distribution is termed the *intrathoracic thermal volume*, which is the sum of the intrathoracic blood volume and extravascular lung water. The intrathoracic blood volume comprises the end-diastolic volumes of all four cardiac chambers (global end-diastolic volume) and the pulmonary blood volume.

The pulse contour analysis-based systems are capable of measuring and deriving the pulse-continuous CO, systemic vascular resistance, stroke volume variation, and pulse pressure variation, apart from arterial pressure and heart rate. Aside from these parameters, the systems needing TDCO with calibration also reflect global end-diastolic volume, intrathoracic volume, and extravascular lung water derived from the TDCO data. However, these parameters are not measured in real time.

The electrical impedance cardiography-based systems calculate CO from the stroke volume and heart rate. They can also measure thoracic fluid content, left ventricular ejection time, systemic vascular resistance, and left cardiac work index.

Table 8.1. Comparison of various modalities of measuring cardiac output

System	Technique	Degree of Invasiveness	Arterial cannulation	Calibration by another method required	Continuous real-time	Remarks
Fick's principle	Direct Fick's	Face mask	No	No	No	Experimental
	Differential carbon dioxide partial rebreathing	Endotracheal tube/face mask	No	No	Yes	Measures only CO
Indicator dilution	Dye dilution	Central vein	Yes	No	No	Repeated measurements not possible
	Intermittent TDCO	Pulmonary artery	No	No	No	Clinical gold standard
	Continuous TDCO	Pulmonary artery	No	No	Yes	Special catheters available for mixed venous oximetry and end-diastolic volume estimation in addition
Pulse contour	Diastolic contour	Pulmonary artery	Yes	Yes	Yes	
	Systolic contour	Pulmonary artery/central vein	Yes	Yes	Yes	
	Pulse pressure	Pulmonary artery*	Yes	Yes*	Yes	*Lithium dilution to calibrate in LiDCO. No calibration in Flotrac
	Modelflow	Pulmonary artery	Yes	Yes	Yes	Only trend monitoring if not calibrated
	Pressure recording analytical method	No	Yes	No	Yes	
Electric impedance cardiography	Thoracic	No	No	No	Yes	
	Endotracheal	Endotracheal tube	No	No	Yes	
Doppler ultrasound	Esophageal	Esophageal	No	No	No	
	Transtracheal	No	No	No	Yes	
	TEE	Esophageal	No	No	No	

Table 8.2. Cardiac performance– and intravascular volume–related parameters measured by the different cardiac output techniques

Parameter	Differential CO_2 partial rebreathing	Thermodilution cardiac output	Arterial pulse contour analysis	Electrical impedance cardiography	Doppler ultrasound
Cardiac performance–related					
Continuous cardiac output	Yes	Yes	Yes	Yes	Yes
Pulmonary artery pressures	No	Yes	No	No	No
Left/right ventricular stroke work/volume	No	Yes	Yes	Yes	Yes
Systemic/pulmonary vascular resistance	No	Yes	Yes	Yes	No
Intravascular volume related					
Central venous pressure	No	Yes	No	No	No
Global end-diastolic volume	No	Yes	Yes*	Yes	No
Intrathoracic volume	No	Yes	Yes*	Yes	No
Extravascular lung water	No	Yes	Yes*	Yes	No
Stroke volume/pulse pressure variation	No	No	Yes	No	Yes
Right ventricular end-diastolic volume	No	Yes	No	No	Yes
Left ventricular end-diastolic area	No	No	No	No	Yes

* Parameters measured not in real-time but only during calibration, using thermodilution technique.

Measurements of most real-time Doppler ultrasound-based systems are limited to cardiac output; they give no indication of other hemodynamic variables, such as pressure measurements, vascular resistance, or stroke work calculations. TEE monitoring provides multiple data apart from cardiac output and intravascular-related parameters but has the disadvantage of not being a continuous real-time monitor. The left ventricular end-diastolic area index can be estimated by TEE, which is a sensitive parameter for intravascular volume assessment.

Evidence of utility

Clinically, CO should be measured in patients with unstable cardio–circulatory status and those dependent on the administration of catecholamines. The measured CO and the derived values serve as the basis for therapeutic decisions. If such decisions are made based on incorrect information, the result may prove fatal for the patient.[80] A number of studies in critical care have shown the unreliability of clinical and radiological signs to evaluate hemodynamic status.[81,82]

The value of more comprehensive cardiovascular monitoring, especially with new noninvasive devices for estimating CO, is well documented.[1,83] There is sufficient evidence to show that CO monitoring-directed hemodynamic management is beneficial, at least in patients at risk of – rather than having – established organ failure, such as high-risk surgical patients.[84]

The outcome benefit from hemodynamic manipulation using either invasive or noninvasive monitoring techniques has been demonstrated in high-risk surgery, severe heart failure, and sepsis.[85–88] However, few studies have demonstrated outcome benefit in critically ill patients in whom metabolic, inflammatory, and cellular processes are often too far advanced for benefit to be gained from hemodynamic manipulations that prevent and/or reverse tissue hypoxia.[84,89] A study in patients in cardiogenic shock also found that the PAC provided hemodynamic information that cannot be obtained by clinical evaluation.[90]

A landmark study by Connors and coworkers[91] in the mid-1990s suggested a rise in mortality rates in patients receiving a Swan-Ganz catheter, leading to a call for a moratorium on the catheter's use.[92] The outcomes of this study were later questioned, as most ICUs during that period had adopted Shoemaker's "supra-normalized oxygen delivery philosophy" to raise the cardiac index and oxygen delivery and consumption by fluid loading and dobutamine infusion.[85] This led to the calling of a Pulmonary Artery Catheter Consensus Conference, which reaffirmed the likely worth of the PAC and acknowledged the lack of conclusive data showing benefit or harm.[93]

The role of the PAC in improving outcome and reducing mortality and morbidity still remains under a cloud, with several large published studies (in critically ill patients, high-risk surgical patients, patients with lung injury, and heart failure patients) showing either no benefit or actual harm with the use of the PAC.[94–97] A meta-analysis of 13 studies, including more than 5000 critically ill patients, recently concluded that the use of the PAC is not associated with improved survival or reduced hospitalization.[98]

Putting it all together

Accurate assessment of the intravascular status is important to improve patient outcomes, especially in the critically ill. Recent guidelines for the hemodynamic management of critically ill patients have emphasized the importance of adequate volume resuscitation in predicting favorable outcomes.[3,99,100] Only 40 percent to 72 percent of ICU patients with hemodynamic instability are able to respond to fluid loading by a significant increase in stroke volume or CO, emphasizing the need for predictive factors to select patients who might benefit from volume expansion and to avoid ineffective, or even deleterious, volume expansion.[3,101,102] A number of studies in surgical and medical intensive care and cardiac surgical patients, using pulse contour analysis–based systems, have consistently demonstrated that the magnitude of respiratory variation of surrogates of stroke volume allows accurate prediction of fluid responsiveness.[103–106]

When comparing evidence on dynamic measurements of fluid responsiveness, pulse contour analysis remains the simplest and the most accurate way to predict response to a fluid challenge.[102] Automatic real-time monitoring of pulse pressure variation using pulse contour analysis-based systems allows a beat-to-beat measurement of left ventricular stroke volume and quantification of its variation during a short period of a few seconds.[107] Monitoring and minimizing pulse pressure variation by volume loading during high-risk surgery improves postoperative outcome and decreases the length of hospital stay.[108]

Doppler recording of aortic blood flow also has been used to quantify the respiratory variation in aortic peak velocity or in velocity time integral at the level of the aortic annulus or in the descending aorta.[109]

In cardiac surgery, the esophageal Doppler ultrasound-based system has been shown to assist in optimizing gut perfusion and to decrease perioperative complications.[87] When used to guide intraoperative intravascular volume loading to optimize stroke volume in orthopedic surgery, it has been credited with a more rapid postoperative recovery and reducing hospital stay significantly.[88] These studies, however, demonstrated greater sensitivity of stroke volume over CO, as compensatory tachycardia tended to maintain CO in the milieu of mild-to-moderate hypovolemia. Left ventricular end-diastolic area obtained using TEE has been demonstrated to be a reliable indicator of preload, but not of fluid responsiveness.

Complications

Complications associated with CO monitoring are mostly related to the use of PAC and can be classified as those

1. Related to central venous access: unintentional trauma (to nearby vessels, pleura, and nerves) and air embolism.[110]
2. Related to catheterization procedure: transient dysrhythmias (usually during advance or withdrawal of the

catheter), conduction blocks, knotting of PAC, and pulmonary artery trauma (most serious adverse effect, with an incidence of 0.1%–1.5% and associated with a 53% mortality rate).[111,112]

3. Related to catheter residence: venous/pulmonary thromboembolism/infarct, cardiac valve trauma, infection, and pulmonary artery rupture.[113]

4. Related to mismanagement: based on faulty data acquisition and incorrect interpretation.[114]

Complications with the pulse contour analysis-based systems are related to peripheral arterial cannulation and local infection/thromboembolism. Complications with devices, based on the indirect Fick's principle, are airway-related. Complications with use of bioimpedence devices have not been reported.

Complications with Doppler ultrasound devices are limited to devices involving insertion of esophageal probes. They are classified as

1. Probe-related: failure of introduction, thermal/pressure injuries of esophagus and vocal cords

2. Procedure-related: respiratory compromise (hypoxia, bronchospasm, laryngospasm), cardiovascular compromise (arrhythmia, hypotension, cardiac arrest, angina pectoris), infection, dysphagia, and nausea/vomiting

Credentialing

The placement of a PAC and the correct interpretation of the CO and derived data from TDCO have a fairly long learning curve. The authors are not aware of any specific approved credentialing process for TDCO measurement; however, a few national bodies consider PAC insertion as a core procedural skill of an anesthesiologist.

Pulse contour analysis-based systems have a short learning curve, as the devices are almost totally automated and little intervention is required. Accreditation activities are available for these devices with a contact process of one hour. Other minimally invasive techniques, such as the indirect Fick's principle and the bioimpedance-based systems, are also automated and have short learning curves.

CO measurement by TEE has a long learning curve. Certificate courses in basic and advanced conventional TEE are run by a number of professional bodies around the world. For example, an experience of six months of using TEE, after attending the basic course, has been described as minimal training for competence by the National Credentialing Committee of Malaysia.

In the United States, there are several pathways to board certification in TEE. For anesthesiologists, board certification in perioperative TEE is most commonly achieved through serving a 12-month fellowship devoted to the anesthetic care of cardiothoracic surgical patients (i.e. a cardiac anesthesia fellowship). During this time, the trainee must receive specific training in TEE and must report a minimum of 300 intraoperative

TEE exams (a minimum of 150 of which must be performed and personally reported by the trainee, and an additional 150 of which must be studied under appropriate supervision but not personally reported). In addition, the trainee must achieve a passing grade on an exam administered by the National Board of Echocardiography.

All Doppler ultrasound-based systems are operator-dependent and need frequent manipulation of the probe to obtain accurate data.[115–117] Some instruction and practice are required to acquire the skill for Doppler ultrasound systems other than TEE, but this training time and cost is negligible compared with that of mastering conventional TEE.

Conclusions

To date, PAC remains the primary clinical diagnostic and monitoring tool used to diagnose cardiac dysfunction and low cardiac output and to monitor their treatment. The accuracy and validity of the new modes of monitoring CO and measuring derived data, using less-invasive monitors based on the indirect Fick's principle and arterial pulse contour analysis, bioimpedance, and Doppler ultrasound-based systems, has been elucidated. However, the technique used to validate the newer modes of CO has been TDCO, using PAC, an "imperfect gold standard," which is often used imperfectly.[84]

In cardiac surgery, TDCO measurement, using PAC, remains the monitoring modality of choice, as other modes of CO measurement are erroneous in the presence of valvular regurgitation, shunts, balloon counterpulsation, and the like. The essential parameters monitored to guide therapy are CO, pulmonary artery pressures, pulmonary capillary wedge pressure, and the systemic/pulmonary vascular resistances. Computed parameters from the collected data help assess the cardiovascular status more comprehensively.

In settings of intensive care and noncardiac surgery, use of minimally invasive devices, such as bioimpedance, pulse contour analysis, and Doppler ultrasound-based systems, is preferable, as real-time trends, rather than absolute values, have more value in guiding therapy. These devices dynamically assess the intravascular volume status. To predict fluid responsiveness in critically ill patients, dynamic parameters should be used preferentially to static parameters. The dynamic parameters that predict fluid responsiveness best are stroke volume variation and pulse pressure variation.

References

1. Dueck R. Noninvasive cardiac output monitoring. *Chest* 2001;120:339–40.

2. Pinsky MR, Teboul JL. Assessment of indices of preload and volume responsiveness. *Curr Opin Crit Care* 2005;11:235–9.

3. Michard F, Teboul JL. Predicting fluid responsiveness in ICU patients. A critical analysis of the evidence. *Chest* 2002;121:2000–8.

4. Kumar A, Anel R, Bunnell E, Habet K, et al. Pulmonary artery occlusion pressure and central venous pressure fail to predict ventricular filling volume, cardiac performance, or the response

to volume infusion in normal subjects. *Crit Care Med* 2004;32:419–28.

5. Fick A. Ueber die Messung des Blutquantums in der Herzenventrikeln. *Sitzung der Phys Med Gesell zu Wurzburg.* 1870;16.

6. Ganz, W, Donoso R, Marcos H, Forrester J, Swan HJC. A new technique for measurement of cardiac output by thermodilution in man. *Am J Cardiol* 1971;27:392–5.

7. Ehlers KC, Mylrea KC, Waterson CK, Calkins JM. Cardiac output measurements. A review of current techniques and research. *Ann Biomed Eng* 1986;14:219–39.

8. Botero M, Lobato EB. Advances in noninvasive cardiac output monitoring: an update. *J Cardiothorac Vasc Anesth* 2001;15:631–40.

9. Jaffe MB, Partial CO_2 rebreathing cardiac output – operating principles of the NICO system. *J Clin Monit* 1999;15:387–401.

10. Haryadi DG, Orr JA, Kuck K, McJames S, Westenskow DR. Partial CO_2 rebreathing indirect Fick technique for non-invasive measurement of cardiac output. *J Clin Monit Comput* 2000;16:361–74.

11. Russell AE, Smith SA, West MJ, et al. Automated non-invasive measurement of cardiac output by the carbon dioxide rebreathing method: Comparison with dye-dilution and thermodilution. *Br Heart J* 1990;63:195–9.

12. Van Heerden PV, Baker S, Lim SI, et al. Clinical evaluation of the non-invasive cardiac output (NICO) monitor in the intensive care unit. *Anaesth Intensive Care* 2000;28:427–30.

13. Tachibana K, Imanaka H, Takeuchi M, Takauchi Y, Miyano H, Nishimura M. Noninvasive cardiac output measurement using partial carbon dioxide rebreathing is less accurate at settings of reduced minute ventilation and when spontaneous breathing is present. *Anesthesiology* 2003;98:830–7.

14. Ng JM, Chow MY, Ip-Yam PC, Goh MH, Agasthian T. Evaluation of partial carbon dioxide rebreathing cardiac output measurement during thoracic surgery. *J Cardiothorac Vasc Anesth* 2007;21:655–8.

15. Kotake Y, Moriyama K, Innami Y, et al. Performance of noninvasive partial CO_2 rebreathing cardiac output and continuous thermodilution cardiac output in patients undergoing aortic reconstruction surgery. *Anesthesiology* 2003;99:283–8.

16. Mielck F, Buhre W, Hanekop G, Tirilomis T, Hilgers R, Sonntag H. Comparison of continuous cardiac output measurements in patients after cardiac surgery. *J Cardiothorac Vasc Anesth* 2003;17:211–6.

17. Stewart GN. Researches on the circulation time and on the influences which offset it. IV. The output of the heart. *J Physiol* 1897;22:159–83.

18. Moore FA, Haenel JB, Moore EE. Alternatives to Swan-Ganz cardiac output monitoring. *Surg Clin North Am* 1991;71:699–721.

19. Burchell SA, Yu M, Takiguchi SA, Ohta RM, Myers SA. Evaluation of a continuous cardiac output and mixed venous oxygen saturation catheter in critically ill surgical patients. *Crit Care Med* 1997;25:388–91.

20. Gardner PE, Bridges ET. Hemodynamic monitoring. In Woods SL, Sivarajan-Froelicher ES, Halpenny CJ, Motzer SU, eds. Cardiac Nursing. 3rd ed. Philadelphia: J. B. Lippincott, 1995, pp. 424–58.

21. Pearl RG, Rosenthal MH, Nielson L, Ashton JPA, Brown BW Jr. Effect of injectate volume and temperature on thermodilution cardiac output determination. *Anesthesiology* 1986;64:798–801.

22. Vennix CV, Nelson DH, Pierpont GL. Thermodilution cardiac output in critically ill patients: comparison of room temperature and iced injectate. *Heart Lung* 1984;13:574–8.

23. Greim CA, Roewer N, Thiel H, Laux G, Schulte am Esch J. Continuous cardiac output monitoring during adult liver transplantation: Thermal filament technique versus bolus thermodilution. *Anesth Analg* 1997;85:483–8.

24. Yelderman M. Continuous measurement of cardiac output with the use of stochastic system identification techniques. *J Clin Monit* 1990;6:322–32.

25. Thrush D, Downs JB and Smith RA. Continuous thermodilution cardiac output: agreement with Fick and bolus thermodilution methods. *J Cardiothorac Vasc Anesth* 1995;9:399–404.

26. Michard F, Alaya S, Zarka V, et al. Global end-diastolic volume as an indicator of cardiac preload in patients with septic shock. *Chest* 2003;124:1900–8.

27. Goldwyn RM, Watt T. Arterial pressure pulse contour analysis via a mathematical model for the clinical quantification of human vascular properties. *IEEE Trans Biomed Eng* 1967;14:11–17.

28. Watt T, Burrus C. Arterial pressure contour analysis for estimating human vascular properties. *J Appl Physiol* 1976;40:171–6.

29. Michard F. Changes in arterial pressure during mechanical ventilation. *Anesthesiology* 2005;103:419–28.

30. Bendjelid K, Suter PM, Romand JA. The respiratory changes preejection period: a new method to predict fluid responsiveness. *J Appl Physiol* 2004;96:337–42.

31. De Backer D, Heenen S, Piagnerelli M, Koch M, Vincent JL. Pulse pressure variations to predict fluid responsiveness: influence of tidal volume. *Intensive Care Med* 2005;31:517–23.

32. Berkenstadt H, Friedman Z, Preisman S, et al. Pulse pressure and stroke volume variations during severe haemorrhage in ventilated dogs. *Br J Anaesth* 2005;94:721–6.

33. van Leishout JJ, Wesselling KH. Continuous cardiac output by pulse contour analysis? *Br J Anaesth* 2001;86:467–9.

34. Manecke GR Jr. Cardiac output from the arterial catheter: deceptively simple. *Cardiothorac Vasc Anesth* 2007;21:629–31.

35. Wesseling KH, de Wit B, Weber JAP, Ty Smith N. A simple device for continuous measurement of cardiac output. *Adv Cardiovasc Physiol* 1983;5:16–52.

36. Wesseling KH, Jansen JRC, Settels JJ, Schreuder JJ. Computation of aortic flow from pressure in humans using a nonlinear, three-element model. *J Appl Physiol* 1993;74:2566–73.

37. Rodig G, Prasser C, Keyl C, Liebold A, Hobbhahn J. Continuous cardiac output: pulse contour analysis vs. thermodilution technique in cardiac surgical patients. *Br J Anaesth* 1999;82:525–30.

38. Maus TM, Lee DE. Arterial pressure–based cardiac output assessment. *J Cardiothorac Vasc Anesth* 2008;22:468–73.

39. Yamashita K, Nishiyama T, Yokoyama T, Abe H, Manabe M. The effects of vasodilation on cardiac output. *J Cardiothorac Vasc Anesth* 2008;22:688–92.

40. Della Rocca G, Costa MG, Pompei L, Coccia C, Pietropaoli P. Continuous and intermittent cardiac output measurement: pulmonary artery catheter versus aortic transpulmonary technique. *Br J Anaesth* 2002:88:350–6.

41. Della Rocca G, Costa MG, Coccia C, et al. Cardiac output monitoring: aortic transpulmonary thermodilution and pulse contour analysis agree with standard thermodilution methods in patients undergoing lung transplantation. *Can J Anesth* 2003;50:707–11.

42. Jansen JRC, Schreuder JJ, Mulier JP, Smith NT, Settels JJ, Wesseling KH. A comparison of cardiac output derived from the arterial pressure wave against thermodilution in cardiac surgery patients. *Br J Anaesth* 2001;87:212–22.

43. Langewouters GJ, Wesseling KH, Goedhard WJ. The pressure-dependant dynamic elasticity of 35 thoracic and 16 abdominal human aortas invitro described by a five component model. *J Biomech* 1985;18:613–20.

44. Langewouters GJ, Wesseling KH, Goedhard WJ. The static elastic properties of 45 human thoracic and 20 abdominal aortas in vitro and the parameters of a new model. *J Biomech* 1984;17:425–35.

45. Remmen JJ, Aengevaeren WR, Verheugt FW, et al. Finapres arterial pulse wave analysis with Modelflow is not a reliable noninvasive method for assessment of cardiac output. *Clin Sci (Lond)* 2002;103:143–9.

46. Azabji Kenfack M, Lador F, Licker M, et al. Cardiac output by Modelflow method from intra-arterial and fingertip pulse pressure profiles. *Clin Sci (Lond)* 2004;106:365–9.

47. Tam E, Azabji Kenfack M, Cautero M, et al. Correction of cardiac output obtained by Modelflow from finger pulse pressure profiles with a respiratory method in humans. *Clin Sci (Lond)* 2004;106:371–6.

48. de Vaal JB, de Wilde RBP, Van Den Berg PCM, Schreuder JJ, Jansen JRC. Less invasive determination of cardiac output from the arterial pressure by aortic diameter-calibrated pulse contour. *Br J Anaesth* 2005;95:26–31.

49. Rhodes A, Sunderland R. Arterial pulse power analysis, the LiDCO™ plus system. In Pinsky MR, Pyen D, eds. Functional Hemodynamics. Berlin: Springer Verlag, 2005, pp. 183–92.

50. Button D, Weibel L, Reuthebuch O, Genoni M, Zollinger A, Hofer CK. Clinical evaluation of the FloTrac/Vigileo™ system and two established continuous cardiac output monitoring devices in patients undergoing cardiac surgery. *Br J Anaesth* 2007; 99:329–36.

51. Chakravarthy M, Patil TA, Jayaprakash K, Kalligudd P, Prabhakumar D, Jawali V. Comparison of simultaneous estimation of cardiac output by four techniques in patients undergoing off-pump coronary artery bypass surgery – a prospective observational study. *Ann Card Anaesth* 2007;10:121–6.

52. Della Rocca G, Costa MG, Chiarandini P, et al. Arterial pulse cardiac output agreement with thermodilution in patients in hyperdynamic conditions. *J Cardiothorac Vasc Anesth* 2008;22:681–7.

53. Lorsomradee S, Lorsomradee S, Cromheecke S, De Hert SG. Uncalibrated arterial pulse contour analysis versus continuous thermodilution technique: effects of alterations in arterial waveform. *J Cardiothorac Vasc Anesth* 2007;21:636–43.

54. Breukers RMBGE, Sepehrkhouy S, Spiegelenberg SR, Groeneveld ABJ. Cardiac output measured by a new arterial pressure waveform analysis method without calibration compared with thermodilution after cardiac surgery. *J Cardiothorac Vasc Anesth* 2007;21:632–5.

55. Scolletta S, Romano SM, Biagioli B, Capannini G, Giomarelli P. Pressure recording analytical method (PRAM) for measurement of cardiac output during various haemodynamic states. *Br J Anaesth* 2005;95:159–65.

56. Kubicek WG. Development and evaluation of an impedance cardiac output system. *Aerospace Med* 1966;12:1208–12.

57. Sramek B. Cardiac output by impedance. *Med Electronics* 1982;4:93–7.

58. Atallah MM, Demain AD. Cardiac output measurement. Lack of agreement between thermodilution and thoracic electric bioimpedance in two clinical settings. *J Clin Anesth* 1995;7:182–5.

59. Young JD, McQuillan P. Comparison of thoracic electrical bioimpedance and thermodilution for the measurement of cardiac index in patients with severe sepsis. *Br J Anaesth* 1993;70:58–62.

60. Weiss S, Calloway E, Cairo J, Granger W, Winslow J. Comparison of cardiac output measurements by thermodilution and thoracic electrical bioimpedance in critically ill versus non-critically ill patients. *Am J Emerg Med* 1995; 13:626–31.

61. Critchley LA, Critchley JA. Lung fluid and impedance cardiography. *Anaesthesia* 1998; 53:369–72.

62. Easterling TR, Benedetti TJ, Carlson KL, Watts DH. Measurement of cardiac output in pregnancy by thermodilution and impedance techniques. *Br J Obstet Gynaecol* 1989;96: 67–9.

63. Weiss SJ, Kulik JP, Calloway E. Bioimpedance cardiac output measurements in patients with presumed congestive heart failure. *Acad Emerg Med* 1997;4:568–73.

64. Critchley LA, Leung DH, Short TG. Abdominal surgery alters the calibration of bioimpedance cardiac output measurement. *Int J Clin Monit Comput* 1996; 13:1–8.

65. Wallace AW, Salahieh A, Lawrence A, Spector K, Owens C, Alonso D. Endotracheal cardiac output monitor. *Anesthesiology* 2000; 92:178–89.

66. Spiess BD, Patel MA, Soltow LO, Wright IH. Comparison of bioimpedance versus thermodilution cardiac output during cardiac surgery: evaluation of a second-generation bioimpedance device. *J Cardiothorac Vasc Anesth* 2001;15:567–73.

67. Sageman WS, Riffenburgh RH, Spiess BD. Equivalence of bioimpedance and thermodilution in measuring cardiac index after cardiac surgery. *J Cardiothorac Vasc Anesth* 2002;16: 8–14.

68. Bein B, Worthmann F, Tonner PH, et al. Comparison of esophageal Doppler, pulse contour analysis and realtime pulmonary artery thermodilution for the continuous measurement of cardiac output. *J Cardiothorac Vasc Anesth* 2004;18:185–9.

69. Singer M, Bennet ED. Noninvasive optimization of left ventricular filling using esophageal Doppler. *Crit Care Med* 1991;19:1132–7.

70. Cheung AT, Savino JS, Weiss SJ, Aukburg SJ, Berlin JA. Echocardiographic and hemodynamic indexes of left ventricular preload in patients with normal and abnormal ventricular function. *Anesthesiology* 1994;81:376–87.

71. Perrino AC Jr. Cardiac output monitoring by echocardiography: Should we pass on Swan-Ganz catheters? *Yale J Biol Med* 1993;66:397–413.

72. Tan HL, Pinder M, Parsons R, Roberts B and van Heerden PV. Clinical evaluation of USCOM ultrasonic cardiac output monitor in cardiac surgical patients in intensive care unit. *Br J Anaesth* 2005;94:287–91.

73. List W, Gravenstein N, Banner T, et al. Interaction in sheep between mean arterial pressure and cross-sectional area of the descending aorta: implications for esophageal monitoring. *Anesthesiology* 1987;67:A178.

74. Perrino AC, Fleming J, LaMantia KR. Transesophageal cardiac output monitoring: Performance during aortic reconstructive surgery. *Anesth Analg* 1991;73:705–10.

75. Seigel LC, Fitzgerald DC, Engstom RH. Simultaneous intraoperative measurement of cardiac output by thermodilution and transtracheal Doppler. *Anesthesiology* 1991;74:664–9.

76. Perrino AC, Harris SN, Luther MA. Intraoperative determination of cardiac output using multiplane transesophageal echocardiography: a comparison to thermodilution. *Anesthesiology* 1998;89:350–357.

77. Critchley LA, Peng ZY, Fok BS, Lee A, Phillips RA. Testing the reliability of a new ultrasonic cardiac cutput monitor, the USCOM, by using aortic flowprobes in anesthetized dogs. *Anesth Analg* 2005;100:748–53.

78. Phillips RA. Transcutaneous continuous-wave Doppler monitoring is feasible producing reliable and reproducible signals. *J Am Coll Cardiol* 2002; 39(Suppl B):283.

79. Spahn DR, Schmid ER, Tornic M, et al. Noninvasive versus invasive assessment of cardiac output after cardiac surgery: clinical validation. *J Cardiothorac Anesth* 1990;4:46–59.

80. Zimmermann A, Kufner C, Hofbauer S, et al. The accuracy of the Vigileo/FloTrac continuous cardiac output monitor. *J Cardiothorac Vasc Anesth* 2008;22:388–93

81. Eisenberg PR, Jaffe AS, Schuster DP. Clinical evaluation compared to pulmonary artery catheterisation in the haemodynamic assessment of critically-ill patients. *Crit Care Med* 1984;12:549–53

82. Bayliss J, Norell M, Ryan A, et al. Bedside haemodynamic monitoring: experience in a general hospital. *Br Med J* 1983;287:187–90.

83. Gan TJ, Soppitt A, Maroof M, et al. Goal-directed intraoperative fluid administration reduces length of hospital stay after major surgery. *Anesthesiology* 2002;97:820–826.

84. Singer M. Cardiac output in 1998. *Heart* 1998;79:425–8.

85. Shoemaker WC, Appel PL, Kram HB, et al. Prospective trial of supranormal values of survivors as therapeutic goals in high-risk surgical patients. *Chest* 1988;94:1176–86.

86. Boyd O, Grounds RM, Bennett ED. A randomized clinical trial of the effect of deliberate perioperative increase of oxygen delivery on mortality in high-risk surgical patients. *JAMA* 1993;270:2699–707.

87. Mythen MG, Webb AR. Peroperative plasma volume expansion reduces the incidence of gut mucosal hypoperfusion in cardiac surgery. *Arch Surg* 1995;130:423–9.

88. Sinclair S, James S, Singer M. Intraoperative intravascular volume optimisation and length of hospital stay after repair of proximal femoral fracture: randomised, controlled trial. *BMJ* 1997;315:909–12.

89. Mimoz O, Rauss A, Rekik N, et al. Pulmonary artery catheterization in critically ill patients: a prospective analysis of outcome changes associated with catheter-prompted changes in therapy. *Crit Care Med* 1994;22:573–9.

90. Linton RAF, Linton NWF, Kelly F. Is clinical assessment of the circulation reliable in postoperative cardiac surgical patients? *J Cardiothorac Vasc Anesth* 2002;16:4–7.

91. Connors AF Jr, Speroff T, Dawson NV, et al. The effectiveness of right heart catheterization in the initial care of critically ill patients. SUPPORT Investigators. *JAMA* 1996;276:889–97.

92. Dalen JE, Bone RC. Is it time to pull the pulmonary artery catheter? *JAMA* 1996;276:916–18.

93 Pulmonary artery catheter consensus conference: consensus statement. *Crit Care Med* 1997;25:910–25.

94. Harvey S, Harrison DA, Singer M, et al. Assessment of the clinical effectiveness of pulmonary artery catheters in management of patients in intensive care (PAC-Man): a randomized controlled trial. *Lancet* 2005;366:472–7.

95. Sandham JD, Hull, RD, Brant RF, et al. A randomized, controlled trial of the use of pulmonary-artery catheters in high-risk surgical patients. *N Engl J Med* 2003;348:5–14.

96. The National Heart, Lung, and Blood Institute Adult Respiratory Distress Syndrome (ARDS) Clinical Trial Network: Pulmonary-artery vs central venous catheter to guide treatment of acute lung injury. *N Engl J Med* 2006;354:2213–24.

97. The ESCAPE Investigators and ESCAPE Study Coordinators: Evaluation study of congestive heart failure and pulmonary artery catheterization effectiveness. The ESCAPE trial. *JAMA* 2005;294:1625–33.

98. Shah MR, Hasselblad V, Stevenson LW, et al. Impact of the pulmonary artery catheter in critically ill patients. *JAMA* 2005;294:1664–70.

99. Rivers E, Nguyen B, Havstad S, et al. Early goal-directed therapy in the treatment of severe sepsis and septic shock. *N Engl J Med* 2001;345:1368–77.

100. Monnet X, Teboul JL. Volume responsiveness. *Curr Opin Crit Care* 2007;13:549–53.

101. Hadian H, Pinsky MR. Functional hemodynamic monitoring. *Curr Opin Crit Care* 2007;13:318–23.

102. Auler JOC Jr, Galas FRBG, Sundin MR, Hajjar LA. Arterial pulse pressure variation predicting fluid responsiveness in critically ill patients. *Shock* 2008;30(Suppl 1):18–22.

103. Feissel M, Teboul JL, Merlani P, Badie J, Faller JP, Bendjelid K. Plethysmography dynamic indices predict fluid responsiveness in septic ventilated patients. *Intensive Care Med* 2007;33: 993–9.

104. Hofer CK, Muller SM, Furrer L, Klaghofer R, Genoni M, Zollinger A. Stroke volume and pulse pressure variation for prediction of fluid responsiveness in patients undergoing off-pump coronary artery bypass grafting. *Chest* 2005;128:848–54.

105. Feissel M, Badie J, Merlani PG, Faller JP, Bendjelid K. Preejection period variations predict the fluid responsiveness of septic ventilated patients. *Crit Care Med* 2005;33:2534–9.

106. Natalini G, Rosano A, Taranto M, Faggian B, Vittorielli E, Bernardini A. Arterial versus plethysmographic dynamic indices to test responsiveness for testing fluid administration in hypotensive patients: a clinical trial. *Anesth Analg* 2006;103:1478–84.

107. Auler JO, Galas F, Hajjar L, Santos L, Carvalho T, Michard F. Online monitoring of pulse pressure variation to guide fluid therapy after cardiac surgery. *Anesth Analg* 2008;106: 1201–6.

108. Lopes MR, Oliveira MA, Pereira VOS, Lemos IPB, Auler JOC Jr, Michard F. Goal-directed fluid management based on pulse pressure variation monitoring during high-risk surgery: a pilot randomized controlled trial. *Crit Care* 2007, 11:R100.

109. Cannesson M, Slieker J, Desebbe O, Farhat F, Bastien O, Lehot JJ. Prediction of fluid responsiveness using respiratory variations in left ventricular stroke area by transoesophageal echocardiographic automated border detection in mechanically ventilated patients. *Crit Care* 2006;10:R171.

110. Boyd KD, Thomas S, Gold J, et al. A prospective study of complications of pulmonary artery catheterizations in 500 consecutive patients. *Chest* 1983;84:245–9.

111. Abreu AR, Campos MA, Krieger BP. Pulmonary artery rupture induced by a pulmonary artery catheter: A case report and review of the literature. *J Intensive Care Med* 2004;19:291–6.

112. Arnau JG, Montero CG, Luengo C, et al. Retrograde dissection and rupture of pulmonary artery after catheter use in pulmonary hypertension. *Crit Care Med* 1982;10:694–5.

113. Damen J, Verhoef J, Bolton DT, et al. Microbiologic risk of invasive hemodynamic monitoring in patients undergoing open-heart operations. *Crit Care Med* 1985;13: 548–55.

114. Iberti TJ, Fischer EP, Leibowitz AB, et al. A multicenter study of physicians' knowledge of the pulmonary artery catheter. *JAMA* 1990;264:2928–32.

115. Mark JB, Steinbrook RA, Gugino LD, et al. Continuous noninvasive monitoring of cardiac output with esophageal Doppler ultrasound during cardiac surgery. *Anesth Analg* 1986;65:1013.

116. Freund PR. Transesophageal Doppler scanning versus thermodilution during general anesthesia. *Am J Surg* 1987;153:490–503.

117. Spahn DR, Schmid ER, Tornic M, et al. Noninvasive versus invasive assessment of cardiac output after cardiac surgery: Clinical validation. *J Cardiothorac Anesth* 1990;4:46–59.

Gastric tonometry

Elliott Bennett-Guerrero

Background

The gut is one of the most susceptible organs to hypoperfusion during conditions of trauma or stress.[1–3] More than three decades ago, Price and colleagues removed 15 percent of the blood volume from healthy volunteers, causing a 40 percent reduction in splanchnic blood volume.[2] In this study, cardiac output (CO), blood pressure (BP), and heart rate (HR) did not change from baseline. A more recent study was conducted by Hamilton-Davies and associates, in which 25 percent of the blood volume was removed from six healthy volunteers.[4] Gastric mucosal perfusion, as measured by saline gastric tonometry, was the first variable to decline (in five of the six subjects). Stroke volume (SV) also decreased; however, routinely measured cardiovascular variables such as HR, BP, and CO did not change significantly enough from baseline values to cause suspicion of a hypovolemic state. These studies suggest that during periods of hypovolemia, the gut vasoconstricts, thus shunting blood toward "more vital organs," such as the heart and brain.[1–3] Gut hypoperfusion can progress to ischemia, which may result in complications that take place many hours and days following an episode of hypovolemia.[5]

Technical concepts

Until recently, an FDA-approved monitor (the gastrointestinal tonometer) was available to measure gut hypoperfusion (Tonocap; GE Healthcare, Barrington, IL). The tonometer is a naso/orogastric tube that is modified to include a silicone balloon into which air or saline is introduced (Figure 9.1). The most recent commercially available method of tonometry involved the introduction of air into the tonometer's balloon. Following a brief period of equilibration (<15 minutes), air in the balloon is assayed for PCO_2 by the monitor's accompanying infrared analyzer. This newer method allowed for the determination of gastric mucosal PCO_2 every five minutes.

The gastric mucosal bed is similar to the overall splanchnic mucosa in its propensity to become hypoperfused during periods of physiologic stress. Hypoperfused areas of tissue develop regional hypercapnia (elevated PCO_2), which diffuses into the tonometer balloon, allowing for an indirect measurement of gastric mucosal PCO_2. Hypoperfusion is manifested by a positive gap between the gastric mucosal PCO_2 and the arterial PCO_2 (gastric mucosal PCO_2 > arterial PCO_2). A gap greater than 8 mmHg is considered to reflect splanchnic hypoperfusion.[6] In theory, any gap is abnormal; however, the use of a higher cutoff value appears to improve the specificity of this monitor without significantly decreasing its sensitivity.

Initially, early studies reported "pHi," which is a calculated measure that takes into account both the level of CO_2 in the stomach and the plasma bicarbonate concentration. However, Schlichtig and colleagues correctly reported that the gastric–arterial PCO_2 difference is a better and more specific measure of gastric ischemia, because pHi can be low in the setting of a metabolic acidosis even if gastric PCO_2 is not elevated.[7]

Evidence of utility
Observational studies

Several studies have observed a high incidence of splanchnic hypoperfusion during cardiac surgery, with some showing an association between abnormal gut perfusion during cardiac surgery and postoperative complications.[8–15] Fiddian-Green and Baker used saline tonometry to measure gastric mucosal perfusion in 85 cardiac surgical patients.[11] Half (49%) of these patients developed evidence of abnormal perfusion, and all serious postoperative complications (eight patients, including five deaths) developed in this group. Gastric tonometry was shown in this and in other studies to be a more sensitive predictor of adverse postoperative outcome compared with more routinely used global measures such as CO, BP, HR, and urine output.[12, 14]

Several studies have demonstrated an association between gastric ischemia, as manifested by elevated gastric PCO_2, and adverse outcome after routine elective cardiac surgery.[14,15] Studies that have failed to demonstrate an association between splanchnic hypoperfusion and adverse postoperative outcome are limited in part by small sample size, insensitive measures of postoperative morbidity, and deviation from validated methodology of tonometry.[9,10] In addition, tonometric measurements of gastric mucosal perfusion during hypothermic cardiopulmonary bypass (CPB) have not been validated in terms of their ability to predict postoperative morbidity.

In addition to studies involving cardiac surgery, there are several observational studies showing an association between

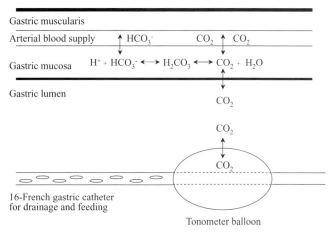

Figure 9.1. Diagram of operation of gastric tonometer in gastric lumen. Tonometer balloon is filled with either saline solution or air. Protons (H^+) are generated in the gastric mucosa from anaerobic metabolism (tissue acidosis). Protons then combine with bicarbonate (HCO^-_3) to form carbonic acid (H_2CO_3), which dissociates into carbon dioxide (CO_2) and water (H_2O). Carbon dioxide diffuses freely into the gastric lumen and tonometer balloon.

abnormal tonometric variables and adverse outcome in ICU,[16] trauma,[17] and noncardiac surgical patients.[18]

Randomized clinical trials

Observational studies cannot prove that the use of the monitor "causes" or results in better outcome. Unfortunately, there are few published randomized clinical trials of gastric-tonometry–guided care versus the standard-of-care therapy.

Gutierrez and associates randomized ICU patients to standard of care versus gastric-tonometric–guided care, in which apparent splanchnic ischemia was treated with strategies aimed at optimizing oxygen delivery.[19] For patients who were admitted to the ICU with normal pHi (no apparent ischemia), those randomized to the tonometric-guided care exhibited higher survival (58% vs 42%; $p < 0.01$). In contrast, for patients with evidence of gastric ischemia on admission to the ICU, there was no apparent benefit to this experimental intervention (survival 37% vs 36%).

Ivatury and coworkers randomized ICU patients to gastric-tonometric–guided care versus maintenance of oxygen delivery.[20] There was no apparent benefit to the tonometric-guided care, although the comparison group was not a true standard-of-care group. The study did, however, show an association between splanchnic ischemia using tonometry and adverse outcomes consistent with previous studies.

Therefore, at the current time, there are scant data from randomized clinical trials to address the question of whether gastric tonometry can be used to improve outcome.

Complications

Gastric tonometry is minimally invasive and carries few risks. It should not be used in patients for whom instrumentation of the stomach or esophagus would be contraindicated.

Credentialing

Gastric tonometry is not currently available; however, no specific credentialing process or training have been required.

Practice parameters

Gastric tonometry is not currently available. There is a large body of observational studies that provide a theoretical justification for its use, but there are scant data from randomized clinical trials, so its use cannot be strongly recommended at this time.

References

1. Mythen MG, Webb AR. The role of gut mucosal hypoperfusion in the pathogenesis of post-operative organ dysfunction. *Intensive Care Med* 1994;20:203–9.
2. Price HL, Deutsch S, Marshall BE, Stephen GW, Behar MG, Neufeld GR. Hemodynamic and metabolic effects of hemorrhage in man, with particular reference to the splanchnic circulation. *Circ Res* 1966;18:469–74.
3. Lundgren O. Physiology of intestinal circulation. In Martson A, et al., eds. *Splanchnic Ischemia and Multiple Organ Failure*. St. Louis: Mosby, 1989, pp. 29–40.
4. Hamilton-Davies C, Mythen MG, Salmon JB, Jacobson D, Shukla A, Webb AR. Comparison of commonly used clinical indicators of hypovolaemia with gastrointestinal tonometry. *Intensive Care Med* 1997;23:276–81.
5. Fink MP. Effect of critical illness on microbial translocation and gastrointestinal mucosa permeability. *Semin Respir Infect* 1994;9:256–60.
6. Mythen MG, Faehnrich J. Monitoring gut perfusion. In Rombeau JL, Takala J, eds. *Gut Dysfunction in Critical Illness*. Heidelberg: Springer-Verlag, 1996, pp. 246–63.
7. Schlichtig R, Mehta N, Gayowski TJ. Tissue-arterial PCO2 difference is a better marker of ischemia than intramural pH (pHi) or arterial pH-pHi difference. *J Crit Care* 1996;11:51–6.
8. Berendes E, Mollhoff T, Van Aken H, et al. Effects of dopexamine on creatinine clearance, systemic inflammation, and splanchnic oxygenation in patients undergoing coronary artery bypass grafting. *Anesth Analg* 1997;84:950–7.
9. Andersen LW, Landow L, Baek L, Jansen E, Baker S. Association between gastric intramucosal pH and splanchnic endotoxin, antibody to endotoxin, and tumor necrosis factor-alpha concentrations in patients undergoing cardiopulmonary bypass. *Crit Care Med* 1993;21:210–7.
10. Riddington DW, Venkatesh B, Boivin CM, et al. Intestinal permeability, gastric intramucosal pH, and systemic endotoxemia in patients undergoing cardiopulmonary bypass. *JAMA* 1996;275:1007–12.
11. Fiddian-Green RG, Baker S. Predictive value of the stomach wall pH for complications after cardiac operations: comparison with other monitoring. *Crit Care Med* 1987;15:153–6.
12. Mythen MG, Webb AR. Intra-operative gut mucosal hypoperfusion is associated with increased post-operative complications and cost. *Intensive Care Med* 1994;20:99–104.
13. Mythen MG, Webb AR. Perioperative plasma volume expansion reduces the incidence of gut mucosal hypoperfusion during cardiac surgery. *Arch Surg* 1995;130:423–9.
14. Bennett-Guerrero E, Panah MH, Bodian CA, et al. Automated detection of gastric luminal partial pressure of carbon dioxide

during cardiovascular surgery using the Tonocap. *Anesthesiology* 2000;92:38–45.

15. Kavarana MN, Frumento RJ, Hirsch AL, Oz MC, Lee DC, Bennett-Guerrero E. Gastric hypercarbia and adverse outcome after cardiac surgery. *Intensive Care Med* 2003;29:742–8.

16. Levy B, Gawalkiewicz P, Vallet B, Briancon S, Nace L, Bollaert PE. Gastric capnometry with air-automated tonometry predicts outcome in critically ill patients. *Crit Care Med* 2003;31:474–80.

17. Calvete JO, Schonhorst L, Moura DM, Friedman G. Acid-base disarrangement and gastric intramucosal acidosis predict outcome from major trauma. *Rev Assoc Med Bras* 2008;54: 116–21.

18. Lebuffe G, Vallet B, Takala J, et al. A European, multicenter, observational study to assess the value of gastric-to-end tidal PCO_2 difference in predicting postoperative complications. *Anesth Analg* 2004;99:166–72.

19. Gutierrez G, Palizas F, Doglio G, et al. Gastric intramucosal pH as a therapeutic index of tissue oxygenation in critically ill patients. *Lancet* 1992;339:195–9.

20. Ivatury RR, Simon RJ, Islam S, Fueg A, Rohman M, Stahl WM. A prospective randomized study of end points of resuscitation after major trauma: global oxygen transport indices versus organ-specific gastric mucosal pH. *J Am Coll Surg* 1996;183:145–54.

Chapter

10

Oxygen delivery, oxygen transport, and tissue oxygen tension

Critical monitoring in the ICU

Jayashree Raikhelkar and Peter J. Papadakos

Introduction

A continuous supply of oxygen is essential for aerobic metabolism and maintenance of natural functioning in all cells. When metabolic needs of an organ exceed supply, tissue and organ dysfunction result and a state of shock ensues. This overview focuses on the fundamental concepts of oxygen delivery (DO_2) and utilization by tissues as well as special emphasis on monitoring of DO_2 and tissue perfusion in the critically ill.

Oxygen transport and delivery variables

Global DO_2 is dependent on an intact respiratory system. Respiratory failure can lead to inadequate oxygen delivery, tissue hypoxia, and organ injury. The availability of oxygen to tissues can be quantified by a number of measured variables. The partial pressure of oxygen in the plasma (PaO_2) and the arterial oxygen saturation (SaO_2) are some of the principal components for assessment of adequacy of oxygen transport and delivery. Although regularly used to monitor respiratory function, PaO_2 is largely dependent on ventilation/perfusion matching.[1] PaO_2 and SaO_2 may be normal in cases of anemia and low cardiac output states. The alveolar PO_2-to-PaO_2 gradient (A–a gradient) is a better indicator of integrity of oxygen transport from the alveoli to the blood.[2] Arterial O_2 content of blood is given as

$$CaO_2 = (1.39 \times Hb \times SaO_2) + (0.0031 \times PaO_2),$$

where CaO_2 is the oxygen content of arterial blood and Hb is the hemoglobin concentration. The total concentration of oxygen in arterial blood in an average-sized adult is approximately 200mL per liter. More than 98 percent of this oxygen is bound to hemoglobin, and the remaining 1.5 percent is dissolved in the plasma. This underscores the significance of hemoglobin in the transport of oxygen within the body.

The concentration of O_2 in venous blood (CvO_2) is calculated in a similar fashion to CaO_2, with the use of venous O_2 saturation (SvO_2) and PO_2 (PvO_2):

$$CvO_2 = (1.34 \times Hb \times SvO_2) + (0.003 \times PvO_2).$$

The rate at which oxygen is delivered to the peripheral tissues by cardiac output can be derived by the Fick equation:

$$DO_2 = 10 \times Qt \times CaO_2,$$

where Qt is cardiac output. DO_2 is the volume of oxygen (mL) that reaches the peripheral capillary bed every minute. From the equation, one can easily deduce that the most effective way to increase global DO_2 to the tissues is by increasing hemoglobin concentration and by secondarily increasing cardiac output (3).

The plateau of the oxygen equilibrium curve (OEC) is attained at an oxygen saturation of 90 percent (Figure 10.1). Above this level, additional oxygen does not significantly enhance DO_2. Shifting of the ODC affects SaO_2 and, consequently, DO_2. Shifts to the right occur with increased 2,3-diglycerophosphate, acidosis, and hyperthermia. In contrast, decreased 2,3-diglycerophophate, alkalosis, and hypothermia shift the curve to the left, increasing hemoglobin saturation for any given PO_2.

The rate at which delivered oxygen is metabolically consumed is oxygen uptake (VO_2) and is presented in a variation of the Fick equation:

$$VO_2 = 10 \times CO(CaO_2 - CvO_2).$$

Further modified, the equation can be stated as:

$$VO_2 = Qt \times 13.4 \times Hb \times (SaO_2 - SvO_2).$$

The Fick equation does not take into oxygen consumption by the lung. Normal lung VO_2 accounts for less than 5 percent of total VO_2. In the critically ill, this fraction may increase to up to 20 percent (4). Direct measurement of VO_2 involves measurement of whole-body VO_2 and is therefore a more accurate measurement of VO_2 (5).

Another important measure of oxygen transport is oxygen extraction ratio (O_2ER). It is defined as the fraction of oxygen delivered to the capillaries that is taken up by the tissues:

$$O_2ER = VO_2/DO_2.$$

Under resting conditions, 25 percent of the total oxygen delivered is extracted by the tissues. Individual organ O_2ERs vary, with metabolically active organs such as the heart and brain having higher values.

Critical DO_2

In healthy individuals, as VO_2 increases with physiologic stress, oxygen delivery will increase simultaneously. After a certain point, the O_2ER will increase to maintain oxygen delivery. Critical DO_2 is the level of oxygen transport at which VO_2 begins

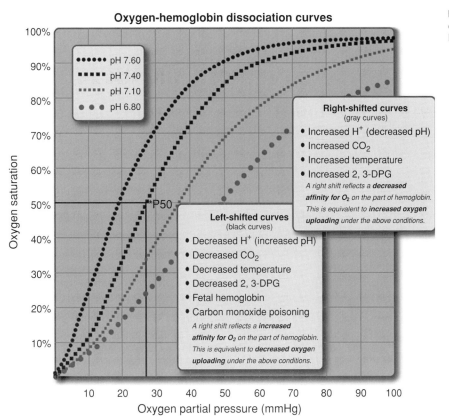

Figure 10.1. The hemoglobin–oxygen dissociation curve with factors known to increase and decrease hemoglobin's affinity for oxygen.

*Hemoglobin P50 is the partial pressure of oxygen where hemoglobin is 50% saturated; normally about 26.8 mmHg.

to decline, becoming a supply-dependent variable (6) (Figure 10.2). In critical illness, there is a reduced ability for tissues to extract oxygen. As the slope of O_2ER continues to increase, oxygen debt and anaerobic glycolysis result and shock ensues (7, 8).

Multiple clinical trials comparing optimum versus normal resuscitation endpoints in severely critically ill patients have been inconclusive. Velmahos and colleagues found no difference in the rate of death, organ failure, and ICU stay (9). Kern and associates' meta-analysis evaluating hemodynamic goals in acute, critically ill patients and evaluation of outcomes of

resuscitation therapy showed that optimization of hemodynamic variables prior to the onset of multiorgan failure significantly reduced mortality as compared with doing so after the onset of multisystemic dysfunction (10). Rivers and coworkers also concluded that early goal-directed therapy in cases of severe sepsis and septic shock results in less-severe organ failure (11,12). These studies may suggest that timely therapeutic intervention and optimization, not supranormalization of hemodynamic variables, is the key to successful management of shock and avoidance of multiorgan dysfunction. The normal ranges for oxygen transport variables are given in Table 10.1.

Monitoring of DO₂ (global and regional)
Metabolic indicators of tissue perfusion

The assessment of intravascular volume and adequacy of resuscitation presents unique clinical challenges. Clinical indicators

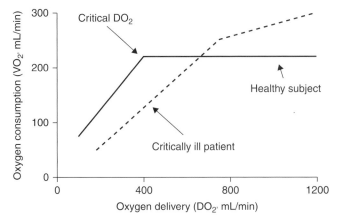

Figure 10.2. Schematic representation of the relationship between DO₂ and VO₂ in healthy and critically ill individuals.[2] (Reproduced from reference. 3, with permission from BMJ Publishing Group Ltd.)

Table 10.1. Oxygen transport variables

Parameters	Normal range (size-adjusted)
1. Oxygen delivery (DO₂)	520–570 mL/min/m²
2. Oxygen uptake (VO₂)	110–160 mL/min/m²
3. Oxygen extraction ratio (O₂ER)	20%–30%
4. Mixed venous oxygen saturation (SvO₂)	70%–75%
5. Cardiac output (CO)	2.4–4.0 L/min/m²

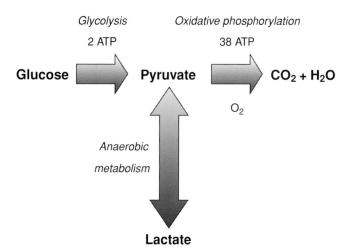

Glycolysis ... Oxidative phosphorylation

Figure 10.3. Aerobic and anaerobic metabolic pathways.

of tissue perfusion have been extensively studied and used to guide resuscitative efforts in shock. Conventional markers, such as heart rate, blood pressure, and urine output, have been disappointing measures of ongoing tissue hypoxia (13) and have failed to predict diminished oxygen delivery or correlate with the various stages of shock (14). Serum lactate and base deficit have proved to be reliable indicators in resuscitation. These metabolic indicators of tissue perfusion are global measures of total body oxygen debt.

Serum lactate

Abnormalities in lactate metabolism are a common occurrence in the critically ill and are a direct result of systemic hypoperfusion and ongoing tissue hypoxia. Lactate is a byproduct of anaerobic metabolism after glycolysis. At the tissue level, as a result of uncoupling of oxygen demands and supply, pyruvate cannot enter the Krebs cycle; instead, pyruvate is converted to lactate. If there continues to be an insufficient cellular oxygen supply, lactic acidosis ensues. Anaerobic glycolysis leads to the production of two molecules of adenosine triphosphate (ATP) per molecule of glucose, rather than 38 molecules of ATP from aerobic glycolysis (Figure 10.3).

Initial serum lactate levels are normally used to direct resuscitative efforts and do correlate with mortality (15,16). The monitoring of lactate concentrations over time appears to be more predictive of mortality than monitoring of initial lactate concentrations. Multiple studies have indicated that the time required for clearance of lactate or normalization of lactate during resuscitation from shock can be used as an index of outcome (17–19). The use of lactate as a marker of tissue perfusion has limitations. Hyperlactatemia can be produced in type B lactic acidosis in the absence of tissue malperfusion. Also, for blood lactate levels to increase, lactate must accumulate and leak outside a tissue into the systemic circulation, and its rate of production must surpass its rate of uptake by other organs (20).

The anion gap is a commonly used screening test for the presence of lactic acidosis. A study in surgical ICU patients

concluded, however, that in patients with peak blood lactate levels greater or equal to 2.5 mmol/L, the anion gap is an insensitive screen for elevated lactate in a critically ill, hospitalized population (21). Fifty-seven percent of the patients with elevated lactate levels did not have an elevated anion gap, suggesting that hyperlactatemia should be included in the differential diagnosis of nonanion gap acidosis. Acidosis (pH <7.30) was not found to alter mortality.

Base deficit

Base deficit is a derived variable, and is defined as the amount of additional base (mmol) required to normalize the pH of 1 L of whole blood. It is calculated from the blood gas analyzer from the PCO_2, pH, and HCO_3^- values applied to a standard nomogram.

$$\text{Base deficit} = -[(HCO_3) - 24.8 + (16.2 \times (pH - 7.4))]$$

An elevated base deficit has been a proven marker of mortality from many studies, and has been shown to have direct correlation with lactate levels (22,23). The severity of this deficit has been directly linked to the volume of fluid replacement within the first 24 hours of resuscitation. Husain and colleagues reported that initial base deficit values are poor predictors of mortality and do not correlate with lactate levels in the surgical intensive care population (24). Base deficit measurements have proved usefulness in trauma populations. In a prospective observational study conducted by Schmelzer and associates (25), the measurement of central venous base deficit was predictive of survival past 24 hours. Paladino and colleagues concluded that the additional information derived from metabolic parameters such as lactate and base deficit with traditional vital signs increases the sensitivity of the ability to distinguish major and minor injury by 76 percent (26).

Metabolic derangements, such as hyperchloremic acidosis from the administration of normal saline, renal failure, or diabetic ketoacidosis, can produce a metabolic acidosis distinct to tissue malperfusion and alter base deficit values. Furthermore, the administration of sodium bicarbonate can confound the utility of base deficit during resuscitation (27, 28).

Mixed venous oxygen saturation (SvO$_2$)

SvO_2 measurement is considered a gold standard in determining adequacy of oxygen delivery and global tissue perfusion. Blood is aspirated from the distal port of a pulmonary artery catheter. It represents the saturation of blood returning to the pulmonary artery after mixing in the right ventricle. The formula for the SvO_2 calculation can be derived by modification of the Fick equation:

$$SvO_2 = SaO_2 - VO_2/CO \times 1.34 \times Hb$$

A decrease in the SvO_2 is indicative of a reduction in total oxygen delivery. This may include one or more of the following situations: (a) decreased CO; (b) increased oxygen consumption; (c) decreased arterial oxygen saturation; or (d) decreased hemoglobin concentration. Normal values range from 70 percent to 75 percent. SvO_2 values below 60 percent may be a sign of cellular oxidative impairments; values consistently below 50 percent are indicative of anaerobic metabolism (29).

Central venous oxygen saturation (ScvO₂)

SvO_2 is a very useful monitoring in the management of shock, but it requires the placement of PAC, which is less routinely used in modern day critical care. Recent literature has focused on the sampling of central venous oxygen saturation ($ScvO_2$) in the resuscitation in septic shock with impressive results (12). $ScvO_2$ is the oxygen saturation of venous blood measured near the junction of the superior vena cava and the right atrium. Advantages of $ScvO_2$ sampling include the need for only a central venous catheter and its ability to be used for patients in whom a PAC cannot be inserted, such as in pediatric patients. $ScvO_2$ values are usually less than the corresponding SvO_2 by about 2percent to 3 percent because of the higher extraction ratio of the brain (30, 31). Much controversy has arisen regarding whether $ScvO_2$ is an actual surrogate to SvO_2. The differences between the absolute values of $ScvO_2$ and SvO_2 changes with the degree of shock and the type of shock (32, 33).

The SvO_2 and $ScvO_2$ parallel has been studied extensively. Yazigi and coworkers evaluated the correlation between the two in 64 consecutive postcardiac surgical patients. The study revealed a large discrepancy in $ScvO_2$ and SvO_2 values sampled. It was concluded that in patients after coronary artery surgery, $ScvO_2$ could not be used as a direct alterative to SvO_2 (34). Chawla and associates studied paired samplings of $ScvO_2$ and SvO_2 in a mixed medical and surgical population requiring a PAC to guide fluid therapy. They concluded that measurements of $ScvO_2$ and SvO_2 were not equivalent in this sample of critically ill patients and that $ScvO_2$ was not a reliable surrogate for SvO_2 (35). However, Dueck and colleagues recently performed a prospective clinical trial sampling $ScvO_2$ and SvO_2 measurements in patients undergoing elective neurosurgical procedures. In this sample of patients, the absolute values of $ScvO_2$ were not equivalent to those of SvO_2 in varying hemodynamic conditions, but the trend of $ScvO_2$ may be substituted for the trend of SvO_2 (36). Tahvanainen and coworkers found similar results (37). Further studies are required for evaluation and validation of $ScvO_2$ during resuscitation for specific patient populations.

Regional indicators of tissue perfusion

Regional endpoints are intended for the early detection of tissue ischemia and hypoxia in the microvasculature; when compared with global endpoints of resuscitation, they have been superior predictors of outcome (38).

Near-infrared spectroscopy

Near-infrared spectroscopy (NIRS) has emerged in recent years as a potentially valuable way of monitoring hypoperfusion noninvasively and optimizing oxygen delivery and consumption specifically at the tissue level. NIRS uses computer analysis of spectra in the near-infrared range, 700 nm to 2500 nm, to determine the oxidation state of hemoglobin in tissues. Light is absorbed by the various derivatives of hemoglobin, such as oxyhemoglobin (HbO_2), deoxyhemoglobin (Hob), and myoglobin, which differ in near-infrared wavelengths (39). Tissue oxygen saturation (StO_2) is calculated from an intricate algorithm of the ratio of absorption of wavelengths of the individual hemoglobins. This developing technology is allowing for swift, noninvasive approximation of local tissue oxygen saturation (40).

McKinley and colleagues (41) compared changes in StO_2 with a series of clinical indices of resuscitation in trauma patients. This study demonstrated changes in skeletal muscle StO_2 paralleled oxygen delivery during the resuscitation of severely injured trauma patients who were at risk of developing multiple-organ failure. Multiple studies have been done with NIRS technology in patients with various degrees of sepsis. Measurements comparing muscle StO_2 values in resuscitated sepsis patients and healthy volunteers were found to be inconsistent. In some studies, StO_2 measurements between the two groups were found to be comparable (42, 43).

Creteur and associates established that there are frequent alterations in muscle StO_2 in a large population of critically ill sepsis patients and that these alterations are more prevalent in the presence of shock (44). Mulier and colleagues (45) concluded that NIRS measurements of StO_2 correlated with invasive hemodynamic measurements in patients with severe sepsis but did not correlate with severity of illness. These findings suggest that NIRS may be clinically useful in measurement and monitoring of patients with severe sepsis. Additional studies are required for the evaluation of NIRS technology in the early resuscitation phase of sepsis. (See Chapter 21 for a more extensive discussion of NIRS.)

Tissue CO₂ monitoring

Tissue hypoperfusion in the gastrointestinal tract in the face of disturbed hemodynamics is well documented. Gastric tonometry and sublingual capnometry are based on the premise that tissue CO_2 levels escalate in conditions in which gut tissue perfusion is impaired (46–48). CO_2 is liberated when excess hydrogen ions are formed from the breakdown of high-energy phosphate compounds during tissue hypoperfusion, which are then buffered by bicarbonate (49). Gastric tonometric measurements of gastric intramucosal pH (pHi) correlate with splanchnic vascular blood flow, with pHi decreasing in value as splanchnic perfusion diminishes. Although pHi is the first to be affected during the onset of shock (50), it has been shown to correlate poorly with lactate and base deficit (51, 52). In the critical care arena, gastric tonometry has been used to titrate vasopressor agents to improve perfusion of the gastrointestinal tract in the critically ill (53, 54). Various studies have demonstrated its usefulness in predicting weaning outcomes in patients being

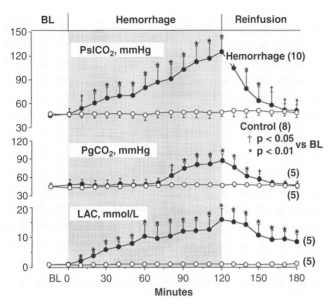

Figure 10.4. Comparison of sublingual PCO_2 ($PslCO_2$), gastric PCO_2 ($PgCO_2$), and arterial lactate (LAC) before, during, and after reversal of hemorrhage. All values represent mean ± standard deviation. $P < 0.05$, *$p < 0.01$ versus baseline. (From reference 59. Copyright American Thoracic Society.)

liberated from mechanical ventilation (55, 56). Limitations of gastric tonometry include the requirement of placement of specialized nasogastric tubes, excluding pediatric patients; slow calibration time; and the inability to provide enteral nutrition while measurements are being taken (49). (See Chapter 9 for a more complete description of gastric tonometry.)

Sublingual capnometry, on the other hand, is an easily accessible method to evaluate perfusion of the splanchnic circulation. A sensor placed beneath the tongue measures the partial pressure of carbon dioxide ($PslCO_2$) generated. Several studies have confirmed that an increase in sublingual PCO_2 correlated with reductions in mean arterial pressure – and, thus, cardiac output – during hemorrhagic and septic shock (57–60). Nakagawa and colleagues investigated sublingual tissue PCO_2 during hemorrhagic and septic shock in rats. In both forms of shock, highly significant linear correlations were observed among end-tidal PCO_2, sublingual PCO_2, and arterial blood lactate levels (Figure 10.4) (59).

A $PslCO_2$ value of 70 mmHg or more has been linked to elevated arterial lactate levels and is predictive of decreased hospital survival (61). Limitations of sublingual capnography include the fact that sublingual mucosa is not perfused by splanchnic blood flow; therefore, elevations in $PslCO_2$ may be delayed compared with pHi levels in progressive shock states. Therefore, it may not serve as a "canary" of the body (62).

Both Marik (63) and Rackow (64) found higher differences between $PslCO_2$ and $PaCO_2$ values ($\Delta Psl–aCO_2$) in hemodynamically unstable nonsurvivors versus survivors admitted to the ICU. This suggests that $\Delta Psl-aCO_2$ is a better prognostic indicator than $PslCO_2$ alone.

Orthogonal polarization spectral imaging

Orthogonal polarization spectral (OPS) imaging employs polarized light to directly visualize the microcirculation. Polarized light is transmitted to hemoglobin molecules in the microcirculation, which in turn absorbs and reflects the light to a videomicroscope (65). The functional density of the capillaries imaged has been shown to be a sensitive marker of tissue perfusion (66). De Backer and coworkers reported that the density, as well as the total number, of sublingual vessels diminished significantly in patients with sepsis compared with controls (67). Other tissues evaluated with OPS imaging include oral, sublingual, rectal, and vaginal mucosa. Currently, OPS imaging remains an investigational method of monitoring (68).

Transcutaneous oxygen tension

Direct measurements of oxygen and carbon dioxide tension within the skin with the help of heated probes is a monitoring modality that was first developed 30 years ago. In a state of shock, similar to the splanchnic circulation, the skin and skeletal muscle blood flow is restricted. Measurements of oxygen and carbon dioxide tension may be indicative of tissue hypoperfusion. Tatevossian and associates have demonstrated an increased mortality rate in patients with low oxygen or high carbon dioxide values (69). This technology is limited by the potential for thermal burns from the heated probes and tissue trauma from probe insertion (66).

Metabolic positron emission tomography

Metabolic positron emission tomography (PET) is another noninvasive method for measuring oxygen transport and regional tissue oxygenation. With PET scanning, an isotope tracer is used to highlight blood flow and estimate oxygen delivery. Mintun and coworkers noted that oxygen levels in the brains of nine healthy volunteers had no correlation with blood flow (70). Regional oxygenation of the liver and myocardium have also been calculated (71, 72). The lack of transportability and cost of PET are the major deterrents to its implementation in the ICU setting.

Conclusions

To prevent shock-related multiorgan failure, there is an urgent need to develop methods to accurately and rapidly recognize oxygen delivery and tissue hypoxia in the critically ill. Despite the large number of technologies available to clinicians, none individually is universally applicable or has been demonstrated to improve survival when resuscitative efforts are under way. Measurement of CaO_2 and CO for the calculation of oxygen delivery is currently the most familiar approach for assessment of global DO_2. Regional assessments of tissue oxygenation, such as tissue goniometry, have yet to influence outcome. Newer methods, such as NIRS and OPS imaging, have allowed for continuous monitoring of oxygenation of individual organs. More research is necessary in the future to provide useful clinical devices for the quantification of adequacy of regional tissue oxygenation in the critically ill.

References

1. Levy MM. Pathophysiology of oxygen delivery in respiratory failure. *Chest* 2005;128:547S–553S.
2. Greene KE, Peters JI. Pathophysiology of acute respiratory failure. *Clin Chest Med* 1994;15:1–12.
3. Leach RM, Treacher DF. Oxygen delivery and consumption in the critically ill. *Thorax* 2002;57:170–177.
4. Jolliet P, Thorens JB, Nicod L, et al. Relationship between pulmonary oxygen consumption, lung inflammation, and calculated venous admixture in patients with acute lung injury. *Intensive Care Med* 1996;22:277–285.
5. Marino PL. Oxygen and carbon dioxide transport. In *The ICU Book*, Third Edition. Philadelphia: Lippincott Williams & Wilkins, 2007, pp. 28–31.
6. Huang Y. Monitoring oxygen delivery in the critically ill. *Chest* 2005;128:554S–560S.
7. Schumacher PT, Cain SM. The concept of a critical DO_2. *Intensive Care Med* 1987;13:223.
8. Bihari D, Smithies M, Gimson A, et al. The effect of vasodilation with prostacyclin on oxygen delivery and uptake in critically ill patients. *N Engl J Med* 1987;317:397–403.
9. Velmahos GC, Demetriades D, Shoemaker WC, et al. Endpoints of resuscitation of critically injured patients: normal or supranormal? A prospective randomized trial. *Ann Surg* 2000;232(3):409–18.
10. Kern JW, Shoemaker WC. Meta-analysis of hemodynamic optimization in high-risk patients. Review. *Crit Care Med* 2002;30(8):1686–92.
11. Rivers EP, Coba V, Whitmaill M. Early goal-directed therapy in severe sepsis and septic shock: a contemporary review of the literature. *Curr Opin Anaesthesiol* 2008;21(3):424.
12. Rivers E, Nguyen B, Haystad S, et al. Early goal-directed therapy in the treatment of severe sepsis and septic shock. *N Engl J Med* 2001 Nov 8;345(19):1368–77.
13. Abou-Khalil B, Scalea TM, Trooskin SZ, et al. Hemodynamic responses to shock in young trauma patients: need for invasive monitoring. *Crit Care Med* 1994;22:633–9.
14. De Backer D, Creteur J, Dubois MJ, et al. The effect of dobutamine on microcirculation alterations in patients with septic shock are are independent of systemic effects. *Crit Care Med* 2006;34:403–8.
15. Peretz DI, Scott HM, Duff J, et al. The significance of lactic academia in the shock syndrome. *Ann NY Acad Sci* 1965;119:1133–41.
16. Vincent J-L, Dufaye P, Berre J, et al. Serial lactate determinations during circulatory shock. *Crit Care Med* 1983;11:449–51.
17. Falk JL, Rackow EC, Leavy J, et al. Delayed lactate clearance in patients surviving circulatory shock. *Acute Care* 1985;11:212–5.
18. Abramson D, Scalea TM, Hitchcock R, et al. Lactate clearance and survival following injury. *J Trauma* 1993;35:584–9.
19. McNeilis J, Marini A, Jurkiewicz A, et al. Prolonged lactate clearance is associated with increased mortality in the surgical intensive care unit. *Am J Surg* 2001;182:481–2.
20. Mizock BA, Falk JL. Lactic acidosis in critical illness. *Crit Care Med* 1992;20:80.
21. Iberti TJ, Leibowitz AB, Papadakos PJ, et al. Low sensitivity of the anion gap as a screen to detect hyperlactatemia in critically ill patients. Crit Care Med 1990 Mar;18(3):275–7.
22. Davis JW. The relationship of base deficit to lactate in porcine hemorrhagic shock and resuscitation. *J Trauma* 1994;36:168–72.
23. Bannon MP, O'Neill CM, Martin M, et al. Central venous oxygen saturation, arterial base deficit, and lactate concentration in trauma patients. *Am Surg* 1995;61:738–45.
24. Husain FA, Martin MJ, Mullenix PS, et al. Serum lactate and base deficit as predictors of mortality and morbidity. *Am J Surg* 2003;185(5):485–91.
25. Schmelzer TM, Perron AD, Thomason MH, et al. A comparison of central venous and arterial base deficit as a predictor of survival in acute trauma. *Am J Emerg Med* 2008;26(2):119–23.
26. Paladino L, Sinert R, Wallace D, et al. The utility of base deficit and arterial lactate in differentiating major from minor injury in trauma patients with normal vital signs. *Resuscitation* 2008;77(3):363–8.
27. Brill SA, Stewart TR, Brundage SI, et al. Base deficit does not predict mortality when secondary to hyperchloremic acidosis. *Shock* 2002;17:459–62.
28. Englehart MS, Schreiber MA. Measurement of acid-base resuscitation endpoints: lactate, base deficit, bicarbonate or what? *Curr Opin Crit Care* 2006;12:569–74.
29. Miller MJ, Cook W, Mithoefer J. Limitations of the use of mixed venous pO_2 as an indicator of tissue hypoxia. *Clin Res* 1979;27:401.
30. Marx G, Reinhart K. Venous oximetry. *Curr Opin Crit Care* 2006;12:263–68.
31. Polanco PM, Pinsky MR. Practical issues of hemodynamic monitoring at the bedside. *Surg Clin North Am.* 2006;86(6):1431–56.
32. Lee J, Wright F, Barber R, et al. Central venous oxygen saturation in shock: study in man. *Anesthesiology* 1972;36:472–478.
33. Reinhart K, Kuhn HJ, Hartog C, et al. Continuous central venous and pulmonary artery oxygen saturation monitoring in the critically ill. *Intensive Care Med* 2004;30:1572–8.
34. Yazigi A, Khoury CE, Jebara S, et al. Comparison of central venous to mixed venous oxygen saturation in patients with low cardiac index and filling pressures after coronary artery surgery. *J Cardiothorac Vasc Anesth* 2008;22:77–83.
35. Chawla LS, Zia H, Gutierrez G, et al. Lack of equivalence between central and mixed venous oxygen saturation. *Chest* 2004;126:1891–6.
36. Dueck MH, Klimek M, Appenrodt S, et al. Trends but not individual values of central venous oxygen saturation agree with mixed venous oxygen saturation during varying hemodynamic conditions. *Anesthesiology* 2005;13:249–57.
37. Tahvanainen J, Meretoja O, Nikki P. Can central venous blood replace mixed venous blood samples? *Crit Care Med* 1982;10:758–61.
38. Poeze M, Solberg BC, Greve JW, et al. Monitoring global volume-related hemodynamic or regional variables after initial resuscitation: what is a better predictor of outcome in critically ill septic patients? *Crit Care Med* 2005;33:2494–2500.
39. Salman M, Glantzounis GK, Yang W, et al. Measurement of critical lower limb tissue hypoxia by coupling chemical and optical techniques. *Clin Sci* 2005;108:159–65.
40. Crookes BA, Cohn SM, Buton EA, et al. Noninvasive muscle oxygenation to guide fluid resuscitation after traumatic shock. *Surgery* 2004;135:662–70.
41. McKinley BA, Marvin RG, Cocanour CS, et al. Tissue hemoglobin O_2 saturation during resuscitation of traumatic shock monitored using near infrared spectroscopy. *J Trauma* 2000;48:637–42.

42. Pareznik R, Knezevic R, Voga G, et al. Changes in muscle tissue oxygenation during stagnant ischemia in septic patients. *Intensive Care Med* 2006;32:87–92.

43. De Blasi RA, Palmisani S, Alampi D, et al. Microvascular dysfunction and skeletal muscle oxygenation assessed by phase modulation near-infrared spectroscopy in patients with septic shock. *Intensive Care Med* 2005;31:1661–1668.

44. Creteur J, Carollo T, Soldati G, et al. The prognostic value of muscle StO2 in septic patients. *Intensive Care Med* 2007;33:1549–56.

45. Mulier KE, Skarda DE, Taylor JH, et al. Near-infrared spectroscopy in patients with severe sepsis: correlation with invasive hemodynamic measurements. *Surg Infect* 2008;9(5):515–9.

46. Marik PE, Bankov A. Sublingual capnometry versus traditional markers of tissue oxygenation in critically ill patients. *Crit Care Med* 2003;31:818–22.

47. Fink MP. Tissue capnometry as a monitoring strategy for critically ill patients: just about ready for prime time. *Chest* 1998;114:667–70.

48. Weil MH, Nakagawa Y, Tang W, et al. Sublingual capnometry: a new noninvasive measurement for diagnosis and quantitation of severity of circulatory shock. *Crit Care Med.* 1999;27:1225–9.

49. Marik PE. Regional carbon dioxide monitoring to assess the adequency of tissue perfusion. *Curr Opin Crit Care* 2005;11:245–51.

50. Porter J. Splanchnic circulation in shock. *Trauma* 1996;12:205–18.

51. Chang MC, et al. Gastric tonometry supplements information provided by systemic indicators of oxygen transport. *J Trauma* 1994;37:488–94.

52. Ivatury RR, et al. A prospective randomized study of end points of resuscitation after major trauma:global oxygen transport indices versus organ-specific gastric mucosal pH. *J Am Coll Surg* 1996;183:145–54.

53. Marik PE, Mohedin M. The contrasting effects of dopamine and norepinephrine on systemic and splanchic oxygen utilization in hyperdynamic sepsis. *JAMA* 1994;272(17):1354–7.

54. Duranteau J, Sitbon P, Teboul JL. Effects of epinephrine, norepinephine, or the combination of norepinephrine and dobutamine on gastric mucosa in septic shock. *Crit Care Med* 1999;27:2166–77.

55. Bouachour G, Guiraud MP, Gouello JP, et al. Gastric intramucosal pH and intraluminal PCO_2 during weaning from mechanical ventilation in COPD patients. *Eur Respir J* 1996;9:1868–73.

56. Hurtado FJ, Beron M, Olivera W, et al. Gastric intramucosal pH and intraluminal PCO_2 during weaning from mechanical ventilation. *Crit Care Med* 2001;29:70–76.

57. Jin X, Weil MH, Sun S, et al. Decreases in organ blood flows associated with increases in sublingual PCO_2 during hemorrhagic shock. *J Appl Physiol* 1998;85:2360–64.

58. Pernat A, Weil MH, Tang W, et al. Effects of hyper- and hypoventilation on gastric and sublingual PCO_2. *J Appl Physiol* 1999;87:933–7.

59. Nakagawa Y, Weil MH, Tang W, et al. Sublingual capnometry for diagnosis and quantitation of circulatory shock. *Am J Respir Crit Care Med* 1998;157:1838–43.

60. Povoas HP, Weil MH, Tang W, et al. Comparisons between sublingual and gastric tonometry during hemorrhagic shock. *Chest* 2000;118:1127–32.

61. Weil MH, Nakagawa Y, Tang W, et al. Sublingual capnometry: a new noninvasive measurement for diagnosis and quantification of severity of circulatory shock. *Crit Care Med* 1999;27(7):1225–9.

62. Dantzker DR. The gastrointestinal tract: the canary of the body? *JAMA* 1993;270:1247–48.

63. Marik PE. Sublingual capnography: a clinical validation study. *Chest* 2001;120:923–7.

64. Rackow EC, O'Neil P, Astiz ME, Carpati CM. Sublingual capnometry and indexes of tissue perfusion in patients with circulatory failure. *Chest* 2001;120:1633–8.

65. Wilson M, Davis DP, Coimbra R. Diagnosis and monitoring of hemorrhagic shock during the initial resuscitation of multiple trauma patients: a review. *J Emerg Med* 2003;24(4):413–22.

66. Winters ME, McCurdy MT, Zilberstein J. Monitoring the critically ill emergency department patient. *Emerg Med Clin North Am* 2008;26:741–57.

67. De Backer D, Creteur J, Preiser JC et al. Microvascular blood flow is altered in patients with sepsis. *Am J Respir Crit Care Med* 2002;166:98–104.

68. Lima A, Bakker J. Noninvasive monitoring of peripheral perfusion. *Intensive Care Med* 2005;31:1316–26.

69. Tatevossian RG, Wo CC, Velmahos GC, et al. Transcutaneous oxygen and CO_2 as early warning of tissue hypoxia and hemodynamic shock in critically ill emergency patients. *Crit Care Med* 2000;28:2248–53.

70. Mintun MA, Lundstrom BN, Snyder AZ, et al. Blood flow and oxygen delivery to human brain during functional activity: theoretical modeling and experimental data. *Proc Natl Acad Sci USA* 2001;98:6859–64.

71. Piert M, Machulla HJ, Becker G, et al. Dependency of the 18F fluoromisonidazole uptake on the oxygen delivery and tissue oxygenation in the porcine liver. *Nucl Med Biol* 2000;27:693–700.

72. Porenta G, Cherry S, Czernin J, et al. Noninvasive determination of myocardial blood flow, oxygen consumption and efficiency in normal humans by carbon-11 acetate positron emission tomography imaging. *Eur J Nucl Med* 1999;26:1465–74.

Transesophageal echocardiography

Ronald A. Kahn and Gregory W. Fischer

Technical concepts

Physics of ultrasound

In ultrasonography, the heart and great vessels are insonated with ultrasound, which is sound above the human audible range. The ultrasound is sent into the area of interest and is partially reflected by the structures. From these reflections, distance, velocity, and density of objects are derived.

Wavelength, frequency, and velocity

An ultrasound beam is a continuous or intermittent train of sound waves emitted by a transducer or wave generator. It is composed of density or pressure waves and can exist in any medium, with the exception of a vacuum. Ultrasound waves are characterized by their wavelength, frequency, and velocity. *Wavelength* is the distance between the two nearest points of equal pressure or density in an ultrasound beam, and *velocity* is the speed at which the waves propagate through a medium. As the waves travel past any fixed point in an ultrasound beam, the pressure cycles regularly and continuously between a high and a low value. The number of cycles per second (hertz) is called the *frequency* of the wave. Ultrasound is sound with frequencies above 20,000 Hz, which is the upper limit of the human audible range. The relationship among the frequency (f), wavelength (λ), and velocity (v) of a sound wave is defined by the formula

$$v = f \times \lambda. \qquad (11.1)$$

The velocity of sound varies with the properties of the medium through which it travels. For soft tissues, this velocity approximates 1540 m/sec. Because the frequency of an ultrasound beam is determined by the properties of the emitting transducer, and the velocity is a function of the tissues through which the sound travels, wavelengths vary according to the relationship expressed in Equation 11.1.

Piezoelectric crystals convert between ultrasound and electrical signals. When presented with a high-frequency electrical signal, these crystals produced ultrasound energy, which is directed toward the areas to be imaged. Commonly, a short ultrasound signal is emitted from the piezoelectric crystal. After ultrasound wave formation, the crystal "listens" for the returning echoes for a given period of time and then pauses prior to

repeating this cycle. This cycle length is known as the *pulse repetition frequency* (PRF). This cycle length must be long enough to provide enough time for a signal to travel to and return from a given object of interest. Typically, PRFs vary from 1 to 10 kHz, which results in 0.1 to 1 msec between pulses. When reflected ultrasound waves return to these piezoelectric crystals, they are converted into electrical signals, which may be appropriately processed and displayed. Electronic circuits measure the time delay between the emitted and received echoes. Because the speed of ultrasound through tissue is a constant, this time delay may be converted into the precise distance between the transducer and tissue.

Attenuation, reflection, and scatter

Waves interact with the medium in which they travel and with one another. Interaction among waves is called *interference*. The manner in which waves interact with a medium is determined by its density and homogeneity. When a wave is propagated through an inhomogeneous medium (and all living tissue is essentially inhomogeneous), it is partly reflected, partly absorbed, and partly scattered.

Ultrasound waves are reflected when the width of the reflecting object is larger than one-fourth of the ultrasound wavelength. To visualize smaller objects, ultrasound waves of shorter wavelengths must be used. Because the velocity of sound in soft tissue is approximately constant, shorter wavelengths are obtained by increasing the frequency of the ultrasound beam. In addition, ultrasound impedance of the object must be significantly different from the ultrasonic impedance in front of the object. The ultrasound impedance of a given medium is equal to the medium density multiplied by the ultrasound propagation velocity. Air has a low density and propagation velocity, so it has a low ultrasound impedance. Bone has a high density and propagation velocity, so it has a high ultrasound impedance. Because the ultrasound impedances of air or bone are significantly different from that of blood, ultrasound is strongly reflected from these interfaces, limiting the availability of ultrasound to deeper structures. Echo studies across lung or other gas-containing tissues are not feasible, nor are those across bone.

Reflected echoes, also called *specular echoes*, are usually much stronger than scattered echoes. A grossly inhomogeneous medium, such as a stone in a water bucket or a cardiac valve in a blood-filled heart chamber, produces strong specular reflections at the water–stone or blood–valve interface because of the significant differences in ultrasound impedances. Conversely, media that are inhomogeneous at the microscopic level, such as muscle, produce more scatter than specular reflection, because the differences in adjacent ultrasound impedances are low and the objects are small. Although smaller objects can be visualized with higher frequencies, more scatter is produced by insignificant inhomogeneities in the medium, confusing signals are generated, ultrasound beams are attenuated, and the depth of ultrasound penetration is limited.

Attenuation refers to the loss of ultrasound power as it traverses tissue. Tissue attenuation is dependent on ultrasound reflection, scattering, and absorption. The absorption occurs as a result of the conversion of ultrasound energy into heat. The greater the ultrasound reflection and scattering, the less ultrasound energy is available for penetration and resolution of deeper structures; this effect is especially important during scanning with higher frequencies. Whereas water, blood, and muscle have low ultrasound attenuation, air and bone have very high tissue ultrasound attenuation, limiting the ability of ultrasound to traverse these structures.

Image formation

M mode

The most basic form of ultrasound imaging is M-mode echocardiography. In this mode, the density and position of all tissues in the path of a narrow ultrasound beam (i.e. along a single line) are displayed as a scroll on a video screen. The scrolling produces an updated, continuously changing time plot of the studied tissue section, several seconds in duration. Because this is a timed *motion display* (normal cardiac tissue is always in motion), it is called M mode. Because only a very limited part of the heart is being observed at any one time and because the image requires considerable interpretation, M mode is not currently used as a primary imaging technique.

2D mode

By rapid, repetitive scanning along many different radii within an area in the shape of a fan (sector), echocardiography generates a two-dimensional (2D) image of a section of the heart. This image, which resembles an anatomic section and, thus, can be more easily interpreted, is called a *2D scan*. Information on structures and motion in the plane of a 2D scan is updated 30 to 60 times per second. This repetitive update produces a live (real-time) image of the heart. Scanning 2D echo devices image the heart by using either a mechanically steered transducer or, as is common in most devices, an electronically steered ultrasound beam (phased-array transducer).

Doppler techniques

Most modern ultrasound scanners combine Doppler capabilities with their 2D imaging capabilities. After the desired view

has been obtained by 2D ultrasonography, the Doppler beam, represented by a cursor, is superimposed on the 2D image. The operator positions the cursor as parallel as possible to the assumed direction of blood flow and then empirically adjusts the direction of the beam to optimize the audio and visual representations of the reflected Doppler signal. At the present time, Doppler technology can be used in at least four different ways to measure blood velocities: pulsed, continuous-wave, and color-flow.

The Doppler effect

Information on blood flow dynamics can be obtained by applying Doppler frequency shift analysis to echoes reflected by the moving red blood cells. Blood flow velocity, direction, and acceleration can be instantaneously determined. This information is different from that obtained in 2D imaging and hence complements it.

The Doppler principle, as applied in echocardiography, states that the frequency of ultrasound reflected by a moving target (red blood cells) will be different from the frequency of the reflected ultrasound. The magnitude and direction of the frequency shift are related to the velocity and direction of the moving target. The velocity of the target is calculated with the Doppler equation:

$$v = (c f_d)/(2 f_0 \cos \theta), \qquad (11.2)$$

where v = the target velocity (blood flow velocity), c = the speed of sound in tissue, f_d = the frequency shift, f_0 = the frequency of the emitted ultrasound, and θ = the angle between the ultrasound beam and the direction of the target velocity (blood flow).

The only ambiguity in Equation 11.2 is that, theoretically, the direction of the ultrasonic signal could refer to either the transmitted or the received beam; however, by convention, Doppler displays are made with reference to the received beam. Thus, if the blood flow and the reflected beam travel in the same direction, the angle of incidence is zero degrees and the cosine is +1. As a result, the frequency of the reflected signal will be higher than the frequency of the emitted signal.

Equipment currently used in clinical practice displays Doppler blood flow velocities as waveforms. The waveforms consist of a spectral analysis of velocities on the ordinate and time on the abscissa. By convention, blood flow toward the transducer is represented above the baseline. If the blood flows away from the transducer, the angle of incidence will be 180 degrees, the cosine will equal –1, and the waveform will be displayed below the baseline. When the blood flow is perpendicular to the ultrasonic beam, the angle of incidence will be 90 or 270 degrees, the cosine of either angle will be zero, and no blood flow will be detected. Because the cosine of the angle of incidence is a variable in the Doppler equation, blood flow velocity is measured most accurately when the ultrasound beam is parallel or antiparallel to the direction of blood flow. In clinical practice, a deviation from parallel of up to 20 degrees can be tolerated, because this results in an error of only 6 percent or less.

Pulsed-wave Doppler

In pulsed-wave (PW) Doppler, blood flow parameters can be determined at precise locations within the heart by emitting repetitive short bursts of ultrasound at a specific frequency (the PRF) and analyzing the frequency shift of the reflected echoes at an identical sampling frequency (f_s). A time delay between the emission of the ultrasound signal burst and the sampling of the reflected signal determines the depth at which the velocities are sampled. The delay is proportional to the distance between the transducer and the location of the velocity measurements. To sample at a given depth (D), sufficient time must be allowed for the signal to travel a distance of $2 \times D$ (from the transducer to the sample volume and back). The time delay, T_d, between the emission of the signal and the reception of the reflected signal is related to D and to the speed of sound in tissues (c) by the following formula:

$$D = c\,T_d/2. \tag{11.3}$$

The operator varies the depth of sampling by varying the time delay between the emission of the ultrasonic signal and the sampling of the reflected wave. In practice, the sampling location or *sample volume* is represented by a small marker, which can be positioned at any point along the Doppler beam by moving it up or down the Doppler cursor. On some devices, it is also possible to vary the width and height of the sample volume.

The tradeoff for the ability to measure flow at precise locations is that ambiguous information is obtained when flow velocity is very high. A simple reference to Western movies will clearly illustrate this point. When a stagecoach gets under way, its wheel spokes are observed as rotating in the correct direction. As soon as a certain speed is attained, rotation in the reverse direction is noted because the camera frame rate is too slow to correctly observe the motion of the wheel spokes. In PW Doppler, the ambiguity exists because the measured Doppler frequency shift (f_D) and the sampling frequency (f_s) are in the same frequency (kilohertz) range. Ambiguity will be avoided only if the f_D is less than half the sampling frequency.

The expression $f_s/2$ is also known as the Nyquist limit. Doppler shifts above the Nyquist limit will create artifacts described as "aliasing" or "wraparound," and blood flow velocities will appear in a direction opposite to the conventional one. Blood flowing with high velocity toward the transducer will result in a display of velocities above and below the baseline. This artifact can be avoided by increasing the f_s, but this then limits the time available for a pulse to travel to the sample volume and back, thus limiting the range.

Continuous-wave Doppler

The continuous-wave (CW) Doppler technique uses continuous, rather than discrete, pulses of ultrasound waves. As a result, the region in which flow dynamics are measured cannot be precisely localized. Blood flow velocity is measured with great accuracy, however, even at high flows. CW Doppler is particularly useful for the evaluation of patients with valvular lesions or congenital heart disease. It is also the preferred technique when attempting to derive hemodynamic information from Doppler signals.

Color-flow mapping

During color-flow Doppler (CFD) mapping, real-time blood flow within the heart as colors, along with 2D images in black and white, are displayed. In addition to showing the location, direction, and velocity of cardiac blood flow, the images produced by these devices allow estimation of flow acceleration and differentiation of laminar and turbulent blood flow. CFD echocardiography is based on the principle of multigated PW Doppler, in which blood flow velocities are sampled at many locations along many lines covering the entire imaging sector. At the same time, the sector is also scanned to generate a 2D image.

A location in the heart in which the scanner has detected flow toward the transducer (the top of the image sector) is assigned the color red. Flow away from the direction of the top is assigned the color blue. This color assignment is arbitrary and determined by the equipment's manufacturer and the user's color mapping. In the most common color-flow coding scheme, the faster the velocity, the more intense the color. Flow velocities that change by more than a preset value within a brief time interval (flow variance) have another color added to either the red or the blue. Both rapidly accelerating laminar flow (change in flow speed) and turbulent flow (change in flow direction) satisfy the criteria for rapid changes in velocity. In summary, the brightness of the red or blue colors at any location and time is usually proportional to the corresponding flow velocity, and the hue is proportional to the temporal rate of change of the velocity.

Technical concepts of 3D echocardiography

Two different technological approaches are available for acquiring three-dimensional (3D) images. The first technique requires the acquisition of multiple, gated image planes using ECG and respiratory gating to limit the amount of motion artifacts. Once a region of interest is identified, the probe rotates from zero to 180 degrees acquiring different 2D images every few degrees. After all 2D images are acquired and stored, they are postprocessed and integrated into a 3D image that can further be optimized. Real-time, instantaneous imaging can never be obtained using this technology because of the sequential acquisition of the different planes. Additionally, the gating requirements of this technology (e.g. 90 or more 2D planes) frequently result in motion artifacts. The gated technique uses the same technology that is currently employed for standard 2D scanning. One-dimensional arrays, consisting of 128 piezoelectric crystals that are interconnected electronically, generate an acoustic beam that can be steered in a flat scanning plane (axial and

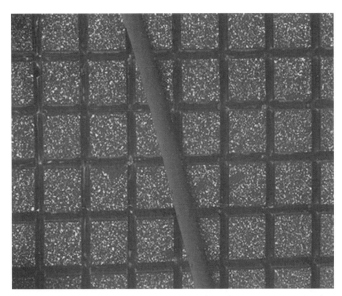

Figure 11.1. Matrix array with 2500 independent elements representing the basis for real-time 3D scanning. Human hair is shown to better demonstrate dimensions. (See Color Plate I.)

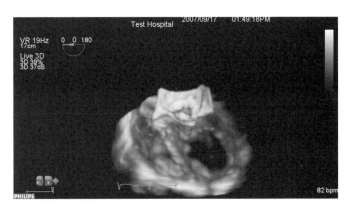

Figure 11.2. Live 3D real-time scanning showing a 3D volume pyramid. (See Color Plate II.)

lateral planes). This to-and-fro sweeping motion of the acoustic beam across the sector represents the basis of any phased array transducer system. This technology is available for both transthoracic and transesophageal acquisition and is supported by multiple platforms.

The second technology is based on a matrix array design of the piezoelectric crystals within the transducer head, allowing for real-time volumetric scanning (Figure 11.1). The matrix array, as opposed to the standard 1D array, is a 2D array, consisting of 50 rows and 50 columns of elements. Whereas in a 1D array only 128 elements need to be controlled independently of one another, the matrix technology requires independence of the 2500 elements all in the confined space of the head of a sonographic probe. This 2D array enables the generation of scan line that can be steered not only in the axial and lateral dimensions, but also in the elevational dimension.

Even though one would expect that imaging the heart in three dimensions should result in better understanding of the topographical anatomy of different intracardiac structures and how they interact with one another during the cardiac cycle, it must be emphasized that the same constraints of 1D and 2D echocardiography apply for 3D echocardiography. Sector size, resolution, and frame rate interact with one another. Increasing the requirements of one will lead to deterioration in either or both. Three-dimensional echocardiography is subject to the same laws of acoustic physics as 2D echocardiography. Artifacts such as ringing, reverberations, shadowing, and attenuation occur in 3D as well as in 2D and M-mode.

Two platforms currently support this technology for transthoracic scanning; however, only one has a fully functional real-time 3D transesophageal echocardiography (TEE) probe.

Display of 3D images

Classical views acquired in 2D echocardiography are not required in 3D echocardiography, because entire volumetric datasets are acquired that can be spatially oriented at the discretion of the echocardiographer. The electronically steered 3D TEE has two modes of operation. The first is a live mode in which the system scans in real-time 3D. The second integrates only four to eight gated beats (as opposed to >90), which enables wider volumes to be generated while maintaining frame rate and resolution.

Live 3D – real time

In this mode, a 3D volume pyramid is obtained. The image shown in this mode is in real time. The 3D image changes as the transducer is moved, just as in the live 2D imaging case. Manipulations of the TEE probe (e.g. rotation, change in position) lead to instantaneous changes in the image seen on the monitor (Figure 11.2).

3D zoom – real time

Besides the superior acquisition of ventricular volumes and function, the main advantage of the 3D TEE compared with conventional 2D transducers lies in its ability to obtain real-time images of the mitral valve (MV) apparatus. The best way to image the MV live is with the 3D zoom mode. This mode displays a small magnified pyramidal volume of the MV which may vary from $20° \times 20°$ up to $90° \times 90°$, depending on the density setting. This small dataset can be spatially oriented at the discretion of the echocardiographer, enabling views of the MV from both the left atrium (LA) and left ventricle (LV) perspectives. The real-time (RT) 3D images are devoid of rotational artifacts, as are commonly encountered with ECG gated 3D acquisitions (Figure 11.3).

Full volume – gated

Three-dimensional imaging is limited not by computer and circuit processing power, but simply by the speed of sound. There is insufficient time for sound to travel back and forth in large

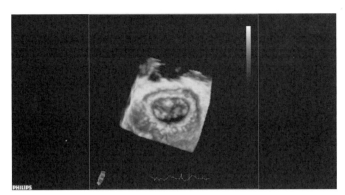

Figure 11.3. 3D zoom mode. En face view of mitral valve after repair and annuloplasty. This view is real-time and devoid of ECG artifacts. (See Color Plate III.)

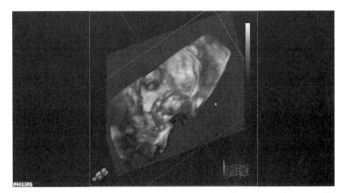

Figure 11.5. Same image as shown in Figure 11.4. The operator has spatially reoriented the dataset and started to crop with the intent to better expose a region of interest. (See Color Plate V.)

volumes while maintaining a frame rate of >20 Hz and reasonable resolution in live scanning modes. One maneuver to overcome this limitation entails stitching four to eight gates together to create a full-volume mode. These gated slabs or subvolumes represent a pyramidal 3D dataset, as would be acquired in the live 3D mode. This technique can generate >90-degree scanning volumes at frame rates greater than 30Hz. Increasing the gates from four to eight creates smaller 3D slabs; this can be used to maintain frame rates and/or resolution as the volumes (pyramids) become larger (Figure 11.4).

Gating refers to the ability to analyze ECG RR intervals, discarding errant subvolumes if the intervals are too irregular. As with any conventional gating techniques, patients with arrhythmias are prone to motion artifacts when the individual datasets are combined. As long as the RR intervals fall within a reasonable range, a full-volume dataset can still be reconstructed (e.g. atrial fibrillation, electrocautery artifact). The acquired RT 3D dataset can subsequently be cropped, analyzed, and quantified using integrated software in the 3D operating system (QLAB; Philips Healthcare, Andover, MA) (Figures 11.5 and 11.6).

3D color Doppler – gated

CFD requires obtaining multiple samples along a common scan line. Tissue or blood velocity is determined by analyzing frequency shifts among these transmited pulses. Structures that do not move maintain the same Doppler frequency spectrum. Unfortunately, firing more events along a stationary scan line deteriorates the frame rate. To increase the frame rate, a gating method must be used, similar to that of the full-volume mode; however, because of the large amount of data required, eight to eleven beats are needed to be combined to create an image. Jet direction, extent, and geometry can easily be recognized using this technique. Reports started emerging a decade ago showing that the strength of this methodology lies in its ability to quantify the severity of regurgitant lesions. Three-dimensional quantification of mitral regurgitation correlates better than 2D imaging, when using angiography as the gold standard.[1] In an experimental setting, 3D quantification was more accurate (2.6% underestimation) than 2D or M-mode methods, which had the tendency to underestimate regurgitant volumes (44.2% and 32.1%, respectively)[2] (Figure 11.7).

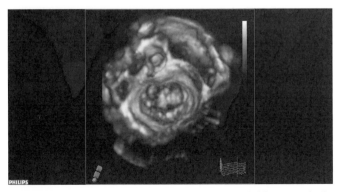

Figure 11.4. Full volume image. Four to eight ECG gated slabs are stitched together, enabling the acquisition of a larger volume without loss of frame rate or resolution. (See Color Plate IV.)

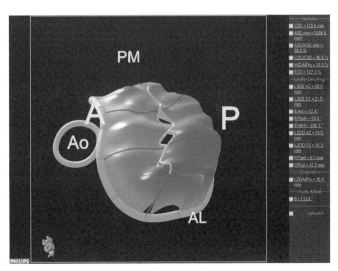

Figure 11.6. The 3D dataset can be quantified using semiautomatic software. The model created shows the relationship of the leaflet to the annular plane (red above, blue below). True volumes and unforeshortened distances can be measured. (See Color Plate VI.)

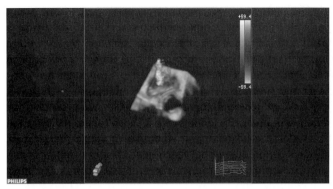

Figure 11.7. 3D color Doppler gated. Concentric jet originating from P2. Valve viewed from anterior to posterior. (See Color Plate VII.)

Parameters monitored

Twenty standard American Society of Echocardiography views

Transgastric midpapillary short axis

The probe is advanced into the stomach and slightly anteroflexed until the posterolateral and anterolateral papillary muscles are visualized at their attachment to the ventricular wall (Figure 11.8). It is important to image the insertion of the papillary muscles to ensure accurate intra- and inter-observer examinations. The LV is centered on the screen. If the MV apparatus is visualized, the probe should be either further advanced or posteroflexed. Similarly, if the ventricular apex is visualized, the probe should be either withdrawn or anteroflexed. All six middle segments of the ventricle are visualized, which represents perfusion from each of the three coronary arteries. The size and function of both the right and left ventricle may be evaluated. Although qualitative evaluation of right ventricular function may be performed, quantitative measurement of left ventricular fractional area of shortening may be calculated. Regional wall motion abnormalities may be visualized, which may represent myocardial ischemia.

Transgastric two chamber

From the transgastric midpapillary short axis view with the ventricle centered in the screen, the array is rotated to 90° (Figure 11.9). The length of the LV should be optimized to avoid foreshadowing. The apical, middle, and basal segments of both the anterior and inferior walls of the LV may be evaluated. The anterior and posterior leaflets of the MV can be visualized. The base of anterolateral aspect of the anterior MV leaflet (A1) through the tip of posteriomedial aspect of the anterior leaflet (A3) may be visualized, as it coapts with the posteriomedial scallop of the posterior leaflet (P3). The subvalvular MV apparatus may be evaluated even in the presence of heavy mitral valvular calcification. The left atrial appendage can be evaluated for thrombus.

Transgastric long axis

As the array is rotated to approximately 120°, the long axis of the left ventricular outflow is visualized (Figure 11.10). The angle of the array should be optimized to included the left ventricular apex, the left ventricular outflow tract, aortic valve, and the proximal aspect of the ascending aorta. The apical, middle, and basal aspects of the anteroseptal and inferolateral (posterior) left ventricular walls can be seen. The direction of left ventricular outflow through the aortic valve may be parallel to the ultrasonic beam, to allow for calculation of gradient across the aortic valve and calculation of aortic valve area. CFD may be used to evaluate the severity of aortic regurgitation.

Transgastric right ventricular inflow

From the transgastric long axis view, the probe is rotated right to visualize the right atrium and ventricle (Figure 11.11). The anterior and posterior leaflets of the tricuspid valve may be seen. Right ventricular size and function can be evaluated, as well as the severity of the tricuspid regurgitation.

Deep transgastric long axis

The array is rotated back to 0° and is advanced further into the stomach to the ventricular apex (Figure 11.12). The probe is

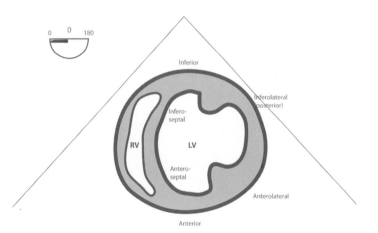

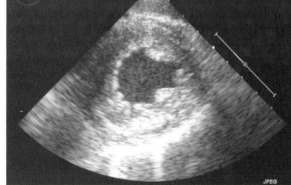

Figure 11.8. Transgastric midpapillary short axis. RV = right ventricle, LV = left ventricle.

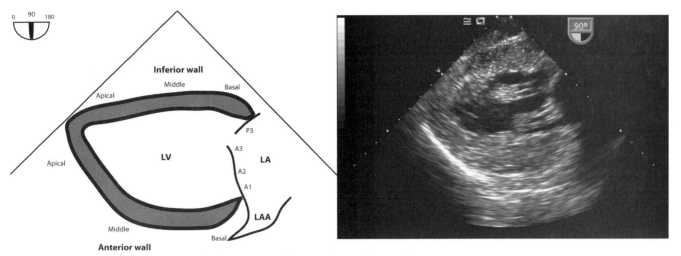

Figure 11.9. Transgastric two chamber. LA = left atrium, RV = right ventricle, LV = left ventricle.

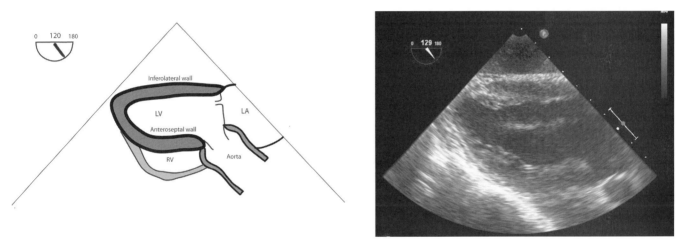

Figure 11.10. Transgastric long axis. LA = left atrium, LV = left ventricle, LAA = left atrial appendage.

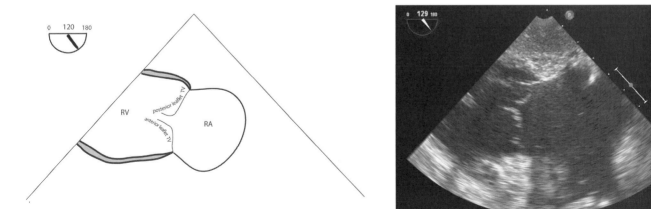

Figure 11.11. Transgastric right ventricular inflow. RA = right atrium, LA= left atrium.

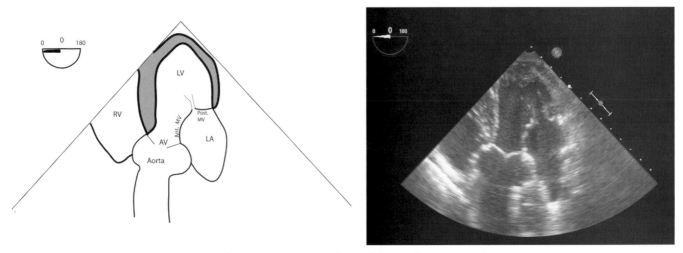

Figure 11.12. Deep transgastric long axis. LA = left atrium, RV = right ventricle, LV = left ventricle, AV = aortic valve.

severely anteroflexed and directed toward the ventricular base. As in the transgastric long axis view, the anteroseptal and inferolateral wall may be visualized. The axis of left ventricular outflow is usually optimized with the direction of the ultrasonic beam, allowing for accurate estimations of both aortic stenosis and regurgitation. The subvalvular apparatus of the mitral valve may be evaluated for severity of calcification.

Transgastic basal short axis

As the probe is withdrawn from the deep transgastric long axis view, though the transgastric midpapillary view, the transgastric basal short axis view may be obtained (Figure 11.13). The basal aspects of the walls of the LV may be visualized. Both the anterior and posterior MV leaflet tips are seen, allowing for visualization of the MV leaflet tips. Restriction of leaflet opening may be visualized and localized if mitral stenosis is present. If CFD is used, spatial localization of MV regurgitation may be identified within the opening of the MV; however, localization of

pathology to the anterior or posterior leaflet is usually not possible with this view.

Midesophageal four chamber

Maintaining the probe at approximately 0°, the probe is withdrawn into the mid-esophagus (Figure 11.14). Slight anteroflexion is usually necessary to avoid foreshortening of the LV. The array may need to be rotated approximately 10° to avoid imaging the left ventricular outflow tract and optimize visualization of the basal aspect of the inferoseptal left ventricular wall. In this view, the basal, middle, and apical aspects of the anterolateral and inferoseptal LV walls may be evaluated. Left and right atrial sizes may be evaluated by measuring atrial diameter; left atrial size may be further described by the measurement of the distance between the MV annular plane and the left atrial dome. The presence of left atrial spontaneous echo contrast ("smoke") may be observed in patients with left atrial stasis, and the left atrial appendage may be examined for evidence of thrombus.

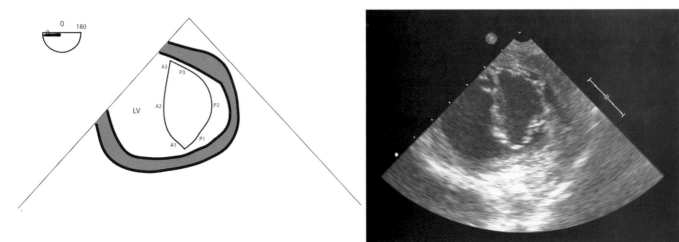

Figure 11.13. Transgastric basal short axis. LV = left ventricle.

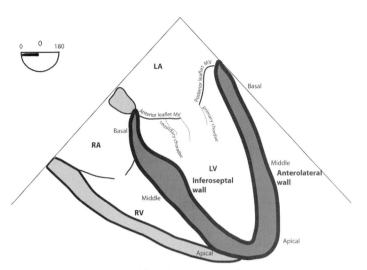 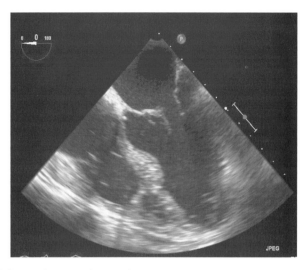

Figure 11.14. Midesophageal four chamber. LA = left atrium, RA = right atrium, LV = left ventricle, RV = right ventricle.

Right ventricular size and function may evaluated. Whereas estimation of right ventricular ejection fraction is limited by the complex geometric shape of the right ventricle, changes in the distance between the tricuspid annulus and the right ventricular apex may be used as a measurement of right ventricular function.

Both anterior and posterior leaflets of the MV may be imaged and evaluated for motion and pathology. With the echo probe optimally retroflexed with full visualization of the left ventricular apex, the most posteriomedial aspects of the anterior and posterior MV leaflets are usually imaged. As the probe is either slowly anteroflexed or withdrawn, the middle and, finally, anterolateral apects of these leaflets may be imaged. The septal and posterior tricuspid valve leaflets are usually visualized; however, if the probe is withdrawn too far or is too far anteroflexed, the anterior tricuspid valve leaflet may be visualized instead of the posterior leaflet. Pulse wave Doppler at the level of the MV leaflet tips may be used to evaluate diastolic

function and the severity of mitral stenosis. With moderate to severe mitral stenosis, continuous wave Doppler will probably need to be employed. Tissue Doppler measurements of the MV annulus, as well as color M-mode imaging of left ventricular inflow, may be used to evaluate left ventricular diastolic function. CFD may be used to evaluate the severity of mitral and tricuspid regurgitation as well as the presence of an atrial septal defect. Because of the low expected gradients between the atria, a low CFD setting will need to be employed to appreciate interatrial flow if it is present.

Midesophageal mitral commissural

The posterior leaflet is shaped like a crescent, whereas the anterior leaflet has an oblong shape as it coapts within this crescent (Figure 11.15). In the commissural view, the MV is imaged across this commissural opening with the anterolateral (P1) and posteromedial (P3) scallops of the posterior leaflet at either side of the image, with the middle aspect of the anterior leaflet (A2)

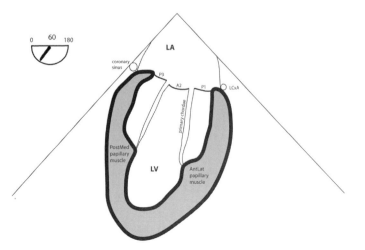 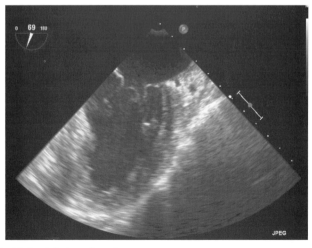

Figure 11.15. Midesophageal mitral commissural. LA = left atrium, LV = left ventricle, LCxA = left circumflex artery.

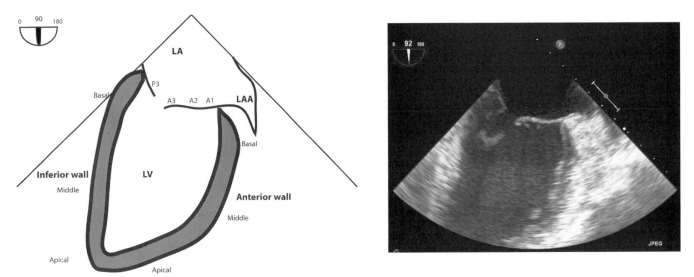

Figure 11.16. Midesophageal two chamber. LA = left atrium, LV = left ventricle, LAA = left atrial appendage.

in the middle of the MV opening. With the MV centered in the image and the apex of the LV imaged, the array is rotated to approximately 60°, so both the posteromedial scallop of the posterior leaflet (P3) and P1 are visualized. A2 will be seen between these two leaflet scallops. This view provides a high degree of confidence that both P1 and P3 are being imaged accurately. P3 restriction may be observed with ischemic mitral regurgitation. The MV commissural opening may be visualized, and the motion of these leaflet segments may be evaluated. Color Doppler is helpful in the localization of the site of MV regurgitation (i.e. anterolateral versus posteromedial commissure) as well as the severity of mitral regurgitation.

Midesophageal two-chamber

Further rotation of the transducer array to 90° will develop the midesophageal two-chamber view (Figure 11.16). Similar to the transgastric view, all segments of the anterior and inferior left ventricular walls may be evaluated for thickness and contractility. The anterior and posterior leaflets of the MV are imaged,

and evidence of stenosis and regurgitation may be obtained. The left atrial size may be measured and smoke may be imaged if present. The left atrial appendage can be examined for thrombus, which is not uncommon with left atrial stasis. Withdrawal of the probe will allow for imaging of both the upper and lower pulmonary veins; their Doppler evaluation will allow qualitative estimates of left atrial pressure and severity of mitral regurgitation.

Midesophageal long axis

Similar to the midesophageal two-chamber view, this midesophageal view of the left ventricular long axis usually provides better resolution than its transgastric equivalent (Figure 11.17). Further rotation to 120° develops the long axis view. A single axis from the left ventricular apex to the left ventricular outflow tract to the aortic valve to the ascending aorta should be developed. Further rotation to 130° or 140° may be necessary to obtain this axis alignment with cardiac rotation. In this view, both segments (basal and middle) of the anteroseptal and

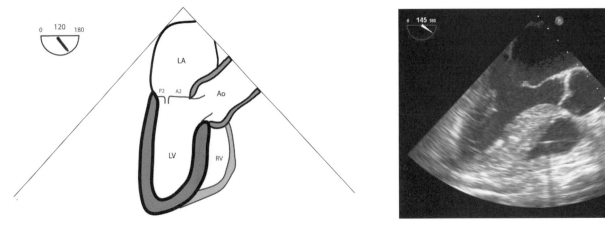

Figure 11.17. Midesophageal long axis. LA = left atrium, RV = right ventricle, LV = left ventricle, Ao = aorta.

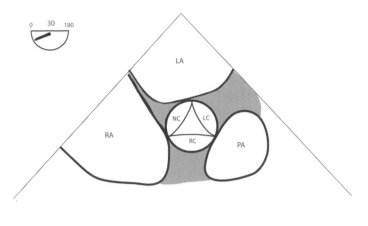
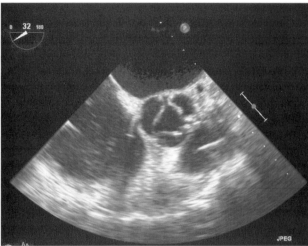

Figure 11.18. Midesophageal aortic valve short axis. LA = left atrium, RA = right atrium, PA = pulmonary artery, NC = noncoronary cusp, RC = right coronary cusp, LC = left coronary cusp.

inferolateral walls may be seen and evaluated. The A2 and P2 segments of the mitral valve may be seen and evaluated for motion. P2 restriction may be seen with ischemic cardiac disease, and systolic anterior motion of the anterior MV leaflet may be easily appreciated with hypertrophic obstructive cardiomyopathy in this view. The severity of mitral regurgitation may be estimated by CFD.

Midesophageal aortic valve short axis

Attention is now directed toward the aortic valve (Figure 11.18). The aortic valve is centered on the screen and the array is rotated to approximately 30°. The three cusps of the aortic valve (right, left, and noncoronary) may be visualized, along with its triangular opening. Evidence of pathology on the aortic valve cusps may be appreciated. Aortic valve stenosis may be estimated qualitatively by observing the aortic valve leaflet opening. Quantization of aortic stenosis by planimetry may

be attempted in this view; however, its use may be limited by shadowing caused by valvular calcification. CFD may be used to identify the site of aortic valve regurgitation, but quantification using this view may be difficult. The left main coronary artery may be imaged as it emerges adjacent to the left coronary cusp. Its bifurcation into the left anterior descending and circumflex artery is occasionally appreciated.

Midesophageal aortic valve long axis

The transducer array is rotated to 120° to develop the midesophageal aortic valve long axis view (Figure 11.19). The orientation of the image is similar to that of the midesophageal long axis. The right coronary cusp of the aortic valve may be visualized anteriorly; the posterior cusp is either the right or the noncoronary cusp. Rightward (clockwise) rotation of the probe will favor visualization of the right coronary cusp, whereas leftward (counterclockwise) rotation will favor visualization of the

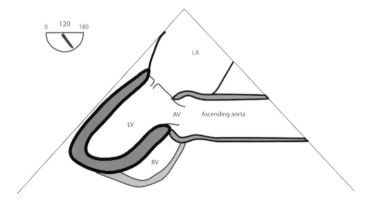
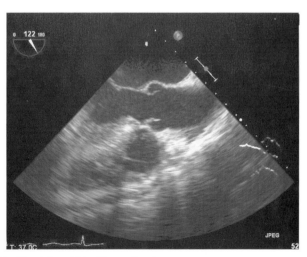

Figure 11.19. Midesophageal aortic valve long axis. LA = left atrium, RV = right ventricle, LV = left ventricle, AV = aortic valve.

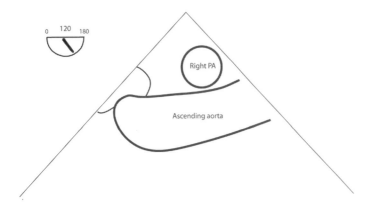
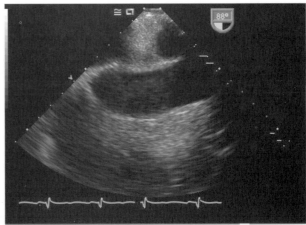

Figure 11.20. Midesophageal ascending aortic long axis. PA = pulmonary artery.

noncoronary cusp. The diameters of the aortic valve annulus, sinus of Valsalva, and the sinotubular junction may be measured. The severity of aortic regurgitation may be evaluated by examining the size of the aortic regurgitant jet as it extends into the left ventricular outflow tract. The right coronary artery can be visualized as it exits the aorta anteriorly. Proximal ascending aortic pathology may be evaluated.

Midesophageal ascending aortic long axis

The probe is further withdrawn to visualize the ascending aorta (Figure 11.20). Because of the interposition of the esophagus and either the trachea or bronchus, the distal ascending aorta usually cannot be visualized. The proximal and middle sections of the aorta can usually be seen and examined for atherosclerotic disease up to the crossing of the right pulmonary artery. More detailed examination of the ascending aorta at potential aortic cannulation and cross-clamp sites for cardiac surgery

require epiaortic imaging, which is a sensitive modality for the detection of atherosclerotic disease.

Midesophageal right ventricular inflow–outflow

The transducer array is returned to 0° and the four-chamber view is redeveloped (Figure 11.21). The tricuspid valve is centered on the screen and the array is rotated to approximately 60°. In addition to the left atrium, the right atrium, tricuspid valve, right ventricle, right ventricular outflow tract, pulmonary valve, and proximal pulmonary artery may be visualized. The septal and anterior leaflets of the tricuspid valve may be seen. CFD may be superimposed, evaluating the severity of tricuspid regurgitation. Moving the color Doppler field to the pulmonary valve allows estimation of pulmonary regurgitation. If there is tricuspid regurgitation, continuous-wave Doppler may be used to estimate systolic pulmonary artery pressure.

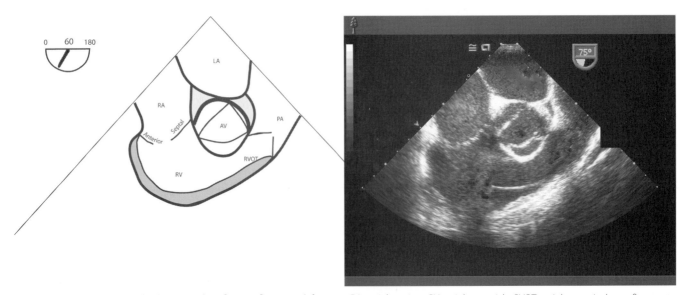

Figure 11.21. Midesophageal right ventricular inflow–outflow. LA = left atrium, RA = right atrium, RV = right ventricle, RVOT = right ventricular outflow tract, AV = aortic valve, PA = pulmonary artery.

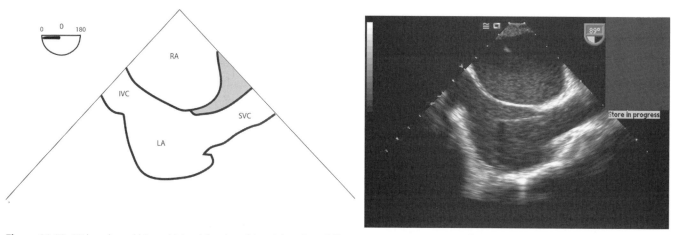

Figure 11.22. Midesophageal bi-caval. LA = left atrium, RA = right atrium, SVC = superior vena cava, IVC = inferior vena cava.

Midesophageal bi-caval

If the array is rotated to approximately 90° and rotated clockwise, the bi-caval view may be obtained (Figure 11.22). The superior and inferior vena cava may be visualized as they enter the right atrium. The eustachian valve may be seen as a fibrinous structure at the junction of the inferior vena cava with the right atrium. Septum secundum may be visualized as it extends from the inferior aspect of the right atrium superiorly, and the septum primum may be visualized as it extends from the superior aspect of the right atrium. Low-velocity CFD may be used to visualize atrial septal defects, which are usually left-to-right flows. The intravenous injection of contrast (such as agitated saline) with the release of Valsalva may reveal right-to-left flow through a patent foramen ovale. Further rightward rotation allows visualization of the right upper and lower pulmonary veins as they enter the left atrium.

Midesophageal ascending aortic short axis

The array probe is returned to 0° and the aortic valve is once again centered on the screen (Figure 11.23). The probe is withdrawn through the base of the heart until the pulmonary artery and its bifurcation are imaged. The severity of proximal and middle ascending aortic atherosclerosis and pathology may be evaluated. If a clear view of the ascending pulmonary artery is obtained, Doppler imaging may be used to estimate stroke volume.

Descending aortic short axis and upper esophageal aortic arch long axis

The probe is turned leftward toward the descending thoracic aorta. Because the probe is severely rotated, the orientation of the images will have changed. The top of the image is now the anteromedial aortic wall, and the bottom of the image is the posterolateral wall. The probe is advanced toward the stomach until the image is lost. The probe is withdrawn slowly, thus imaging the entire descending aorta. The presence of atherosclerotic disease should be noted. The probe is withdrawn until the level of the upper esophagus, where a long axis view of the aortic arch may be seen.

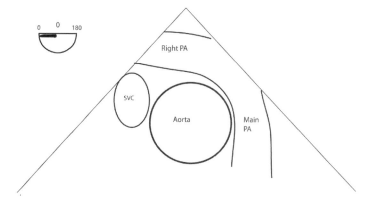
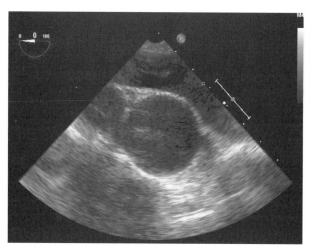

Figure 11.23. Midesophageal ascending aortic short-axis. SVC = superior vena cava, PA = pulmonary artery.

Descending aortic long axis and upper esophageal aortic arch short axis

The probe is returned to the stomach and the array is rotated to 90° to develop a long axis view of the descending aorta. Once again, the probe is withdrawn slowly. It may be necessary to rotate the probe right and left to optimize this long axis visualization. The arch is visualized in the upper esophageal area when a cross-sectional image is developed. At this point, the probe generally does not need to be withdrawn further. The probe is rotated anteriorly, allowing for visualization of the left subclavian, left carotid, and right innominate arteries as they exit the aortic arch. The left and main pulmonary arteries may be visualized. The left innominate vein may be seen anteriorly and superiorly to the aortic arch, which may be misdiagnosed as an aortic dissection.

Derived information
Evaluation of right and left ventricular size and function

The ability to assess ventricular function noninvasively is one of the most commonly posed questions to the echocardiographer. Assessment of ventricular function is unfortunately not as straightforward as one might think. The ideal measurement would be simply obtainable, reproducible, and independent of loading conditions placed on the ventricle. As surrogates, echocardiographers use a vast array of measurements.

One-dimensional measurements (linear)

M-mode has the advantage of high frame rates, leading to exceptional temporal resolution. A disadvantage to this method is the fact that the ventricle is being interrogated solely along a single line (ice pick). Although geometric assumptions can be made that correlate well with normal ventricular size and function, limitations are quickly reached once regional wall motion abnormalities or deviations from normal ventricular size appear.

Fractional shortening

A common measurement representing LV function is fractional shortening (FS). This measurement is derived by measuring the LV internal diameter in diastole and subtracting it from the LV internal diameter (LVID) measured in systole:

$$((LVIDd - LVIDs)/LVIDd) \times 100.$$

A transgastric two-chamber view is ideal for obtaining this measurement. LV diameters are measured from the endocardium of the inferior wall to the endocardium of the anterior wall in a line perpendicular to the long axis of the ventricle at the junction of the basal and middle segments of the anterior and inferior walls. Normal values are 25 percent to 43 percent in men and 27 percent to 45 percent in women.[3] It is important not to confuse FS with fractional area change or ejection fraction.

Left ventricular wall thickness

Left ventricular wall thickness is measured to diagnose ventricular hypertrophy. Normal values are less than 10 mm for men and less than 9 mm for women.[3] The TG midpapillary short axis view is acquired at end-diastole and the thickness of the septum and posterior wall measured.

Derived from these two measurements: relative wall thickness

The relative wall thickness (RWT) is used to subdivide the different forms of ventricular hypertrophy (eccentric vs. concentric):

$$RWT = (PWTd + SWTd)/LVIDd.$$

RWT > 0.42 is indicative for concentric hypertrophy, whereas RWT < 0.42 is typically found in eccentric hypertrophy.

Left ventricular mass

Left ventricular mass is the parameter most commonly used to evaluate the success of treatment trials in epidemiologic studies.[4] Mass is derived by subtracting left ventricular cavity volume from the volume of the LV in its entirety. This shell volume is then converted to mass by multiplying by myocardial density.

The American Society of Echocardiography (ASE) recommends the use of the following formula to calculate LV mass:

$$LVmass = 0.8 \times (1.04[(LVIDd + PWTd + SWTd)^3 - (LVIDd)^3]) + 0.6g,$$

where LVIDd = left ventricular internal diastolic diameter in diastole, PWT = posterior wall thickness, and SWT = septal wall thickness.[3]

This formula was found to have a high level of correlation with LV mass found at autopsies ($r = 0.9$, $p = 0.001$).[5]

Two-dimensional assessment of ventricular function
Fractional area change

The fractional area change (FAC) is the parameter most often requested from the echocardiographer. Although this measurement is dependent on loading conditions, it is frequently used to guide clinical management of patients with cardiovascular disease. This measurement is conceptionally simple and reproducible. The LV cavity is imaged in a transgastric midpapillary SAX view, and the area measured in end-systole and end-diastole. The difference divided by the area in end-diastole represents the FAC:

$$FAC (\%) = [(LVAd - LVAs)/LVAd] \times 100$$

Normal values are 56 percent to 63 percent in men and 59 percent to 65 percent in women.[3]

The FAC should not be confused with the ejection fraction (EF) or fractional shortening. The FAC is a change in area, whereas the EF is a change in volume and fractional shortening is a change in length. In normal hearts there is a good correlation between the FAC and EF; however, in the setting of abnormal ventricular geometry (e.g. aneurysm), the relationship no longer applies.

3D assessment of LV function

Geometric assumptions applied to the LV allow estimation of volumetric measurements based on 2D measurements. The most commonly used formula is the biplane method of disks or Simpson's modified rule. The LV volume is calculated by summing a stack of elliptical disks that are superimposed along the long axis of the LV. Two views that are orthogonal to each other are recommended; most commonly, the four-chamber and two-chamber views are used for this purpose (Figure 11.24). Unfortunately, there are multiple shortcomings when volumes are calculated based on these geometric assumptions. First, the LV must be elliptical in shape. This is true only for normal ventricles. Patients who have impaired ventricular function (where EF is of great interest) are the ones with altered geometry. Second, the placement of the 2D plane can be subject to positioning errors, which may lead to chamber foreshortening. Although these errors were accepted in the past as unavoidable, the emergence of 3D imaging will most likely change the playing field, as 3D echocardiography does not rely on geometric assumptions for volume and/or mass calculations. Studies comparing LV volumes and mass measured by 3D echocardiography, 2D echocardiography, and magnetic resonance imaging (MRI), which is the gold standard, showed significantly better

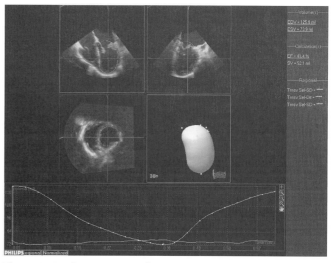

Figure 11.25. Semiautomatic software with endocardial border detection capability enabling the measurement of true ventricular volumes and calculation of a true ejection fraction. (See Color Plate VIII.)

correlation between 3D echocardiography and MRI than between 2D echocardiography and MRI (Figure 11.25).[6–8]

Right ventricle

The right ventricle (RV) is a complex crescent-shaped structure that does not lend itself as easily to geometric assumptions as its left ventricular counterpart. This thin-walled ventricle wraps itself around the left ventricle and is most commonly assessed in a qualitative fashion by integrating multiple views (RV inflow–outflow, four-chamber, RV inflow, and transgastric (TG) SAX view). Despite this apparent nonscientific approach to RV function, numerous reports have emerged linking RV function to prognostic outcome in a variety of cardiopulmonary diseases.[9]

The RV is ideally configured to pump large volumes against a low resistance system. Normal RV measurements can be obtained from a midesophageal four-chamber view at end-diastole (Figure 11.26). Basal measurements at the level of the tricuspid annular plane are normally between 2.0 cm and 2.8 cm, midcavity diameter should not exceed 3.3 cm, and its long axis, measured between the apex and the tricuspid annular plan, should be less than 8 cm.[10] RV wall thickness is physiologically less than 5 mm. As opposed to the LV, acute increases in right ventricular afterload are poorly tolerated, leading to RV distension, tricuspid regurgitation, and, ultimately, circulatory collapse. Chronic increases in afterload are compensated by concentric hypertrophy.

A semiquantitive method of examining RV function is by interrogating the displacement of the tricuspid annulus toward the RV apex during systole. Under normal circumstances, a descent of 1.5 cm to 2.0 cm should be observed. 3D echocardiography may allow better quantification of RV function. Software programs are emerging showing promising results for their ability to identify the RV endocardial border.

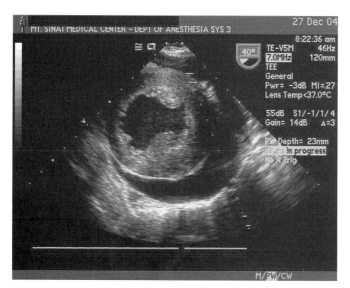

Figure 11.24. Transgastric short axis view of left ventricle. Large pericardial effusion seen surrounding the LV.

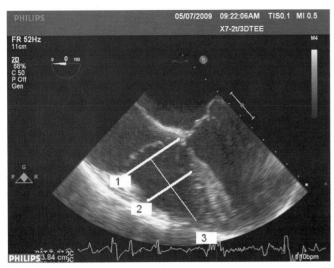

Figure 11.26. Midesophageal four-chamber of RV: (1) annular plane measurement, (2) mid-chamber measurement, and (3) long-axis measurement from apex to annular plane.

Assessment of coronary ischemia

The ability to reliably detect regional wall motion abnormalities (RWMAs) is clinically relevant because of its diagnostic and therapeutic implications. Not every RWMA detected by TEE is diagnostic for myocardial ischemia. Myocarditis, ventricular pacing, and bundle branch blocks can easily lead to wall motion abnormalities that can potentially lead to mismanagement of the patient.

Common classifications should be used to describe the anatomic localization and degree of dysfunction in RWMA, so that communication is possible between echocardiographer and nonechocardiographer, as well as documentation of ongoing disease course. The ASE has published guidelines using a sixteen-segment model of the LV to aid in this communication.[11] This model subdivides the LV into three zones (basal, mid, and apical). The basal (segments 1–6) and midventricular zones (segments 7–12) are further subdivided into six segments each, whereas the apical zone consists of only four segments (segments 13–16). Another model, published by the American Heart Association Writing Group on Myocardial Segmentation and Registration for Cardiac Imaging, uses a seventeen-segment model. The seventeenth segment merely represents the apical cap of the previously described sixteen-segment model[12] (Figure 11.27)

The coronary distribution related to the individual segments can be assessed, enabling the echocardiographer to make assumptions regarding the localization of a potential coronary lesion. Segments 1, 2, 7, 13, 14, and 17 are in the distribution territory of the left anterior descending artery. Segments 5, 6, 11, 12, and 16 are associated with the circumflex artery, and segments 3, 4, 9, 10, and 15 belong to the right coronary artery (Figure 11.28). This segmental distribution can be variable among patients owing to the variability of the coronary arteries. In addition to defining a system that defines anatomical

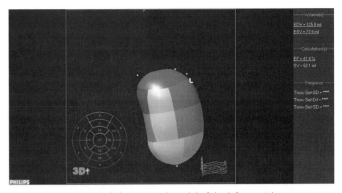

Figure 11.27. Myocardial segmental model of the left ventricle as reconstructed by software from a 3D dataset. (See Color Plate IX.)

segments of the LV, it is important to grade segment thickening and excursion.

Wall motion

The simplest assessment is achieved by the echocardiographer eyeballing the motion of the ventricle and classifying its motion as being either normal, hypokinetic, akinetic, dyskinetic, or aneurysmal. Subsequently, a numeric score of 1 to 5 can be assigned. A wall motion index can then be derived by dividing the total score by the number of segments observed. A score of 1 would represent a normal ventricle. The higher the score, the more abnormal the ventricle.

Ventricular thickening

In addition to movement, the normal myocardium thickens during systole. The degree of thickening can also be used to assess overall function of the observed segment. A thickening less than 30 percent is normal, 10 percent to 30 percent represents mild hypokinesia, 0 percent to 10 percent is severe hypokinesia, no thickening is akinesia, and if the segment bulges during systole, dyskinesia would be present.

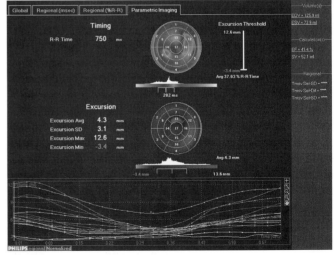

Figure 11.28. Sixteen-segment model showing timing and excursion of the individual segments. (See Color Plate X.)

Assessment of pressures and flow

Doppler echocardiographic measurements may be used to calculate both flow and pressure gradients. A Doppler spectrum consists of a graph of velocity versus time. If one integrates a given Doppler spectrum over a single cardiac cycle, one may determine the distance traversed over that cardiac cycle. This summation of flow velocities in a given period of time is called the *velocity–time integral* (VTI). The VTI is represented by the area enclosed within the baseline and spectral Doppler signal. If this distance traversed is multiplied by the cross-sectional area (CSA) of the structure interrogated, one may determine the stroke volume. The CSA of a cylindrical structure can be estimated by the equation:

$$CSA = \pi r^2, \tag{11.4}$$

where r is the radius of the structure being interrogated.

There are a number of assumptions, including (1) laminar blood flow in the area interrogated; (2) a flat or blunt flow velocity profile, such that the flow across the entire CSA interrogated is relatively uniform; and (3) Doppler angle of incidence between the Doppler beam and the main direction of blood flow is less than 20 degrees, so the underestimation of the flow velocity is less than 6 percent.

The preferred sites for the measurements of stroke volume are (1) the left ventricular outflow tract or aortic annulus, (2) the mitral annulus, or (3) the pulmonary annulus.[13] The major determinant of variability in estimating SV by the use of any technique is the accurate measurement of the CSA. Any error in diameter measurement would be squared in the final results.

A second source of variability in measuring aortic flow involves the proper recording of reproducible Doppler signals. If the left ventricular outflow tract (LVOT) is chosen as the CSA, the VTI should be obtained from the Doppler signal at this level. For this purpose, the systolic forward flow must be obtained from either a deep transgastric or a transgastric long axis view. The sample volume of the pulsed Doppler should be placed in the high portion of the LVOT exactly at the same level as the diameter was measured. Occasionally, the Doppler signal is difficult to obtain, and the morphology of the spectrum may be similar to a triangle with a spike at the peak velocity rather than a round bell-shape flow signal. Under such circumstances, it is inappropriate to estimate the VTI, because under- or overestimations are likely to result. If attention is given to proper recording techniques, the interobserver variability in measuring the aortic VTI in normal subjects should be less than 5 percent.

In an interesting application of echocardiography, various echocardiographic techniques have been used to estimate intracardiac or intravascular pressures. Based on the Doppler shift principle, blood flow velocity can determined. The Bernoulli principle states that an increase in the speed of the fluid occurs simultaneously with a decrease in its pressure or a decrease in the fluid's potential energy. When flow acceleration and viscous friction variables of blood are ignored and

flow velocity proximal to a fixed obstruction is significantly less than flow velocity after the obstruction, the a simplified modified Bernoulli equation may be defined as:

$$\Delta P = 4v^2, \tag{11.5}$$

where ΔP is the pressure difference between two structures, and v is the velocity across the structures.

With this formula, the pressure gradient across a fixed orifice can be calculated.

The velocity of a regurgitant valve is a direct application of pressure gradient calculations, as it represents the pressure drop across that valve and therefore can be used to calculate intracardiac pressure. For example, tricuspid regurgitation (TR) velocity reflects systolic pressure differences between the RV and right atrium (RA). RV systolic pressure can be obtained by adding RA pressure (estimated or measured) to (TR velocity)$^2 \times 4$. In the absence of right ventricular outflow tract obstruction, PA systolic pressure will be the same as right ventricular end systolic pressure (RVESP). For example,

If TR velocity = 3 m/s and right atrial pressure (RAP) = 10 mmHg, then,

$$RVESP = (TR\ VEL)^2 \times 4 + RAP \tag{11.6}$$

RVESP = PA systolic = $4(3)^2$ = 36 mmHg + 10 mmHg = 46 mm Hg.

Valvular stenosis and regurgitation
Aortic valve evaluation

Two-dimensional transesophageal echocardiographic interrogation provides information on valve area, leaflet structure, and mobility. The valve is composed of three fibrous cusps (right, left, and noncoronary) attached to the root of the aorta. Each cusp has a nodule called the *noduli Arantii* in the center of the free edge, at the point of contact of the three cusps. The spaces between the attachments of the cusps are called the *commissures*, and the circumferential connection of these commissures is the *sinotubular junction*. The aortic wall bulge behind each cusp is known as the *sinus of Valsalva*. The sinotubular junction, the sinuses of Valsalva, the valve cusps, the junction of the aortic valve with the ventricular septum, and the anterior mitral valve leaflet comprise the aortic valve complex. The aortic ring is at the level of the ventricular septum and is the lowest and narrowest point of this complex. The three leaflets of the aortic valve are easily visualized, and vegetations or calcifications can be identified on basal transverse imaging or longitudinal imaging.

Aortic stenosis

Aortic stenosis may be caused by congenital unicuspid, bicuspid, tricuspid, or quadricuspid valves, rheumatic fever, or degenerative calcification of the valve in the elderly.[14] Valvular aortic stenosis is characterized by thickened, echogenic, calcified, immobile leaflets and is usually associated with concentric left ventricular hypertrophy and a dilated aortic root. The valve

Table 11.1. Summary of aortic stenosis

	Aortic sclerosis	Mild	Moderate	Severe
Aortic jet velocity (m/sec)	≤ 2.5	2.6–2.9	3.0–4.0	>4.0
Mean gradient (mmHg)		<20	20–40	>40
Aortic valve area (cm^2)		>1.5	1.0–1.5	<1.0

Adapted from ref. 17.

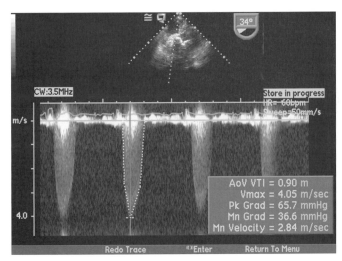

Figure 11.30. Doppler spectrum through a stenotic aortic valve.

leaflets may be domed during systole; this finding is sufficient for a diagnosis of aortic stenosis.[40]

The quantification of aortic stenosis is summarized in Table 11.1. Aortic valve area may be measured by planimetry (Figure 11.29).[15] A cross-sectional view of the aortic valve orifice may obtained by TEE, which corresponds well to measurements of aortic valve area obtained by transthoracic echocardiography and cardiac catheterization, assuming the degree of calcification is not severe. The severity of aortic stenosis may be quantified using Doppler echocardiography (Figure 11.30).[16] The evaluation of severity, however, may be limited by difficulty aligning the ultrasonic beam with the direction of blood flow through the left ventricular outflow tract. This limitation may be overcome by using either a deep transgastric or transgastric long axis view. Normal Doppler signals across the aortic valve have a velocity of less than 1.5 m/sec and have peak signals during early systole. With worsening aortic stenosis, the flow velocities increase and the peak signal is later in systole. These high velocities will limit the use of pulse wave Doppler and necessitate the use of either continuous wave or high pulse repetition frequency Doppler. Aortic velocity allows classification of stenosis as mild (2.6 to 2.9 m/s), moderate (3.0–4.0 m/s), or severe (>4 m/s).[17]

The higher-velocity central jet is characterized by a high-pitched audio sound as well as a fine feathery appearance on the Doppler signal; this is usually less dense than the thicker parajets that are distal to the valve. Peak and mean transvalvular gradients may be calculated using the peak and mean velocities of the signals, respectively. Peak gradients measured by Doppler ultrasonography tend to be higher than those measured in the cardiac catheterization lab, because Doppler-determined peak gradients are instantaneous, whereas those reported by the cardiac catheterization laboratory are peak-to-peak systolic pressure differences. In addition, Doppler determinations of peak gradient may overestimate the gradient because of pressure recovery effects. As blood flows past a stenotic aortic valve, the potential energy of the high-pressure left ventricle is converted into kinetic energy; there is a decrease in pressure with an associated increase in velocity. Distal to the orifice, flow decelerates again with both conversion of this loss of kinetic energy into heat and a reconversion of some kinetic energy into potential energy, with a corresponding increase in pressure. This increase in pressure distal to the stenosis is called the *pressure recovery effect*.[18] Although they are usually minor, these differences in the observed gradient become more significant with a small aorta and moderate aortic stenosis.[19]

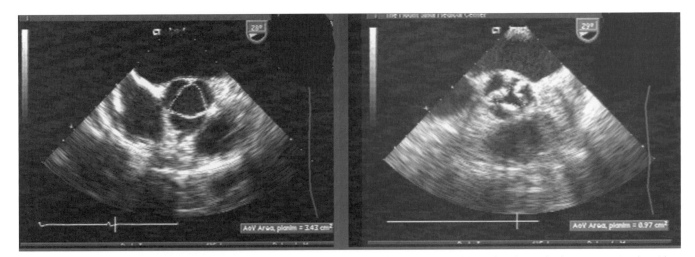

Figure 11.29. Aortic valve stenosis by planimetry. The panel on the left indicates a normal aortic valve and the right-side panel indicates an aortic valve with stenosis. Because there is no significant calcification of the valve, planimetry may be used.

Alternatively, aortic valvular area may be calculated using the continuity equation comparing blood flow through the left ventricular outflow tract with blood through the aortic valve. Stroke volume may be estimated by multiplying the cross-sectional area of a particular orifice by the VTI over one cardiac cycle through that orifice. The continuity equation states that the calculated stroke volume should be equal independent of the site where it is measured; what goes in must come out. When estimating the severity of aortic stenosis, stroke volume through the left ventricular outflow tract and the aortic valve is usually measured. Using either a deep transgastric or transgastric long axis view, the Doppler spectrum of the aortic valve and left ventricular outflow tract are displayed using continuous and pulse wave Doppler, respectively. The VTI through each of these structures is calculated. The diameter of the left ventricular outflow tract is measured in a midesophageal long axis view. Remembering,

$$SV = CSA \times VTI, \tag{11.7}$$

where SV = stroke volume, CSA = cross sectional area, and VTI = velocity time integral, the continuity equation states that

$$SV_{LVOT} = SV_{AV}, \tag{11.8}$$

where LVOT = left ventricular outflow tract and AV = aortic valve.

Substituting the stroke volume equation into the continuity equation,

$$CSA_{LVOT} \times VTI_{LVOT} = CSA_{AV} \times VTI_{AV}. \tag{11.9}$$

Rearranging the terms,

$$CSA_{AV} = CSA_{LVOT} \times VTI_{LVOT}/VTI_{AV}. \tag{11.10}$$

Because the left ventricular outflow tract is essentially cylindrical, the CSA_{LVOT} may be estimated by

$$CSA_{LVOT} = \pi(radius_{LVOT})^2. \tag{11.11}$$

Because CSA_{LVOT}, VTI_{LVOT}, and VTI_{AV} are known, the CSA_{AV} or aortic valve area may be calculated.

Although multiplane TEE planimetric estimations of aortic valve area may be flawed by heavy aortic valvular calcification, measurements using the continuity equation are accurate compared with Gorlin-derived values.[20-21] In a study using TEE, Stoddard and colleagues reported good correlation between aortic valve area measurements using the continuity equation and planimetry; however, they report a steep learning curve for the acquisition of a suitable transgastric long axis view that adequately aligns flow through the aortic valve with the ultrasound beam.[22] Mild aortic stenosis is consistent with a valve area greater than 1.5 cm², whereas severe stenosis has valve areas less than 1 cm².[17,23]

Aortic regurgitation

Aortic regurgitation may be caused by annular dilation, destruction of the annular support, or pathology of the aortic valvular cusps. Regurgitation secondary to annular dilation is characterized by a dilated aortic root, aortic valve leaflets of normal appearance, and a centrally directed retrograde flow through the left ventricular outflow tract. Valvular lesions that may result in aortic regurgitation include leaflet vegetations and calcifications, perforation, or prolapse. These lesions may be seen on transverse imaging across the aortic valve. Signs that may be associated with aortic regurgitation include high-frequency diastolic fluttering of the MV, premature closing of the MV, or reverse doming of the MV.[24-25]

Leaflet movement (excessive, restricted, or normal), origin of jet (central or peripheral), and direction of regurgitant jet (eccentric or central) should be determined to provide insight into the underlying pathology.[26] Bicuspid and tricuspid valve prolapse is associated with excessive valve mobility and eccentric jet direction and origin. Annular dilation, rheumatic disease, sclerosis, and perforation are associated with normal or reduced cusp mobility and a central jet.

Physiological and technical factors may affect estimated severity of aortic regurgitation. Physiological variables may include aortic diastolic pressure, left ventricular end-diastolic pressure, heart rate, and left ventricular compliance.[27] The severity of aortic regurgitation may be underestimated in the presence of eccentrically directed jets. Several technical factors affect perceived severity of regurgitation as well, including severe malalignment of ultrasonic planes with blood flow, the presence of a prosthetic MV interfering with ultrasound penetration, gain settings, and pulse repetition frequency.

Aortic regurgitant flow through the outflow tract is characteristically a high-velocity turbulent jet extending through the left ventricular outflow tract and LV during diastole. The criteria for qualitative grading of mitral regurgitation are summarized in Table 11.2. The severity of aortic regurgitation may be assessed by examining the area, width, and distal extent of the jet by CFD measurements. Unfortunately, determination of the severity of aortic insufficiency by measurements of regurgitant jet areas alone has been questioned and is probably useful only for distinguishing mild from severe regurgitation.[28] A more accurate determination of aortic regurgitation may be made by examination of the width of the origin of regurgitant jet or the ratio of the jet width to the left ventricular outflow tract (w_J/w_{LVOT}).[29-30] A w_J/w_{LVOT} value of 0.25 discriminates mild from moderate regurgitation, and a value of 0.65 discriminates moderate from severe regurgitation.[54] A vena contra diameter less than 0.3 cm is consistent with mild aortic insufficiency, and a diameter greater than 0.6 cm is consistent with severe aortic insufficiency.

Doppler characteristics of the regurgitant flow may be used to estimate the degree of aortic regurgitation using pressure half-time measurements. A normally functioning aortic valve will maintain a large gradient during diastole between the aorta and the left ventricle. With a small degree of aortic insufficiency, there will be a small volume of blood entering the left ventricle through the aortic valve, resulting in a slow increase in left ventricular pressure during diastole. Doppler measurements will

Table 11.2. Quantification of aortic regurgitation

	Mild 1+	Moderate 2+	3+	Severe 4+
Left atrial size	Normal	Normal or dilated		Usually dilated
Aortic cusps	Normal or abnormal	Normal or abnormal		Abnormal/flail or wide coaption defect
Jet width in LVOT*	Small in central jets	Intermediate		Large in central jets; variable in eccentric jets
Continuous wave jet density	Incomplete or faint	Dense		Dense
Jet deceleration rate (pressure half time, ms)	Slow > 500	Medium 200–500		Steep < 200
Vena contracta width (cm)*	< 0.3	0.3–0.60		≥ 0.6
Jet width/LVOT width, %*	< 25	25–45	46–64	≥ 65
Jet CSA/LVOT CSA, %*	< 5	5–20	21–59	≥ 60
Regurgitant orifice area (cm²)	< 0.10	0.10–0.19	0.20–0.29	≥ 0.30

*At Nyquest limits of 50–60 cm/sec
CSA = cross-sectional area
LVOT = left ventricular outflow tract
Adapted from reference 54.

show a regurgitant flow of high velocity, which is maintained during most of diastole (corresponding to a long pressure half-time). As aortic regurgitant flow becomes more severe, there is a more rapid equilibration between aortic and left ventricular diastolic pressure with the nadir of the gradient at end-diastole. As pressures equilibrate, driving pressure across the aortic valve decreases, and Doppler-derived aortic regurgitation velocities decrease over the diastolic period. This pattern of aortic regurgitation flow is characterized by short pressure half-time.

Pressure half-time measurements have been validated as a measure of aortic regurgitation.[31] A pressure half-time of less than 200 milliseconds is consistent with severe aortic regurgitation, whereas a pressure half-time of more than 500 milliseconds is consistent with mild aortic regurgitation.[54] The accuracy of this technique may be influenced by physiologic variables.[32] A higher systemic vascular resistance increases the rate of decline, whereas a reduced ventricular compliance will increase the rate of intraventricular pressure rise, which will also affect the diastolic slope without affecting valvular competence. In a given patient, however, pharmacologic manipulation of afterload or inotropy may result in changes in aortic regurgitant slopes and pressure half-times that are contradictory to other measures of regurgitation.

Mitral valve evaluation

The MV consists of two leaflets, chordae tendineae, two papillary muscles, and a valve annulus. The anterior leaflet is larger than the posterior and is semicircular; however, the posterior MV leaflet has a longer circumferential attachment to the MV annulus.[33] The posterior valve leaflet may be divided into three scallops: lateral (P1), middle (P2), and medial (P3). The leaflets are connected to each other at junctures of continuous leaflet tissue called *commissures*. Primary, secondary, and tertiary chordal structures arise from the papillary muscle, subdividing as they extend and attaching to the free edge and several millimeters from the margin on the ventricular surface of both the anterior and posterior valve leaflets.[34] The annulus of the

MV primarily supports the posterior MV leaflet, whereas the anterior MV leaflet is continuous with the membranous ventricular septum, aortic valve, and aorta.

Mitral stenosis

The most common etiology of mitral stenosis is rheumatic disease; other causes are congenital valvular stenosis, vegetations and calcifications of the leaflets, parachute MV, and annular calcification. In addition to structural valvular abnormalities, mitral stenosis may be caused by nonvalvular etiologies, such as intraatrial masses (myxomas or thrombus) or extrinsic constrictive lesions.[35–36] Generally, mitral stenosis is characterized by restricted leaflet movement, a reduced orifice, and diastolic doming (Figure 11.31).[37] The diastolic doming occurs when the MV is unable to accommodate all the blood flowing from the left atrium into the ventricle, so the bodies of the leaflets separate more than the edges. In rheumatic disease, calcification of the valvular and subvalvular apparatus, as well as thickening, deformation, and fusion of the valvular leaflets at the anterolateral and posteromedial commissures, produce a characteristic

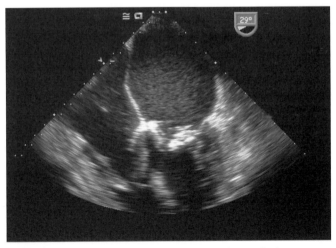

Figure 11.31. Midesophageal four-chamber view. The mitral valve is severely stenotic, with severe calcification of the annulus and leaflets.

Table 11.3. Quantification of mitral stenosis

	Mild	Moderate	Severe
Valve area (cm^2)	>1.5	1.0–1.5	<1.0
Mean gradient (mmHg)	<5	5–10	>10

Adapted from reference 17.

fish-mouth–shaped orifice.[38] Other characteristics that may be associated with chronic obstruction to left atrial outflow include an enlarged left atrium, spontaneous echo contrast or smoke (which is related to low-velocity blood flow with subsequent rouleaux formation by red blood cells[39]), thrombus formation, and RV dilation.

The leaflets, annulus, chordae, and papillary muscles may be assessed in the midesophageal four chamber, commissural, two chamber, and long axis views. If there is significant annular calcification, the transgastric views may be necessary to assess the subvalvular apparatus. Because of the propensity for thrombus formation, the entire left atrium and appendage should be carefully interrogated for thrombus.

The assessment of the severity of mitral stenosis is summarized in Table 11.3. Because planimetry of the mitral valve orifice is not influenced by assumptions of flow conditions, ventricular compliance, or associated valvular lesions, its use is the reference standard for the evaluation of mitral valve area in mitral stenosis.[17] Although it is at times technically difficult, care should be taken to image the orifice at the leaflet tips. Severe calcification of the MV may interfere with MV area determination and, in patients with significant subvalvular stenosis, underestimation of the degree of hemodynamic compromise may occur when determining the MV area by planimetry.[40]

Doppler assessment of mitral valvular stenosis

A transmitral Doppler spectrum is measured along the axis of transmitral blood flow, which may usually be obtained in a midesophageal four-chamber view or two-chamber view (see Figure 11.32). Transmitral valve flow is characterized by two peaked waves of flow away from the transducer. The first wave

(E) represents early diastolic filling, and the second wave (A) represents atrial systole. Transvalvular gradient may be estimated using the modified Bernoulli equation:[41] pressure gradient $= 4 \times$ velocity^2. Because the peak gradient is heavily influenced by left atrial compliance and ventricular diastolic function, the mean gradient is the relevant clinical measurement.[17] The high velocities that may occur with mitral stenosis limit the use of pulse wave Doppler echocardiography; continuous wave Doppler echocardiography should be used.

Normally, with the MV opening during early diastole, there is a torrential increase in transmitral flow, which rapidly decreases to zero during diastasis, when the left atrial and ventricular pressures equilibrate. With mitral stenosis, a gradient between the left atrium and ventricle may be maintained for a longer period of time. This sustained pressure differential maintains flow between the atrium and ventricle, decreasing the slope of this early transmitral flow. The rate of decline of the E-wave velocity may be described by its pressure half-time, which is the time interval from the peak E-wave velocity to the time when the E-wave velocity has declined to half its peak value. The pressure half-time is inversely proportional to the mitral valve area:[42]

$$\text{Mitral valve area} = 220/\text{pressure half-time}. \qquad (11.12)$$

The E wave may have a bimodal characteristic, with an initial rapid decline in transmitral velocity in early diastole compared with the latter aspect of diastole. In these cases, this latter, gentler slope should be measured. The advantage of this technique is that it is independent of valvular geometry. This formula assumes that the mitral valve is at least mildly stenotic. The presence of either mitral regurgitation or aortic regurgitation will decrease the accuracy of pressure half-time measurements for the determination of mitral stenosis.[43] If there is associated aortic regurgitation, care should be taken that the aortic regurgitant jet is not included in the transmitral flow measurement.[44] Inadvertent inclusion of this aortic regurgitant flow may result in a false elevation of transmitral velocity, as well as a false decrease in pressure half-time.[45] Alternatively, aortic insufficiency may result in a rapid increase in diastolic left

Table 11.4. Summary of mitral regurgitation

	Mild	Moderate		Severe
	1+	2+	3+	4+
Left atrial size	Normal	Normal or dilated		Usually dilated
Color flow jet area*	Small central jet (<4 cm^2 or <20% LA area)			Large central jet (>10 cm^2 or >40% LA) or variable-sized wall impinging jet
Pulmonary venous flow	Systolic dominance	Systolic blunting		Systolic flow reversal
Continuous wave jet contour	Parabolic	Usually parabolic		Early peaking triangular
Continuous wave jet density	Incomplete or faint	Dense		Dense
Vena contracta width (cm)	<0.3	0.3–0.69		≥0.7
Regurgitant orifice area (cm^2)	<0.20	0.20–0.29	0.30–0.39	≥0.40

*At Nyquest limits of 50–60 cm/sec
Adapted from reference 54.

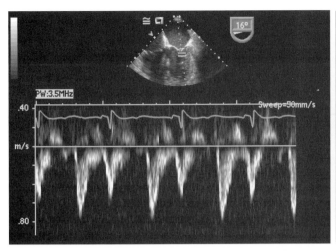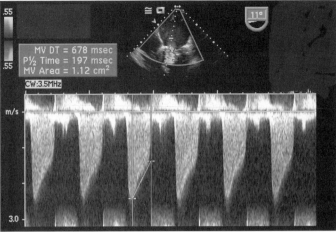

Figure 11.32. Transmitral Doppler spectrum. The panel on the left is the normal transmitral Doppler flow, and the panel on the right is the transmitral flow in the presence of mitral stenosis.

ventricular pressures, hence decreasing transmitral flow velocity. The continuity equation and proximal isovelocity surface area (PISA) method (discussed later) may be used as secondary methods for the evaluation of the severity of mitral stenosis.

Mitral regurgitation

Mitral regurgitation may be caused by disorders of any component of the MV apparatus – specifically, the annulus, the leaflets and chordae, or the papillary muscles. With chronic regurgitation, the annulus and atrium dilate and the annulus loses its normal elliptical shape, becoming more circular.[46] Annular dilation, in turn, leads to poor leaflet coaptation and worsening of valve incompetence. Although increased left atrial and ventricular dimensions may suggest severe mitral regurgitation, smaller dimensions do not exclude the diagnosis.[47] Ischemic mitral regurgitation is usually the result of left ventricle remodeling and enlargement after prior myocardial infarction. Myxomatous degeneration produces ballooning and scalloping of the valve leaflets as well as localized areas of thinning and thickening, which can be seen echocardiographically. In patients with recent endocarditis, vegetations may be attached to the leaflets or chordae. With rheumatic valve disease, thickening and/or calcification of the leaflets, restriction of the leaflets, and a variable degree of shortening and thickening of the subvalvular apparatus may be identified.

Elongated chordae may produce prolapse of one or both attached leaflets; if only one leaflet is affected, leaflet malalignment may occur during systole. Excessively mobile structures near the leaflet tips during diastole may represent elongated chords or ruptured minor chords. These structures do not prolapse into the atrium during systole. In contrast, ruptured major chords are identified as thin structures with a fluttering appearance in the atrium during systole and are associated with marked prolapse of the affected leaflet; in this instance, the valve is said to be *flail*. A flail leaflet generally points in the direction of the left atrium; this directionality of leaflet pointing is

the principal criterion for distinguishing a flailed leaflet from severe valvular prolapse.[48,49] Flail leaflets are most commonly caused by ruptured chordae and less commonly caused by papillary muscle rupture.

Regurgitation may also be caused by papillary muscle infarction in association with infarction of the adjacent left ventricle myocardium, owing to a lack of the normal tethering function performed by these structures. When the adjacent segment is aneurysmal, the dyskinetic wall motion may prevent proper coaptation of the valve by restricting the normal movement of the mitral leaflets during systole.[50] Prior infarctions may be indicated by thinning of the myocardium, atresia of the papillary muscles, and dyskinetic wall segments. Atretic papillary muscles are identified by their diminutive size and increased echocardiographic density on short-axis imaging. This shrinkage in papillary muscle size may result in retraction of chordae and subsequent mitral regurgitation. Papillary muscle rupture typically appears as a mass (papillary muscle head) that prolapses into the left atrium during systole and is connected to the leaflet only by its attached chordae. In addition to these structural abnormalities, mitral regurgitation is suggested by left ventricular volume overload, a dilated hypercontractile left ventricle, a high ejection fraction, and systolic expansion of the left atrium.[51]

Qualitative grading using color flow Doppler

The diagnosis of mitral regurgitation is made primarily by the use of color flow mapping. Multiple user adjustable instrument settings (e.g. color Doppler gain, pulse repetition frequency, and filter cutoffs) also influence the apparent size of the CFD jet for any given degree of valvular regurgitation. These settings must be optimized and ideally should be constant when comparing studies on a given patient. Because flow is best detected when it is parallel to the ultrasonic beam and because some mitral regurgitation jets may be thin and eccentric, multiple views of the left atrium should be interrogated for evidence of mitral

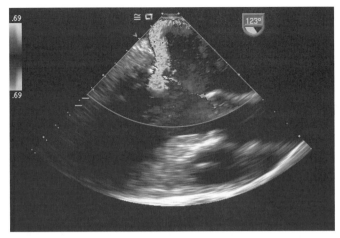

Figure 11.33. Eccentric mitral valve regurgitant jet. (See Color Plate XI.)

regurgitation. It is important to remember that the regurgitant flow disturbances are 3D velocity fields with complex geometry, which must be sampled from multiple imaging planes to provide an accurate estimate of the maximal spatial extent of the CFD signal.

Eccentric jet direction provides corroborative evidence of structural leaflet abnormalities, which may include leaflet prolapse, chordal elongation, chordal rupture, or papillary muscle rupture (Figure 11.33). For example, a jet that is directed laterally along the posterior wall of the left atrium is associated with anterior leaflet prolapse. Similarly, a jet that is directed medially behind the anterior mitral leaflet is associated with prolapse of the posterior leaflet.

It is common to detect trivial degrees of mitral valve regurgitation that extend just superior and posterior to the MV leaflet. Mitral regurgitation is detected more frequently by TEE compared with transthoracic imaging, and the degree of regurgitation is often graded as being more severe using TEE.[52,53]

Atrioventricular valve regurgitation is graded semiquantitatively on a scale of 0 to 4+, where 0 is no regurgitation, 1+ is mild, 2+ is moderate, 3+ is moderate to severe, and 4+ is severe regurgitation. The most common method of grading the severity of mitral regurgitation is CFD mapping of the left atrium. With the Nyquist limits set at 50 to 60 cm/sec, jet areas less than 4 cm^2 or 20 percent of the left atrial size are usually classified as mild, whereas jets greater than 10 cm^2 or 40 percent of the atrial volume are classified as severe.[54] The area of the Doppler jet may be influenced by technical factors such as gain setting, carrier frequency of the transducer, imaging of low-velocity flows, differentiation of regurgitant from displacement flow, complexities in jet geometry such as multiple jets and vortex flow, temporal variation of jet size during systole, and differences between machines in color Doppler display.[55] In addition, jet direction should be considered when grading regurgitation, because eccentric jets that cling to the atrial wall (Coanda effect) have a smaller area than central (free) jets with similar regurgitant volumes and regurgitant fractions.[56–58] An alternative method of grading mitral regurgitation is based on the width of

the narrowest part of the regurgitant jet at its origin or immediate downstream location. This portion of the jet is known as the *vena contracta*.[59] A vena contracta width of less than 0.3 cm is associated with mild mitral regurgitation, whereas a width greater than 0.7 cm is associated with severe mitral regurgitation.

Continuous-wave Doppler integration may also be used in the assessment of the severity of mitral regurgitation.[60] A peak velocity that occurs during early systole and is directed toward the left atrium can be appreciated with mitral regurgitation, and the intensity of this recording may be proportional to the severity of regurgitation.[61] A dense full signal is associated with severe mitral regurgitation, whereas an incomplete and faint signal is associated with less severe regurgitation.

Pulmonary vein flow pattern

Pulmonary vein flow imaged by transesophageal echocardiography provides useful information regarding regurgitant severity.[62] Normally, pulmonary venous flow consists of a phase of retrograde flow during atrial systole, and two phases of antegrade flow during ventricular systole and diastole. Because systolic pulmonary venous flow is augmented by active atrial relaxation, systolic antegrade pulmonary venous flow is usually greater than diastolic antegrade pulmonary venous flow. With mitral regurgitation, there is increased left atrial pressure during ventricular systole, which may either reduce antegrade systolic pulmonary venous flow or cause reversal of systolic flow in cases of severe regurgitation.

It is important to interrogate both the right and the left pulmonary veins. With eccentric jets, flow reversal may be more prominent in the pulmonary veins toward which the jet is directed; however, central mitral regurgitation may also result in discordant pulmonary venous flow patterns.[63] Although discordant flow occurs primarily with eccentric mitral regurgitant jets with systolic reversal primarily in the right upper pulmonary vein, some patients with central regurgitation may also have discordant pulmonary venous flows.

Proximal isovelocity surface area

In addition to these previously discussed indices of mitral regurgitation, regurgitant flow convergence and flow volume also may be used to assess the degree of mitral regurgitation.[64] Quantification of mitral regurgitation by PISA assumes that as blood flows toward a regurgitant lesion, flow converges radially. This convergence occurs along increasing isovelocity hemispheres converging on the lesion. Color Doppler may be used to identify these hemispheres of increasing velocity proximal to the lesion (identified by aliasing), and peak flow may be determined by applying the following equation:

$$\text{peak flow} = 2\pi r^2 v_n, \tag{11.13}$$

where r is the radius of the hemispheric spheres and v_n is the Nyquist limit.

Because flow through these isovelocity spheres equals flow through the regurgitant lesion,

$$2\pi r^2 v_n = \mathrm{ROA}\, V_o, \tag{11.14}$$

where ROA is the area of the regurgitant orifice area and V_o is the maximal velocity. Solving for ROA yields

$$\mathrm{ROA} = 2\pi r^2 v_n / V_o. \tag{11.15}$$

Because the regurgitant volume is equal to the area of the regurgitant lesion multiplied by the velocity time integral of the regurgitant velocity ($\mathrm{VTI_{regurg}}$),

$$\begin{aligned} \text{Regurgitant volume} &= \mathrm{VTI_{regurg}}(\mathrm{ROA}) \\ &= \mathrm{VTI_{regurg}}(2\pi r^2 v_n / V_o). \end{aligned} \tag{11.16}$$

This method of determining mitral regurgitation is time-consuming; however, it has been validated as a method of identifying patients with severe mitral regurgitation.[65] If the Nyquist limits are set for 40 cm/s and assuming that the patient has "normal" systolic blood pressures (the difference between the systolic left ventricular pressure and left atrial pressure is approximately 100 mmHg), the calculation of ROA may be estimated to be

$$\mathrm{ROA} = r^2/2.\text{[66]} \tag{11.17}$$

Tricuspid valve

The tricuspid valve consists of three leaflets, an annular ring, chordae tendineae, and multiple papillary muscles.[67] The anterior leaflet is usually the largest, followed by the posterior and septal leaflets. Chordae arise from a large single papillary muscle, double or multiple septal papillary muscles, and several small posterior papillary muscles, attached to the corresponding walls of the right ventricle.

Intrinsic structural abnormalities of the tricuspid valve that can be well characterized by TEE include rheumatic tricuspid stenosis, carcinoid involvement of the tricuspid valve, tricuspid valve prolapse, flail tricuspid valve, Ebstein anomaly, and tricuspid endocarditis. Rheumatic involvement of the tricuspid valve, which is typically seen with concomitant mitral valve involvement, is characterized by thickening of the leaflets (particularly at their coaptation surfaces), fusion of the commissures, and shortening of the chordal structures, resulting in restricted leaflet motion.[68] Carcinoid syndrome results in a diffuse thickening of the tricuspid valve (and pulmonic valve) and endocardial thickening of right heart structures, which may result in restricted tricuspid valve motion (mixed stenosis and regurgitation) of the tricuspid valve.[69] The bulky and redundant tricuspid leaflet tissue seen in tricuspid valve prolapse is associated with billowing of leaflet tissue superior to the tricuspid annular plane into the right atrium. In patients with an overtly flail tricuspid valve, the disrupted leaflet tissue wildly prolapses into the right atrium, exhibiting high-frequency systolic vibrations. Destructive processes – such as infective endocarditis, valve trauma induced by inadvertent endomyocardial biopsy of the tricuspid apparatus, and spontaneous rupture of chordae – may all result in a partially flail tricuspid valve apparatus.

Supravalvular, valvular, or subvalvular restriction may cause tricuspid stenosis. The most common etiology of tricuspid stenosis is rheumatic heart disease, whereas less common causes include carcinoid syndrome and endomyocardial fibrosis. Tricuspid stenosis is characterized by a domed thickened valve with restricted movement. Tricuspid regurgitation may be secondary to annular or right ventricular dilation or pathology of the leaflets or subvalvular apparatus. Continuous-wave Doppler measurements of the inflow velocities across the tricuspid valve can be employed to estimate the mean diastolic tricuspid valve gradient with the modified Bernoulli equation.[70] Optimal alignment of the Doppler cursor parallel to the tricuspid inflow can be difficult to achieve from transesophageal imaging windows. Alignment can often be achieved, however, by positioning the probe deep within the stomach such that the right ventricular apex is imaged at the top of the sector scan. Alternatively, probe positioning at more rostral levels can display the tricuspid valve adjacent to a basal short axis view of the aortic valve (multiplane crystal orientation $25°$–$30°$), which may be suitable for continuous-wave Doppler interrogation.

Evaluation of the severity of tricuspid regurgitation is frequently required in patients with severe mitral valve disease, severe left ventricular systolic dysfunction and secondary right heart failure, or right ventricular dysfunction resulting from long-standing pulmonary hypertension. The quantification of tricuspid regurgitation is summarized in Table 11.5. The severity of tricuspid regurgitation can be estimated by the apparent size (area in a given imaging plane, volume reconstructed

Table 11.5. Quantification of tricuspid regurgitation

	Mild	Moderate	Severe
Right atrial size	Normal	Normal or dilated	Usually dilated
Tricuspid valve leaflets	Usually normal	Normal or abnormal	Abnormal/flail or wide coaption defect
Jet area – central jets (cm^2)*	<5	5–10	>10
Continuous wave jet density	Soft and parabolic	Dense, variable contour	Dense, triangular with early peaking
Vena contracta width (cm)*	Not defined	Not defined, but <0.7	>0.7
PISA radius (cm)*	≤0.5	0.6–0.9	>0.9
Hepatic vein flow	Systolic dominance	Systolic blunting	Systolic reversal

*At Nyquist limits of 50–60 cm/s.
Adapted from reference 54.

in three dimensions) of the color flow disturbance of tricuspid regurgitation relative to right atrial size.[71] A central jet area of less than 5 cm^2 is consistent with mild regurgitation, whereas a jet area greater than 10 cm^2 is consistent with severe regurgitation.[54] A vena contracta width greater than 0.7 cm is consistent with severe regurgitation.[72] The apparent severity of tricuspid regurgitation is exquisitely sensitive to right heart loading conditions. Thus, during the intraoperative evaluation of tricuspid regurgitation, pulmonary artery and right atrial pressures should be kept near levels observed in the awake resting state. To further assist in the evaluation of the hemodynamic significance of tricuspid regurgitation, the hepatic veins can be interrogated from deep gastric positioning of the transesophageal probe. The presence of blunted systolic hepatic vein flow is associated with moderate regurgitation, and retrograde systolic flow is associated with hemodynamically severe tricuspid regurgitation.

Pericardial disease

The pericardium is a two-layered structure reflecting from a visceral layer to a parietal layer approximately 1 to 2 cm distal to the origin of the great vessels and around the pulmonary veins. Under normal circumstances, 5 to 10 mL of fluid are contained within the pericardial sac, allowing for practically frictionless motion of the heart during the cardiac cycle. The parietal layer of the pericardium is rich in collagen fibers, making it a low-compliance structure confining the volume of the four cardiac chambers. In other words, a volume increase in one chamber requires a reduction of volume within another. Likewise, if an increase in volume is seen within the pericardial sac, a reduction of chamber volumes must occur.

Pericardial effusion

Under normal circumstances, the echocardiographer is unable to visualize the fluid film between the two layers. Under pathologic conditions fluid accumulation can occur, resulting in the development of a pericardial effusion (Figure 11.24) Typical etiologies leading to pericardial effusions are listed in Table 11.6.

Most echocardiographers use a qualitative grading system to characterize the quantity of the pericardial effusion present (minimal, small, moderate, or large). A quantitative score that can be used measures the diameter of the effusion in two dimensions (Table 11.7). Additionally, the effusion can either encompass the entire heart (free effusion) or be loculated. Free effusions are typically seen in medical conditions leading to pericardial effusions, whereas loculated effusions are seen after surgery or inflammatory processes. It is important that the echocardiographer pay attention to the anatomical relationship of the effusion. A loculated effusion found primarily at the inferior aspect of the heart can lead to inadvertent injury of the right ventricle if a subxiphoidal approach is chosen for drainage. For the novice echocardiographer, it can be difficult to differentiate a left-sided pleural effusion from a pericardial effusion. A good clue is to identify the descending thoracic aorta. Because the reflection of the pericardium is typically anterior to the descending thoracic aorta, pericardial effusions are generally seen anterior and to the right of the aorta.

Cardiac tamponade

Cardiac tamponade and pericardial effusion are not synonymous. A pericardial effusion is an anatomic diagnosis that may or may not lead to hemodynamic alterations. Because of the histologic structure of the pericardium characterized by a thick fibrous tissue, a constraint is exerted on the cardiac chambers within the thorax. Rapid fluid accumulation leads to a sharp rise in pressure within the pericardial sac, because of its low compliance. On the other hand, slow accumulation of fluid can go undetected for long periods of time, resulting in volumes exceeding 1 liter.

Under normal circumstances, the respiratory variation of arterial pressure is less than 10 mmHg. During mechanical ventilation, inspiratory positive pressure leads to impeded right-sided filling of the heart. The increase in intrathoracic pressure reduces the capacity of the pulmonary veins and augments the filling of the left side of the heart. During expiration, the exact opposite occurs. As the pressure increases within the pericardial sac, the total blood volume within the heart becomes limited, leading to an exaggerated response to the respiratory cycle. If the pressure of the intrapericardial fluid is not relieved, an equalization will occur among diastolic pressures within the heart. Echocardiographically, this can be identified as a right ventricular collapse during diastole, as well as a right atrial collapse during systole. More subtle signs of pericardial tamponade can be detected with Doppler-based modalities. A respiratory variation of more than 30 percent in peak transmitral or transtricuspid valve flow velocity represents a typical finding.

Table 11.7. Severity of pericardial effusions

Diameter of effusion	Severity
0–0.5 cm	Mild
0.6–2.0 cm	Moderate
>2.1 cm	Severe

Table 11.6. Etiologies of pericardial effusions

Idiopathic	Infections	Inflammatory	Post- myocardial infarction	Systemic disease	Malignancy	Miscellanous
Acute	Viral	Lupus	Dressler syndrome	Uremia	Direct	Posttrauma
Chronic	Bacterial	Rheumatoid arthritis	Acute after transmural infarct	Cirrhosis	Lymphatic obstruction	Postsurgical
	Fungal			Hypothyroidism		CHF

This can be achieved by positioning the pulse wave gate just at the leaflet tips of the mitral or tricuspid valve. Although a large pericardial effusion is frequently associated with pericardial tamponade, other etiologies can also be responsible for respiratory variation in transvalvular flow velocities (e.g. high airway pressures, hematoma).

Aortic disease

Because of the intimate anatomic relationship between the aorta and the esophagus, TEE has proved to be useful in the diagnosis of aortic dissection and aortic atherosclerosis. Detailed reviews of TEE diagnosis of these diseases have recently been published.[73,74]

In the diagnosis of aortic dissection, TEE has overcome some of the major disadvantages of the alternative diagnostic modalities (CT, MRI). In comparison to these modalities, TEE has been shown to have high sensitivity and specificity.[75,76] An examination can be performed within about 15 to 20 minutes, and a diagnosis can usually be obtained at the same time. The diagnosis is based on the presence of an intimal flap. Ideally, the specific locations of the entry and exit sites are also identifiable. Flow in both the true and false lumina can be analyzed with Doppler color flow imaging. TEE is performed in real time, allowing for its unique ability to give functional and hemodynamic information. This enables the detection of the common complications of aortic dissection: aortic valve regurgitation, pericardial tamponade, and left ventricular dysfunction secondary to coronary artery involvement in the dissection process. In addition to the common sequelae of aortic dissection, TEE can also identify a rare but potentially lethal complication of aortic intimal intussusception.[77]

Neurologic injury after cardiopulmonary bypass remains a devastating complication of cardiac surgery. Possible etiologies include hypoperfusion, lack of pulsatile flow, and cerebral embolization of gaseous or particulate matter. The thoracic aorta is a potential source of such emboli, as it often contains atherosclerotic plaques and it may be instrumented multiple times during cardiac operations. TEE can also be used to detect aortic intraluminal thrombi and plaques. One major limitation is that the distal ascending and proximal transverse aortas are not well visualized by TEE.[78] Although the entire ascending aorta is not well visualized, TEE can serve as a screen to detect aortic atherosclerotic debris.[79] The presence of atherosclerotic disease in the visualized portions increases the likelihood of finding atherosclerotic changes in the nonvisualized portion of the aorta. Intraoperatively, this region can be scanned by placing a sterile wrapped probe directly on the aorta to rule out pathology in the locations of planned instrumentation. Once the disease is defined, it can often be avoided during instrumentation and hopefully neurologic injury can be prevented. This epiaortic scanning is more sensitive than digital palpation in the detection of atherosclerotic disease, and its use has modified surgical management during cardiac surgery.[80] Although epiaortic scanning may be justified for all patients presenting

for cardiac surgery, its use should be seriously considered in those patients with increased risk for embolic stroke, including patients with a history of cerebrovascular or peripheral vascular disease or patients with evidence of aortic disease by any modality.[81] Phase array probes are generally used for perioperative aortic scanning. Because of the fan-shaped sector displayed, the most anterior aspect of the aorta cannot be adequately visualized unless a standoff is used between the transducer and the aorta. It is usually most convenient to fill the pericardial cradle with saline and hold the probe approximately 1 cm anterior to the aorta while scanning.

A complete examination will include short axis views of the proximal, middle, and distal ascending aorta and long axis views of both the ascending aorta and arch. These views will allow for evaluation of the twelve areas of the aorta: anterior, posterior, and left and right lateral walls of the proximal, middle, and distal ascending aorta. The proximal ascending aorta is defined as the region from the sinotubular junction to the proximal intersection of the right pulmonary artery. The middle ascending aorta includes the portion of the aorta that is adjacent to the right pulmonary artery. The distal ascending aorta extends from the distal intersection of the right pulmonary artery to the origin of the innominate artery. The severity of atherosclerosis may be graded according to the classification described by Katz and coworkers and is summarized in Table 11.8.[82]

Practice parameters and evidence of utility

An updated report by the American Society of Anesthesiologists (ASA) and the Society of Cardiovascular Anesthesiologists (SCA) Task Force on Transesophageal Echocardiography is currently available on the Internet and should be published shortly.[83] This document updates the 1996 published guidelines for the perioperative use of TEE.[84] The update currently recommends that perioperative TEE should be used in all adult patients who have no contraindications for TEE and present for cardiac or thoracic aortic procedures. A complete TEE exam should be performed in all patients with the following intent: (1) confirm and refine the preoperative diagnosis, (2) detect new or unsuspected pathology, (3) adjust the anesthetic and surgical plan accordingly, and (4) assess results of the surgical intervention.

For patients presenting to the catheterization laboratory, the use of TEE may be beneficial. Especially in the setting of

Table 11.8. Quantification of aortic atherosclerotic disease

Grade	Description
I	Normal to mild intimal thickening
II	Severe intimal thickening without protruding atheroma
III	Atheroma protruding < 5 mm into lumen
IV	Atheroma protruding ≥ 5 mm into lumen
V	Any thickness with mobile component or components

Adapted from reference 82.

catheter-based valve replacement and repair and transcatheter intracardiac procedures, both consultants and ASA members agreed that TEE should be used. In the setting of noncardiac surgery, TEE may be beneficial in patients with known or suspected cardiovascular pathology, which potentially could lead to severe hemodynamic, pulmonary, or neurologic compromise. In life-threatening situations of circulatory instability, TEE remains indicated. A similar viewpoint is taken by the consultants and ASA members in regard to critically ill patients. TEE should be used to obtain diagnostic information that is expected to alter management in the ICU, especially when the quality of transthoracic images is poor or other diagnostic modalities are not obtainable in a timely manner.

The perioperative use of TEE may improve outcome. Eltzschig and associates reported that 7 percent of 12,566 consecutive TEE exams directly influenced surgical decision-making.[85] Combined procedures (CABG, valve) were most commonly influenced by perioperative TEE. In 0.05 percent, the surgical procedure was actually canceled as a direct result of the intraoperative TEE exam. Minhaj and colleagues looked at a much small cohort and found that in 30 percent of patients, the routine use of TEE during cardiac surgery revealed a previously undiagnosed cardiac pathology, leading to change in surgical management in 25 percent of patients studied.[86]

Complications and contraindications

Complications resulting from intraoperative TEE can be separated into two groups: injury from direct trauma to the airway and esophagus, and indirect effects of TEE. In the first group, potential complications include esophageal bleeding, burning, tearing, dysphagia, and laryngeal discomfort. Further confirmation of the low incidence of esophageal injury from TEE is apparent in the few case reports of complications. A study of 10,000 TEE examinations yielded one case of hypopharyngeal perforation (0.01%), two cases of cervical esophageal perforation (0.02%), and no cases of gastric perforation (0%).[87] Kallmayer and associates reported an overall incidences of TEE-associated morbidity and mortality of 0.2 percent and 0 percent, respectively. The most common TEE-associated complications was severe odynophagia, which occurred in 0.1 percent of the study population, followed by dental injury (0.03%), endotracheal tube malpositioning (0.03%), upper gastrointestinal hemorrhage (0.03%), and esophageal perforation (0.01%).[88] Piercy and colleagues have reported a gastrointestinal complication rate of approximately 0.1%, with a greater frequency of injuries among patients more than 70 years old and among women. If resistance is met while advancing the probe, the procedure should be aborted to prevent these potentially lethal complications.

Another possible complication of esophageal trauma is bacteremia. Studies have shown that the incidence of positive blood cultures in patients undergoing upper gastrointestinal endoscopy is 4 to 13 percent,[89,90] and that in patients undergoing TEE it is 0 to 17 percent.[91–93] Even though bacteremia may occur, it does not always cause endocarditis. Antibiotic prophylaxis in accordance with the American Heart Association guidelines is not routinely recommended but is optional in patients with prosthetic or abnormal valves, or who are otherwise at high risk for endocarditis.[94]

The second group of complications that result from TEE includes hemodynamic and pulmonary effects of airway manipulation and, particularly for new TEE operators, distraction from patient care. Fortunately, in the anesthetized patient there are rarely hemodynamic consequences to esophageal placement of the probe, and there are no studies that specifically address this question. More important for the anesthesiologist are the problems of distraction from patient care. There have been instances in which severe hemodynamic and ventilatory abnormalities have been missed because of fascination with the images or the controls of the echocardiograph machine.

To ensure the continued safety of TEE, the following recommendations are made: The probe should be inspected prior to each insertion for cleanliness and structural integrity. If possible, the electrical isolation should also be checked. The probe should be inserted gently and, if resistance is met, the procedure aborted. Minimal transducer energy should be used and the image frozen when not in use. Finally, when not imaging, the probe should be left in the neutral, unlocked position to prevent prolonged pressure on the esophageal mucosa.

Absolute contraindications to TEE in intubated patients include esophageal stricture, diverticula, tumor, recent suture lines, and known esophageal interruption. Relative contraindications include symptomatic hiatal hernia, esophagitis, coagulopathy, esophageal varices, and unexplained upper gastrointestinal bleeding. Despite these relative contraindications, TEE has been used in patients undergoing hepatic transplantation without reported sequelae.[95,96]

Credentialing

This is an era in medicine in which the observance of guidelines for training, credentialing, certifying, and recertifying medical professionals has become increasingly common. Although there have been warnings[97] and objections[98] to anesthesiologists making diagnoses and aiding in surgical decision making, there is no inherent reason that an anesthesiologist cannot provide this valuable service to the patient. The key factors are proper training, extensive experience with TEE, and available backup by a recognized echocardiographer.

In 1990, a task force from the American College of Physicians, the American College of Cardiology (ACC), and the American Heart Association (AHA) created initial general guidelines for echocardiography.[99] The ASE also provided recommendations for general training in echocardiography and has introduced a self-assessment test for measuring proficiency. These organizations recommended the establishment of three levels of performance with a minimum number of cases for each level – level 1: introduction and an understanding of the indications (120 2D and 60 Doppler cases); level 2:

independent performance and interpretation (240 2D and 180 Doppler cases); and level 3: laboratory direction and training (590 2D and 530 Doppler cases).[98,100] However, these guidelines are limited because they are not based on objective data or achievement. Furthermore, because different individuals learn at different rates, meeting these guidelines does not ensure competence, nor does failure to meet these guidelines preclude competence.

Proficiency in echocardiography can be achieved more efficiently in a limited setting (i.e. the perioperative period) with fewer clinical applications (e.g. interpreting wall motion, global function, and mitral regurgitation severity) than in a setting that introduces every aspect of echocardiography. The ASA and the SCA have worked together to create a document on practice parameters for perioperative TEE.[101] The SCA then created a Task Force on Certification for Perioperative TEE to develop a process that acknowledges basic competence and offers the opportunity to demonstrate advanced competence, as outlined by the SCA/ASA practice parameters. This process resulted in the development of the Examination of Special Competence in Perioperative Transesophageal Echocardiography (PTEeXAM). In 1998, the National Board of Echocardiography was formed. Currently, board certification in perioperative transesophageal echocardiography may be granted by meeting the following requirements: (1) the holding of a valid license to practice medicine, (2) board certification in an approved medical specialty (e.g. anesthesiology), (3) training and/or experience in the perioperative care of surgical patients with cardiovascular disease, (4) the study of 300 echocardiographic examinations, and (5) the passing of the PTEeXAM.[102]

References

1. De Simone R, Glombitza G, Vahl CF, et al. Three-dimensional color Doppler: a clinical study in patients with mitral regurgitation. *J Am Coll Cardiol* 1999;33:1646–54.
2. Coisne D, Erwan D, Christiaens L, et al. Quantitative assessment of regurgitant flow with total digital three-dimensional reconstruction of color Doppler flow in the convergent region: in vitro validation. *J Am Soc Echocardiogr* 2002;15:233–40.
3. Lang RM, Bierig M, Devereux RB, et al.; American Society of Echocardiography's Nomenclature and Standards Committee; Task Force on Chamber Quantification; American College of Cardiology Echocardiography Committee; American Heart Association; European Association of Echocardiography, European Society of Cardiology. Recommendations for chamber quantification. *Eur J Echocardiogr* 2006;7(2):79–108.
4. Devereux RB, Wachtell K, Gerdts E, et al. Prognostic significance of left ventricular mass change during treatment of hypertension. *JAMA* 2004;292:1–7.
5. Devereux RB, Alonso DR, Lutas EM, et al. Echocardiographic assessment of left ventricular hypertrophy: comparison to necropsy findings. *Am J Cardiol* 1986;57:450.
6. Gopal AS, Schnellbaecher MJ, Shen Z, Boxt LM, Katz J, King DL. Freehand three-dimensional echocardiography for determination of left ventricular volume and mass in patients with abnormal ventricles: comparison with magnetic resonance imaging. *J Am Soc Echocardiogr* 1997;10:853–61.
7. Takeuchi M, Nishikage T, Mor-Avi V, et al. Measurement of left ventricular mass by real-time three-dimensional echocardiography: validation against magnetic resonance and comparison with two-dimensional and M-mode measurements. *J Am Soc Echocardiogr* 2008;21(9):1001–5.
8. Mor-Avi V, Sugeng L, Lang RM. Three-dimensional adult echocardiography: where the hidden dimension helps. *Curr Cardiol Rep* 2008;10(3):218–25.
9. Samad BA, Alam M, Jensen-Urstad K. Prognostic impact of right ventricular involvement as assessed by tricuspid annular motion in patients with acute myocardial infarction. *Am J Cardiol* 2002;90:778–81.
10. Foale R, Nihoyannopoulos P, McKenna W, et al. Echocardiographic measurement of the normal adult right ventricle. *Br Heart J* 1986;56:33–44.
11. Schiller NB, Shah PM, Crawford M, et al. Recommendations for quantitation of the left ventricle by two-dimensional echocardiography. American Society of Echocardiography Committee on Standards, Subcommittee on Quantitation of Two-Dimensional Echocardiograms. *J Am Soc Echocardiogr* 1989;2:358–67.
12. Cerqueira MD, Weissman NJ, Dilsizian V, et al. Standardized myocardial segmentation and nomenclature for tomographic imaging of the heart: a statement for healthcare professionals from the Cardiac Imaging Committee of the Council on Clinical Cardiology of the American Heart Association. *Circulation* 2002;105: 539–42.
13. Quiñones MA, Otto CM, Stoddard M, et al. Recommendations for quantification of Doppler echocardiography: A report from the Doppler quantification task force of the nomenclature and standards committee of the American Society of Echocardiography. *J Am Soc Echocardiogr* 2002;15:167–84.
14. Rapaport E, Rackley CE, Cohn LH. Aortic valve disease. In Schlant RC, Alexander RW, O'Rourke RA, et al., eds. *Hurst's The Heart: Arteries and Veins.* New York: McGraw Hill, 1994.
15. Stoddard MF, Arce J, Liddell NE, Peters G, Dillon S, Kupersmith J. Two dimensional transesophageal echocardiographic determination of aortic valve area in adults with aortic stenosis. *Am Heart J* 1991;122:1415.
16. Otto CM. Valvular aortic stenosis: disease severity and timing of intervention. *J Am Coll Cardiol* 2006;47: 2141–51.
17. Baumgartner H, Hung J, Bermejo J, et al. Echocardiographic assessment of valve stenosis: EAE/ASE recommendations for clinical practice. *J Am Soc Echocardiogr* 2009;22:1–23.
18. Cape EG, Jones M, Yamada I, et al. Turbulent/viscous interactions control Doppler/catheter pressure discrepancies in aortic stenosis. The role of the Reynolds number. *Circulation* 1996;94:2975.
19. Niederberger J, Schima H, Maurer G, Baumgartner H. Importance of pressure recovery for the assessment of aortic stenosis by Doppler ultrasound. Role of aortic size, aortic valve area, and direction of the stenotic jet in vitro. *Circulation* 1996;15:1934.
20. Cormier B, Iung B, Porte JM, et al. Value of multiplane transesophageal echocardiography in determining aortic valve area in aortic stenosis. *Am J Cardiol* 1996;15:882.
21. Hoffmann R, Flachskampf FA, Hanrath P. Planimetry of orifice area in aortic stenosis using multiplane transesophageal echocardiography. *J Am Coll Cardiol* 1993;22:529.
22. Stoddard MF, Hammons RT, Longaker RA. Doppler transesophageal echocardiographic determination of aortic

valve area in adults with aortic stenosis. *Am Heart J* 1996;132:337.

23. Bonow RO, Carabello BA, Chatterjee K, et al. Focused update incorporated into the ACC/AHA 2006 guidelines for the management of patients with valvular heart disease: a report of the American College of Cardiology/American Heart Association Task Force on Practice Guidelines. *Circulation* 2008;118(15):523–661.

24. Roberson WS, Stewart J, Armstrong WF, Dillon JC, Feigenbaum H. Reverse doming of the anterior mitral leaflet with severe aortic regurgitation. *J Am Coll Cardiol* 1984;3:431.

25. Ambrose JA, Meller J, Teichholz LE, Herman MV. Premature closure of the mitral valve: echocardiographic clue for the diagnosis of aortic dissection. *Chest* 1978;73:121.

26. Cohen GI, Duffy CI, Klein AL, et al. Color Doppler and two-dimensional echocardiographic determination of the mechanism of aortic regurgitation with surgical correlation. *J Am Soc Echocardiogr* 1996;9:508.

27. Perry GJ, Helmcke F, Nanda NC, et al. Evaluation of aortic insufficiency by Doppler color flow mapping. *J Am Coll Cardiol* 1987;9:952–9.

28. Reimold SC, Thomas JD, Lee RT. Relationship between Doppler color flow variables and invasively determined jet variables in patients with aortic regurgitation. *J Am Coll Cardiol* 1992;20:1143.

29. Ishii M, Jones M, Shiota T, et al. Evaluation of eccentric aortic regurgitation by color Doppler jet and color Doppler-imaged vena contracta measurements: an animal study of quantified aortic regurgitation. *Am Heart J* 1996;132:796.

30. Dolan MS, Castello R, St. Vrain JA, et al. Quantification of aortic regurgitation by Doppler echocardiography: a practical approach. *Am Heart J* 1995;129:1014.

31. Grayburn PA, Handshoe R, Smith MD, et al. Quantitative assessment of the hemodynamic consequences of aortic regurgitation by means of continuous wave Doppler recordings. *J Am Coll Cardiol* 1986;8:1341–7.

32. Griffin BP, Flachskampf FA, Siu S, Weyman AE, Thomas JD. The effects of regurgitant orifice size, chamber compliance, and systemic vascular resistance on aortic regurgitant velocity slope and pressure half-time. *Am Heart J* 1991;122:1049.

33. Ranganathan N, Lam JHC, Wigle ED, Silver MD. Morphology of the human mitral valve: II. The valve leaflets. *Circulation* 1970;41:459–67.

34. Perloff JK, Roberts WC. The mitral apparatus: functional anatomy of mitral regurgitation. *Circulation* 1972;46:227–39.

35. Hammer WJ, Roberts WC, deLeon AC Jr. Mitral stenosis secondary to combined massive mitral annular calcific deposits and small, hypertrophied left ventricles: hemodynamic documentation in four patients. *Am J Med* 1978;64:371–6.

36. Pai RG, Tarazi R, Wong S. Constrictive pericarditis causing extrinsic mitral stenosis and a left heart mass. *Clin Cardiol* 1996;19:517.

37. Felner JM, Martin RP. The echocardiogram. In Schlant RC, Alexander RW, O'Rourke RA, et al., eds. *Hurst's The Heart: Arteries and Veins.* New York: McGraw-Hill, 1994, pp. 375–422.

38. Roberts WE. Morphological features of the normal and abnormal mitral valve. *Am J Cardiol* 1983;51:1005–28.

39. Chen YT, Kan MN, Chen JS. et al. Contributing factors to formation of left atrial spontaneous echo contrast in mitral valvular disease. *J Ultrasound Med* 1990;9:151–5.

40. Feigenbaum H. Acquired valvular heart disease. In *Echocardiography.* Philadelphia: Lea & Febiger, 1994, pp. 239–349.

41. Currie PJ, Seward JB, Reeder GS, et al. Continuous-wave Doppler echocardiographic assessment of severity of calcific aortic stenosis: a simultaneous Doppler-catheter correlative study in 100 adult patients. *Circulation* 1985;71:1162.

42. Gorcsan J, Kenny WM, Diana P. Transesophageal continuous-wave Doppler to evaluate mitral prosthetic stenosis. *Am Heart J* 1991;121:911.

43. Chang KC, Chiang CW, Kuo CT, et al. Effect of mitral regurgitation and aortic regurgitation on Doppler-derived mitral orifice area in patients with mitral stenosis. *Chang Keng I Hsueh* 1993;16:217.

44. Moro E, Nicolosi GL, Zanuttini D, et al. Influence of aortic regurgitation on the assessment of the pressure half-time and derived mitral-valve area in patients with mitral stenosis. *Eur Heart J* 1988;9:1010–7.

45. Flachskampf FA, Weyman AE, Gillam L, ChunMing L, Abascal VM, Thomas JD. Aortic regurgitation shortens Doppler pressure half-time in mitral stenosis: Clinical evidence, in vitro simulation, and theoretic analysis. *J Am Coll Cardiol* 1990;16:396.

46. Ormiston JA, Shah PM, Tei C, Wong M. Size and motion of the mitral valve annulus in man. *Circulation* 1981;64:113.

47. Burwash IG, Blackmore GL, Koilpillai CJ. Usefulness of left atrial and left ventricular chamber sizes as predictors of the severity of mitral regurgitation. *Am J Cardiol* 1992;15:774.

48. Mintz GS, Kotler MN, Segal BL, Parry WR. Two-dimensional echocardiographic recognition of ruptured chordae tendineae. *Circulation* 1978;57:244.

49. Ogawa S, Mardelli TJ, Hubbard FE. The role of cross-sectional echocardiography in the diagnosis of flail mitral leaflet. *Clin Cardiol* 1978;1:85.

50. Carpentier A, Loulmet D, Deloche A, Perier P. Surgical anatomy and management of ischemic mitral valve incompetence. *Circulation* 1987;76(suppl IV):II76-II83.

51. Felner JM, Williams BR. Noninvasive evaluation of left ventricular overload and cardiac function. *Prac Cardiol* 1979;5:158–96.

52. Smith MD, Harrison MOR, Pinton R, et al. Regurgitant jet size by transesophageal compared with transthoracic Doppler color flow imaging. *Circulation* 1991;83:79–86.

53. Smith MD, Cassidy J, Gurley JC, et al. Echo Doppler evaluation of patients with acute mitral regurgitation: superiority of transesophageal echocardiography with color flow imaging. *Am Heart J* 1995;129:967.

54. Zoghbi WA, Enriquez-Sarano M, Foster E, et al. Recommendations for evaluation of the severity of native valvular regurgitation with two-dimensional and Doppler echocardiography. *J Am Soc Echocardiogr* 2003;16:777–802.

55. Stevenson JG. Two-dimensional color Doppler estimation of the severity of atrioventricular valve regurgitation: important effects of instrument gain settings, pulse repetition frequency, and carrier frequency. *J Am Soc Echocardiogr* 1989;2:1.

56. Omoto R, Ky S, Matsumura M, et al. Evaluation of biplane color Doppler transesophageal echocardiography in 200 consecutive patients. *Circulation* 1992;85:1237.

57. Sadoshima J, Koyanagi S, Sugimachi M, et al. Evaluation of the severity of mitral regurgitation by transesophageal Doppler flow echocardiography. *Am Heart J* 1992;123:1245.

58. Chen C, Thomas JD, Anconina J, et al. Impact of impinging wall jet on color Doppler quantification of mitral regurgitation. *Circulation* 1991;84:712.

59. Tribouilloy C, Shen WF, Quere JP, et al. Assessment of severity of mitral regurgitation by measuring regurgitant jet width at its origin with transesophageal Doppler color flow imaging. *Circulation* 1992;85:1248–53.

60. Kisanuki A, Tei C, Minagoe S, et al. Continuous wave Doppler echocardiographic evaluations of the severity of mitral regurgitation. *J Cardiol* 1989;19:831.

61. Utsunomiya T, Patel D, Doshi R, Quan M, Gardin JM. Can signal intensity of the continuous wave Doppler regurgitant jet estimate severity of mitral regurgitation? *Am Heart J* 1992;19:831.

62. Klein AL, Obarski TP, Stewart WJ, et al. Transesophageal Doppler echocardiography of pulmonary venous flow: A new marker of mitral regurgitation severity. *J Am Coll Cardiol* 1991;18:518.

63. Mark JB, Ahmed SU, Kluger R, Robinson SM. Influence of jet direction on pulmonary vein flow patterns in severe mitral regurgitation. *Anesth Analg* 1995;80:486.

64. Enriquez-Sarano M, Miller FA Jr, Hayes SN, Bailey KR, Tajik AJ, Seward JB. Effective mitral regurgitant orifice area: clinical use and pitfalls of the proximal isovelocity surface area method. *J Am Coll Cardiol* 1995;25:703–9.

65. Xie G, Berk MR, Hixson CS, et al. Quantification of mitral regurgitant volume by the color Doppler proximal isovelocity surface area method: a clinical study. *J Am Soc Echocardiogr* 1995;8:48.

66. Lambert AS. Proximal isovelocity surface area should be routinely measured in evaluating mitral regurgitation: a core review. *Anesth Analg* 2007;105:940–3.

67. Silver MD, Lam JHC, Ranganathan N, Wigle ED. Morphology of the human tricuspid valve. *Circulation* 1971;43:333–48.

68. Guyer DE et al. Comparison of the echocardiographic and hemodynamic diagnosis of rheumatic tricuspid stenosis. *J Am Coll Cardiol* 1984;3:1135.

69. Lundin L, Landelius J, Andrea B, Oberg K. Transesophaeal echocardiography improves the diagnostic value of cardiac ultrasound in patients with carcinoid heart disease. *Br Heart J* 1990;64:190–4.

70. Perez JE, Ludbrook PA, Ahumada GG. Usefullness of Doppler echocardiography in detecting tricuspid valve stenosis. *Am J Cardiol* 1985;55:601.

71. Miyatake K et al. Evaluation of tricuspid regurgitation by pulsed Doppler and two dimensional echocardiography. *Circulation* 1982;66:777.

72. Tribouilloy CM, Enriquez-Sarano M, Bailey KR, Tajik AJ, Seward JB. Quantification of tricuspid regurgitation by measuring the width of the vena contracta with Doppler color flow imaging: a clinical study. *J Am Coll Cardiol* 2000;36:472–8.

73. Moskowitz D, Reich DL. Aortic dissection: is transesophageal echocardiography the diagnostic method of choice? *Semin Cardiothorac Vasc Anesth* 1997;1:71–80.

74. Shore-Lesserson L, Konstadt SN. Aortic atherosclerosis: should we bother to look for it? *Semin Cardiothorac Vasc Anesth* 1997;1:39–48.

75. Ballal RS, Nanda NC, Gatewood R, et al. Usefulness of transesophageal echocardiography in assessment of aortic dissection. *Circulation* 1991;84:1903–14.

76. Simon P, Owen AN, Havel M, et al. Transesophageal echocardiography in the emergency surgical management of patients with aortic dissection. *J Thorac Cardiovasc Surg* 1992;103:1113–8.

77. Hudak A, Konstadt SN. Aortic intussuception: A rare complication of aortic dissection. *Anesthesiology* 1995;82:1292–4.

78. Konstadt SN, Reich DL, Quintana C, Levy M. The ascending aorta: how much does transesophageal echocardiography see? *Anesth Analg* 1994;78:240–4.

79. Konstadt SN, Reich DL, Kahn R, Viggiani RF. Transesophageal echocardiography can be used to screen for ascending aortic atherosclerosis. *Anesth Analg* 1995;81:225–8.

80. Djaiani G, Ali M, Borger MA, Woo A, et al. Epiaortic scanning modifies planned intraoperative surgical management but not cerebral embolic load during coronary artery bypass surgery. *Anesth Analg* 2008;106:1611–8.

81. Glas KE, Swaminathan M, Reeves ST, et al. Guidelines for the performance of a comprehensive intraoperative epiaortic ultrasonographic examination: recommendations of the American Society of Echocardiography and the Society of Cardiovascular Anesthesiologists; endorsed by the Society of Thoracic Surgeons. Council for Intraoperative Echocardiography of the American Society of Echocardiography; Society of Cardiovascular Anesthesiologists; Society of Thoracic Surgeons. *Anesth Analg* 2008;106:1376–84.

82. Katz ES, Tunick PA, Rusinek H, Ribakove G, Spencer FC, Kronzon I. Protruding aortic atheromas predict stroke in elderly patients undergoing cardiopulmonary bypass: experience with intraoperative transesophageal echocardiography. *J Am Coll Cardiol* 1992;20:70–7.

83. http://www.asahq.org/clinical/TEE_PracticeGuidelinesUpdate. pdf. Accessed May 13, 2009.

84. Practice Guidelines for Perioperative Transesophageal Echocardiography. *Anesthesiology* 199;84(4):986–100.

85. Eltzschig HK, Rosenberger P, Löffler M, Fox JA, Aranki SF, Shernan SK. Impact of intraoperative transesophageal echocardiography on surgical decisions in 12,566 patients undergoing cardiac surgery. *Ann Thorac Surg* 2008;85(3): 845–52.

86. Minhaj M, Patel K, Muzic D, et al. The effect of routine intraoperative transesophageal echocardiography on surgical management. *J Cardiothorac Vasc Anesth* 2007;21(6):800–4.

87. Min JK, Spencer KT, Furlong KT, et al. Clinical features of complications from transesophageal echocardiography: a single-center case series of 10,000 consecutive examinations. *J Am Soc Echocardiogr* 2005;18:925–9.

88. Kallmeyer IJ, Collard CD, Fox JA, et al. The safety of intraoperative transesophageal echocardiography: a case series of 7200 cardiac surgical patients. *Anesth Analg* 2001;92:1126–30.

89. Everett ED, Hirschman JV. Transient bacteremia and endocarditis prophylaxis. *Medicine* 1977;56:61.

90. Botoman VA, Surawicz CM. Bacteremia with gastrointestinal endoscopic procedures. *Gastrointest Endosc* 1986;32:342.

91. Nikutta P, Mantey-Stiers F, Becht I, et al. Risk of bacteremia induced by transesophageal echocardiography: analysis of 100 consecutive procedures. *J Am Soc Echocardiogr* 1992;5:168.

92. Melendez LJ, Kwan-Leung Chan, Cheung PK, et al. Incidence of bacteremia in transesophageal echocardiography: a prospective study of 140 consecutive patients. *J Am Coll Cardiol* 1991;18:1650.

93. Steckelberg JM, Khandheria BK, Anhalt JP, et al. Prospective evaluation of the risk of bacteremia associated with transesophageal echocardiography. *Circulation* 1991;84:177.

94. Dajani AS, Bisno AAL, Chung KJ, et al. Prevention of bacterial endocarditis. *JAMA* 1990;264:2919.

95. Ellis JE, Lichtor JL, Feinstein SB, et al. Right heart dysfunction, pulmonary embolism, and paradoxical embolization during liver transplantation. *Anesth Analg* 1989;68:777.

96. Suriani RJ, Cutrone A, Feierman D, Konstadt S. Intraoperative transesophageal echocardiography during liver transplantation. *J Cardiothorac Vasc Anesth* 1996;10:699–707.

97. Kaplan JA. Monitoring technology: advances and restraints. *J Cardiothorac Anesth* 1989;3:257.

98. Pearlman AS, Gardin JM, Martin RP, et al. Guidelines for physician training in transesophageal echocardiography: recommendations of the American Society of Echocardiography. *J Am Soc Echocardiogr* 1992;5:187.

99. Popp RL, Williams SV, Achord JL, et al. ACP/ACC/AHA Task Force on Clinical Privileges in Cardiology: Clinical competence in adult echocardiography. *J Am Coll Cardiol* 15:1465–1468, 1990.

100. Pearlman AS, Gardin JM, Martin RP, et al. Guidelines for optimal physician training in echocardiography. Recommendations of the American Society of Echocardiography Committee for Physician Training in Echocardiography. *Am J Cardiol* 1987;60:158–63.

101. Thys D, Abel M, Botlen B, et al. Practice parameters for intraoperative echocardiography. *Anesthesiology* 1996;84:986–1006.

102. http://www.echoboards.org/certification/pte/reqs.html. Accessed December 18, 2008.

Chapter 12

Ultrasound guidance of vascular catheterization

Andrew B. Leibowitz and Jonathan Elmer

Technical concepts

The basic principles of ultrasound are covered in Chapter 11, but for the sake of completion they will be re-reviewed here. There are two basic kinds of ultrasound applicable to vascular access, Doppler and B-mode (also known as two-dimensional [2D]).

The Doppler principle may be used to determine the velocity of moving objects, such as red blood cells within a vessel. This velocity information may be displayed as a velocity-versus-time spectrum or may be converted into an audio signal, in which different velocities are rendered as different pitches. Anesthesiologists are most familiar with this technique when it is used to "hear" a pulse to measure blood pressure or the presence or absence of circulation in an extremity (e.g. following vascular bypass). Signals obtained from arteries and veins sound distinctively different and thus can be used to help assist in the identification of vascular structures. Doppler ultrasound can be used alone or combined with 2D ultrasound. With the exception of color Doppler, Doppler ultrasound alone is currently rarely used to assist in vascular catheterization.

B-mode or 2D ultrasound renders reflected ultrasound signals into a 2D gray-scale image. B stands for brightness. Signals returning to the transducer are assigned a gray scale based on amplitude. The device's contrast resolution determines the number of shades of gray that are displayed. Fluid-filled structures (e.g. blood, fluid in collections) are echolucent and are shown as dark gray or black; soft tissue (e.g. muscle) is more echogenic and appears gray; and solid structures (e.g. thick tendons, bone) are very echogenic and appear white (Figure 12.1).

When applied to vascular access, a key use of ultrasound is the identification of and differentiation between arterial and venous structures. Vascular structures can be further assessed by their overall shape and, of greater importance, compressibility. Patent veins are much more compressible and can often be collapsed with the application of pressure, unlike arteries, which retain much of their original shape and appearance. Extrathoracic veins will also enlarge more than arteries with Valsalva maneuvers and Trendelenburg positioning. Finally, the pulsatility of arterial structures can be visualized; however, because this pulsation can be transmitted to adjacent structures, extra care must be taken to avoid confusion.

These devices are used in two main ways: static and dynamic imaging. In static imaging, the anatomy is defined and an "x marks the spot" technique is applied. These authors highly recommend against this technique, because the relative relationship between surface and deep anatomy can change dramatically with minor changes in positioning that may occur between the marking and start of the procedure (Figure 12.2)[1–3]. We recommend dynamic imaging, whereby the transducer is covered in a sterile sheath and held in the nondominant hand and the needle stick is performed with the dominant hand.

Other important technical points that are frequently overlooked include the following:

1. The proper orientation of the transducer should be verified at the beginning of the procedure to ensure that pressure on the left side of the transducer is visualized on the left side of the screen. The recommended transducer orientation is not always clearly marked on the probe.
2. The screen should be positioned in a comfortable place so the operator can see it within a 30-degree glance from the operative field. This positioning will allow almost simultaneous visualization of the surface anatomy and the monitor. When performing an internal jugular catheterization, we prefer the screen to be located on the ipsilateral side of the bed, approximately within arm's reach (Figure 12.3).
3. Ultrasound jelly must be placed within the condom sheath and on the skin to obtain an adequate image.
4. Always start by positioning the vein in the center of the screen and adjust the depth monitored so that the entire needle path can be visualized easily.
5. Pay attention to the actual depth of the vessel by noting the ruler on the screen or the actual size of the image that is rendered, in centimeters. Knowledge of depth will help prevent the operator from accidentally entering the pleural space.

The transducer can be manipulated in several ways to optimize the image and acquire the most information. The four basic maneuvers are pressure, alignment, rotation, and tilting; they can be remembered with the acronym PART. Short axis and long axis techniques may be used (Figure 12.4), but the short axis approach is more commonly preferred. Some devices

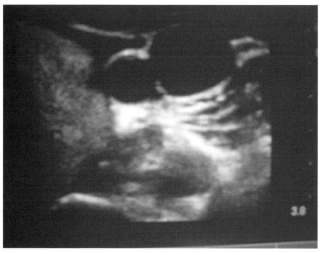

Figure 12.1. Picture obtained from the ultrasound image of the right neck of a patient. The vein lies lateral to the artery in this patient, is larger, and is not as circularly shaped.

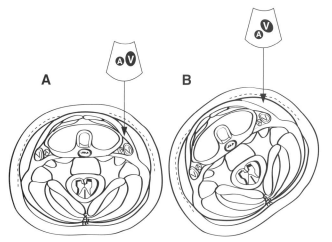

Figure 12.2. Figure demonstrating the effect of change in head position on overlap of the vein and artery. From reference 1, with permission.

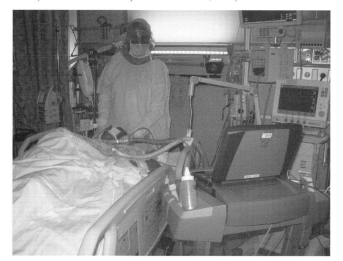

Figure 12.3. Ideal positioning of patient, operator, and monitor. This photo depicts a preprocedure scan of the left internal jugular vein. The transducer is held in the nondominant hand, and the monitor is on the ipsilateral side of the planned procedure, as close to the midline of the operative field as possible.

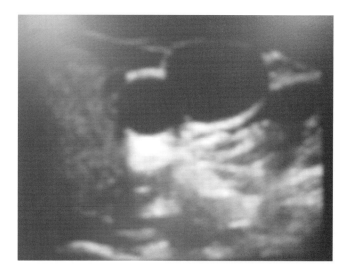

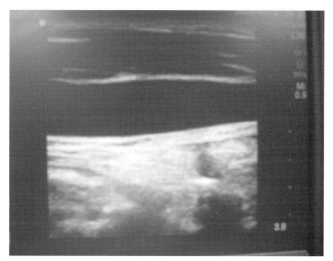

Figure 12.4. Short and long axis views of the internal jugular vein.

allow the simultaneous visualization of both images, which can be quite helpful to the experienced operator, but, in our experience, confuses the novice operator. Long axis views will allow the experienced operator to visualize the entire needle along its plane of passage into the vessel; however, the artery and vein will often not be visualized in the same long axis image. Vigilance must be maintained to avoid confusing the artery with the vein. In contrast, the short axis view almost always allows continuous visualization of both the artery and the vein.

There are many ultrasound machines and transducers available. The larger, more complicated, machines are almost always capable of performing vascular ultrasound if configured properly. Only a few systems are designed specifically for vascular catheterization. The main determinant factor of suitability for vascular imaging is the frequency of the transducer. High frequencies are associated with better resolution of the vascular structures. Vascular ultrasound should generally be performed with a 7.5- to 10-MHz linear array transducer. This transducer

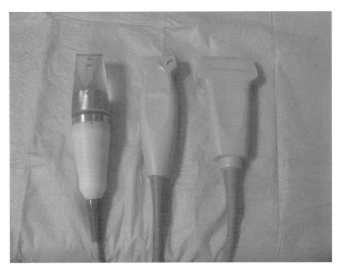

Figure 12.5. Three transducers that the author (ABL) uses. On the left is the Bard Site Rite 3, in the middle is the SonoSite *iLook*, and on the right is the SonoSite S-ICU. Note the differences in shape and width.

has a flat face, resulting in a rectangular image that allows adequate visualization of the vasculature structures of interest, their depth, and their relationship to immediately adjacent structures. Unlike the phase array probes, linear array probes have minimal near-field dropout, which allows for visualization of very superficial structures. Color Doppler will further enhance the ability to differentiate arteries from veins and is now commonly available in several devices, but it is not absolutely necessary. Of note, the color assigned in Doppler views (traditionally, either red or blue) represents only the direction of flow relative to the transducer. Thus, a vein may be depicted as either red or blue, as may an artery, depending on the angulation of the transducer. The transducer should not be too large, as this will interfere with its ability to fit into the operative field, especially in pediatric patients, and in adults if the neck is particularly short and fat. The shape of transducers varies tremendously; the operator should make sure to be comfortable holding it in his or her nondominant hand (Figure 12.5).

When purchasing a vascular ultrasound device, consider several important aspects of the monitor and the stand:

1. The device size and portability, especially the footprint of the stand, will determine whether it can be used in tight quarters. Space requirements may vary greatly from one work area to another.
2. The device should function on alternating current or with a battery. Battery life may be important if the device will travel away from a home base for long periods.
3. Larger screens allow the image to be magnified. This feature is helpful when the vasculature is small.
4. The layout of control functions varies tremendously from device to device. One particularly helpful advance is the presence of controls to adjust gain, image magnification, and depth on the transducer itself, or on a remote control

device that can be sheathed and placed into the operative field. This will allow the operator to work independently.
5. The ability to print or store images will be germane to documentation, performance improvement efforts, and billing.
6. A storage basket on the device pole to hold the sheaths, gels, and other extraneous equipment, such as printer paper, is necessary.

Although devices that incorporate more features almost always appear to be more desirable, the authors feel that if the device will be used only for vascular catheterization, a simpler device with fewer features and controls not only will allow more rapid skill acquisition and acceptance, but will also cost less and be less likely to need repair.

Parameters monitored

We recommend a preprocedure examination before prepping and draping the selected site. Important information obtained from a preprocedure examination should include at least the following:

1. The absolute presence of the intended target vessel is established.
2. The vessel's size should be estimated.
3. The vein's relationship to the artery should be carefully noted, particularly what percentage overlay there is and whether the amount of overlay can be improved by turning the head.
4. The presence of echogenic material within the vessel suggestive of clot or thrombus should be determined. Similarly, complete or nearly complete compressibility of the vessel should be observed to rule out venous thrombosis.
5. How the vessel changes in size with Trendelenburg positioning and Valsalva maneuver should be noted.
6. If any of the previous issues presents concern, then other potential sites should be similarly interrogated.

Prior vascular catheterizations may have scarred, stenosed, or thrombosed the target vessel; a preprocedure examination may immediately lead to change of site. If the vein appears small despite steep Trendelenburg positioning and Valsalva maneuver, or its anatomy relative to the artery is unsatisfactory and arterial puncture is perhaps unavoidable, imaging of the other side should be performed and the comparable risk of the two sides weighed. At the very least, if the first site chosen is unsuccessful, the likelihood of success in the backup site could be estimated a priori. Imaging will help the clinician communicate to the patient the potential for increased difficulty, multiple punctures, and failure. Prior warning of these adverse events seems to increase patient satisfaction.

When the dynamic technique is used, the vessel is visualized in real time. When local anesthetic is injected, the needle should be visualized in the expected plane of approach and the formation of an echogenic local anesthesia bubble anterior to the vessel should be appreciated. If the vessel is small, coaching the patient to Valsalva or steepening the Trendelenburg position will be helpful. The needle should be seen to invaginate the anterior wall of the vessel and usually can be seen to enter the vessel if the relative planes of the transducer and needle tip are correctly oriented. The guidewire may be visualized within the vessel lumen.

If catheterization is unsuccessful, the vessel may disappear and ultrasonic evidence of hematoma formation may be appreciated. This information may lead to the abandonment of that site in a timely fashion, which will reduce time, discomfort, and potential for complications. Preprocedural examination will also have allowed for a thoughtful and orderly progression of attempts at an alternative site or the decision to abort the procedure completely.

Evidence of utility

Traditional approaches

Historically, central venous catheter (CVC) insertion has been performed by blind techniques that rely on anatomic landmarks such as the sternocleidomastoid muscle heads and carotid pulse (internal jugular [IJ] cannulation), the bend of the clavicle (subclavian cannulation), or the inguinal ligament and femoral pulse (femoral cannulation). Such techniques require knowledge of regional anatomy and assume that this anatomy is readily identifiable and invariant from patient to patient. Landmark-based techniques are generally viewed as safe and effective when performed by an experienced operator in optimal conditions. However, historical data show overall noninfectious complication and failure rates as high as 40 percent in adult patients.[2-6] Failure can be attributed to three major factors: patient-related factors, anatomic variability, and operator inexperience.

Numerous patient-related factors have been associated with increased risks of complications from CVC placement. These factors include lack of traditional anatomic landmarks in morbid obesity, extremes of age, or previous radiation or surgery that distorts normal anatomy; factors that increase risk of bleeding with arterial puncture, such as coagulopathy or thrombocytopenia; and factors that limit the patient's ability to tolerate mechanical complications of insertion, such as decreased cardiopulmonary reserve.[4,5] Not surprisingly, pediatric patients are generally at higher risk for almost all major complications.[7,8]

Even in a patient without specific risk factors for difficult cannulation, intrinsic anatomic variability often leads to poor outcomes. This variability is best demonstrated by the example of IJ CVC insertion. The landmark technique for IJ cannulation relies on identification of the two heads of the sternocleidomastoid and/or the carotid pulse; the needle is inserted at the apex of the two heads lateral to the palpated pulse. This technique assumes a lateral location of the jugular vein relative to the carotid artery, an assumption only true in a minority of patients (Figure 12.6).[2] In fact, in most cases, the jugular vein

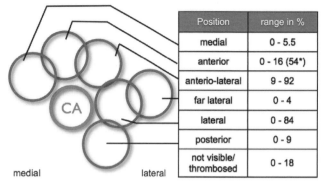

Position	range in %
medial	0 - 5.5
anterior	0 - 16 (54*)
anterio-lateral	9 - 92
far lateral	0 - 4
lateral	0 - 84
posterior	0 - 9
not visible/ thrombosed	0 - 18

Figure 12.6. Figure demonstrating the relative position of the vein to the carotid artery (CA) compiled from several studies. From reference 2, with permission.

overlaps the carotid artery anteriorly to at least some extent, and may even lie medial to the artery.

Operator experience also plays a significant role in the complication and failure rates of the landmark technique.[5,9] We suggest that approximately 50 line placements are required before an operator can be deemed competent to place CVCs independently. Operators who have placed more than 50 lines have half the complication rate of those who have placed fewer than 50.

Ultrasound guidance

Because of the relatively high complication rate of landmark-based CVC placement, as discussed previously, the development of ultrasound-guided techniques for CVC was greeted with considerable excitement. As discussed elsewhere in this chapter, three broad categories of ultrasound guidance for central venous catheterization exist: Doppler, 2D static, and 2D dynamic. Doppler, although initially thought to be promising, proved to be inferior to 2D ultrasound guidance and equivalent to landmark techniques in a majority of studies in both adult and pediatric populations.[10-13] As a consequence, the technique has largely been abandoned.

Static ultrasound has been compared with dynamic ultrasound and landmark techniques in several moderate-sized randomized controlled trials in recent years (Table 12.1). Because of the few studies that directly compare static ultrasound to another technique, conclusions about its utility are limited; however, static ultrasound was demonstrated to be superior to landmark in one adult and one pediatric study.[14,15] Data comparing dynamic ultrasound with static ultrasound are equivocal, with dynamic ultrasound appearing to be superior to static ultrasound in several studies, and equivalent in others.[15-17] Of note, to date there are no studies suggesting statistical or nonsignificant trend toward superiority of static ultrasound. However, additional studies are required to elucidate significant differences between the two.

In contrast with static ultrasound, numerous clinical trials have demonstrated the efficacy of dynamic ultrasound guidance in CVC placement in a variety of clinical settings and patient populations, both adult (Table 12.2) and pediatric (Table 12.3). In the overwhelming majority of studies, dynamic

Table 12.1. Studies of static ultrasound prelocation in adult and pediatric populations

First Author/ Year	Study Type Comparison	Patient type	n	Total success	Mean Attempts	Complications[1]	Conclusions
Chuan 2005[14]	RCT SUS vs LM	Infants <12 kg	62	80% vs 100%	2.55 vs 1.57	26.7% vs 3.1%	Benefit to SUS over LM in peds
Hosokawa 2007[16]	RCT DUS vs SUS	Infants <7.5 kg	60	89% vs 100%[NS]	NR	4% vs 0%[NS]	NS trend favoring DUS over SUS in peds
Milling 2005[15]	RCT DUS vs SUS vs LM	Adults	201	64% vs 82% vs 98%	5.2 vs 2.9 vs 2.3[2]	13% vs 3% vs 3% [NS]	DUS better than SUS better than LM in adults
Hayashi 2002[17]	RCT DUS vs SUS	Adults w/ VAD	188	96.9% vs 97.6%[NS]	NR	1% vs 3.3%[NS]	DUS equivalent to SUS if VAD
Hayashi 2002[17]	RCT DUS vs SUS	Adults w/o VAD	53	78.3% vs 97.6%	NR	13% vs 0%	DUS superior to SUS if no VAD

Abbreviations: RCT = randomized controlled trial; LM = landmark; SUS = static ultrasound prelocation; DUS = real-time dynamic ultrasound; VAD = ventilator-associated venodilation; NR= not reported; Peds = pediatrics; NS, not significant.
[1] Major complications unless otherwise noted (arterial puncture, pneumothorax, hemothorax).
[2] All significant except DUS vs SUS.

ultrasound use increased overall success rates, decreased the number of attempts required for cannulation, and reduced the number of mechanical complications associated with CVC placement. In addition to these general studies, the limitations of landmark techniques described previously have prompted several investigators to examine the safety and efficacy of dynamic ultrasound in a variety of high-risk patient populations (Table 12.4). In each of these patient populations, dynamic ultrasound has been demonstrated to be safe, effective, and superior to landmark techniques.

Table 12.2. Studies of dynamic ultrasound use compared with landmark technique in adult populations

First author/Year	Study type Site (if not IJ)	Setting Patient population	n	Total success	Mean attempts	Complications
Gualtieri 1995[36]	RCT Subclavian	ICU	53	44% vs 92%	2.5 vs 1.4	0% vs 0%[NS]
Karakitsos 2006[37]	RCT	ICU	900	94.4% vs 100%	2.6 vs 1.1	6.7% vs 1.1%
Leung 2006[38]	RCT	ED	130	78.5% vs 93.9%	3.5 vs 1.6	7.7% vs 1.5%
Mallory 1990[39]	RCT	ICU	29	65% vs 100%	3.12 vs 1.75	NR
Milling 2006[40]	RCT	ED + MICU	201	64% vs. 98%	5.2 vs 2.3	13% vs 3%
Troianos 1991[41]	RCT	ORs	160	96% vs 100% [NS]	2.8 vs 1.4	8.43% vs 1.39%[NS]
Hilty 1997[42]	Randomized case-control Femoral	ED PEA arrest	40	65% vs 90%	5.0 vs 2.3	20% vs 0%
Miller 2002[43]	Prospective quasi-random[3]	ED	122	NR	3.52 vs 1.55	14% vs 12% [NS,4]
Cajozzo 2004[44]	Prospective quasi-random[5]	NR	196	98.1% vs 91.2%	NR	9.7% vs 0%
Hrics 1998[45]	Prospective case series	ED	40	62.5% vs 81.3%	2.0 vs 2.0[NS]	0% vs 0%
Wigmore 2007[46]	Prospective case series	OR	284	93.9% vs 99.4%	1.31 vs 1.23[NS]	4.3% vs 1.8% [NS]
Augoustides 2002[47]	Prospective case series	OR	462	86.2% vs 97.9%	NR	8.1% vs 5.9%[NS]
Martin 2004[48]	Prospective case series	ICU	484	NR	NR	9% vs 11%[NS,3]
Cajozzo 2004[49]	Retrospective chart review	Wards Pts >65 y/o	72	98.7%	NR	0%

$P < 0.05$ unless otherwise noted.
Abbreviations: RCT= randomized controlled trial; ICU = intensive care unit; ED = emergency department; PEA = pulseless electrical activity; NR = not reported; NS, not significant.
[3] Alternating days.
[4] Including hematoma.
[5] Based on operator availability.

Table 12.3. Studies of dynamic ultrasound use in pediatric populations

First author/Year	Study type	Patient population	n	Total success	Mean attempts	Complications[6]
Verghese 2000[50]	RCT	Pts <10 kg for OHS	45	81% vs 94%	2 vs 1[7]	19% vs 6%
Leyvi 2004[51]	Retrospective	Peds pts for OHS	149	72.5% vs 91.5%	NR	4.9% vs 6.4%

Abbreviations: RCT = randomized controlled trial; LM = landmark; pts, patients; OHS = open heart surgery; NR = not reported; Peds = pediatrics.
[6]Major complications unless otherwise noted (arterial puncture, pneumothorax, hemothorax).
[7]Study-reported medians.

To date, three major meta-analyses have been published, each of which confirmed these findings. Randolph and colleagues[18] reviewed the eight randomized controlled trials available at the time, finding that ultrasound use significantly decreased the risk of failed catheter placement regardless of site of insertion (RR 0.32, 95% CI 0.18–0.55), reduced mechanical complications of placement (RR 0.22, 95% CI 0.10–0.45), and reduced the number of attempts required for successful cannulation (RR 0.60, 95% CI 0.45–0.79), although there was no significant change in the time to successful placement (95% CI 80.1–62.2 sec). Of note, the authors did not distinguish between studies using audio Doppler, static ultrasound, and dynamic ultrasound. However, as noted earlier, subsequent data suggest that restriction to dynamic ultrasound would only be expected to increase the magnitude of the observed benefit. Additionally, the analysis included studies with varied definitions of failure, potentially clouding their conclusions.

Keenan[19] evaluated eighteen randomized controlled trials, including a total of 2092 patients. The analysis differentiated dynamic ultrasound from Doppler and included studies comparing both to landmark techniques. Once again, this meta-analysis confirmed that dynamic ultrasound use reduced the risk of failure (RR 0.40), number of attempts (absolute risk reduction 1.41), and arterial punctures (RR 0.299) when compared with landmark techniques. The study also concluded that dynamic ultrasound was superior to Doppler in all major parameters studied. Again, the studies included had variable definitions of what constituted failed placement, potentially confounding their analysis.

Most recently, in a study commissioned by the British National Institute for Clinical Excellence (NICE), Hind and associates[20] reviewed the 18 randomized controlled trials of dynamic ultrasound available in 2003, including a total of 1646 patients. This meta-analysis differentiated among technique (dynamic ultrasound vs Doppler), patient population (adult

Table 12.4. Traditionally high-risk patient populations in which dynamic ultrasound use has been demonstrated to be safe and effective

Significant coagulopathy[52]
Hematology/oncology patients[53]
Anatomic contraindications to LM insertion (venous stenosis, extremely low CVP, etc.)[54]
History of difficult or failed cannulation[55]
Geriatric patients[49]
Pulseless patients undergoing CPR[47]
Unable to tolerate Trendelenburg positioning[56]

vs pediatric), and insertion site (IJ, subclavian, or femoral). As expected, this study confirmed that dynamic ultrasound use reduces failure rates of IJ cannulation in pediatric patients (RR 0.15, 95% CI 0.03–0.64) and adult patients (RR 0.14, 95% CI 0.06–0.33), and reiterated the limited data that support dynamic ultrasound over landmark in subclavian and femoral cannulation.

In addition to being superior for patient-related outcomes, dynamic ultrasound may be cost-effective from an economic standpoint. However, limited studies exist to support this claim. Calvert and coworkers[21] analyzed data from 20 randomized controlled trials and confirmed the superiority of dynamic ultrasound over landmark techniques. They went on to calculate the cost-effectiveness of dynamic ultrasound use, including initial equipment costs, training costs, and maintenance costs in their analysis as compared with the cost of complications and delayed cannulation. Based on conservative estimates, the authors calculate that for every 1000 CVC placements, dynamic ultrasound use would save approximately £2000 (about $4000 in 2008).

Future directions

Significant data support the superiority of dynamic ultrasound in terms of patient outcomes, and some data suggest cost-effectiveness. However, there is limited evidence of the level of training or operator experience required to achieve optimal outcomes using ultrasound guidance. The majority of studies cited previously included a one- to six-hour training period on ultrasound use prior to randomization to the ultrasound wing of the study. In comparison with historical data on landmark CVC placement, which suggested that up to 50 procedures were necessary to obtain optimal results, some authors have suggested that because of the rapid learning curve observed anecdotally for ultrasound-guided CVC placement, four hours of training in general ultrasound and its application to CVC placement, and only five to ten proctored examinations, are sufficient for competence.[22] However, this assertion has yet to be validated. Several models, including cadaveric models[23] and inexpensive homemade systems using materials such as gelatin and latex tubing,[24,25] are described in the literature to facilitate training in ultrasound techniques. Use of these models increases ultrasound use by participants, presumably because of increased familiarity of the technique, but quality outcome data are lacking.

Despite the data supporting its use, several surveys conducted as recently as 2007 have demonstrated that implementation of dynamic ultrasound for CVC placement remains limited, with between 11 percent and 20 percent of respondents using ultrasound most of the time.[26-29] The most significant barriers to implementation were the availability of adequate ultrasound equipment and perceived usefulness of dynamic ultrasound among respondents. However, three of the four published surveys were conducted in Britain, and may not reflect current trends in the United States. Further studies aimed at identifying and overcoming specific barriers to ultrasound use are needed to facilitate its widespread implementation.

Additionally, and of note, to our knowledge no study at this time has demonstrated that ultrasound use significantly alters rates of CVC infection or catheter sepsis, nor has it been demonstrated to reduce ICU length of stay or overall patient morbidity or mortality parameters. If these analyses are conducted and prove to be favorable, they may encourage use of ultrasound and decrease barriers to its implementation.

Several recent studies have expanded the traditional role of dynamic ultrasound as a guide for initial puncture of the target vein. These studies suggest that, as practitioners become more comfortable with ultrasound use, dynamic ultrasound may be used effectively to confirm correct guidewire placement within the vein during the cannulation procedure[30,31] and to rapidly detect the presence of a pneumothorax after the procedure before portable chest X-ray is possible.[32] However, additional studies confirming the reproducibility and reliability of these techniques are needed before use becomes widespread.

Credentialing

In preparation of this chapter, an informal survey of several anesthesiology departments revealed that not a single one required separate credentialing for use of ultrasound to assist in CVC insertion. However, the American Medical Association states that ultrasound imaging privileging should be specifically delineated by department based on background and training, although this recommendation may have been written without the specific consideration of the very narrow scope of ultrasound for vascular access. Various professional societies have mandated incorporation of ultrasound training in their residency programs, most notably the American College of Emergency Physicians and the American College of Surgeons, but again, the narrow scope of ultrasound solely for vascular access is not the main intent of this mandated training.

Given that ultrasound does require skill acquisition and that incorrect use (e.g. failure to distinguish right from left, recognize intravascular thrombus) can be associated with an increase in morbidity, we recommend that basic documented training and credentialing should become standard. Given that training and credentialing of central line insertion are already ubiquitous, perhaps simply adding ultrasound use for this procedure in the training and credentialing process makes the most sense. This will be more important if the technique is adopted widely as the standard of care, or even if there is only agreement that, at least, it should always be available.

Practice parameters

Compelling data from numerous randomized controlled trials and multiple meta-analyses support the superiority of dynamic ultrasound use for CVC placement when compared with landmark techniques. Both intuitively and from the literature, there are a variety of situations in which landmark techniques place the patient at particularly high risk for failure and mechanical complication. In these high-risk scenarios, we feel strongly that ultrasound guidance should be considered the standard of care. One such situation is a known or anticipated lack of traditional landmarks such as in morbid obesity, prior neck surgery or radiation, or cannulation of sites such as the deep brachial vein, which lack definite anatomic landmarks. Other scenarios in which we feel strongly that dynamic ultrasound guidance represents standard of care are (1) patients who have had multiple prior access procedures (e.g. hematology/oncology patients), because the vein might be thrombosed or stenosed; (2) patients who should be put at the lowest risk of a carotid puncture (e.g. prior vascular intervention or known large plaque); and (3) patients who are at higher than usual risk of complication from vascular mishap (e.g. anticoagulated or thrombocytopenic patients).

Based on the data discussed earlier, governmental organizations have recognized the potential benefit of ultrasound guidance. In 2002, NICE recommended that this be made the standard of care, stating, "Two-dimensional (2-D) imaging ultrasound guidance is recommended as the preferred method for insertion of central venous catheters (CVCs) into the internal jugular vein (IJV) in adults and children in elective situations. The use of two-dimensional (2-D) imaging ultrasound guidance should be considered in most clinical circumstances where CVC insertion is necessary either electively or in an emergency situation."[33] This recommendation was reviewed, updated, and confirmed in 2005. In the United States, the Agency for Healthcare Research and Quality (AHRQ) recommended in 2001 that ultrasound guidance be one of eleven procedures that "were rated most highly in terms of strength of the evidence supporting more widespread implementation."[34]

Despite the existing evidence and governmental recommendations, it remains controversial whether use of ultrasound guidance should be considered standard of care in all situations, and, as discussed earlier, multiple barriers exist to its widespread adoption. Many anesthesiologists and hospitals do not have ultrasound devices at their disposal, are not adequately trained or do not routinely employ these devices, and/or have not recognized similar improvements in procedural outcome as demonstrated in the published literature. Benefits of ultrasound guidance may not be realized until operators who are comfortable with traditional techniques gain experience and comfort with ultrasound guidance. Furthermore, the meta-analyses that have been published to date are limited by the data available at the time of analysis, and because of the rapid evolution of ultrasound availability and use, may no longer be applicable.

At the time of writing, there is an active Cochrane review that will attempt to determine more definitively the efficacy and generalizability of ultrasound guidance for central venous cannulation. We expect this study to confirm what has been previously demonstrated in randomized controlled trials and meta-analyses, which will facilitate a more widespread adoption of ultrasound use in central line placement.[35]

References

1. Troianos CA, Kuwik R, Pasqual P, et al. Internal jugular vein and carotid artery anatomic relation as determined by ultrasound. *Anesthesiology* 1996;85:43–48.

2. Maecken T, Grau T. Ultrasound imaging in vascular access. *Crit Care Med* 2007;35:S178–85.

3. Eisen L, Narasimhan M, Berger J, et al. Mechanical complications of central venous catheters. *J Intensive Care Med* 2006;21:40–46.

4. Merrer J, De Jonghe B, Golliot F, et al. Complications of femoral and subclavian venous catheterization in critically ill patients: A randomized controlled trial. *JAMA* 2001;286:700–7.

5. Mansfield P, Hohn D, Fornage B, et al. Complications and failures of subclavian-vein catheterization. *N Engl J Med* 1994; 331:1735–8.

6. Sznajder J, Zveibil F, Bitterman H, et al. Central vein catheterization: failure and complication rates by three percutaneous approaches. *Arch Intern Med* 1986;146:259–61.

7. Johnson E, Saltzman D, Suh G, et al. Complications and risks of central venous catheter placement in children. *Surgery* 1998;124:911–6.

8. Casado-Flores J, Barja J, Martino R, et al. Complications of central venous catheterization in critically ill children. *Pediatr Crit Care Med* 2001;2:57–62.

9. Bernard RW, Stahl WM. Subclavian vein catheterizations: a prospective study. I. Noninfectious complications. *Ann Surg* 1971;173:184–90.

10. Bold RJ, Winchester DJ, Madary AR, Gregurich MA, Mansfield PF. Prospective, randomized trial of Doppler-assisted subclavian vein catheterization. *Arch Surg* 1998;133:1089–93.

11. Gilbert TB, Seneff MG, Becker RB. Facilitation of internal jugular venous cannulation using an audio-guided Doppler ultrasound vascular access device: results from a prospective, dual-center, randomized, crossover clinical study. *Crit Care Med* 1995;23:60–65.

12. Verghese ST, McGill WA, Patel RI, Sell JE, Midgley FM, Ruttimann UE. Comparison of three techniques for internal jugular vein cannulation in infants. *Paediatr Anaesth* 2000;10:505–11.

13. Arai T, Yamashita M. Central venous catheterization in infants and children – small-caliber audio-Doppler probe versus ultrasound scanner. *Paediatr Anaesth* 2005;15:858–61.

14. Chuan WX, Wei W, Yu L. A randomized-controlled study of ultrasound prelocation vs anatomical landmark-guided cannulation of the internal jugular vein in infants and children. *Paediatr Anaesth* 2005;15:733–8.

15. Milling TJ Jr, Rose J, Briggs WM, et al. Randomized, controlled clinical trial of point-of-care limited ultrasonography assistance of central venous cannulation: the Third Sonography Outcomes Assessment Program (SOAP-3) Trial. *Crit Care Med* 2005;33:1764–9.

16. Hosokawa K, Shime N, Kato Y, Hashimoto S. A randomized trial of ultrasound image-based skin surface marking versus real-time ultrasound-guided internal jugular vein catheterization in infants. *Anesthesiology* 2007;107:720–4.

17. Hayashi H, Amano M. Does ultrasound imaging before puncture facilitate internal jugular vein cannulation? Prospective randomized comparison with landmark-guided puncture in ventilated patients. *J Cardiothorac Vasc Anesth* 2002;16: 572–5.

18. Randolph AG, Cook DJ, Gonzales CA, Pribble CG. Ultrasound guidance for placement of central venous catheters: a meta-analysis of the literature. *Crit Care Med* 1996;24:2053–8.

19. Keenan SP. Use of ultrasound to place central lines. *J Crit Care* 2002;17:126–37.

20. Hind D, Calvert N, McWilliams R, et al. Ultrasonic locating devices for central venous cannulation: meta-analysis. *BMJ* 2003;16:327–61.

21. Calvert N, Hind D, McWilliams RG, Thomas SM, Beverley C, Davidson A. The effectiveness and cost-effectiveness of ultrasound locating devices for central venous access: a systematic review and economic evaluation. *Health Technol Assess* 2003;7:1–84.

22. Feller-Kopman D. Ultrasound-guided internal jugular access: a proposed standardized approach and implications for training and practice. *Chest* 2007;132:302–9.

23. Nip IL, Haruno MM. A systematic approach to teaching insertion of a central venous line. *Acad Med* 2000;75:552.

24. Di Domenico S, Santori G, Porcile E, Licausi M, Centanaro M, Valente U. Inexpensive homemade models for ultrasound-guided vein cannulation training. *J Clin Anesth* 2007;19:491–6.

25. Kendall JL, Faragher JP. Ultrasound-guided central venous access: a homemade phantom for simulation. *CJEM* 2007;9: 371–3.

26. Bailey PL, Glance LG, Eaton MP, Parshall B, McIntosh S. A survey of the use of ultrasound during central venous catheterization. *Anesth Analg* 2007;104:491–7.

27. Tovey G, Stokes M. A survey of the use of 2D ultrasound guidance for insertion of central venous catheters by UK consultant paediatric anaesthetists. *Eur J Anaesthesiol* 2007;24:71–5.

28. Girard TD, Schectman JM. Ultrasound guidance during central venous catheterization: a survey of use by house staff physicians. *J Crit Care* 2005;20:224–9.

29. Jefferson P, Ogbue MN, Hamilton KE, Ball DR. A survey of the use of portable ultrasound for central vein cannulation on critical care units in the UK. *Anaesthesia* 2002;57:365–8.

30. Stone MB. Identification and correction of guide wire malposition during internal jugular cannulation with ultrasound. *CJEM* 2007;9:131–2.

31. Howes B, Dell R. Ultrasound to detect incorrect guidewire positioning during subclavian line insertion. *Anaesthesia* 2006;61:615

32. Maury E, Guglielminotti J, Alzieu M, Guidet B, Offenstadt G. Ultrasonic examination: an alternative to chest radiography after central venous catheter insertion? *Am J Respir Crit Care Med* 2001;164:403–5.

33. National Institute for Clinical Excellence. *Guidance on the Use of Ultrasound Locating Devices for Placing Central Venous Catheters.* London: National Institute for Clinical Excellence, September 2002, reviewed August 2005. Available online at http://www.nice. org.uk/nicemedia/pdf/Ultrasound_49_GUIDANCE.pdf.

34. Rothschild, JM. Ultrasound guidance of central vein catheterization. In *Making Health Care Safer: A Critical Analysis of Patient Safety Practices*. Evidence Report/Technology Assessment, No. 43. AHRQ Publication No. 01-E058, July 2001. Rockville, MD: Agency for Healthcare Research and Quality, http://www.ahrq.gov/clinic/ptsafety.

35. Brass P, Hellmich M, Kolodziej, L, et al. Traditional landmark versus ultrasound guidance for central vein catheterization. Cochrane Database Syst Rev 1: CD0069262, 2008.

36. Gualtieri E, Deppe SA, Sipperly ME, Thompson DR. Subclavian venous catheterization: greater success rate for less experienced operators using ultrasound guidance. *Crit Care Med* 1995;23:692–7.

37. Karakitsos D, Labropoulos N, De Groot E, et al. Real-time ultrasound-guided catheterisation of the internal jugular vein: a prospective comparison with the landmark technique in critical care patients. *Crit Care* 2006;10:R162.

38. Leung J, Duffy M, Finckh A. Real-time ultrasonographically guided internal jugular vein catheterization in the emergency department increases success rates and reduces complications: a randomized, prospective study. *Ann Emerg Med* 2006;48: 540–7.

39. Mallory DL, McGee WT, Shawker TH, et al. Ultrasound guidance improves the success rate of internal jugular vein cannulation. A prospective, randomized trial. *Chest* 1990;98:157–60.

40. Milling T, Holden C, Melniker L, Briggs WM, Birkhahn R, Gaeta T. Randomized controlled trial of single-operator vs. two-operator ultrasound guidance for internal jugular central venous cannulation. *Acad Emerg Med* 2006;13: 245–7.

41. Troianos CA, Jobes DR, Ellison N. Ultrasound-guided cannulation of the internal jugular vein. A prospective, randomized study. *Anesth Analg* 1991;72:823–6.

42. Hilty WM, Hudson PA, Levitt MA, Hall JB. Real-time ultrasound-guided femoral vein catheterization during cardiopulmonary resuscitation. *Ann Emerg Med* 1997;29: 331–6.

43. Miller AH, Roth BA, Mills TJ, Woody JR, Longmoor CE, Foster B. Ultrasound guidance versus the landmark technique for the placement of central venous catheters in the emergency department. *Acad Emerg Med* 2002;9:800–5.

44. Cajozzo M, Quintini G, Cocchiera G, et al. Comparison of central venous catheterization with and without ultrasound guide. *Transfus Apher Sci* 2004;31:199–202.

45. Hrics P, Wilber S, Blanda MP, Gallo U. Ultrasound-assisted internal jugular vein catheterization in the ED. *Am J Emerg Med* 1998;16:401–3.

46. Wigmore TJ, Smythe JF, Hacking MB, Raobaikady R, MacCallum NS. Effect of the implementation of NICE guidelines for ultrasound guidance on the complication rates associated with central venous catheter placement in patients presenting for routine surgery in a tertiary referral centre. *Br J Anaesth* 2007;99(5):662–5.

47. Augoustides JG, Diaz D, Weiner J, Clarke C, Jobes DR. Current practice of internal jugular venous cannulation in a university anesthesia department: influence of operator experience on success of cannulation and arterial injury. *Cardiothorac Vasc Anesth* 2002;16:567–71.

48. Martin MJ, Husain FA, Piesman M, et al. Is routine ultrasound guidance for central line placement beneficial? A prospective analysis. *Curr Surg* 2004;61:71–4.

49. Cajozzo M, Cocchiara G, Greco G, et al. Ultrasound (US) guided central venous catheterization of internal jugular vein on over 65-year-old patients versus blind technique. *J Surg Oncol* 2004;88:267–8.

50. Verghese ST, McGill WA, Patel RI, Sell JE, Midgley FM, Ruttimann UE. Ultrasound-guided internal jugular venous cannulation in infants: a prospective comparison with the traditional palpation method. *Anesthesiology* 1999;91:71–7.

51. Leyvi G, Taylor DG, Reith E, Wasnick JD. Utility of ultrasound-guided central venous cannulation in pediatric surgical patients: a clinical series. *Paediatr Anaesth* 2005;15:953–8.

52. Tercan F, Ozkan U, Oguzkurt L. US-guided placement of central vein catheters in patients with disorders of hemostasis. *Eur J Radiol* 2008;65:253–6.

53. Mey U, Glasmacher A, Hahn C, et al. Evaluation of an ultrasound-guided technique for central venous access via the internal jugular vein in 493 patients. *Support Care Cancer* 2003;11:148–55.

54. Fry WR, Clagett GC, O'Rourke PT. Ultrasound-guided central venous access. *Arch Surg* 1999;134:738–40.

55. Hatfield A, Bodenham A. Portable ultrasound for difficult central venous access. *Br J Anaesth* 1999;82:822–6.

56. Schummer W, Schummer C, Tuppatsch H, Fuchs J, Bloos F, Hüttemann E. Ultrasound-guided central venous cannulation: is there a difference between Doppler and B-mode ultrasound? *J Clin Anesth* 2006;18:167–72.

Chapter 13

Ultrasound guidance for regional anesthesia procedures

Christina L. Jeng and Meg A. Rosenblatt

Introduction

Peripheral nerve blocks have traditionally been performed employing anatomic landmarks to locate sensory and motor nerves. Over the past two decades, nerve stimulation (NS) techniques have increased in popularity, using concentrated electrical impulses to depolarize, stimulate, and thus identify specific nerves. In recent years, the application of ultrasound (US) to visualize nerves and the spread of local anesthetic has revolutionized the practice of regional anesthesia.

US-guided regional anesthesia requires knowledge of the anatomy as well as basic ultrasound principles, which will allow practitioners to choose their equipment wisely. A number of linear and curved array US probes are available, and newer echogenic needles with distance markers continue to improve visualization. Portable US machines are available that will provide diagnostic-quality images for block performance.

Generally, linear array probes provide excellent near-field visualization. The higher-frequency ultrasound waves provide the best image resolution but are limited by depth penetration. Greater penetration requires lower-frequency ultrasound waves; however, these lower frequencies result in poorer image resolution. For superficial targets, including most peripheral nerves, the high-frequency linear array US probes are sufficient; they provide excellent near-field visualization with high resolution. US imaging for upper extremity blocks is straightforward, because the brachial plexus and peripheral nerves are superficial (within centimeters of the skin) even in patients with high body mass indexes (Figures 13.1, 13.2). For these blocks, a linear array 38-mm high-frequency (10–15 MHz) US probe is ideal, and a smaller probe (25 mm) should be considered for most upper extremity blocks secondary to the limited anatomic space. For deeper structures, such as the the infraclavicular region, a lower-frequency probe ($\leq$7 MHz) may be necessary to obtain better ultrasound penetration. Imaging of nerves in the lower extremities can be more challenging because the target structures are deeper within muscle and adipose tissue (Figure 13.3). For these blocks, a phased array lower-frequency (5–7 MHz) probe will provide greater penetration and is necessary to scan a wider anatomic area, thus facilitating imaging.[1] Therefore, the probes chosen should have the highest possible frequency and still allow adequate tissue penetration for imaging of the target nerve and surrounding structures.[2]

Needle visualization may be optimized by minimizing refraction and maximizing reflection. This is accomplished by maintaining the needle perpendicular to the US beam. There are two options available for needle visualization: in-plane and out-of-plane techniques. With the in-plane technique, the needle is advanced in-line and parallel to the transducer. Both the needle and the shaft of the needle may be visualized within the entire US sector. In the out-of-plane technique, the needle is placed perpendicular to the transducer. The needle is visualized as a single point in the US image. For deeper targets, the out-of-plane technique is preferable. For more superficial nerve targets, the in-plane technique is preferred because the entire needle may be visualized as it approaches its target.[2]

Needle choice for optimal US image is controversial. Echogenic, insulated, B-bevel needles are most commonly used for peripheral nerve blocks. Klein and colleagues describe the use of a piezoelectric vibrating needle and catheter for enhancing the US image and confirming the location of the needle or catheter tip.[3] Using a synthetic phantom, Deam and associates improved visibility under ultrasound with echogenic "textured" needles.[4] After investigating 12 needles, Maecken and coworkers concluded that there is yet no ideal choice and that the improvement of needles for use under US guidance is necessary.[5]

Evidence of utility

Ultrasound has allowed practitioners to determine the sensitivity of traditional localization techniques. Perlas and associates studied 103 patients who were undergoing forearm or hand surgery.[6] During the performance of an US-guided axillary

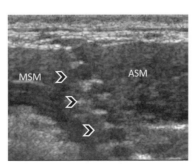

Figure 13.1. Anatomy of the interscalene groove. ASM: anterior scalenus muscle, MSM: middle scalenus muscle; arrows: nerves within interscalene groove.

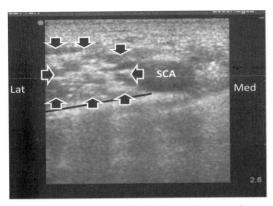

Figure 13.2. Anatomy requisite for the performance of a supraclavicular block. SCA: subclavian artery. Arrows identify the nerves of the brachial plexus at the level of the divisions, lateral to the artery.

block, a 22-gauge insulated needle was placed in direct contact with one of the nerve branches. A paresthesia perceived by the patients and then a motor response to nerve stimulation at 0.5 mA were sought. Paresthesia was 38 percent sensitive and motor response 74.5 percent sensitive for needle nerve contact. To elicit a paresthesia, the needle must be in contact with a sensory nerve, just as a motor response requires contact with a motor nerve. Urmey and colleagues and Bollini and coworkers were unable to correlate the elicitation of a sensory paresthesia to the ability to elicit a motor response with peripheral nerve stimulation in immobile needles while performing interscalene blocks.[7,8] Neither paresthesia nor NS are reliable techniques for the performance of neuronal blockade.

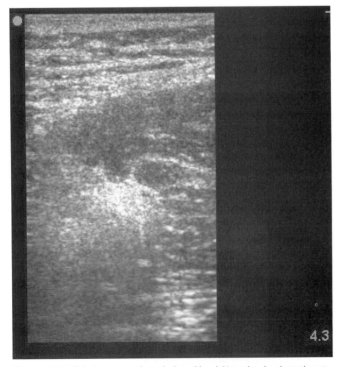

Figure 13.3. Sciatic nerve at the subgluteal level. Note the depth marker at 4.3 cm.

For both upper and lower extremity blocks, US decreases the time to successful placement, improves quality, and increases the duration of blocks. Comparing 56 patients who were undergoing elective hand surgery under either transarterial axillary (TA) or US-guided perivascular block, Sites and colleagues found that whereas eight of the patients (28%) in the TA group required conversion to general anesthesia, none in the US group did.[9] The time needed to perform the block using the US technique was also significantly shorter (7.9 $\pm$ 3.9 min vs 11.1 $\pm$ 5.7 min, $P = 0.05$).

Not only did Williams and associates demonstrate a significant decrease in the execution time to perform supraclavicular blocks when US is added to a NS technique (5.0 min vs 9.8 min, $P = 0.0001$), but they also found that the quality of the block, particularly of the ulnar nerve distribution, was significantly improved with the use of US.[10] When comparing an US group with a NS group for interscalene block, Kapral and associates demonstrated that surgical anesthesia (sensory, motor, and extent of blockade) was significantly better in the US group (99% vs 91%, $P < 0.01$).[11] For lower-extremity blocks, Marhofer and colleagues showed that US guidance improved the quality of sensory block and the onset time of three-in-one blocks in patients undergoing hip surgery after trauma.[12] Perlas and coworkers found a statistically significantly higher block success rate when US was used to place sciatic nerve blocks in the popliteal fossa than when NS was employed (89.2% vs 60.6%, $P = 0.005$).[13]

The addition of NS does not appear to increase the effectiveness of US techniques. One hundred eighty patients undergoing elective hand surgery were randomized to receive an axillary block performed one of three ways, using (1) three motor response endpoints elicited with NS, (2) real-time in-plane US visualization of the injection of local anesthetic around the three nerves, or (3) nerve stimulation to confirm the US localization of the nerves and readjusting the needles to ensure that stimulation was achieved at 0.5 mA prior to injecting. Block success was higher in the US and US–NS groups (82.9% and 80.7%) than in the NS-alone group (62.9%), but the difference between the US and US–NS groups was not statistically significant.[14] The role of nerve stimulation as an adjunct may be limited. Evaluation of 94 consecutive patients for surgery below the elbow under supraclavicular block demonstrated that for adequately US-imaged blocks, confirmation with motor response at less than 0.5 mA did not increase the success rate of the block.[15]

The use of US may allow successful peripheral nerve block placement in patients in whom traditional methods of nerve localization are limited. Van Geffen and colleagues described several cases of successful neuronal block placement in patients with extensive previous surgery in the region of the planned blocks or demylinating polyneuropathy.[16] Blocks were performed for surgical anesthesia and/or postoperative analgesia only with the use of US guidance. In addition, US-guided blocks for surgical anesthesia have been made possible for patients with abnormal coagulation. Khelemsky and associates reported a supraclavicular block in a patient anticoagulated with the direct thrombin inhibitor argatroban, and Bigeleisen described an infraclavicular brachial plexus block in a patient on a heparin infusion.[17,18]

In an editorial in the journal *Anesthesiology*, Hebl discussed the possibility that US-guided regional anesthesia might prevent neurologic injury.[19] He speculated that although there will be no effect on surgical risk factors (intraoperative trauma or stretch, vascular compromise, hematoma formation, tourniquet ischemia, or improperly applied immobilizers or casts) or on patient risk factors (male sex, increasing age, preexisting neurologic deficit), the use of US may be able to decrease the anesthesia risk factors of mechanical trauma and local anesthesia toxicity. In fact, the use of US guidance has been shown to provide a 42 percent reduction ($P = 0.002$) in the volume of ropivacaine required to block the femoral nerve compared with the use of NS to perform the same block.[20] Two recent case reports of accidental intravascular injection of local anesthetic resulting in seizures after properly performed US guided blocks, though, have highlighted the need to continually employ safe techniques, including slow injection of small aliquots with aspiration between them, even when blocks are performed under US visualization.[21,22]

The use of ultrasound has enabled regionalists to diagnose nonneural pathology. Sites and colleagues reported three cases in which vascular lesions – clots in the femoral vein, femoral artery, and carotid artery – were diagnosed on scanning to perform anesthetic blocks, and ultimately resulted in therapeutic and anesthetic management changes.[23]

Complications

There are multiple reports of upper-extremity musculoskeletal and back disorders as occupational hazards among ultrasonographers. In a pilot survey of 340 diagnostic medical sonographers, one-third of the responders reported at least one work-related symptom in the upper extremity – most frequently, paresthesia and numbness or finger pain. Carpal tunnel syndrome was diagnosed in 1.5 percent of cases, and more than 60 percent of sonographers experienced neck and low back pain.[24] Schoenfeld and colleagues described "transducer user syndrome" among sonographers in obstetrics and gynecology, which included carpal tunnel syndrome, carpal instability, tendonitis, weakness, motion restriction, and back, shoulder, or neck pain.[25] These same symptoms have also been reported among cardiac sonographers.[26] It is possible that these types of complications could be expected for regionalists using US in busy practices.

US causes tissue injury by thermal and nonthermal mechanisms. Because normal variations in core temperature of several degrees Celsius occur naturally, the temperature increase secondary to US exposure for short periods of time has no significant biological effects.[27] Unlike other imaging modalities, diagnostic US induces mechanical strain on tissues, especially those containing dissolved gas. However, any damage heals quickly and completely with no clinically significant effect. In tissues not containing gas, there is no evidence of adverse effect. Acceleration of bone healing and auditory or tactile sensation may also occur. None of these effects poses a risk to the health of the patient.[28]

Credentialing

Learning US-guided regional anesthesia is challenging. It requires an intimate knowledge of anatomy as well as the ability to interpret ultrasound images. The operator must be able to use each hand independently while continuously looking at the screen. Sites and associates studied the learning curve associated with a simulated US-guided interventional task by inexperienced anesthesia residents.[29] Using US guidance, the residents were asked to place a 22-gauge B-bevel needle into an olive buried inside a turkey breast. Upon successive trials, the time for each subject to perform the task was reduced and accuracy improved. However, this trial also identified a "concerning novice pattern" in which subjects advanced the needle without adequate visualization, resulting in excessive depth of penetration of the needle. The researchers then studied six anesthesia residents on a dedicated one-month US-regional anesthesia rotation as the residents performed a total of 520 nerve blocks.[30] Again, speed and accuracy improved throughout the rotation, but five "quality-compromising patterns of behavior" were identified: (1) failure to recognize maldistribution of local anesthesia, (2) failure to recognize inappropriate needle tip location, (3) operator fatigue, (4) incorrectly correlating sidedness of patient with sidedness of US image, and (5) poor choice of needle-insertion site and angle, resulting in difficult or absent needle visualization. Although errors continued to occur, they seemed to reach a consistent nadir after approximately 71 to 80 blocks were performed.

Is credentialing necessary to use US for procedures that have been for years performed blindly? Is not any visualization likely to be an improvement or be potentially safer than traditional techniques? In response to the World Health Organization's recommendations, in its report on training in diagnostic US, that professional associations should be actively involved in developing training programs,[31] the American Society of Regional Anesthesia (ASRA) has taken a leadership role in providing lectures and workshops at its annual meetings. Currently the ASRA, in association with the European Society of Regional Anesthesia (ESRA), has recommended guidelines for education and training in US-guided regional anesthesia. The ASRA and ESRA have defined a list of 10 common skills that should be acquired during US training. They appear in Table 13.1.

Proficiency in US-guided regional anesthesia can be divided into four major categories, each with a defined skill set. The first skill set involves understanding US image generation and operation – basic principles of image generation, selection of appropriate transducer, depth and focus settings, use of time gain compensation and overall gain, use and application of color Doppler, and orientation of screen to patient. Image

Table 13.1. ASRA–ESRA recommended skills

1. Ability to visualize key landmark structures (i.e. blood vessels, muscles, fascia, and bone)
2. Identification of nerves/plexus on short axis imaging
3. Confirmation of normal anatomy and recognizing anatomic variations
4. Plans for needle approach avoiding unnecessary tissue trauma
5. Maintenance of aseptic technique
6. Ability to follow needle to target in real time
7. Consideration of confirmation of proper needle placement (e.g. nerve stimulation)
8. Test injection of local anesthetic and visualization
9. Proper needle adjustment to visualize appropriate local anesthetic spread through entirety of injection
10. Maintenance of traditional safety guidelines (i.e. immediate availability of resuscitation equipment, standard monitoring, frequent aspiration for blood to avoid intravascular injection, and acknowledgment of patient response)

Source: Sites BD, Chan VW, Neal JM, et al. The American Society of Regional Anesthesia and Pain Medicine and the European Society of Regional Anaesthesia and Pain Therapy Joint Committee Recommendations for Education and Training in Ultrasound-Guided Regional Anesthesia. *Reg Anesth Pain Med* 2009;34:40–6.

optimization (not related to the US device) and image interpretation constitute the second and third skill sets. Image optimization includes learning to apply appropriate transducer pressure, alignment, rotation, and tilting. Image interpretation incorporates the ability to identify nerves, muscles and fascia, blood vessels (distinguishing artery from vein), bone, and pleura, as well as common acoustic and anatomic artifacts. The final set of skills important in determining proficiency consists of proper needle insertion and injection of local anesthetic. In-plane and out-of-plane techniques should be mastered, and the benefits and limitations of each technique should be recognized. Familiarity with correct local anesthetic spread, minimization of unintentional transducer movement, proper ergonomics, and ability to identify intraneural needle location are all skills within this category.[32] There are still no specific recommendations for credentialing of individual practitioners to perform US-guided regional anesthesia; however, each institution should have its own individualized credentialing process.

Conclusions

The application of US to the practice of regional anesthesia has not only advanced our knowledge but has also decreased the time to perform blocks, increased their success, allowed the provision of blocks for those who may not otherwise be candidates, and may ultimately prove to improve safety. Hopkins hopes that the use of US will not be "paralyzed by an inability to satisfy the lust for the highest levels of evidence-based medicine," because this technology is such a significant "step-change" in the way regional anesthesia is practiced.[33] With appropriate training and experience, US-guided regional anesthesia has proved itself a safe and effective technology.

References

1. Marhofer P, Chan VW. Ultrasound-guided regional anesthesia: current concepts and future trends. *Anesth Analg* 2007;**104**:1265–9.
2. Sites BD, Brull R, Chan VW, et al. Artifacts and pitfall errors associated with ultrasound-guided regional anesthesia. Part I: understanding the basic principles of ultrasound physics and machine operations. *Reg Anesth Pain Med* 2007;**32**:412–8.
3. Klein SM, Fronheiser MP, Reach J, Nielsen KC, Smith SW. Piezoelectric vibrating needle and catheter for enhancing ultrasound-guided peripheral nerve blocks. *Anesth Analg* 2007;**105**:1858–60.
4. Deam RK, Kluger R, Barrington MJ, McCutcheon CA. Investigation of a new echogenic needle for use with ultrasound peripheral nerve blocks. *Anaesth Intensive Care* 2007;**35**:582–6.
5. Maecken T, Zenz M, Grau T. Ultrasound characteristics of needles for regional anesthesia. *Reg Anesth Pain Med* 2007;**32**:440–7.
6. Perlas A, Niazi A, McCartney C, et al. The sensitivity of motor response to nerve stimulation and paresthesia for nerve localization as evaluated by ultrasound. *Reg Anesth Pain Med* 2006;**31**:445–50.
7. Urmey WF, Stanton S. Inability to consistently elicit a motor response following sensory paresthesia during interscalene block administration. *Anesthesiology* 2002;**96**:552–4.
8. Bollini CA, Urmey WF, Vascello L, Cacheiro F. Relationship between evoked motor response and sensory paresthesia in interscalene brachial plexus block. *Reg Anesth Pain Med* 2003;**28**(5):384–8.
9. Sites BD, Beach ML, Spence BC, Wiley CW, Hartman GS Gallagher JD. Ultrasound guidance improves the success rate of perivascular axillary plexus block. *Acta Anaesthesiol Scand* 2006;**50**:687–84.
10. Williams SR, Chouinard P, Arcand G, et al. Ultrasound guidance speeds execution and improves the quality of supraclavicular block. *Anesth Analg* 3003;**97**:1518–23.
11. Kapral S, Greher M, Huber G, et al. Ultrasonographic guidance improves the success rate of interscalene brachial plexus blockade. *Reg Anesth Pain Med* 2008;**33**(3):253–8.
12. Marhofer P, Schrogendorfer K, Konig H, et al. Ultrasonographic guidance improves sensory block and onset time of three-in-one blocks. *Anest Analg* 1997;**85**:854–7.
13. Perlas A, Brull R, Chan VWS, et al. Ultrasound guidance improves the success of sciatic nerve block at the popliteal fossa. *Reg Anesth Pain Med* 2008;**33**:259–65.
14. Chan VWS, Perlas A, McCartney CJL, Brull R, Xu D. Ultrasound guidance improves success rate of axillary brachial plexus block. *Can J Anesth* 2007;**54**:176–82.
15. Beach ML, Sites BD, Gallagher JD. Use of a nerve stimulator does not improve the efficacy of ultrasound-guided supraclavicular nerve blocks. *J Clin Anesth* 2006;**18**:580–4.
16. Van Geffen GJ, McCartney CJL, Gielen M, Chan VWS. Ultrasound as the only nerve localization technique for peripheral nerve block. *J Clin Anesth* 2007;**19**:381–5.
17. Khelemsky Y, Rosenblatt MA. Ultrasound-guided supraclavicular block in a patient anticoagulated with argatroban. *Pain Pract* 2008;**8**(2):152.
18. Bigeleisen PE. Ultrasound-guided infraclavicular block in an anticoagulated and anesthetized patient. *Anesth Analg* 2007;**104**(5):1285–7.

19. Hebl JR. Ultrasound-guided regional anesthesia and the prevention of neurologic injury: fact or fiction? *Anesthesiology* 2008;**108**:186–88.

20. Casati A, Baciarello M, Di Cianni S, et al. Effects of ultrasound guidance on the minimum effective anaesthetic volume required to block the femoral nerve. *Br J Anaesth* 2007;**98**:823–7.

21. Loubert C, Williams SR, Helie F, Acand G. Complication during ultrasound-guided regional block: accidental intravascular injection of local anesthetic. *Anesthesiology* 2008;**108**:759–60.

22. Zetlaoui PJ, Labbe J, Benhamou D. Ultrasound guidance for axillary plexus block does not prevent intravascular injection. *Anesthesiology* 2008;**108**:761.

23. Sites BD, Spence BC, Gallagher JD, Beach ML. On the edge of the ultrasound screen: regional anesthesiologists diagnosing nonneural pathology. *Reg Anesth Pain Med* 2006;**31**:555–62.

24. Mirk P, Magnavita N, Masini L, Bazzocchi M, Fileni A. Frequency of musculoskeletal symptoms in diagnostic medical sonographers. Results of a pilot survey. *Radiol Med (Torino)* 1999;**98**:236–41.

25. Schoenfeld A, Goverman J, Weiss DM, Meizner I. Transducer user syndrome: an occupational hazard of the ultrasonographer. *Eur J Ultrasound* 1999;**10**:41–5.

26. Vanderpool HE, Friis EA, Smith BS, Harms KL. Prevalence of carpal tunnel syndrome and other work-related musculoskeletal problems in cardiac sonographers. *J Occup Med* 1993;**35**:604–10.

27. O'Brien WD, Deng CX, Harris GR, et al. The risk of exposure to diagnostic ultrasound in postnatal subjects – thermal effects. *J Ultrasound Med* 2008;**27**:517–35.

28. Church CC, Carstensen EL, Nyborg WL, Carson PL, Frizzell LA, Bailey MR. The risk of exposure to diagnostic ultrasound in postnatal subjects – nonthermal mechanisms. *J Ultrasound Med* 2008;**27**:565–92.

29. Sites BD, Gallagher JD, Cravero J, Lundberg J, Blike G. The learning curve associated with a simulated ultrasound-guided interventional task by inexperienced anesthesia residents. *Reg Anesth Pain Med* 2004;**29**:544–8.

30. Sites BD, Spence BC, Gallagher JD, et al. Characteristic novice behavior associated with learning ultrasound-guided peripheral regional anesthesia. *Reg Anesth Pain Med* 2007;**32**:107–15.

31. World Health Organization. Training in diagnostic ultrasound: essentials, principles and standards. WHO Technical Report Series, No. 875, Geneva: World Health Organization, 1998.

32. Sites BD, Chan VW, Neal JM, et al. The American Society of Regional Anesthesia and Pain Medicine and the European Society of Regional Anaesthesia and Pain Therapy Joint Committee Recommendations for Education and Training in Ultrasound-Guided Regional Anesthesia. *Reg Anesth Pain Med* 2009;**34**(1):40–6.

33. Hopkins PM. Ultrasound guidance as a gold standard in regional anesthesia. *Br J Anaesth* 2007;**98**:299–301.

Chapter

14

Respiratory gas monitoring

James B. Eisenkraft

Introduction

Gases of interest to the anesthesia caregiver include oxygen, carbon dioxide, nitrous oxide, and the potent inhaled anesthetic agents. Other gases that may be relevant in certain situations are nitrogen, helium, and nitric oxide. Although gas monitors from different manufacturers may appear to offer various options to the user, ultimately, these monitors use one or more of a limited number of technologies to make the analysis and present the data.

The monitoring of respired gases has evolved considerably over the past few years. Contemporary systems are reliable and accurate, have rapid response times, and are becoming less expensive as a result of competition among manufacturers. The early gas monitoring systems were large stand-alone units that were usually placed on a shelf on the anesthesia machine (Figure 14.1). Modern technology has facilitated the miniaturization of these monitors so that on some contemporary anesthesia workstations, the analysis is performed in one component module of a modular physiologic monitoring system

(Figure 14.2). This aim of this chapter is to provide a framework for the understanding of the methods whereby respiratory gases are analyzed, as well as clinical applications, limitations, and pertinent standards of care.

Gas sampling systems

For a respired gas mixture to be analyzed, either the gas must be brought to the analyzer or the analyzer must be brought to the gas in the airway. A fuel cell oxygen analyzer located in the breathing system by the inspiratory unidirectional valve is one example of bringing the analyzer to the gas in the circuit. Figure 14.3 shows two different mainstream analyzer modules. Gas is not removed from the circuit for analysis elsewhere, so this is termed a *nondiverting* or *mainstream* analyzer. Alternatively, the gas to be analyzed can be sampled continuously from the vicinity of the patient's airway and conducted via fine-bore tubing (Figure 14.4) to the analyzer unit. Such a design is termed a *diverting*, or *sidestream sampling*, system because the gas is diverted from the airway for analysis elsewhere.

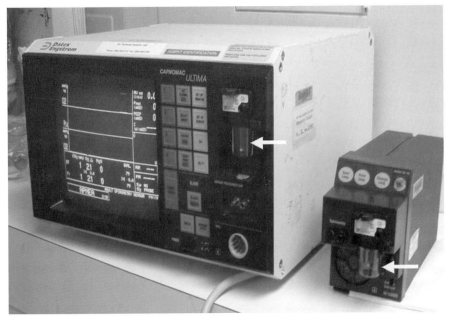

Figure 14.1. Left: Datex Capnomac Ultima stand-alone multigas analyzer (circa 1991) that uses infrared analysis for CO_2, N_2O, and anesthetic agents, and paramagnetic analysis for O_2. Right: the much smaller GE Compact Airway module (circa 2001), which uses the same technologies to perform the same functions. White arrows indicate water traps.

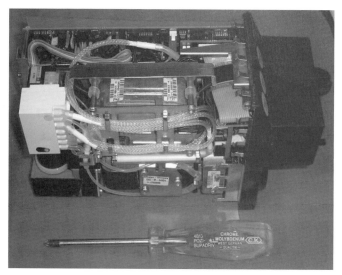

Figure 14.2. GE Compact Airway Module shown in Figure 14.1, opened to show miniaturization of gas monitoring technology.

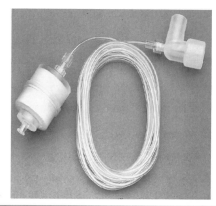

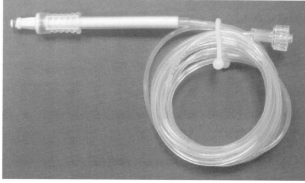

Figure 14.4. (A) Gas sampling tubing and airway adapter for sidestream sampling gas analyzer. (B) Nomoline™ gas sampling line that incorporates a water and water vapor removal system (Phasein AB Medical Technologies, Danderyd, Sweden).

Sidestream (diverting) systems

Compared with mainstream analyzers, the advantages of the diverting types of analyzers are that because they are remote from the patient, they can be of any size and therefore offer more versatility in terms of monitoring capabilities. The sampled gas is continuously drawn from the breathing circuit via an adapter placed between the circuit and the patient's airway (the Y-piece in a circle breathing system) and passes through a water trap (see arrows in Figure 14.1) before entering the analyzer. The gas sampling flow rate is usually about 200 mL/min, with a range of 50 to 250 mL/min. Disadvantages include problems with the catheter sampling system, such as clogging with secretions or water, kinking, failure of the sampling pump, slower response time (although usually <3 sec), and artifacts when the gas sampling rate is poorly matched with the patient's inspiratory and expiratory gas flow rates. Thus, if a diverting system is used with a very small patient (e.g. a neonate) and the gas sampling rate exceeds the patient's expiratory gas flow rate, spurious readings may result. Similarly, if an uncuffed tracheal tube is used and

there is a leak between the tube and the trachea, the gas sampling pump may draw room air into the tracheal tube and into the analyzer.

Ideally, the gas sampling flow rate should be appropriate for the patient and for the breathing circuit used. Thus the sampling flow rate may limit the ability to use low-flow or closed-circuit anesthesia techniques. If the gas sampling rate exceeds the fresh gas inflow rate, negative pressures potentially can be created in the breathing system.[1] Once the sampled gas has been analyzed, it should be directed to the waste gas scavenging system or returned to the patient's breathing system.

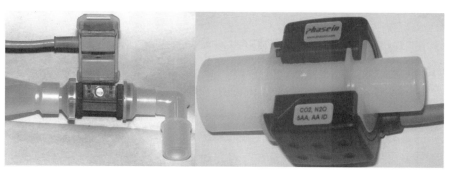

Figure 14.3 (A) Mainstream infrared CO_2 analyzer (Hewlett-Packard). (B) Mainstream lightweight infrared multi-agent (CO_2, N_2O, anesthetic agent) analyzer (Phasein AB Medical Technologies, Danderyd, Sweden).

In multigas analyzers that incorporate paramagnetic oxygen sensors, simultaneous room air sampling (10 mL/min) is required to provide a reference. This air is therefore added (at a rate of 10 mL/min) to the waste gas exiting the monitor and then may be returned to the patient circuit. This might create a problem during closed-circuit anesthesia, because nitrogen (albeit at a rate of about 8 mL/min) would be added to the breathing circuit (see the section on paramagnetic oxygen analyzer).

Mainstream (nondiverting) systems

Until recently, all multigas analyzers were of the diverting or sidestream sampling type. The alternative to a diverting system is a mainstream, or nondiverting, system. Other than for monitoring oxygen by fuel cell, mainstream analysis has, until recently, been available only for carbon dioxide, using infrared technology (Figure 14.3A). By miniaturizing components, mainstream multigas analysis is now available, and a mainstream infrared CO_2, N_2O, and anesthetic agent analyzer is being marketed (Figure 14.3B). Although mainstream analyzers overcome the gas sampling problem, they require a special airway adapter and analysis module to be placed in the breathing system by the patient's airway. From this location, the mainstream carbon dioxide analyzers produce a sharp capnogram in real time but are vulnerable to damage and add dead space. New designs are light in weight (one ounce), have small dead space, and use solid-state technology (Figure 14.3B). Waste gas scavenging is not required with mainstream gas analysis.

Carbon dioxide mainstream analyzer modules placed in the airway are subject to interference by water vapor, secretions, and blood. Because condensed water blocks all infrared wavelengths, leaving too little infrared source intensity to make a measurement, the cuvette's window is heated (usually to 41°C) to prevent such condensation and interference.

Gas analysis systems

The respiratory tract and the anesthesia delivery system contain respired gases in the form of molecules. These molecules are in constant motion. When the molecules strike the boundaries of their container, they give rise to pressure (defined as force per unit area); the greater the number of gas molecules present, the greater is the pressure exerted for a given temperature. Dalton's law of partial pressures states that the total pressure exerted by a mixture of gases is equal to the arithmetic sum of the partial pressures exerted by each gas in the mixture. The total pressure of all gases in the anesthesia system at sea level is equivalent to approximately 760 mmHg (per unit of area). Although anesthetic gas monitors may display data expressed in millimeters of mercury (mmHg) or as volumes percent (vols%), it is important to understand how the measurement was made in principle. The reader should understand the difference between partial pressure (mmHg), which is an absolute term, and volumes percent, which is an expression of a proportion, or ratio.

If the partial pressure of one component of a gas mixture is known, a reading in volumes percent can be computed as follows:

$$Volumes\ \% = \frac{Partial\ pressure\ of\ the\ component\ gas\ (mmHg)}{Total\ pressure\ of\ all\ gases\ (mmHg)} \times 100$$

Number of molecules (partial pressure)

An analysis method that is based on quantifying a specific property of a gas molecule in effect determines in absolute terms the number of molecules of that gas that are present – that is, mmHg. Gas molecules that are composed of two or more dissimilar atoms (e.g. CO_2, N_2O, potent inhaled anesthetics) have bonds between their component atoms. Certain wavelengths of infrared radiation excite these molecules, stretching or distorting the bonds, which also absorb the radiation. Carbon dioxide molecules absorb infrared radiation at a wavelength of 4.3 μm. The greater the number of molecules of carbon dioxide present, the more radiation at 4.3 μm that is absorbed. This property of the carbon dioxide molecule is applied in the infrared carbon dioxide analyzer. Because the amount of infrared radiation absorbed is a function of the *number* of molecules present, it is, therefore, also a function of partial pressure. Thus, infrared analyzers measure partial pressure.

In the analysis of gases by Raman spectroscopy (as was used in the now obsolete Ohmeda RASCAL II analyzer), a helium–neon laser emits monochromatic light at a wavelength of 633 nm. When this light interacts with the intramolecular bonds of specific gas molecules, it is scattered and re-emitted at wavelengths different from that of the incident monochromatic light. Each re-emission wavelength is characteristic of a specific gas molecule present in the gas mixture and therefore is a function of its partial pressure. Thus, Raman spectroscopy also measures partial pressures.

A sufficient number of molecules of the gas(es) to be analyzed (i.e. adequate partial pressures) must be present to facilitate gas analysis by the infrared and Raman technologies. These systems must also be pressure-compensated if analyses are being made at ambient pressures other than those used for the original calibration of the systems.[2]

Measurement of proportion (volumes percent)

Another approach to gas analysis is to separate the molecular component species of a gas mixture and determine what proportion (percentage) each gas contributes to the total (100%). This approach is applied in mass spectrometry. Thus, if in a sample of gas containing 100 molecules there were 21 molecules of oxygen, oxygen would represent 21 percent of the gas sample and therefore might reasonably be assumed to represent 21 percent of the original gas mixture. The result is expressed as 21 volumes percent, or as a fractional concentration (0.21). This technology does not measure partial pressures; it measures only proportions. If the system is provided with an absolute pressure reading that is equivalent to 100 percent, the basic measured proportions can be converted to readings in mmHg. In the preceding example, if 100 percent were made equivalent to 760 mmHg, oxygen would have a calculated partial pressure of $(760 \times 21\%) = 159$ mmHg.

These fundamental differences in the approaches to gas analysis and their basic units of measurement are important, particularly when the data displayed by these monitors are interpreted in a clinical setting and may affect patient management.

Gas analysis technologies

Contemporary respiratory multigas analyzers use infrared spectroscopy to measure CO_2, N_2O, halothane, enflurane, isoflurane, desflurane, and sevoflurane. Oxygen is measured by a paramagnetic (rapid responding) analyzer or by a slow or fast responding fuel cell. Although certain technologies are no longer in common clinical use, it is worthwhile to briefly review some of them to appreciate their principles of operation.

Mass spectrometry

For many anesthesia caregivers, the term "mass spec" is used as if it were synonymous with gas analysis. Indeed, many anesthetic record forms still (incorrectly) include the term MASS SPEC, but this technology has not been in routine clinical use for some years. It was, however, the first multigas monitoring system in widespread clinical use, following a description by Ozanne and colleagues in 1981.[3]

The mass spectrometer is an instrument that allows the identification and quantification, on a breath-by-breath basis, of up to eight of the gases commonly encountered during the administration of an inhalational anesthetic. These gases include oxygen, nitrogen, nitrous oxide, halothane, enflurane, and isoflurane; other agents, such as helium, sevoflurane, argon, and desflurane, could sometimes be added or substituted if desired. Although the technology of mass spectrometry had been available for many years, analyzer units dedicated to a single patient were too expensive for routine use in each operating room. In 1981, the concept of a shared, or multiplexed, system was introduced.[3] This arrangement allowed one centrally located analyzer to function as part of a computerized multiplexed system that could serve up to 31 patient sampling locations (ORs and recovery room or intensive care unit beds) on a time-shared basis. The two multiplexed systems that became widely used were the Perkin-Elmer (later the Marquette Advantage System), and SARA (System for Anesthetic and Respiratory Analysis).

Principles of operation

The mass spectrometer analyzer unit separates the components of a stream of charged particles (ions) into a spectrum according to their mass/charge ratios. The relative abundance of ions at certain specific mass/charge ratios is determined and is related to the fractional composition of the original gas mixture. The creation and manipulation of ions is carried out in a high vacuum (10^{-5} mmHg) to avoid interference by outside air and to minimize random collisions among the ions and residual gases.

The most common design of mass spectrometer was the magnetic sector analyzer, so called because it uses a permanent magnet to separate the ion beam into its component ion spectra (Figure 14.5). A stream of the gas to be analyzed is continuously drawn by a sampling pump from an airway connector via a long nylon catheter. During transit through the sampling catheter, the pressure decreases from atmospheric (usually 760 mmHg) in the patient circuit to approximately 40 mmHg by the inlet of the analyzer unit. A very small amount of the gas actually sampled from the circuit (approximately 10^{-6} mL/sec) enters the analyzer unit's high-vacuum chamber through the molecular inlet leak. The gas molecules are then bombarded by an electron beam, which causes some of the molecules to lose one or more electrons and become positively charged ions. Thus an oxygen molecule (O_2) might lose one electron and become an oxygen ion (O_2^+) with one positive charge. The mass/charge ratio (often termed m/z) would therefore be 32/1, or 32. If the oxygen molecule lost two electrons, it would gain two positive charges and the resulting ion (O_2^{2+}) would have an m/z of 32/2, or 16. The process of electron bombardment also causes large molecules (e.g. halothane, enflurane, isoflurane) to become fragmented, or cracked, into smaller, positively charged ions.

The positive ions created in the analyzer are then focused into a beam by the electrostatic fields in the ion source, directed through a slit to define an exact shape for the beam, and accelerated and directed into the field of the permanent magnet. The magnetic field influences the direction of the ions, causing each ion species to curve in a trajectory whose arc is related to its m/z. The effect is to create several separate ion beams exiting the magnetic field. The separated beams are directed to individual collectors, which detect the ion current and transmit it to amplifiers that create output voltages in relation to the abundance of the ion species detected by each collector. The collector plates are positioned so that an ion with a specific m/z ratio strikes a specific collector. The heaviest ions are deflected the least and travel the farthest before striking a collector (Figure 14.5). Collectors for these heavy ions are therefore located furthest from the ion source.

Summing and other computer software measures the total voltage from all of the collector circuits as well as the individual voltages from each collector. Total voltage is considered equivalent to 100 percent of the analyzed gas mixture. Individual gas collector circuit voltages are expressed as percentages of the total voltage and displayed as percentages of the sampled gas mixture. Thus, if the voltage from the oxygen collector circuit (m/z 32) represented 30 percent of the total voltage from all of the collector circuits, oxygen would be read as constituting 30 percent of the total gas mixture analyzed. The Marquette Advantage and SARA systems used magnetic sector analyzers

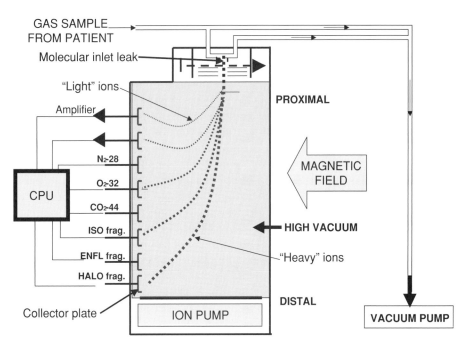

GAS SAMPLE FROM PATIENT

Molecular inlet leak

"Light" ions

Amplifier

PROXIMAL

N₂-28

O₂-32

MAGNETIC FIELD

CO₂-44

ISO frag.

HIGH VACUUM

ENFL frag.

"Heavy" ions

HALO frag.

Collector plate

DISTAL

CPU

ION PUMP

VACUUM PUMP

Figure 14.5. Schematic of a magnetic sector respiratory mass spectrometer. The respiratory gas is sampled and drawn over a molecular leak. Gas molecules enter a vacuum chamber (through the molecular inlet leak), in which they are ionized and electrically accelerated. A magnetic field deflects the ions. The mass and charge of the ions determine their trajectory, and metal dish collectors are placed to detect them. The electrical currents produced by the ions impacting the collectors are processed, the composition is computed, and the results are displayed.

that had up to eight collectors and therefore were able to detect and analyze up to eight different ion species, and thereby, parent gases.

The mass spectrometer functions as a proportioning system for the components of a gas mixture. When it displays each of the components of the mixture as a percentage of the total, it makes the assumption that all the gases present have been detected. If ambient (atmospheric) pressure information is entered into the software, the measured percentages or proportions can be converted to readings in mmHg (i.e. partial pressures). Remember that the mass spectrometer does not measure partial pressures; it calculates them from the measured proportions and the atmospheric pressure information that must be supplied to it. Thus:

$$\text{Partial pressure (mmHg)} = \text{fractional concentration} \\ \times \text{total pressure.}$$

Usually, because the mass spectrometer was sampling respired gases from the patient circuit, the total pressure entered into the computer was ambient minus 47 mmHg, the latter representing the saturated vapor pressure of water at body temperature (37°C). Thus, at sea level (760 mmHg), a pressure of 713 mmHg would be entered into the mass spectrometer software to be apportioned among the gases present. The mass spectrometer readings, when displayed in mmHg, represent somewhat of a compromise because inspired gas is usually not fully saturated with water vapor, whereas expired gas usually is. If an incorrect value for total ambient pressure is entered into the mass spectrometer software, all readings in mmHg will be incorrect, but the readings in volumes percent will be correct. By way of an example, assume that the end-tidal carbon dioxide is measured as 5 percent by the mass spectrometer and that

ambient pressure is 760 mmHg. The reading in mmHg will be 35.65 [i.e. (760 − 47) × 5%]. If a value of 500 mmHg is entered instead of 713 mmHg, the reading in mmHg will be 25 (i.e. 500 × 5%). In any case of doubt, the astute clinician would revert to the reading in volumes percent.

Shared (multiplexed) mass spectrometry systems

Multiplexing permitted the sharing of one (expensive) mass spectrometer among up to 31 sampling locations or stations. In a shared system, the gas from each sampling location is directed in sequence by the multiplexing valve system to the mass spectrometer for analysis. The time between analyses at any particular location therefore depends on (1) the number of breaths analyzed from each sampling location (i.e. dwell time); (2) the number of sampling locations in use; (3) the priority settings; and (4) in the case of stat samples, the distance between sampling locations and the analyzer (up to 300 feet in some installations).

Use of multiplexed mass spectrometry systems led anesthesia caregivers to appreciate the value of respiratory gas monitoring, as well as the limitations, the main one being that they were shared and that the data were updated only intermittently.

In October 1986, the American Society of Anesthesiologists (ASA) first approved standards for basic intraoperative monitoring. As the standards evolved, the requirement for continuous capnometry was not met by a shared mass spectrometry system. The systems were expensive to install and maintain, and were not always easily upgradable when the new agents desflurane and sevoflurane were introduced. In addition, the long sampling catheters, combined with rapid respiratory rates, led to significant artifacts; the sampling pump could cause significant negative pressure in the breathing system, and when the system failed, all of the monitored sites were affected.[4,5]

Practitioners demanded continuous gas monitoring. The most important functions of a multiplexed mass spectrometry system could be served by other dedicated gas monitors, and the multiplexed mass spectrometer-based systems became extinct.

Dedicated (stand-alone) mass spectrometry systems

A number of smaller stand-alone mass spectrometers were developed (e.g. Ohmeda 6000; Ohmeda, Madison, WI) for dedicated single-patient use. The Ohmeda 6000 Multigas Analyzer was a quadrupole filter type of mass spectrometer. It worked on the principle that a controlled electrostatic field can prevent all but a narrow range with regard to mass/charge ratio of charged particles (ions) from reaching a target. In the Ohmeda 6000 unit, the gas sampling rate was fixed at 30 mL/min. One potential advantage of a quadrupole system is that it could be adapted to measure new or additional agents by changes in software only. A number of other stand-alone quadrupole filter mass spectrometers were marketed but, owing to cost and reliability issues, their production was discontinued.

Infrared analysis

The infrared (IR) spectrum ranges between wavelengths 0.40 and 40 μm. Measurement of the energy absorbed from a narrow band of wavelengths of IR radiation as it passes through a gas sample can be used to measure the concentrations of certain gases. Asymmetric, polyatomic, polar molecules, such as carbon dioxide, nitrous oxide, water, and the potent volatile anesthetic agents absorb IR energy when their atoms rotate or vibrate asymmetrically, resulting in a change in dipole moment (i.e. the charge distribution within the molecule). The nonpolar molecules argon, nitrogen, helium, xenon, and oxygen do not absorb IR energy. Because the number of gas molecules in the path of the IR energy beam determines the total absorption, IR analyzers measure the partial pressure.

Carbon dioxide, nitrous oxide, and anesthetic gases exhibit absorption of radiation at unique bands in the IR spectrum (Figure 14.6). Carbon dioxide molecules absorb strongly between 4.2 and 4.4 μm, whereas nitrous oxide molecules absorb strongly between 4.4 and 4.6 μm and less strongly at 3.9 μm. The potent volatile anesthestic agents have strong absorption bands at 3.3 μm and throughout the range of 8 to 12 μm.

The close proximity of the nitrous oxide and carbon dioxide absorption bands may cause some carbon dioxide analyzers to be affected by high concentrations of nitrous oxide.[6,7] This phenomenon is called *collision* or *pressure broadening* because molecular collisions result in a change in the dipole moment of the gas being analyzed. Thus the IR absorption band is broadened and the apparent absorption at the measurement wavelength may be altered. In a typical IR carbon dioxide analyzer, 95 percent oxygen causes a 0.5 percent decline in the measured carbon dioxide. Nitrous oxide causes a more substantial increase of about 0.1 percent carbon dioxide per 10 percent

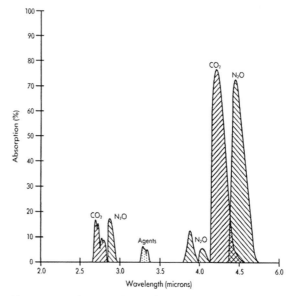

Figure 14.6. Absorption bands of respiratory gases in the infrared spectrum. (From Raemer DB. Monitoring respiratory function. In Rogers MC, Tinker JH, Covino BG, Longnecker DE, eds. *Principles and Practice of Anesthesiology*, St. Louis: Mosby-Year Book,1992, with permission.)

nitrous oxide because of collision broadening. Contemporary multigas analyzers automatically compensate for the effect of collision broadening by measuring the concentrations of interfering gases.

A simple IR analyzer (Figure 14.7) consists of a heated black body radiator that is the source of IR radiation, a sample cell (or cuvette) through which the gas to be analyzed is drawn by a sampling pump, and a detector that generates an output signal related to the intensity of the IR radiation that is detected. (A black body radiator is a theoretical object that is totally absorbent to all thermal energy that falls on it; thus, it does not reflect any light and so appears black. As it absorbs energy, it heats up and reradiates the energy as electromagnetic

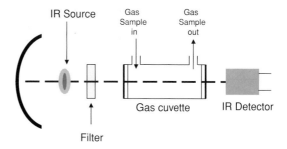

Single-beam single filter infrared analyzer

Figure 14.7. Diagram of a simple single-wavelength IR respiratory gas analyzer. An IR source emits a beam that passes through a filter, which passes only the wavelength absorbed by the gas of interest. The respiratory gas from the patient is sampled and passes through the gas cell in the optical path. An IR detector measures intensity of the IR wavelength that has passed through the gas sample. The intensity is inversely related to the partial pressure of that gas in the sample cell. The electrical signal from the detector is processed to report the gas composition in mmHg (or in kilopascals, abbreviated kPa; 1 kPa is equivalent to 7.5 mmHg). This value can be converted (automatically) to a reading in volumes percent if the ambient pressure is known.

radiation.) A narrow bandpass filter, which allows only radiation at the wavelength of interest to pass through, is interposed between the IR source and the cuvette, or between the cuvette and the detector. The intensity of radiation reaching the detector is inversely related to the concentration of the specific gas being measured.

A number of sources of IR radiation can be used to produce a broad spectrum of IR radiation. Light sources made of tungsten wires or ceramic resistive materials heated to 1500 to 4000 K emit energy over a broad wavelength range that includes the absorption spectra of the respiratory gases. The radiation may be pulsed electronically, or if constant, may be made intermittent by being interrupted ("chopped") mechanically. Because energy output of IR light sources tends to drift, optical systems have been designed to stabilize the analyzers. Three common designs are distinguished by their use of single or dual IR beams and by their use of positive or negative filtering.[8]

Single-beam positive filter

In one single-beam positive filter design, precision optical bandpass filters mounted on a chopper wheel spinning at 40 to 250 revolutions per minute sequentially interrupt a single IR beam. The beam retains energy at a narrow band of wavelengths during each interruption. For each gas of interest, a pair of bandpass filters are selected at an absorption peak and at a reference wavelength where relatively little absorption occurs. The chopped IR beam then passes through a cuvette containing the sample gas. The ratio of intensity of the IR beam for each pair of filters is proportional to the partial pressure of the gas and is insensitive to changes in the intensity of the IR source.

Single-beam negative filter

In the single-beam negative filter design, the filters are usually gas-filled cells mounted in a spinning wheel. During each interruption, the IR beam retains energy at all wavelengths except those absorbed by the gas. The chopped IR beam then passes through a cuvette containing the sample gas. Analogous to the positive filter design described previously, the ratio of IR beam intensity for each pair of filter cells is proportional to the partial pressure of the gas and is insensitive to changes in intensity of the IR source.

Dual-beam positive filter

In the dual-beam positive filter design, the IR energy from the source is split into two parallel beams. One beam passes through the sample gas, and the other passes through a reference gas. A spinning blade passes through the beams and sequentially interrupts one, the other, then both. The two beams are optically focused to a single point, at which a bandpass optical filter selected at the absorption peak of the gas of interest is mounted over a single detector. As before, the ratios of the intensities of the sample and reference beams are proportional to the partial pressure of the gas.

Detectors of infrared radiation

To measure carbon dioxide, nitrous oxide, and sometimes anesthetic agents, a radiation-sensitive solid state material, lead selenide, is commonly used as a detector. Lead selenide is quite sensitive to changes in temperature; therefore, it is usually thermostatically cooled or temperature-compensated.

Anesthetic agents, carbon dioxide, and nitrous oxide are sometimes measured with another detector type, the Luft cell. This detector uses a chamber filled with gas that expands as IR radiation enters the chamber and is absorbed. A flexible wall of the chamber acts as a diaphragm that moves as the gas expands, and a microphone converts the motion to an electrical signal.

The signal processor converts the measured electrical currents to display gas partial pressure. First, the ratios of detector currents at various points in the spinning wheel's progress (or from multiple detectors) are computed. Next, electronic scaling and filtering are applied. Finally, linearization, according to a look-up table containing the point-by-point conversion from electrical voltage to gas partial pressure, is accomplished by a microprocessor. Compensation for cross-sensitivity or interference between gases can be accomplished by the microprocessor following linearization.

Infrared wavelength and anesthetic agent specificity

Infrared analyzers must use a specific wavelength of radiation according to the absorbance peak of each gas to be measured. Thus, carbon dioxide is measured using a wavelength of 4.3 μm and nitrous oxide using 3.9 μm. Older agent analyzers (e.g. the Datex Capnomac)[9] used a wavelength of 3.3 μm to measure the potent inhaled anesthetics, but use of a single wavelength did not permit differentiation among the agents. When such a system is used, the analyzer must be programmed by the user for the particular agent being administered. This action sets the appropriate gain in the software program, and the displayed reading will be accurate for the one agent in use. Obviously, programming such an analyzer for the wrong agent, or use of mixed agents, leads to erroneous readings of anesthetic agent concentration.

Modern IR analyzers are agent-specific (i.e. they have the facility to both identify and quantify mixed agents in the presence of one another) by measuring each agent at a separate specific wavelength. Contemporary analyzers that can identify and quantify anesthetic agents incorporate individual wavelength filters in the range of 8 to 12 μm. An example is the Datex-Ohmeda Compact Airway Module (GE Healthcare) (Figures 14.1, 14.2, and 14.8), which is a nondispersive (i.e. with no provision for dispersing the emitted radiation into its

Nondispersive IR analyzer

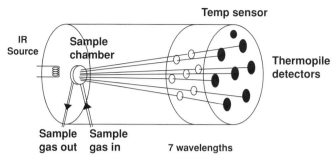

Figure 14.8. Principles of GE/Datex-Ohmeda IR analyzer in the Compact Airway Module. In this design, the IR beam is interrupted electronically rather than mechanically by a "chopper" wheel. From ref. 10, by permission of GE Datex-Ohmeda.

IR absorbance of AAs

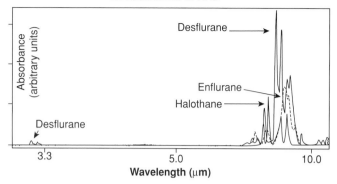

Figure 14.10. Principles of GE/Datex-Ohmeda IR analyzer in Compact Airway Module. Absorbance bands for the potent inhaled anesthetic agents. From ref. 10, by permission of GE Datex-Ohmeda.

component wavelengths) IR analyzer that measures the absorption of the gas sample at seven different wavelengths, which are selected using optical narrow band filters. The IR radiation detectors are thermopiles. Carbon dioxide and N_2O are calculated from absorption measured at 3 to 5 μm (Figure 14.9). Identification and calculation of the concentrations of anesthetic agents are made by measuring absorption at five wavelengths in the 8 to 9 μm band and solving for the concentrations from a set of five equations (Figure 14.10).[10] A schematic of a multiwavelength analyzer in which the beam of radiation is interrupted mechanically (chopped) is shown in Figure 14.11.

Sampling systems and infrared analysis

Sidestream sampling analyzers continuously withdraw between 50 and 250 mL/min from the breathing circuit through narrow-gauge sample tubing to the optical system, where the measurement is made. One of the disadvantages of sidestream monitors is the need to deal with liquid water and water vapor. Water vapor from the breathing circuit condenses on its way to the sample cuvette and can interfere with optical transmission. Nafion tubing (PermaPure, Toms River, NJ), a semipermeable

Absorbances of CO_2 and N_2O

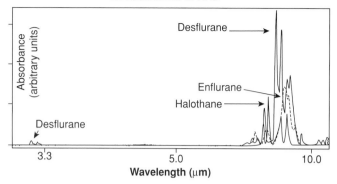

Figure 14.9. Principles of GE/Datex-Ohmeda IR analyzer in Compact Airway Module. Absorbance bands used for CO_2 and N_2O. From ref. 10, by permission of GE Datex-Ohmeda.

polymer that selectively allows water vapor to pass from its interior to the relatively dry exterior, is commonly used to eliminate water vapor. In addition, a water trap is usually interposed between the patient sampling catheter and the analyzer to protect the optical system from liquid water and body fluids (Figure 14.1). One design of sampling tubing (Nomoline, see Figure 14.4) incorporates a water separation section and bacterial filter that removes both water and liquid water from the sampled gas flow.

Infrared photoacoustic spectrometer

The photoacoustic spectrometer (Figure 14.12) is similar to the basic IR spectrometer. Infrared energy is passed through optical filters that select narrow-wavelength bands corresponding to the absorption characteristics of the respired gases. Carbon dioxide is measured at a wavelength of 4.3 μm, nitrous oxide at 3.9 μm, and the potent inhaled agents at a wavelength between 10.3 and 13.0 μm.[11] Evenly spaced windows are located along the circumference of a rotating wheel. The optical components are located astride the wheel along one of its radii. A series of IR beams pulse on and off at particular frequencies, according to the rate of rotation of the wheel and the spacing of the windows. The gas flowing through the measurement cuvette is exposed to the pulsed IR beams. As each gas absorbs the pulsating IR energy in its absorption band, it expands and contracts at that frequency. The resulting sound waves are detected with a microphone. The partial pressure of each gas in the sample is then proportional to the amplitude (or volume) of the measured sound.

The photoacoustic technique has the distinct advantage over other IR methods in that a simple microphone detector can be used to measure all the IR-absorbing gases. However, this device is sensitive to interference from loud noises and vibration. Also, because only one wavelength is used to measure the potent inhaled anesthetics, this monitor is unable to distinguish among the agents and requires that it be programmed for the one that is in use. Erroneous readings might arise in the presence of mixed anesthetic agents. This technology was used in the

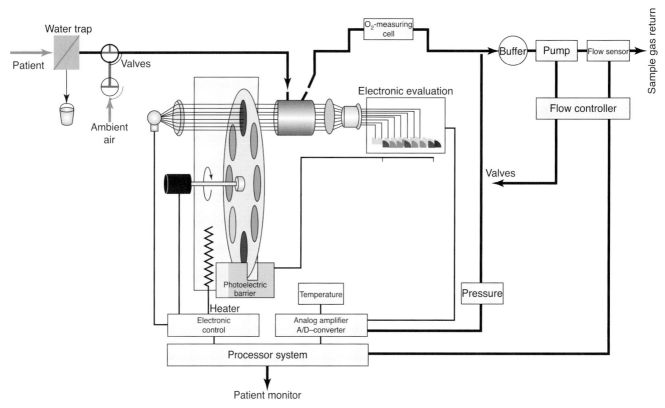

Figure 14.11. Schematic of multiwavelength IR analyzer with mechanical interruption ("chopping") of IR beam. Courtesy of Dräger Medical, Telford, PA.

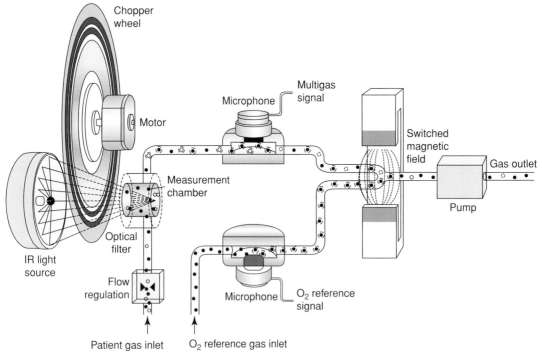

Figure 14.12. Schematic diagram of a photoacoustic spectrometer. An IR source emits a beam which passes through a spinning chopper wheel that has several rows of circumferential slots. The interrupted IR beams then pass through optical filters that select specific wavelengths of light chosen to be at the absorption peaks of the gases to be measured. Each interrupted IR light beam impinges on its respective gas in the measurement chamber, causing vibration of the gas as energy is absorbed and released from the molecules. The vibration frequency of each gas depends on the spacing of its slots on the chopper wheel. A microphone converts the gas vibration frequencies and amplitudes into electrical signals that are converted to the gas concentrations for display. (From Raemer DB. Monitoring respiratory function. In Rogers MC, Tinker JH, Covino BG, Longnecker DE, eds. *Principles and Practice of Anesthesiology*, St. Louis: Mosby-Year Book, 1992, with permission.)

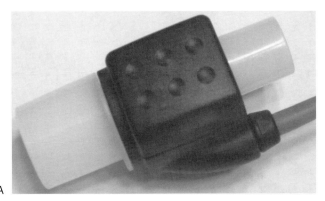

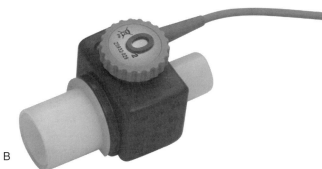

Figure 14.13. (A) Mainstream multigas analyzer module that measures CO_2, N_2O, and anesthetic agents. (B) Same as (A) but with additional ultrafast oxygen sensor. IRMA Phasein AB, Danderyd, Sweden.

Bruel and Kjaer Anesthetic Gas Monitor 1304. It is the technology that is currently used in the Innova 1412 Field Gas Monitor used for monitoring traces gases (Luma Sense Technologies, California Analytical Instruments, Orange, CA).

Mainstream multigas analysis

Mainstream multigas IR analysis has recently been introduced by Phasein (Danderyd, Sweden) in its IRMA series of multigas analyzers. The entire IRMA mainstream probe weighs only 30 g and measures IR light absorption at ten different wavelengths to precisely determine gas concentrations in the mixture (Figure 14.13A). A selection of disposable airway adapters is available for different clinical applications. The probe comprises all the necessary components required for advanced signal processing, along with a comprehensive digital RS232 interface. The probes are universally calibrated and deliver processed data for display on the screen of any display monitor. The same miniaturized technology is used in Phasein's EMMA Emergency Capnometer, a device that displays respiratory rate and incorporates apnea, high CO_2, and low CO_2 audible and visual alarms (Figure 14.14).

Raman spectroscopy

When light strikes gas molecules, most of the energy scattered is absorbed and re-emitted in the same direction and at the same wavelength as the incoming beam (Rayleigh scattering).[12] At room temperature, about one-millionth of the energy is scattered at a longer wavelength, producing a so-called red-shifted spectrum. This Raman scattering can be used to measure the constituents of a gas mixture. Unlike IR spectroscopy, Raman scattering is not limited to gas species that are polar. Carbon dioxide, oxygen, nitrogen, water vapor, nitrous oxide, and the potent volatile anesthetic agents all exhibit Raman activity. Monatomic gases such as helium, xenon, and argon, which lack intramolecular bonds, do not exhibit Raman activity.

The medical Raman spectrometer uses a helium–neon laser (wavelength 633 nm, or 0.633 μm) to produce the incoming monochromatic light beam. The Raman scattered light is of low intensity and measured perpendicular to the laser beam. The measurement cuvette is located in the cavity of the laser so the gas molecules are struck repeatedly by the beam (Figure 14.15). This results in enough Raman scattering to be collected and processed by the optical detection system. Photomultiplier tubes count the scattered photons at the characteristic Raman-shifted wavelength for each gas. Thus the Raman spectrometer measures the partial pressures of the gases in its measurement cuvette. Measurements are converted electronically to the desired units of measure and displayed on the screen. Raman spectroscopy is the principle of operation of the Ohmeda RASCAL II monitor (Ohmeda; Boulder, CO).

The RASCAL II Raman spectrometer had the same capabilities as the mass spectrometer. In particular, it was able to measure nitrogen for detection of air embolism. Unfortunately, despite its obvious versatility, this monitor is no longer in production, although many are still in use.

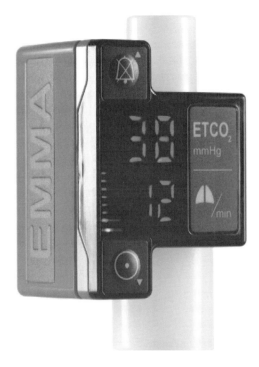

Figure 14.14. EMMA Capnocheck Mainstream capnometer Plug-in and Measure Multigas Technologies, Phasein AB, Danderyd, Sweden.

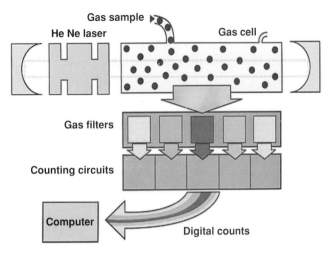

Figure 14.15. Diagram of a Raman scattering respiratory gas analyzer. A laser tube generates a monochromatic (633 nm) light beam that is contained within a cavity by mirrors. The respiratory gas from the patient is sampled and passes through the laser beam. The gas molecules scatter a small amount of light at wavelengths different from that of the incoming beam. The wavelength shift is characteristic of the gas species. The scattered light is detected, and the gas composition is computed and displayed to the user in the appropriate units of measure.

Microstream capnography technology

Microstream is a relatively new approach to capnometry that uses a novel laser-based technology called molecular correlation spectroscopy (MCS) as the infrared emission source.[13] This produces a highly efficient and selective emission of a spectrum of discrete wavelengths that exactly match those for CO_2 absorption. One of the major problems of conventional nondispersive IR technology is that the black body emitter produces a very broad IR spectrum, most of which is redundant to CO_2 monitoring, and must be removed using optical interference filters. Such filters are limited in their ability to remove radiation that falls between the discrete absorbing lines.

Microstream technology uses an MCS source that operates at room temperature (unlike the black-body emitters) and emits only CO_2-specific radiation of approximately 100 discrete lines in the region of 4.2 to 4.35 μm. This permits use of a smaller sample cell (15 μL) and a gas sampling flow rate of 50 mL/min. The technology was initially developed by Oridion (Oridion Microstream; Needham, MA) but is now used (through licensing partnerships) in many other brands of capnograph (e.g. Spacelabs, Dräger, Philips). The small size, low power requirement, small sample cell size, low gas sampling flow rate, rapid response time, short warmup time, CO_2 specificity, and no need for routine calibration make this technology particularly useful in portable carbon dioxide monitors.[14]

Water vapor and accuracy of capnometers

Water vapor may be an important factor in the accuracy of a carbon dioxide analyzer. Most sidestream carbon dioxide analyzers report ambient temperature and pressure, dry (ATPD) values for PCO_2 by using a water trap and Nafion (water vapor permeable) tubing to remove water vapor from the sample. It has been recommended that carbon dioxide analyzers report their results at body temperature and pressure, saturated (BTPS), so end-tidal values are close to conventionally reported alveolar gas partial pressure.[15] The error in reporting PCO_2 at ATPD when it should be reported at BTPS is about 2.5 mmHg.

Carbon dioxide values reported in ATPD can be converted to BTPS by decreasing the dry gas reading by the fraction $(P_{ATM} - 47)/P_{ATM}$, where P_{ATM} is the atmospheric pressure in mmHg and 47 mmHg is the vapor pressure of water at $37°$C.

Mainstream sampling analyzers naturally report readings near BTPS. Depending on breathing circuit conditions, a small decrease from body temperature may result in the analyzer reading slightly less than BTPS values. Condensation of water can affect the windows of the mainstream airway adapter and cause erroneous readings. These adapters are therefore heated or otherwise designed to prevent condensation.

Colorimetric carbon dioxide detectors

Carbon dioxide in solution is acidic; therefore, pH-sensitive dyes can be used to detect and measure its presence. A colorimetric carbon dioxide detector is designed to be interposed between the tracheal tube and the breathing circuit. Respired gas passes through a hydrophobic filter and a piece of filter paper that is visible through a plastic window. The originally described detector (FENEM FEF CO_2 Detector) consisted of a piece of filter paper permeated with an aqueous solution containing metacresol purple, a pH-sensitive dye. Carbon dioxide from the exhaled breath dissolves in the aqueous solution, changing the color of the dye from purple to yellow. The degree of color change is dependent on the concentration of carbon dioxide. On inspiration of carbon dioxide-free gas, carbon dioxide leaves the solution and the color of the indicator returns to its resting (purple) state.[16]

A number of colorimetric devices are now commercially available for use in adult and pediatric patients. They may use other CO_2-sensitive dyes and are calibrated to provide an approximate indication of expired carbon dioxide concentration that can be discerned by comparison of the indicator color with a graduated color scale printed on the device's housing. For example, the Easy Cap II (Covidien-Nellcor, Boulder, CO) color changes from purple to yellow, indicating 2 percent to 5 percent (15–38 mmHg) carbon dioxide with each exhaled breath. On inspiration, the color should change back to purple, indicating absence of CO_2 in the inspired gas (Figure 14.16). A permanent change in color may mislead the uneducated user;[17,18] hence the following caution in the directions for use from the manufacturer of the Easy Cap II CO_2 detector: "Interpreting results before confirming six breath cycles can yield false results. Gastric distension with air prior to attempted intubation may introduce CO_2 levels as high as 4.5% into the Easy Cap detector if the endotracheal tube is misplaced in the esophagus. Initial Easy Cap detector color (yellow) may be interpreted as a false positive if read before delivery of six breaths." The warnings also

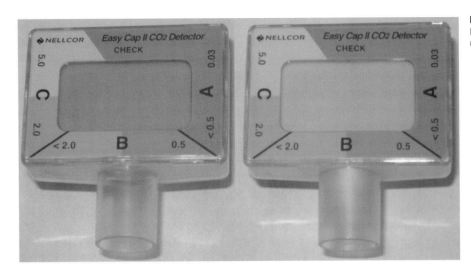

Figure 14.16. Nellcor Easy Cap II CO₂ detector. Left: Purple = No. little CO₂; Right: Yellow = 5% CO₂. Tyco Healthcare, Boulder, CO.

further include a statement, "Reflux of gastric contents, mucus, edema fluid, or intratracheal epinephrine into the Easy Cap can yield persistent patchy yellow or white discoloration *which does not vary with the respiratory cycle*. Contamination of this type may also increase airway resistance and affect ventilation. Discard device if this occurs."

This type of detector is intended to be used to confirm clinical signs of tracheal intubation when conventional capnography is not available. Both adult and pediatric versions are commercially available. The newest FENEM CO₂ indicator is designed to be attached to the exhalation port (30 mm or 19 mm) of a self-inflating resuscitator bag, where it does not add dead space or resistance to flow.

Another version of the colorimetric CO₂ detector, the CO2NFIRM NOW CO₂ Detector (Kendall, Tyco Healthcare; Mansfield, MA), is marketed as a device to confirm intragastric placement of an orogastric or nasogastric tube to prevent intratracheal placement.

Oxygen analyzers

In all contemporary anesthesia delivery systems, the fraction of inspired oxygen (FIO₂) in an anesthesia breathing circuit is monitored by an oxygen analyzer. Two types of oxygen analyzers are in common use for monitoring: those based on a fuel or galvanic cell principle, and paramagnetic (Pauling) sensors. In the past, in addition to these methods, multigas analyzers using mass spectroscopy or Raman spectroscopy to measure oxygen were also used as oxygen monitors (see previous discussion).

Fuel cell

The fuel cell or galvanic cell is basically an oxygen battery consisting of a diffusion barrier, a noble metal (gold mesh or platinum) cathode, and a lead or zinc anode in a basic (usually potassium hydroxide) electrolyte bath (Figures 14.17 and 14.18). The sensor, covered by an oxygen-permeable membrane, is exposed to the breathing circuit. Oxygen diffusing into the

Figure 14.17. Fuel cell oxygen analyzer. GE Datex-Ohmeda, Madison, WI.

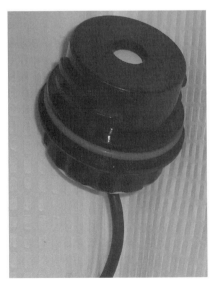
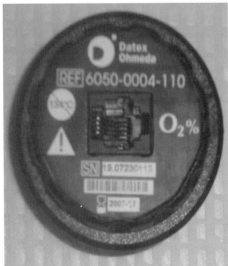

Fuel cell

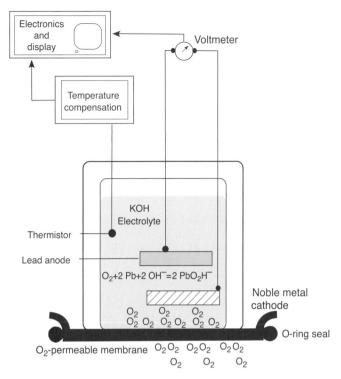

Figure 14.18. Principles of fuel cell oxygen analyzer. Oxygen in the gas sample permeates a membrane and enters a potassium hydroxide electrolyte solution. An electrical potential is established between a lead anode and noble metal cathode as oxygen is supplied to the anode. The measured voltage between the electrodes is proportional to the oxygen tension of the gas sample. Temperature compensation is required for accurate measurement. (From Raemer DB. Monitoring respiratory function. In Rogers MC, Tinker JH, Covino BG, Longnecker DE, eds. *Principles and Practice of Anesthesiology*, St. Louis: Mosby-Year Book, 1992, with permission.)

sensor is reduced to hydroxyl ions at the cathode, according to the following reaction:

$$O_2 + 2\,H_2O + 4\,e^- \rightarrow 4\,OH^-$$

The hydroxyl ions then oxidize the lead (or zinc) anode, and the following reaction occurs at the anode:

$$2\,Pb + 6\,OH^- \rightarrow 2\,PbO_2H^- + 2\,H_2O + 4\,e^-$$

The flow of current depends on the uptake of oxygen at the cathode (according to Faraday's first law of electrolysis), and the voltage developed is proportional to the oxygen partial pressure. No polarizing potential is needed because the cell produces its own. The fuel cell sensor voltage is measured and electronically scaled to units of partial pressure or equivalent concentration (in volumes percent) and displayed as a readout. Similar to any battery, the fuel cell has a limited lifespan, depending on its period of exposure to oxygen. For this reason, machine manufacturers have recommended that the cell be removed from the breathing system when not in use. The response time of conventional fuel cell O_2 analyzers is slow; therefore, they are best

used to monitor the average oxygen concentration in the inspiratory limb of the breathing system. An ultrafast galvanic oxygen sensor will be available for the mainstream multigas analyzer (Figure 14.13B). This is specified to have a response time of <300 msec, enabling breath-by-breath oxygen analysis.

Paramagnetic oxygen analyzer

The oxygen molecule has two electrons in unpaired orbits, which makes it paramagnetic (i.e. susceptible to attraction by a magnetic field). Most other gases are weakly diamagnetic and repelled. The paramagnetic oxygen sensor uses the strong, positive magnetic susceptibility of oxygen in a pneumatic bridge configuration to determine oxygen concentration by measuring a pressure differential between a stream of reference gas (room air at about 10 mL/min) and one of the measured gas as the two streams are exposed to a changing magnetic field (Figure 14.19). An electromagnet is rapidly switched off and on (at a frequency of 165 Hz in the GE compact airway module[10]), creating a rapidly changing magnetic field between its poles. The electromagnet is designed to have its poles in close proximity, forming a narrow gap. The streams of sample and reference gas have different oxygen partial pressures, and the pressure between the entrance and exit of the respective gas streams differs slightly because of the magnetic force on the oxygen molecules. This generates sound waves from each gas stream. A sensitive pressure transducer (i.e. a microphone) is used to convert the sound waves to an electrical signal. The output signal is proportional to the oxygen partial pressure difference between the two gas streams and should be displayed as the PO_2 but is more usually displayed as the equivalent concentration in volumes percent. Paramagnetic oxygen analysis is used in most contemporary multigas analyzers.

The main advantage of paramagnetic analysis over the standard fuel cell is that it has a very rapid response, permitting continuous breath-by-breath monitoring of the respired oxygen

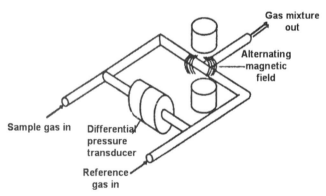

Figure 14.19. Paramagnetic oxygen analyzer. The sample and reference gas streams converge in a rapidly changing magnetic field. Because the two streams have different oxygen tensions (i.e. different numbers of oxygen molecules), a pressure differential is created across a sensitive pressure transducer. The transducer converts this force to an electrical signal that is displayed as oxygen partial pressure or converted to a reading in volumes percent.

CAPNOGRAM

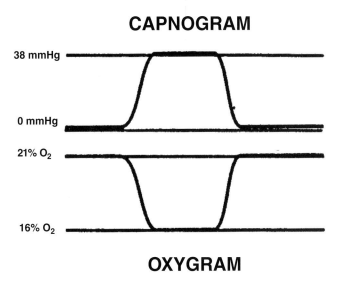

OXYGRAM

Figure 14.20. Capnogram (above) and oxygram (below). The latter is almost a mirror image of the capnogram.

concentration. The graphical representation of this can be displayed as the oxygram, which is essentially a mirror image of the capnogram (Figure 14.20).

Normally, the gas exiting the multigas analyzer is directed to the waste gas scavenging system of the anesthesia delivery system. If a low-flow or closed-circuit anesthesia technique is being used, the gas exiting the analyzer is usually returned to the breathing system. In this case, it must be remembered that nitrogen from the room air reference gas stream is also being added, albeit at a low rate (8 mL/min), and will accumulate in the breathing circuit.

Calibration of oxygen analyzers

Oxygen analyzers require periodic calibration. Because all analyzers produce an electrical signal that is proportional to oxygen partial pressure, the constant of proportionality (gain) must be determined. Generally, the electrical signal in the presence of 0 percent oxygen is known to be near zero; therefore, no offset correction is required. In the fuel cell, the gain changes over time because of changes in the electrolyte, electrodes (the anode is sacrificial), and membrane. The anesthesia caregiver must therefore calibrate it to read 21 percent by removing it from the breathing system and allowing equilibration in room air. It must be remembered that the fuel cell is actually measuring the ambient PO_2 (normally 159 mmHg in dry air at sea level) but for convenience displays 21 volumes percent. Therefore, if a fuel cell that has been calibrated to read 21 percent at sea level is then used at a much higher altitude, the readout will show less than 21 percent (because the ambient PO_2 is lower), even though the composition of the atmosphere is still 21 percent oxygen by volume.

The gain of the paramagnetic sensor changes with temperature, humidity, and pneumatic factors. The contemporary paramagnetic oxygen analyzers perform their own periodic computer-controlled automated calibration process.

Gases in the anesthesia delivery system can be analyzed via a number of modern technologies, each of which is based on application of some specific physical property of the gas molecule. The analysis methods and their applications are summarized in Table 14.1. In interpreting gas analysis data, it is important to understand the principles of how the data were obtained so erroneous data can be identified and, if necessary, rejected.

Balance gas

Contemporary multigas analyzers measure the partial pressure of each gas of interest in a dry gas mixture. The PO_2 is measured by paramagnetic analysis, and PN_2O, PCO_2, and Panesthetic agent by IR technology. If the sum of these partial pressures is subtracted from the ambient barometric pressure, the result is the partial pressure(s) of unmeasured gas(es) and may be displayed as balance gas (Figure 14.21). In most cases, the balance gas is nitrogen; in the absence of a specific nitrogen gas analyzer (i.e. Raman or mass spectrometer), it has been described as the "poor man's nitrogen." However, if a heliox (75% helium/25% oxygen) mixture were being analyzed, helium would be read as the balance gas.

Nitric oxide

Inhaled nitric oxide (NO) is used to treat hypoxemia and pulmonary hypertension associated with acute respiratory failure. A number of NO delivery systems are commercially available, and incorporate or require contemporaneous use of a nitric oxide analyzer.

Table 14.1. Gas monitoring technologies

Technology	Gas O₂	CO₂	N₂O	AA specific	N₂	He	Ar
Mass spec	x	x	x	x	x	x	x
Raman	x	x	x	x	x		
IR light		x	x	x			
IR acoustic		x	x	x			
Fuel cell	x						
Paramagnetic	x						
Moleculare correlation spectroscopy	x						

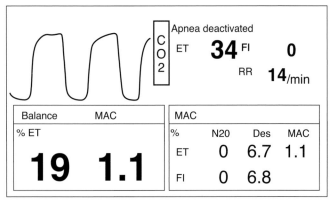

Figure 14.21. Screen of GE Datex-Ohmeda S5 monitor showing balance gas concentration and MAC value.

The INOvent delivery system (GE/Datex-Ohmeda) delivers NO in concentrations of 0 to 40 ppm. Circuit gas is sampled at a rate of 230 mL/min and analyzed electrochemically (amperometric approach) when NO reacts with an electrode to induce a current or voltage change. The measurement ranges are 0 to 100 ppm for NO, and 0 to 15 ppm for nitrogen dioxide, NO_2.

The concentration of NO can also be determined using a simple chemiluminescent reaction involving ozone.[19] Chemiluminescence is the emission of light with limited emission of heat (luminescence), as the result of a chemical reaction. A sample containing nitric oxide is mixed with a large quantity of ozone. The nitric oxide reacts with the ozone to produce oxygen and nitrogen dioxide. This reaction also produces light (chemiluminescence), which can be measured with a photodetector. The amount of light produced is proportional to the amount of nitric oxide in the gas sample.

$$NO + O_3 \rightarrow NO_2 + O_2 + light$$

To determine the amount of nitrogen dioxide (NO_2) in a sample (containing no NO), it must first be converted to nitric oxide (NO) by passing the sample through a converter before the ozone activation reaction is applied. The ozone reaction produces a photon count proportional to NO, which is proportional to NO_2 before it was converted to NO. In the case of a mixed sample containing both NO and NO_2, the preceding reaction yields the amount of NO and NO_2 combined in the gas sample, assuming that the sample is passed through the converter. If the mixed sample is not passed through the converter, the ozone reaction produces activated NO_2 only in proportion to the NO in the sample. The NO_2 in the sample is not activated by the ozone reaction. Although unactivated NO_2 is present with the activated NO_2, photons are emitted only by the activated species, which is proportional to the original NO. The final step is to subtract NO from (NO + NO_2) to yield NO_2.[19]

Applications of gas monitoring
Oxygen

The qualitative and quantitative oxygen-specific analyzer in the anesthesia breathing system is probably the most important of all the monitors on the anesthesia workstation. Prior to the general use of an oxygen analyzer in the anesthesia breathing system, a number of adverse outcomes resulting from unrecognized delivery of a hypoxic gas were reported.[20]

To be used correctly, the oxygen analyzer must be calibrated and appropriate low and high audible and visual concentration alarm limits set. This analyzer, sampling gas in the inspiratory limb of the breathing system or at the Y-piece, is the only means of ensuring that oxygen is actually being delivered to the patient. In the event that a hypoxic gas or gas mixture is delivered, the alarm will sound. Such situations can occur if there is a pipeline crossover (e.g. O_2 for N_2O), an incorrectly filled oxygen storage tank or cylinder, or failure of a proportioning system intended to prevent delivery of a gas mixture containing less than 25 percent oxygen. The high oxygen concentration alarm limit is important when caring for patients for whom a high oxygen concentration may be harmful, such as premature infants and patients treated with chemotherapeutic drugs (e.g. bleomycin), who are more susceptible to oxygen toxicity.

Continuous monitoring of inspired and end-expired oxygen is very helpful in assuring completeness of preoxygenation of the lungs before a rapid-sequence induction of anesthesia or in patients at increased risk for hypoxemia during induction of anesthesia, such as the morbidly obese. During preoxygenation, nitrogen is washed out of the lungs and is replaced by oxygen.[21] Preoxygenation is ideal when the inspired oxygen concentration is 100 percent and the end-tidal O_2 is 95 percent, the difference of 5 percent being the exhaled CO_2.

The rapid-response oxygen analyzer makes possible the display of the oxygram, a continuous real-time display of oxygen concentration on the y-axis, against time on the x-axis (Figure 14.20). Now that it is possible to accurately measure inspiratory and expiratory gas flows and, therefore, volumes (i.e. flow = volume/time), by the airway, the oxygram can be combined with these flow signals to plot inspired and expired oxygen concentrations against volume.[10] In theory, the integral of simultaneous flow and oxygen concentration during inspiration and expiration is the inspired and expired volume of oxygen. From the difference between these two amounts, oxygen consumption can be estimated. Barnard and Sleigh used this method (with a Datex Ultima monitor) to measure oxygen consumption in patients under general anesthesia and compared it with that obtained simultaneously using a metabolic monitor.[22] These authors concluded that the Datex Ultima may be used with moderate accuracy to measure oxygen uptake during anesthesia. The analogous plot for the capnogram allows measurement of carbon dioxide production.

The application of this concept is termed *indirect calorimetry* and is used in the GE bedside metabolic module.[23] By monitoring flow and measuring the gas concentrations, this module

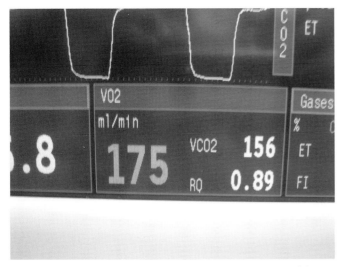

Figure 14.22. Screen of GE Datex-Ohmeda S5 Compact Airway Module monitor showing metabolic monitoring data (VO2, VCO2, RQ) from integrating concentration and flow signals.

Table 14.2.	Capnogram abnormalities
Abnormality	**Possible causes**
1. Absent	Capnograph line disconnect No ventilation, circuit obstructed Esophageal intubation, tube misplaced
2. End-tidal increased Inspired CO_2 zero	**Increased production** (fever, MH, tourniquet or X-clamp release, bicarbonate, CO_2 administration)
Inspired CO_2 increased	**Decreased removal** (hypoventilation) Rebreathing (exhausted absorbent, channeling, incompetent unidirectional valves, CO_2 delivered to circuit in fresh gas flow)
3. End-tidal decreased	Hyperventilation, decreased CO_2 production/delivery to lungs, low CO, V/Q mismatch, increased alveolar dead space, pulmonary embolism, artifactual (rapid shallow breaths, gas sampling rate>expiratory flow rate, miscalibration of analyzer, air leak into sampling system

Source: By permission of Jaffee MB and Novametrix Inc., Wallingford, CT. Courtesy of Philips-Respironics.

provides measurements of O_2 consumption (VO2) and CO_2 production (VCO2), and calculates respiratory quotient and energy expenditure (Figure 14.22).[24] Although the applications may be more pertinent to patients in the intensive care unit, some have found it useful during liver transplantation surgery in predicting the viability of the organ once in the recipient. It might also be useful in the early detection of a hypermetabolic state in a patient under general anesthesia (e.g. malignant hyperthermia) and distinguishing it from insufflation of CO_2 during a laparoscopy procedure.

Carbon dioxide

The introduction of CO_2 monitoring into clinical practice is one of the major advances in patient safety. Prior to its introduction, many cases of esophageal intubation were unrecognized, leading to adverse outcomes, not to mention increases in malpractice premiums. Detection of CO_2 on a breath-by-breath basis is considered to be the best method to confirm endotracheal intubation.[25] The applications of CO_2 monitoring (capnography) are numerous; entire textbooks have been devoted to this subject.[26,27]

A normal capnogram is depicted in Figure 14.23. The normal capnogram is divided into four phases. Phase I (A–B) is the inspiratory baseline, which is normally zero. Phase II (B–C) is the expiratory upstroke. This is normally steep. As the

patient exhales, fresh gas in the anatomic dead space (with no carbon dioxide) is gradually replaced by carbon dioxide-containing gas from the alveoli. Phase III (C–D) is the expiratory plateau, which normally has a slight upward gradient. This is because there is not perfect matching of ventilation and perfusion throughout the lungs. Alveoli with lower V/Q ratios – and, therefore, higher carbon dioxide concentrations – tend to empty later during exhalation than those with high V/Q ratios. When exhalation is complete, the plateau continues because exhaled carbon dioxide from the alveoli remains at the gas sampling site until the next inspiration. The end-tidal carbon dioxide concentration ($PE'CO_2$) is considered to be the same as the alveolar concentration ($PACO_2$). Phase IV (D–E) is the inspiratory downstroke, as fresh gas replaces alveolar gas at the sampling site. The presence of a normal capnogram indicates that the lungs are being ventilated. The ventilation may be spontaneous, assisted, or controlled. The inspired CO_2 concentration is normally zero, and the end-tidal normally between 34 and 44 mmHg. Table 14.2 shows some of the possible causes for values outside the normal ranges. Abnormalities by phases of the capnogram are shown in Table 14.3.

Observation of the shape of the capnogram may also be helpful in alerting the caregiver to certain conditions. Examples of abnormal capnograms are shown in Figures 14.24 through 14.31.

The end-tidal CO_2 concentration is commonly used as a surrogate for alveolar CO_2 tension, which in turn is used to track arterial CO_2, a value that must be obtained invasively. There is normally an arterial-to-end-tidal CO_2 tension difference of about 4 mmHg. This difference is not constant and is affected by the alveolar dead space (DSA), which is the portion of the alveolar ventilation (VA) that is wasted.[28] Consider the following example of a patient whose lungs are being ventilated:

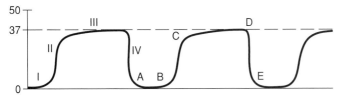

Figure 14.23. Normal capnogram; see text for details. Capnograms by permission of Jaffe MB and Novametrix Inc., Wallingford, CT. Courtesy of Philips-Respironics.

Table 14.3. Capnogram abnormalities by phase

Abnormality	Possible Causes
Phase I Increased FICO₂	Rebreathing of CO_2 (exhausted absorbent, channeling, incompetent inspiratory/expiratory unidirectional valve(s), CO_2 delivered to circuit in fresh gas flow (some machines have CO_2 flowmeters), CO_2 gas being delivered via N_2O pipeline, inadequate fresh gas flow in Mapleson (rebreathing) circuit, Bain circuit inner tube disconnect, capnograph analyzer not calibrated
Phase II Slow/slanted	Exhalation gas flow obstruction (mechanical or in patient), kinked tracheal tube, bronchospasm, gas sampling rate poorly matched to exhalation flow rate, exhaled CO_2 becomes more quickly diluted by fresh gas.
Phase III Irregular	Mechanical impingement on chest or abdomen by surgeons; patient attemping to breathe sponataeously while lungs are being mechanically ventilated ("curare cleft")
Regular	Cardiac oscillations; after exhalation complete, blood pulsating in chest moves gas forward and backward past sampling site. Slow decay of end-tidal gas sampling during expiratory pause causes CO_2 to be gradually diluted by fresh gas.
Phase IV	Widened, slurred downstroke, not reaching baseline Incompetent inspiratory valve; CO_2 accumulated in inspiratory limb mixed with fresh gas gradually replaced by fresh gas.

Source: By permission of Jaffe MB and Novametrix, Inc., Wallingford, CT. Courtesy of Philips-Respironics.

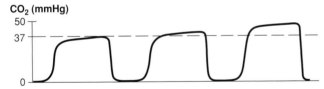

Figure 14.24. Abnormal capnogram: CO_2 increasing. Courtesy of Philips-Respironics.

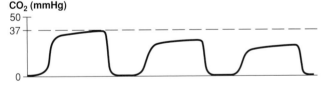

Figure 14.25. Abnormal capnogram: CO_2 decreasing. Courtesy of Philips-Respironics.

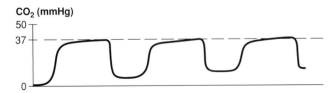

Figure 14.26. Abnormal capnogram: rebreathing of CO_2 Courtesy of Philips-Respironics.

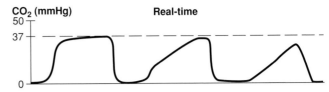

Figure 14.27. Abnormal capnogram: expiratory obstruction or bronchospasm. Courtesy of Philips-Respironics.

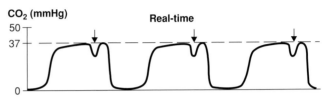

Figure 14.28. Abnormal capnogram: spontaneous efforts of breathing during positive-pressure ventilation ("curare clefts"). Courtesy of Philips-Respironics.

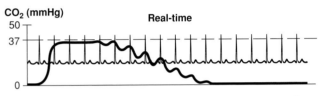

Figure 14.29. Abnormal capnogram: cardiac oscillations. Courtesy of Philips-Respironics.

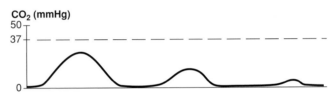

Figure 14.30. Abnormal capnogram: esophageal intubation. Courtesy of Philips-Respironics.

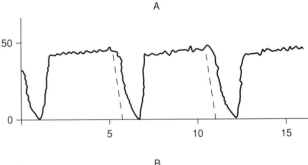

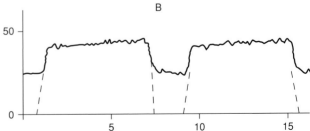

Figure 14.31. Abnormal capnogram: circle breathing system with (A) incompetent inspiratory valve; (B) incompetent expiratory valve. Note that there is more rebreathing of CO_2 with an incompetent expiratory valve. Courtesy of Philips-Respironics.

$PaCO_2$ 40 mmHg, end-tidal (alveolar, PA) CO_2 36 mmHg, tidal volume 500 mL, anatomical dead space 150 mL; therefore, alveolar tidal ventilation (VA) is $(500 - 150) = 350$ mL.

$$DSA/VA = (PaCO_2 - PACO_2)/PaCO_2$$
$$= (40 - 36)/40 = 10\%$$

Thus, $350 \times 10\% = 35$ mL of the alveolar tidal ventilation is alveolar dead space or wasted ventilation.

In addition to its use for confirming tracheal rather than esophageal intubation, and to make adjustments to ventilator settings, end-tidal CO_2 monitoring has been found to correlate well with cardiac output during low flow states. This has been applied in the evaluation of the efficacy of resuscitation efforts in cardiac arrest victims. Several studies have found that a low end-tidal CO_2 is associated with a poorer prognosis.[29,30]

Nitrogen

When available, measurement of nitrogen is useful in following preoxygenation (nitrogen washout) and detecting venous air embolism and air leaks into the anesthesia breathing system. Fortunately, alternative means are now available to perform these functions.

Potent inhaled anesthetic agents and nitrous oxide

Contemporary multigas analyzers measure the inspired and end-tidal concentrations of N_2O as well as the potent agents desflurane, enflurane, halothane, isoflurane, and sevoflurane in the presence of one another. Although no study has established the value of this monitoring modality, the possible applications make the potential benefits of its use obvious. Thus it makes possible the monitoring of anesthetic uptake and washout, as well as setting high and (if desired) low alarm limits for agent concentrations.

By adding the minimum alveolar concentration (MAC) values for N_2O and the potent agents to the analyzer software, and because MAC values are additive, once the composition of the gas mixture is known, a (total) MAC value can be displayed (Figure 14.21). This may be useful as an indication of anesthetic depth and a form of awareness monitoring.

Monitoring agent levels during uptake permits a safer and more intelligent use of the anesthesia vaporizer to reach target end-tidal concentrations in the patient. A high fresh gas flow and vaporizer concentration dial setting will ensure that the gas composition in the circuit changes rapidly; the technique of overpressure can be used to speed anesthetic uptake. When the desired end-tidal concentration has been attained, the vaporizer concentration dial setting can be decreased. When equilibrium has been reached – that is, inspired and end-tidal agent concentrations are almost equal – the fresh gas flow can be decreased to maintain the equilibrium and conserve anesthetic agent. Monitoring of the anesthetic concentration during elimination provides information as to the state of its washout. The washout rate might then be increased by increasing the fresh gas flow, and hence removal into the waste gas scavenging system.

The anesthetic agent high-concentration alarm can be used to alert to potential anesthetic overdosing. The ASA Closed Claims Project includes several adverse outcomes resulting from anesthetic overdose, and there are other reports of vaporizer malfunction leading to higher-than-intended output concentrations.[31,32] The low-concentration alarm can be used to help prevent awareness by maintaining an anesthetic agent concentration that exceeds MAC_{awake}. The latter is the average of the concentrations immediately above and below those permitting voluntary response to command.[33] MAC_{awake} is approximately one-third of MAC.[34] The anesthetic agent low-concentration alarm will also serve as a late sign that the vaporizer is becoming empty. An agent analyzer may also alert to an air leak into the breathing system that is causing an unintended low agent concentration.[35]

Assuming that the analyzer has been calibrated according to the manufacturer's instructions, it can be used to check the calibration of a vaporizer, as well as detect mixed agents in a vaporizer.

Monitoring of N_2O concentrations may be helpful when one is discontinuing or avoiding its administration. This may apply in patients who have closed air spaces that might expand with the use of N_2O.

The continuous analysis of all of the respired gases by a multigas monitor also facilitates recording of the data by an automated anesthesia information management system. Many anesthesia caregivers find it useful to record end-tidal concentrations of the gases administered. Monitoring of agent concentration, fresh gas flow, and time facilitates calculation of the consumption of the potent agents, both in liters of vapor or in milliliters of liquid agent. Attention to these data might be used to promote the more economical use of the more expensive anesthetics.

Complications

The complications associated with respiratory gas monitoring can be divided into two categories: pure equipment failure and use(r) error.[31]

As with any mechanical or electronic piece of equipment, failure can occur but, overall, the devices are very reliable if properly maintained. This includes any recommended maintenance and calibration procedures. Use(r) error is a much more common problem. The user must understand respiratory physiology, as well as the monitoring technology; otherwise, he or she may not recognize a spurious reading or may misinterpret data. This can lead to an inappropriate change in patient management. A simple example is that a low end-tidal CO_2 reading may cause the user to assume that the cause is hyperventilation and to decrease ventilation, when the problem is really a low cardiac output state.

In the event of total failure of the capnograph (electrical, mechanical, optical, and so forth) one should always keep a colorimetric CO_2 detector as an immediate backup. Because these devices have an expiration date shown on the packaging, they should be checked routinely and replaced as necessary. For greater accuracy, an arterial blood sample can be drawn for analysis in a blood gas analyzer.

Credentialing

At the time of writing, there is no specific credentialing requirement associated with the use of gas monitoring. All users should receive in-service training when a new monitor is introduced, and, in particular, they should understand and use the alarm features. Unfortunately, this is often not the case. There is no doubt that an educated user will derive more benefit than one who has less understanding of the equipment. In this regard, the Anesthesia Patient Safety Foundation (APSF) has sponsored a technology training initiative to promote critical training on new, sophisticated, or unfamiliar devices that can directly affect patient safety. [36]

Practice parameters

In 1986, the ASA first approved its Standards for Basic Anesthesia Monitoring. These have undergone periodic review and modification, the most recent being on October 20, 2010 with an effective date of July 1, 2011.[37]

The following bolded sections are quoted directly from Standard II of the ASA Standards for Basic Anesthetic Monitoring, and pertain to the contents of this chapter.

STANDARD II

During all anesthetics, the patient's oxygenation, ventilation, circulation and temperature shall be continually evaluated.

OXYGENATION
OBJECTIVE

To ensure adequate oxygen concentration in the inspired gas and the blood during all anesthetics.

METHODS

l) Inspired gas: During every administration of general anesthesia using an anesthesia machine, the concentration of oxygen in the patient breathing system shall be measured by an oxygen analyzer with a low oxygen concentration limit alarm in use.*

[† Note that "continual" is defined as "repeated regularly and frequently in steady rapid succession" whereas "continuous" means "prolonged without any interruption at any time."]

• Under extenuating circumstances, the responsible anesthesiologist may waive the requirements marked with an asterisk (*); it is recommended that when this is done, it should be so stated (including the reasons) in a note in the patient's medical record.]

The requirement to monitor the FIO_2 in the breathing system is not only one of the ASA standards, but it is also included in the health code regulations of some states, including New York[38] and New Jersey. The standard does not demand use of any specific technology to make the measurement, nor does it specify where in the inspiratory path oxygen must be monitored. Thus it is common to have a fuel cell located in the inspiratory unidirectional valve housing, but downstream (on the patient side) of the valve. It is also acceptable to sample gas from a connector by the patient's airway at the Y-piece for oxygen analysis in a multigas analyzer.

VENTILATION
OBJECTIVE

To ensure adequate ventilation of the patient during all anesthetics.

METHODS

l) Every patient receiving general anesthesia shall have the adequacy of ventilation continually evaluated. Qualitative clinical signs such as chest excursion, observation of the reservoir breathing bag and auscultation of breath sounds are useful. Continual monitoring for the presence of expired carbon dioxide shall be performed unless invalidated by the nature of the patient, procedure or equipment. Quantitative monitoring of the volume of expired gas is strongly encouraged.*

When an endotracheal tube or laryngeal mask is inserted, its correct positioning must be verified by clinical assessment and by identification of carbon dioxide in the expired gas. Continual end-tidal carbon dioxide analysis, in use from the time of endotracheal tube/laryngeal mask placement, until extubation/removal or initiating transfer to a postoperative care location, shall be performed using a quantitative method such as capnography, capnometry or mass spectroscopy.* When capnography or capnometry is utilized, the end tidal CO_2 alarm shall be audible to the anesthesiologist or the anesthesia care team personnel.*

3) When ventilation is controlled by a mechanical ventilator, there shall be in continuous use a device that is capable of detecting disconnection of components of the breathing system. The device must give an audible signal when its alarm threshold is exceeded.

4) During regional anesthesia (with no sedation) or local anesthesia (with no sedation), the adequacy of ventilation shall be evaluated by continual observation of qualitative clinical signs. During moderate or deep sedation the adequacy of ventilation shall be evaluated by continual observation of qualitative clinical signs and monitoring for the presence of exhaled carbon dioxide unless precluded or invalidated by the nature of the patient, procedure, or equipment.

The ASA standards applicable to CO_2 monitoring have evolved considerably since they were first written. In particular, they have been revised to include use of the laryngeal mask airway (a supraglottic airway device), as well as use in regional anesthesia and monitored anesthesia care. Note that in item 3, the capnograph could be considered a disconnect detection device and as such must be used with an audible alarm activated. Catastrophes have been reported when state-of-the-art monitoring has been used, but with the alarms silenced.[39]

At the time of this writing, there is no ASA standard that requires monitoring of N_2O and the potent inhaled anesthetics. However, as use of this monitoring becomes more widespread, it may become a de facto standard.[40] The manufacturers of anesthesia workstations anticipate this trend; the most recent American Society for Testing and Materials (ASTM) voluntary consensus standard requires that the anesthesia workstation be provided with a device to monitor the concentration of anesthetic vapor in the inspired gas.[41]

The ASA standards for postanesthesia care (last updated in 2004)[42] do not require monitoring of gas concentrations.

ASA STANDARDS FOR POSTANESTHESIA CARE

STANDARD IV

THE PATIENT'S CONDITION SHALL BE EVALUATED CONTINUALLY IN THE PACU.

1. The patient shall be observed and monitored by methods appropriate to the patient's medical condition. Particular attention should be given to monitoring oxygenation, ventilation, circulation, level of consciousness and temperature. During recovery from all anesthetics, a quantitative method of assessing oxygenation such as pulse oximetry shall be employed in the initial phase of recovery.* This is not intended for application during the recovery of the obstetrical patient in whom regional anesthesia was used for labor and vaginal delivery.

In many postanesthesia care units (PACUs), however, capnometry is used in patients who are tracheally intubated. If a patient requires reintubation, means to confirm tracheal placement of the tube should be available and its use documented.

Acknowledgment

The author is grateful to Dr. Daniel Raemer and Dr. Michael Jaffe for reviewing this chapter and for their valuable contributions.

References

1. Mushlin PS, Mark JB, Elliott WR et al. Inadvertent development of subatmospheric airway pressure during cardiopulmonary bypass. *Anesthesiology* 1989;**71**:459–62.
2. Pattinson K, Myers S, Gardner-Thorpe C. Problems with capnography at high altitude. *Anaesthesia* 2004;**59**:69–72.
3. Ozanne GM, Young WG, Mazzei WJ, et al. Multipatient anesthetic mass spectrometry. *Anesthesiology* 1981;**55**:62-7.
4. Eisenkraft JB, Raemer DB. Monitoring gases in the anesthesia delivery system. In Ehrenwerth J, Eisenkraft JB, eds. *Anesthesia Equipment: Principles and Applications*. St. Louis: Mosby-Year Book, 1993, p. 210.
5. Steinbrook RA, Elliott WR, Goldman DB, Philip JH. Linking mass spectrometers to provide continuing monitoring during system failure. *J Clin Monit* 1991;**7**:271–3.
6. Severinghaus JW, Larson CP, Eger EI. Correction factors for infrared carbon dioxide pressure broadening by nitrogen, nitrous oxide, and cyclopropane. *Anesthesiology* 1961;**22**:429–32.
7. Nielsen JR, Thornton V, Dale EB. The absorption laws for gases in the infrared. *Rev Mod Physics* 1944;**16**:307–24.
8. Raemer DB, Philip JH. Monitoring anesthetic and respiratory gases. In Blitt CD, ed. *Monitoring in Anesthesia and Critical Care Medicine*, New York: Churchill-Livingstone, 1990, pp. 373–86.
9. PB 254 Owners Manual. Puritan-Bennett Corp., Wilmington, MA, 1985.
10. Datex-Ohmeda Compact Airway Modules Technical Reference Manual. Document 800 1009–5. Datex-Ohmeda Division, Instrumentarium Corp., Finland, 2003 (accessed February 20, 2011).
11. Møllgaard K. Acoustic gas measurement. *Biomed Instr Technol* 1989;**23**:495–7.
12. Westenskow DR, Smith KW, Coleman DL, et al. Clinical evaluation of a Raman scattering multiple gas analyzer for the operating room. *Anesthesiology* 1989;**70**:350–5.
13. Colman Y, Krauss B. Microstream capnography technology: a new approach to an old problem. *J Clin Monit Comput* 1999;**15**:403–9.
14. Casati A, Gallioli A, Passarretta P, Borgi B, Torri G. Accuracy of end-tidal carbon dioxide monitoring using the NPB 75 Microstream capnometer. A study in intubated, ventilated and spontaneously breathing nonintubated patients. *Eur J Anaesthesiol* 2000;**17**:622–6.
15. Severinghaus JW. Water vapor calibration errors in some capnometers: respiratory conventions misunderstood by manufacturers? *Anesthesiology* 1989;**70**:996–8.
16. Sum Ping ST, Mehta MP, Symreng T. Accuracy of the FEF CO_2 detector in the assessment of endotracheal tube placement. *Anesth Analg* 1992;**74**:415–9.
17. Srinivasa V, Kodali BS. Caution when using colorimetry to confirm endotracheal intubation. *Anesth Analg* 2007;**104**: 738.
18. Brackney SM, Bennett NP. Caution when using colorimetry to confirm endotracheal intubation. *Anesth Analg* 2007;**104**:739.
19. Fontijn A, Sabadell AJ. Ronco RJ. Homogeneous chemiluminescent measurement of nitric oxide with ozone. *Analyt Chem* 1979;**42**:575–9.
20. Holland R. Wrong gas disaster in Hong Kong. *APSF Newsletter* 1989;**4**:25–36.
21. Berry CB, Myles PS. Preoxygenation in healthy volunteers: a graph of oxygen "washin" using end-tidal oxygraphy. *Br J Anaesth* 1994;**74**:116–8.
22. Barnard JP, Sleigh JW. Breath-by-breath analysis of oxygen uptake using the Datex Ultima. *Br J Anaesth* 1995;**74**: 155–8.
23. Takala J. Meriläinen P. *Handbook of Indirect Calorimetry and Gas Exchange*. Helsinki, Finland: Datex-Ohmeda, 876710–01, 2001, p. 30.
24. Takala J. Appliguide. *Clinical application guide of gas exchange and indirect calorimetry*. Helsinki, Finland: Datex-Ohmeda 895143–1, 2000.
25. Birmingham PK, Cheney FW, Ward RJ. Esophageal intubation: a review of detection techniques. *Anesth Analg* 1986;**65**:886–91.
26. Gravenstein JS, Jaffe MB, Paulus DA. *Capnography: Clinical Aspects*. New York: Cambridge University Press, 2004.
27. Smalhout B, Kalenda Z. *An Atlas of Capnography*. 2nd ed. Utrecht, The Netherlands: Kerkebosche Zeist, 1981.
28. Nunn JF. *Applied Respiratory Physiology*. Boston: Butterworths, 1977, p. 226.
29. Sanders AB, Kern KB, Otto CW Milander MM, Ewy GA. End-tidal CO_2 monitoring during CPR. A prognostic indicator for survival. *JAMA* 1989;**262**:1347–51.
30. Wayne ME, Levine RL, Miller CC. Use of end-tidal CO_2 to predict outcome in pre-hospital cardiac arrest. *Ann Emerg Med* 1995;**25**:762–7.
31. Caplan RA, Vistica MF, Posner KL, Cheney FW. Adverse anesthetic outcomes arising from gas delivery equipment: a closed claims analysis. *Anesthesiology* 1997;**87**:741–8.

32. Geffroy JC, Gentili ME, Le Pollès R, Triclot P. Massive inhalation of desflurane due to vaporizer dysfunction. *Anesthesiology* 2005;**103**:1096–8.

33. Stoelting RK, Longnecker DE, Eger EI II. Minimal alveolar concentrations on awakening from methoxyflurane, halothane, ether and fluroxene in man: MAC awake. *Anesthesiology* 1970;**33**:5–9.

34. Eger EI II, Weisskopf RB, Eisenkraft JB. *The Pharmacology of Inhaled Anesthetics*. San Antonio, TX: Dannemiller Memorial Educational Foundation, 2002, p. 27.

35. Sandberg WS, Kaiser S. Novel breathing system architecture: new consequences of old problems. *Anesthesiology* 2004;**100**: 755–6.

36. Olympio MA. Formal training and assessment before using advanced medical devices in the OR. *APSF Newsletter* 2007;**22**:63–65.

37. American Society of Anesthesiologists. *Standards for Basic Anesthetic Monitoring*. http://www.asahq.org/publications AndServices/standards/02.pdf (accessed February 20, 2011).

38. NY State Laws and regulations,section 405.13. Anesthesia services (b)(2)(iii)(d).

39. $16 million settlement. Monitoring devices turned off/down: patient suffers irreversible brain damage. *Anesthesia Malpractice Prevention Newsletter* 1997;**2**(3)1.

40. Eichhorn JH. Pulse oximetry as a standard of practice in anesthesia. *Anesthesiology* 1993;**78**:423–5.

41. *Standard Specification for Particular Requirements for Anesthesia Workstations and their Components ASTM F1850–2005*. West Conshohocken, PA: American Society for Testing and Materials, 2005.

42. ASA Standards for postanesthesia care. http://www.asahq.org/ publicationsAndServices/standards/36.pdf.

Monitoring pressure, volume, and flow in the anesthesia breathing system

James B. Eisenkraft

Introduction

The anesthesia breathing system is an enclosed environment with which the patient makes respiratory gas exchange. By controlling the composition of the gases in the breathing circuit, as well as ventilatory parameters, the anesthesia caregiver can control the tensions of oxygen, carbon dioxide, nitrogen, and the inhaled anesthetics in the patient's arterial blood. Monitoring of the respired gases has been discussed in Chapter 14. This chapter addresses the monitoring of pressures, volumes, and gas flows in the breathing system. Monitoring of these parameters is important in enhancing the safety of ventilation and verifying the appropriateness of ventilatory settings.

Measurement of respiratory pressures, volumes, and flows

Pressure

Pressure is defined as force per unit area (e.g. pounds per square inch), although the units of the denominator are often omitted, as they are assumed to be understood (as in mmHg or cmH_2O). Pressures are usually measured using either a simple mechanical device or an electromechanical transducer.

Simple analog gauges have been commonly used to measure and display breathing system pressure. These gauges are termed *aneroid* (meaning without fluid) gauges. The gauge may be based on a Bourdon tube (Figure 15.1), diaphragm, or bellows (Figure 15.2). In the Bourdon tube design, an indicator needle mechanism is attached to the closed, free end of a curved piece of flattened soft metal tubing. The open end of the tubing is in communication with the breathing circuit. Pressure in the circuit causes the flattened tubing to become more circular. This causes the tubing to uncoil and move the indicator needle mechanism (Figure 15.1). A small adjustment screw is often used to align the indicator needle to the zero-pressure mark when the gauge is exposed to atmosphere. A high-quality Bourdon tube is accurate and reliable, and requires no mechanical stop at zero. Excessive pressures can bend the malleable tubing or indicator needle mechanism, thus rendering the device inoperable, but such pressures are unlikely to be encountered in a breathing system. The gauge is usually calibrated to measure negative as well as positive pressures.

The principle of the bellows pressure gauge is that the volume of a bellows changes according to the pressure that is applied to it. If the bellows is sealed, its volume is a function of the ambient or surrounding pressure (Figure 15.2A). If the interior of the bellows is in communication with the breathing system, the volume of the bellows is determined by the difference in pressures across the bellows (Figure 15.2B), and is termed *gauge pressure*.

The advantage of the analog pressure gauge is that it is simple and mechanical, and requires no warmup time or electrical energy to function. Such gauges were widely used on traditional anesthesia machines. Disadvantages are that they cannot be interfaced with electronic anesthesia care stations or to trigger alarms. Although modern electronic anesthesia care stations use sophisticated electronic pressure transducers to measure pressures, some manufacturers still offer a mechanical analog gauge as an optional extra.

Contemporary anesthesia workstations use electromechanical transducers to measure pressure. When used in combination with pneumotachometers, Pitot tubes, or variable orifices, the pressure measurements can be used to measure gas flows and volumes. The most common electromechanical transducer is the metal or semiconductor strain gauge. When a metal wire or thin segment of semiconductor material is stretched within its elastic limit, its resistance is altered because of dimensional changes and a change in the material's resistivity. The change in

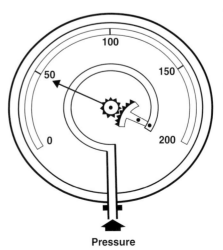

Figure 15.1. Bourdon tube pressure gauge. From Davis PD, Parbrook GD, Kenny GNC. *Basic Physics and Measurement in Anesthesia*, 4th ed. Boston: Butterworth Heinemann, 1995, with permission.

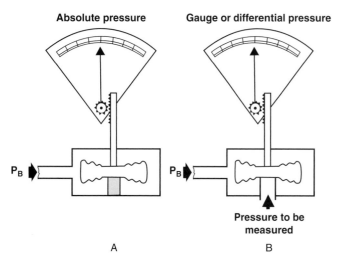

Figure 15.2. Bellows-based pressure gauges. A: The bellows is sealed and therefore measures absolute or atmospheric pressure (P_B). B: The bellows is connected to the system whose pressure is to be measured and therefore measures pressure in relation to ambient (P_B). From Davis PD, Parbrook GD, Kenny GNC. *Basic Physics and Measurement in Anesthesia*, 4th ed. Boston: Butterworth Heinemann, 1995, with permission.

resistivity is called the *piezoresistive effect*. Fine wires made from such alloys as constantan, nichrome, and karma are particularly appropriate for metal strain gauges. In one common design, the bonded-wire strain gauge, the wires are cemented to a backing (Figure 15.3). A flexible diaphragm attached to the bonded-wire strain gauge is exposed to the pressure to be measured on one side and the ambient pressure on the other. As the diaphragm bends, the wires are stretched and the change in resistance corresponding to the change in pressure is measured.

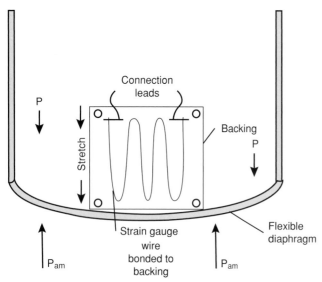

Figure 15.3. Bonded wire strain gauge. A length of metal strain gauge wire is cemented to a backing that is fixed at one end. As pressure is applied to the flexible diaphragm, the backing and strain gauge wire are stretched. The change in resistance of the wire is measured and displayed as a change in pressure. P, applied pressure; P_{am}, ambient pressure. From Raemer DB. Monitoring ventilation. In Ehrenwerth J, Eisenkraft JB. *Anesthesia Equipment: Principles and Applications*. St. Louis: Mosby Year Book, 1993.

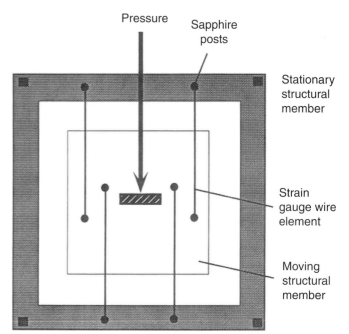

Figure 15.4. Top view of an unbonded-wire strain gauge. Lengths of strain gauge wire are stretched between posts on two supporting structural members. The outer structural member is stationary. When pressure is applied in the direction of the arrow, the center structural member moves incrementally. One pair of strain gauge wires is stretched further, and the other is relaxed. The resulting change in resistance of the four elements is measured using a Wheatstone bridge circuit and displayed as pressure. From Raemer DB. Monitoring ventilation. In Ehrenwerth J, Eisenkraft JB. *Anesthesia Equipment: Principles and Applications*. St. Louis: Mosby Year Book, 1993, with permission.

In another design (Figure 15.4), two pairs of wires are attached to posts of two structural members that can move with respect to each other. One of the structural members is mechanically attached to a pressure-sensing diaphragm. When the diaphragm moves as a response to applied pressure, two of the wires are stretched and the other pair is relaxed. The changes in the resistances of the four wires are then measured using a Wheatstone bridge circuit.

In the semiconductor strain gauge, the materials used are usually crystals of silicon or germanium. A flexible diaphragm is etched into the crystal by integrated circuit techniques. A system of four silicon elements is produced in the diaphragm in such a way that the elements change predictably in resistance value as the diaphragm is deformed. During manufacture, the resistance elements are trimmed dimensionally with a laser, and so no further calibration is required.

The advantage of semiconductor materials is that they exhibit 50 to 100 times the change in resistance per unit of strain compared to metals.[1] However, the temperature sensitivity is substantially greater in semiconductor gauges, and accurate compensation is a major factor in their design.

In both the metal and semiconductor strain gauges, the change in resistance of the elements is measured via an electrical circuit called a Wheatstone bridge (Figure 15.5). This arrangement is particularly useful for several reasons. First, the Wheatstone bridge allows the simultaneous measurement of resistance

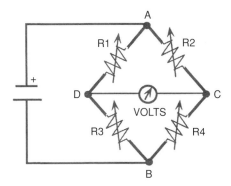

Figure 15.5. Wheatstone bridge circuit used for strain gauge transducers. Voltage from a battery is applied between points A and B. One or more of the variable resistors shown (R1–R4) are resistance elements of the transducer. The remaining resistor values are selected so that the voltage difference measured between points C and D is very small, or "balanced," when zero pressure is applied to the transducer. As the pressure applied to the transducer changes, the bridge becomes "unbalanced," and a voltage appears between points C and D. Appropriate selection of resistance elements and temperature-sensitive elements as resistors in the Wheatstone bridge can result in highly sensitive, temperature-compensated measurement. From Raemer DB. Monitoring ventilation. In Ehrenwerth J, Eisenkraft JB. *Anesthesia Equipment: Principles and Applications.* St. Louis: Mosby Year Book, 1993, with permission.

changes in multiple elements when they are used as legs of the bridge. Second, temperature compensation can be incorporated directly into the bridge by way of metal or semiconductor elements that are sensitive to temperature but not exposed to the strain. Third, a small change in resistance can be measured as a relative change in voltage near zero between the two balance points of the bridge.

Volume and flow

Flow is defined as volume per unit of time; therefore, measurement of flow and time permits calculation of volume. Like pressure, flow can be measured using a simple mechanical device or by electronic means.

Mechanical

The simplest flow measurement device is the vane anemometer. This was originally introduced into respiratory measurement by B. Martin Wright in England.[2] Using adaptors, this is a freestanding device that can be inserted into the breathing system, where it is commonly used to measure tidal volume and minute ventilation. This device uses a low-mass rotating vane in the gas stream (Figure 15.6). Gas molecules colliding with the blades of the vane transfer their momentum in the direction of flow and cause the vane to rotate. In the mechanical version, the rotation of the vane is connected to the dial via a gear mechanism, similar to that in a watch. In an electronic implementation (Figure 15.7), two pairs of light-emitting diodes (LEDs) and silicon photodetectors are used to measure the rate and direction of the vane's rotation. The rotation rate is integrated electronically to determine the volume of gas passing the transducer over time.

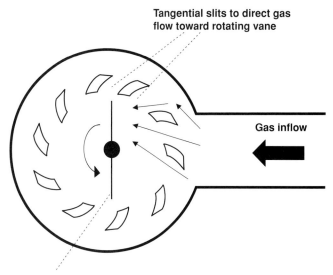

Figure 15.6. Wright's respirometer. Respired gas is directed through oblique slots in a small cylinder enclosing a small vane that is made to rotate. The spindle on which the vane is mounted drives a gear train connected to a pointer that moves over a dial indicating the volume of gas passed. Gases that flow back through the device do not register because they enter along the axis of the vane spindle.

A number of physical factors limit the accuracy of the vane anemometer.[3] Because the principle of operation is momentum, the density of the gas affects the measurement. The gas flow is directed to the blades of the vane by tangential slots; thus, the viscosity of the gas also influences the measurement. Additionally, inertia and momentum of the vane are problematic. Accuracy is poor at low flows because of inertia, and at high flows because of momentum. Pulsatile flows also cause overreading. The accuracy of the Wright respirometer has been shown to be within ± 10 percent during anesthesia. The respirometer is compact and is easily placed between the breathing system and the patient. However, the mechanical version cannot measure bidirectional flow and, because it is mechanical, it has no alarms.

A sealed mechanical volumeter (Figure 15.8) was used by Dräger in some older delivery systems to measure tidal volume and minute ventilation. This device consists of a pair of rotating elements in the gas flow path, configured much like a revolving door at the entrance to a building. A fixed volume of gas is passed across the volumeter with each quarter-rotation of the dumbbell-shaped elements. A seal is formed between the polystyrene rotating elements and the interior wall of the tube. The sealed volumeter provides substantially more resistance to flow than does the vane anemometer. The accuracy of the volumeter is affected by gas density and by the inertia of the rotating elements. However, it is not influenced substantially by the flow pattern of the gas. The number of fixed volumes of gas transferred from inlet to outlet is measured mechanically.

The Dräger Spiromed is an electronic version of the mechanical spirometer. Gas flow through the device determines the rate of rotation of the rotors, which is measured

173

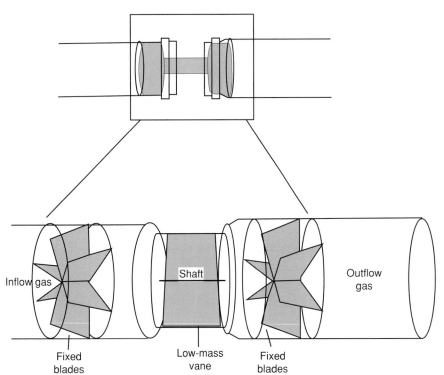

Figure 15.7. Vane anemometer. Gas flow is directed by fixed vanes at the inlet, and the swirling gas causes rotation of a low-mass vane. LEDs are positioned to detect the revolutions of the vane, which are converted into a measurement of flow. This type of anemometer is used in the spirometer on the Ohmeda Modulus anesthesia machines. From Raemer DB. Monitoring ventilation. In Ehrenwerth J, Eisenkraft JB. *Anesthesia Equipment: Principles and Applications.* St. Louis: Mosby Year Book, 1993, with permission.

using an electromagnetic sensing system. The Spiromed is direction-sensitive, and can alert to reversal of gas flow in the circle system. The accuracy of the Spiromed for tidal volumes is ± 40 mL, and for minute ventilation, ± 100 mL or ± 10 percent of the reading.

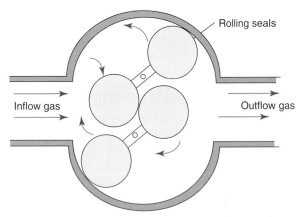

Figure 15.8. Sealed volumeter. Polystyrene rotating elements form a seal against the interior of the volumeter. Gas flow causes rotation of the elements, transferring fixed volumes of gas from the inlet to the outlet. Measured volume is displayed on a gauge that is mechanically connected to the rotating shaft of the volumeter. The device is bidirectional, and can alert to reversed flow. If the number of fixed volumes of gas transferred is measured electronically, measured volume may be read on a remote display, as well as being connected to an alarm system. This is the principle of operation of the Dräger Spiromed. From Raemer DB. Monitoring ventilation. In Ehrenwerth J, Eisenkraft JB. *Anesthesia Equipment: Principles and Applications.* St. Louis: Mosby Year Book, 1993, with permission.

Pneumotachometer

The principle of operation of the pneumotachometer is to measure the loss of energy of the flowing gas as it passes through a resistive element. The resistive element is designed to ensure that the flow of gas is laminar so the energy loss is completely the result of viscosity and the flow is directly proportional to the pressure difference. The energy loss is measured as a pressure difference from the inlet to the outlet of the resistive element. The most common type of resistive element, designed by Fleish,[4] consists of narrow, parallel metal tubes aligned in the direction of the flow (Figure 15.9). Nominally, for laminar flow, the pneumotachometer obeys the Hagen-Poiseuille law:

$$F = [\pi \times r^4 \times (P1 - P2]/[8 \times \eta \times L],$$

where F = gas flow, r and L = radius and length of the element, P1 and P2 = inlet and outlet pressures, and η = viscosity of gas flowing through the device. Measurement of flow is independent of gas density and total pressure.

Fleish pneumotachometers have been used widely in respiratory physiology and pulmonary function studies, and are available in various sizes (resistances) to accommodate the appropriate flow range. The resistance of the element must be chosen so the pressure difference produced in the flow range of interest is large enough to be measured accurately by the available pressure transducer(s). Too resistive an element will impede ventilation. The Fleish pneumotachometer usually uses a heating element to raise the temperature of the device to about 40°C, thus preventing condensation of moisture in expired gas.

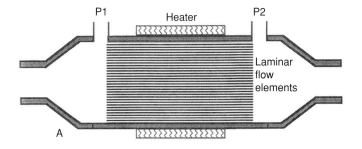

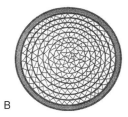

Figure 15.9. Cross-sectional views of a Fleisch pneumotachometer. (A) Longitudinal section showing the parallel paths that constitute the laminar flow resistance element. Ports P1 and P2 are used for measurement of the pressure differential across the resistance element. The device can be used bidirectionally. The heating element surrounds the device and is used to prevent condensation. (B) Cross-sectional view of laminar flow elements. From Raemer DB. Monitoring ventilation. In Ehrenwerth J, Eisenkraft JB. *Anesthesia Equipment: Principles and Applications.* St. Louis: Mosby Year Book, 1993, with permission.

The pressure difference across the resistive element (or head) is measured using a differential pressure transducer with sufficient sensitivity and frequency response. The transducer must be zeroed (nulled) electronically by reserving a measurement made with zero flow. The pressure difference is typically in the range of 2 cmH_2O. Pressure transducer output readings tend to drift, and the measured signal is small; therefore, they must be renulled periodically. For vigorous ventilatory flows, the rate of change in gas flow is great, and the frequency response of the transducer must be adequate to follow these changes.

The respiratory volume is computed by integrating the flow with respect to time (because flow = volume/time). The pneumotachometer is calibrated by setting a gain coefficient according to a volume produced by manually emptying a calibrated (usually 1 L) syringe through the device. Often, the calibration syringe is emptied several times at different rates to simulate the range of gas flows expected during clinical use. In practice, the characteristics of the Fleish pneumotachometer are dependent on the geometry of the tubing on the upstream side of the resistive element. This results in a distinctly nonlinear deviation from the Hagen-Poiseuille law.

The viscosity of gases in the respiratory mixture must be taken into consideration if measurement of flow is to be accurate. Consider that the viscosity of a gas mixture of 88.81 percent oxygen, 1.61 percent nitrogen, and 9.58 percent carbon dioxide is 9.1 percent greater than that of air. Thus, substantial errors can result if gas viscosity is not taken into consideration. Temperature is considered to have a linear effect on the viscosity of

respiratory gases in the range of 20°C to 40°C, although the linear coefficient is different for each gas.

The other disadvantage of the pneumotachometer in an anesthesia circuit is its propensity to accumulate mucus and water in its narrow tubes. It must be repeatedly calibrated because its effective resistance changes with fouling. In addition, the pneumotachometer must be cleaned and sterilized between clinical uses.

Pitot tube flowmeter

The Pitot tube measures the difference in kinetic energy of the gas impinging on a pressure port facing in the direction of the gas flow and on a pressure port perpendicular to the flow.[5] The pressure difference, nominally proportional to the square of the flow rate, is sensitive to the density of the gas. Viscous losses around the pressure ports and small pressure differences at low flows are limitations of the Pitot tube flowmeter (Figure 15.10).

The GE-Datex Sidestream Spirometry system, as used in the GE S/5 Physiologic Monitoring Systems, represents a combination of Pitot tube and pneumotachograph technologies, with gas analysis technology that provides the gas density and viscosity data required for accuracy. This system uses a patented D-Lite adapter (Figure 15.11) that is placed in the breathing system between the Y-piece and the patient's airway. The D-Lite adapter has two Pitot tubes, one facing upstream in the direction of gas flow to measure total pressure (Pt), the other facing downstream in the opposite direction to measure static pressure (Ps; Figure 15.12). The difference (Pt – Ps) is the dynamic pressure, which is proportional to the square of the gas flow rate (see equations that follow).

$$(Pt - Ps) \propto (flow^2 \times density)/4,$$
$$flow^2 \times density \propto 4 \times (Pt - Ps),$$
$$flow \propto 2 \times [(Pt - Ps)/density]^{0.5}.$$

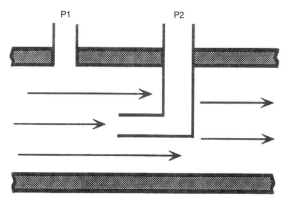

Figure 15.10. Longitudinal cross-section of a Pitot tube flowmeter. The pressure P2 measured at port P2 facing the flow direction is greater than P1 because of the kinetic energy of the gas impinging on the port. The pressure difference (P2-P1) is proportional to the square of the flow rate. From Raemer DB. Monitoring ventilation. In Ehrenwerth J, Eisenkraft JB. *Anesthesia Equipment: Principles and Applications.* St. Louis: Mosby Year Book, 1993, with permission.

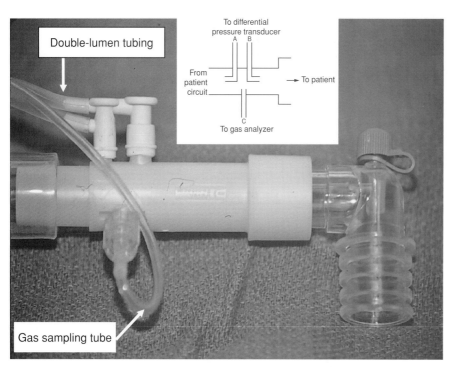

Figure 15.11. D-Lite sidestream spirometry adapter (GE Datex-Ohmeda), placed between the Y-piece of breathing system and the connector to the patient's airway device (tracheal tube, LMA, etc.). The double-lumen tubing connects the Pitot tubes to the differential pressure-sensing elements in the monitoring module.

During inspiration, as gas flows toward the patient's airway, the pressure difference between the two Pitot tubes is measured continuously. During exhalation, gas flow through the adapter is reversed and the pressure difference similarly measured. The D-Lite adapter's two Pitot tubes are connected to the pressure transducers in the monitoring module via a length of noncompliant double-lumen tubing (Figure 15.11). The D-Lite has a third port, to which a gas sampling line that leads to the respiratory gas analyzer in the monitoring module is connected. The continuous analysis of gas composition supplies the density data required for the flow calculation shown earlier.

The Pitot tube flowmeter actually measures gas flow velocity, which can be converted to a volume flow rate if the cross-sectional area of the adapter is known. D-Lite adapters are available in two sizes: the adult (dead space volume 9.5 mL) measures tidal volumes of 150 to 2000 mL; the pediatric (Pedi-Lite, dead space 2.5 mL) measures tidal volumes of 15 to 300 mL. Because the two sizes have different cross-sectional areas, the user must ensure that the compact airway gas monitoring module is set appropriately. Erroneous spirometry data result if the sensor size does not correspond with the appropriate software setting.

Advantages of the sidestream spirometry system are that it provides continuous data of many respiratory parameters (tidal volume, minute ventilation, airway pressures, compliance, and flow-volume and pressure-volume loops) measured at the patient's airway. The readings are therefore not affected by changes in compliance in the breathing system. The adapters are robust and disposable. Disadvantages are that the pressure-sensing (double-lumen) tubes are bulky and may easily become disconnected from the airway adapter, causing a leak. Moisture, condensation, or obstruction in one or both of the tubes results in spurious readings.

Hot wire anemometer

The hot wire anemometer is the technology of the flow sensors used on certain models of Dräger (Fabius, Apollo) and Datascope (Anestar) anesthesia workstations (Figure 15.13). The principle of operation is that the gas whose flow is to be measured flows past a thin wire that is heated to maintain a constant temperature. The flowing gas cools the wire, necessitating an increase in current flow through the wire to maintain a constant temperature. The heating current required is therefore

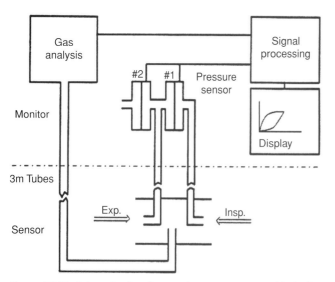

Figure 15.12. Schematic of gas flow sensing arrangement used in the D-Lite airway adapter shown in Figure 15.11. Data from the differential pressure transducers and from the gas analyzer are used to compute flow and volume.

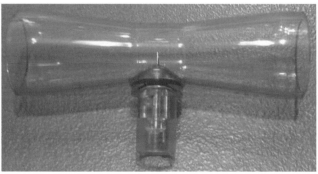 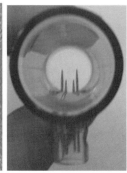

Side view   End-on view

Figure 15.13. Hot wire anemometer sensing adapter as used in the Dräger 6400 anesthesia workstation.

related to gas flow. To make the device sensitive to gas flow direction, two wires are used, one upstream and the other downstream of gas flow. Changes in gas composition (density) affect the accuracy of this design of flowmeter. These data are provided to the measurement system from the gas analysis data. Hot wire anemometry is also used internally in the GE Aisys Carestation to measure fresh gas flow.[6]

Ultrasonic flow sensor

The ultrasonic flow sensor is used on certain models of Dräger anesthesia workstations (e.g. Narkomed 6400). Ultrasonic flow measurement uses the transit time principle, whereby opposite sending and receiving transducers are used to transmit signals through the gas flow. The signal travels faster when moving with the flow stream rather than against the flow stream. The difference between the two transit times is used to calculate the gas flow rate. The device is sensitive to gas flow direction and has no moving parts, and accuracy is independent of gas flow composition.

Variable orifice flow sensor

This design is used on many of the GE (Datex-Ohmeda) delivery systems that are equipped with the 7900 Smartvent series ventilators (e.g., Aestiva, Aespire, Avance, Aisys). As the name implies, the pressure difference across a variable-size orifice is used to infer gas flow (Figure 15.14). The GE workstations use two such flow sensors, one just downstream of the inspiratory unidirectional valve, and the other on the patient side of the expiratory unidirectional valve. Each flow sensor is a plastic tube that has a Mylar (which is MRI compatible) or stainless steel flap (autoclavable) that opens wider as gas flow increases. This creates a pressure difference across the flap. On each side of the flap is a sensor line that is connected to a differential pressure transducer. At very low flows, the flap is in its natural state, forming a small slit orifice. This small orifice allows an easily measurable differential pressure signal to be generated, despite the low flow. As the gas flow increases, the flap opens more, reducing resistance to gas flow. At a given flow rate, the differential pressure across the deflected (more open) flap is lower than at its natural position. There is a one-to-one correspondence between each flow rate and the pressure difference that it creates. This allows the differential pressure measurement to be uniquely converted to the gas flow rate. Furthermore, the variable orifice straightens the pressure-flow characteristic to provide linear and uniform measurement sensitivity through its measured range. The output of the transducer is used to calculate gas flow rate and, thereby, tidal volume. Because movement of the flap is bidirectional, the direction of the pressure gradient is used to determine the direction of gas flow.

The inspiratory flow sensor measures the pressure in the breathing system and the volume of gas entering the inspiratory limb of the circle system during inspiration. If the measured volume differs from that set to be delivered by the ventilator, the information is used to increase or decrease delivered tidal volume. This Smartvent feature ensures a constant tidal volume despite changes in fresh gas flow and I:E ratio.

The expiratory limb flow sensor measures gas flow returning to the machine. The tidal volumes and minute ventilation obtained from this sensor are used to detect and alarm on low minute ventilation and apnea. This flow sensor also acts as a safety check to constantly monitor the appropriate volume delivered by the ventilator; the alarm sounds when the expired gas volume varies significantly from the setting. Such variations may be caused by leaks, or by valve or flow sensor issues.

Moisture is an inherent byproduct of carbon dioxide absorption in the circle breathing system, especially in low flow anesthesia practice. Moisture may cause small beads of water or a foggy appearance in the flow sensor, which does affect performance. Pooled water in the flow sensor or water in the sensing lines could result in false readings.[6]

During the preuse checkout of the GE electronic workstations, the compliance of the breathing system is measured. When this information is stored in the ventilator software, the pressure and flow measurements obtained by the inspiratory flow sensor can be used to display continuous flow-volume and pressure-volume loops, as well as display TV, MV, PEEP, and total thoracic compliance. These flow sensors are reliable, but accuracy may be affected by gas composition. The pressure transducers must be zeroed at the beginning of each day as part of the preuse checkout. Inaccuracies, or even failures, may occur

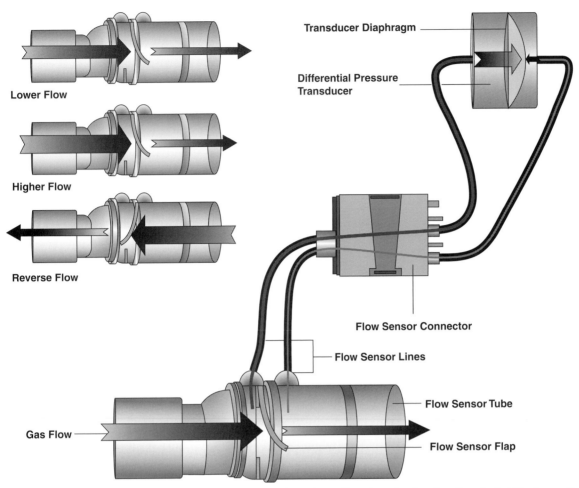

Figure 15.14. Principle of variable orifice flow sensor, as used by the GE Datex_Ohmeda workstations (e.g. Aisys, Aestiva). The flap position changes according to gas flow and gas flow direction. The pressure difference across the flap is used to determine flow. From EXPLORE Aisys (GE Datex Ohmeda) by permission.

when humidity condenses in the pressure transducer tubing. Because the transducers are hidden in the machine, a leak in the breathing system because of a cracked transducer may not be obvious to the caregiver.

Information derived from measuring pressure, flow, and volume

From the preceding discussion it will be recognized that the two basic measurements made on contemporary anesthesia workstations are pressure and flow. Volume is derived from measuring flow and time. Measurement of pressure(s) provides much information.

The simple continuous monitoring of breathing system pressure permits the real-time display of a plot of breathing system pressure against time, as well as numerical display of baseline, peak, and plateau pressures. Appropriate alarm limits can then be set. Breathing system pressure monitors were the original disconnect monitors during positive-pressure ventilation. In the event of a disconnection, pressure fell to zero (atmospheric) and, if the limits had been properly set, an alarm would be annunciated (Figure 15.15). The most important pres-

sure to be monitored is that at the patient's airway. It is therefore important to know the location in the breathing system at which pressure is sensed. If it is at a location remote from the patient, the pressure measured may not truly reflect airway pressure.

Pressure measurements (pneumotachograph, Pitot tube, variable orifice flow meter) are also used to infer gas flow velocity, which, in a fixed-diameter tube, can be read as volume flow rate. Volume measurements by mechanical respirometers (e.g. Spiromed) are old technologies no longer used on contemporary anesthesia workstations. Volume measurements by ultrasonic and hot wire flowmeters are used to provide spirometry data on some contemporary workstations, and are valuable during both spontaneous and controlled ventilation. Spirometry is useful in monitoring the adequacy of spontaneous ventilation during weaning from ventilation. During controlled ventilation, spirometry provides a means to check whether the patient's lungs are receiving the tidal volumes intended. Discrepancies may be caused by ventilator malfunction or leaks. The spirometric volume measurements can be used in combination with pressure measurements to provide pressure-volume and flow-volume plots.

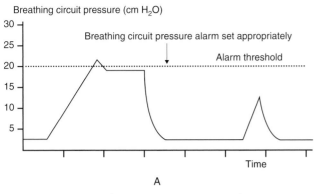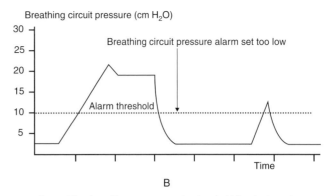

Figure 15.15. Tracing of airway pressure against time during positive pressure ventilation. The dotted line represents the threshold for the low airway pressure alarm. In tracing (A), a partial disconnect in the breathing system results in a smaller pressure increase that does not cross the low-pressure alarm threshold; an alarm is annunciated. In tracing (B), the low-pressure alarm threshold has not been set correctly; that is, just below the normal peak pressure when the circuit is intact. In this case, a partial disconnect results in a lower pressure that does cross the alarm threshold. No alarm is annunciated with this partial disconnect.

Flow measurement has enabled the display of flow-volume and volume-pressure loops, which many practitioners find helpful once they become accustomed to looking at them and recognizing characteristic forms.

The slope of the volume-pressure (volume/pressure) loop represents the total thoracic compliance. Spirometry loops can be frozen or stored for later comparison with newly obtained loops.

Finally, integrating oxygen and carbon dioxide concentrations against inhaled and exhaled tidal volumes permits the continuous real-time calculation of oxygen consumption and carbon dioxide production. Thus, continuous metabolic monitoring is now available by noninvasive means.[7–9]

Utility of pressure, flow, and volume monitoring

Monitoring breathing system pressure and its integration with a prioritized alarm system is one of the most important safety monitors in the anesthesia delivery system. The basic pressure alarm modalities are (1) low peak pressure, (2) continuing pressure, (3) high pressure, and (4) subatmospheric pressure.

Pressure monitoring

Many traditional anesthesia breathing systems incorporate an analog pressure gauge, as well as an electronic pressure monitoring and alarm system. The pressure gauge, if present, is usually mounted on the CO_2 absorber and may measure the pressure at that site (Dräger). In the Ohmeda GMS Absorber System, pressure is sensed on the patient side of the inspiratory unidirectional valve and piloted to the pressure gauge and pressure monitoring system. Depending on circuit configuration, the pressure monitor may fail to detect certain abnormal pressure situations. Thus monitoring pressure at the absorber will not detect positive end-expiratory pressure (PEEP) produced by a free-standing PEEP valve that has been placed between the expiratory limb of the circle system and the expiratory unidirectional valve. Ideally, pressure is monitored at

the patient's airway. Some newer electronic anesthesia workstations use only electronic monitoring and display of pressures, some on a virtual analog flowmeter displayed on the monitor screen.

Low-pressure alarm. Because breathing system disconnects and misconnects are not uncommon occurrences, monitoring of breathing system integrity is essential. Circuit low-pressure monitors have sometimes been referred to as disconnect alarms, but this may be a misnomer because they monitor *pressure*, and the user may infer circuit integrity only if the monitor is used appropriately. They annunciate an audible and visual alarm within 15 seconds when a minimum pressure threshold is not exceeded. The pressure threshold should therefore be set by the user to be just less than the normally expected peak inspiratory pressure (PIP) so any slight decrease will trigger the alarm (Figure 15.15). If the threshold is not bracketed close to the PIP, a circuit leak or disconnect may go undetected if the low-pressure alarm threshold is exceeded. Thus, a small-diameter tracheal tube (e.g. 3.0 mm ID) connected to a circle system might be pulled out of the patient's airway, leaving the lungs unventilated. Because the 3.0-mm tube has high resistance to gas flow, the pressure increase in the circuit with each positive pressure inspiration may exceed the low-pressure alarm threshold. On modern anesthesia workstations, the circuit pressure waveform is displayed, as are the pressure alarm thresholds, so the latter can be suitably adjusted by the user.

Modern delivery systems incorporate low-pressure alarms that are automatically enabled when the ventilator is turned on, but some older designs of alarm systems that must be enabled by the user may be still in use. Because the low-pressure alarm is critical during use of intermittent positive-pressure ventilation (IPPV), the user must be aware of the properties of the monitoring system on the individual machine that he or she is using. If there is any doubt about whether a monitor is interfaced with the ventilator on/off switch, the alarm can be tested by deliberately creating a disconnect.

Although modern breathing system monitors have widely adjustable low-pressure alarm thresholds, older models may provide a choice of only three settings (e.g. 8, 12, and

26 cmH$_2$O), which may limit the sensitivity to detect slight decreases in breathing system pressure. Some low-pressure monitoring alarm systems offer an optional 60-second delay in the event that a slow ventilatory rate – for example, < 4 breaths per minute – is set. A well-thought-out algorithm for responding to the breathing system low-pressure alarm has been described.[10]

Whereas the breathing system low-pressure alarm must be enabled (either automatically or manually) in association with IPPV, the following pressure monitoring modalities are in continuous operation.

Continuing-pressure alarm. Annunciated when circuit pressure exceeds 10 cmH$_2$O for more than 15 seconds, it alerts to more gradual increases in pressure, such as that caused by a ventilator pressure relief valve malfunction (i.e., valve stuck closed) or a scavenging system occlusion. In these situations, fresh gas continues to enter the breathing system from the machine flowmeters, but is unable to leave. The rate of rise of pressure therefore depends on the fresh gas flow rate.[10]

High-pressure alarm. This alarm is annunciated immediately whenever the high-pressure threshold is exceeded. On modern machines, this threshold is adjustable by the user, with a default usually set to 40 cmH$_2$O. Some older pressure monitors are not user-adjustable and have a default setting of +65 cmH$_2$O. This might be too high to detect an otherwise harmful high-pressure condition, such as total obstruction of the tracheal tube, in which the breathing system pressure fails to exceed +65 cmH$_2$O. In contemporary workstations, the ventilator incorporates a high-pressure relief valve, the opening threshold pressure of which is set in conjunction with the high-pressure alarm limit.

Subatmospheric pressure alarm. This annunciates an immediate alarm when pressure is below −10 cm H$_2$O. It should alert to potential negative pressure barotrauma situations owing to suction being applied to the circuit. Negative pressure in the circuit may be caused by spontaneous respiratory efforts by the patient, a malfunctioning waste gas scavenging system, a sidestream sampling gas analyzer when fresh gas flow into the circuit is too low, a suction catheter passed into the airway, or suction via the working channel of a fiberscope passed into the airway via a diaphragm.

Volume monitoring

In traditional anesthesia delivery systems, monitoring of expired tidal and minute volumes is achieved using a spirometer placed in the vicinity of the expiratory unidirectional valve. Spirometry is used to monitor ventilation and circuit integrity. A breathing system disconnect should result in annunciation of the low-volume alarm if an appropriate alarm limit for low volume has been set. Limitations of older spirometers are that the alarm thresholds may not be user-variable. Thus, one older model of machine has a spirometer that has a low-volume alarm threshold fixed at 80 mL. Particularly when a hanging bellows

design of ventilator is used, a circle system disconnection may fail to trigger a low-volume alarm condition because as the weighted bellows descends during exhalation, it may draw a normal tidal volume through the leak site and through the spirometer, thus satisfying the low-volume alarm threshold. A spirometer located by the expiratory unidirectional valve at the absorber does not measure the patient's actual exhaled tidal volume; rather, the volume measured includes both that exhaled by the patient and the gas volume compressed in the breathing system during inspiration.

Although the spirometer low-volume alarm is generally more useful in alerting to a low volume/possible disconnect situation, a high-volume alarm feature may also be useful. Unanticipated increases in tidal volume have resulted from increasing the gas flow into the circuit.[11] This may be from the machine flowmeters, by increasing the I:E ratio, or via a hole in the bellows in a Dräger AV-E ventilator. Thus, any gas entering the patient circuit during inspiration has the potential to be added to the patient's inspired tidal volume. This may be particularly hazardous for the pediatric patient for whom a small tidal volume is intended.

Contemporary workstations measure breathing system compliance during the automated preuse checkout, and use flow sensors located by the inspiratory and expiratory unidirectional valves to accurately monitor inspired (V_I) and expired (V_E) tidal volumes. These values can be used to automatically compensate for small leaks in the breathing system and changes in the fresh gas flow, respiratory rate, and I:E ratio, which otherwise might unintentionally change set tidal volume.

Flow monitoring

Measurement of gas flow is used to measure tidal and minute volumes (because flow = volume/time) and to generate the spirometry loops discussed in the following text. The flow-time signal is used to identify timing of events, such as the beginning and end of inspiration and beginning and end of expiration, duration of breath, and respiratory rate.

Resistance is defined as pressure per unit of flow, so both inspiratory and expiratory airway resistances can be derived from the corresponding pressure and flow signals. The flow-time tracing can be used to recognize the existence of auto-PEEP, when exhalation is incomplete. Auto-PEEP is recognized when the flow tracing does not return to zero at end-exhalation. This may be the result of an expiratory time that is too short, or of lung disease. The ventilator is then reset to eliminate the auto-PEEP.

Spirometry loops

The ability to monitor respiratory physiology continuously in the operating room has long been available but was not routinely used.[12–14] Now that most contemporary anesthesia workstations and physiologic monitoring systems offer the availability of gas flow monitoring, flow-volume and volume-pressure

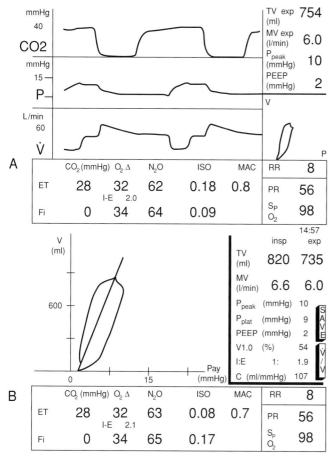

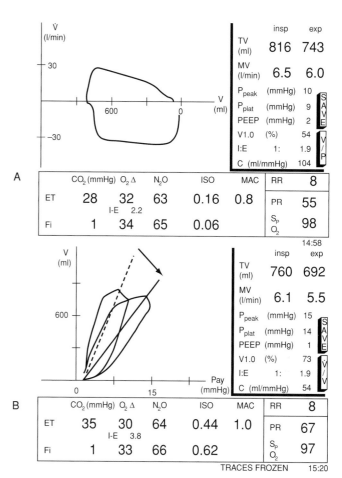

Figure 15.16. Data from sidestream spirometry monitoring. (A) Tracings of CO_2, airway pressure, and gas flow against time. (B) Plot of volume on the *y*-axis vs pressure on the *x*-axis. The slope of the line is the static compliance (shown also numerically as 107 mL/mmHg).

Figure 15.17. (A) flow-volume loop from patient in Figure 15.16, when compliance is 104 mL/mmHg. (B) Saved volume-pressure loop (dotted line), and current volume-pressure loop (solid line) after decrease in compliance owing to endobronchial migration of tracheal tube. Arrow indicates decrease in compliance.

loops are becoming more widely appreciated. (See Figures 15.16–15.20).

Volume-pressure loop

During positive-pressure ventilation, as the pressure in the airway increases, the volume of gas inspired increases (Figure 15.16A, B). The top end of the loop therefore measures tidal volume on the *y*-axis and peak inspiratory pressure on the *x*-axis. Because compliance is defined as change in volume per unit change in pressure, the slope of the line drawn from the origin of the loop to the peak of the loop measures total thoracic compliance. An increase in slope (i.e. more vertical) indicates increased compliance, and vice versa (Figure 15.17B). During exhalation, the expiratory portion of the loop starts at the peak (tidal volume point) and curves back toward the origin. Most monitoring systems allow freezing and saving of a baseline loop for comparison with subsequently obtained loops. Thus changes in compliance can be readily appreciated. The numeric value is also usually displayed digitally.

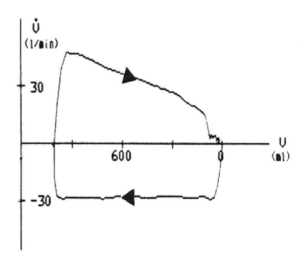

Figure 15.18. Normal flow-volume loop. Inspiratory flow is shown as the tracing below the *x*-axis, and vice versa. The loop is closed, indicating that there is no leak in the system distal to the flow sensor because the inspired and expired volumes are equal.

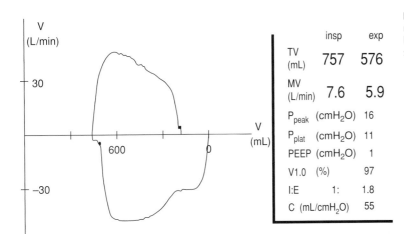

Figure 15.19. Open flow-volume loop, indicating a gas leak of 81 mL (757mL insp. – 576 mL exp.) distal to the flow sensor. This might be the result of a deflated cuff on the tracheal tube, or a poorly seated LMA.

Flow-volume loop

For this loop, flow is displayed on the *y*-axis and volume on the *x*-axis (Figures 15.17A, 15.18). Direction of flow is also indicated by whether the part of the loop is above or below the *x*-axis. In the GE-Datex-Ohmeda monitors, inspiratory flow is indicated in a downward direction. In Dräger displays, the flow axis is inverted so inspiratory flow is indicated above the *x*-axis, and expiratory flow below. Thus, in Figure 15.17A starting at the zero volume point (functional residual capacity [FRC]) which by convention is located at the right hand end of the *x*-axis, during inspiration the loop moves below the *x*-axis, corresponding with inspiratory gas flow. At end-inspiration, the flow slows and then ceases. This point on the *x*-axis corresponds to the inspired tidal volume. As exhalation begins, the loop ascends rapidly above the *x*-axis, corresponding to an initial rapid expiratory flow rate. As exhalation continues, flow slows, and the loop is closed when flow ceases and the lung volume returns to FRC. Storing a loop for later comparison allows the effect of changes in ventilation to be assessed.

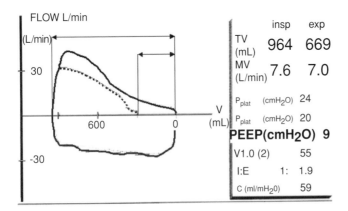

Figure 15.20. Flow-volume loops showing effect on the breath immediately following application of PEEP 9 cmH$_2$O. The solid line shows the saved closed loop from a previous normal breath. The dotted line shows the expiratory part of the current loop, which is now open. In this case, the difference between inspired and expired volumes is the result not of a leak, but of the addition of a volume of 295 mL (964 mL – 669 mL) to the FRC when PEEP was added just before inspiration began. The subsequent flow-volume loops will be closed.

Some applications of spirometry loop monitoring

Spirometry loops provide the anesthesia caregiver with real-time data that are easily interpreted and have proved useful in diagnosing a number of acute problems in the equipment and in the patient. Bardoczky and colleagues described six patients in whom spirometry helped in recognizing or confirming inadequacy of ventilation.[15] These conditions included endobronchial intubation, esophageal intubation, kinking of the tracheal tube, chest compression, double-lumen tube displacement, and bronchospasm.

Breathing system leak detection

During positive-pressure ventilation, the flow-volume loop should be closed; that is, expired volume should be the same as inspired volume. If the loop is open and expired volume is less than inspired, the difference is a measure of the size of the leak distal to the flow sensor (Figure 15.19). In the case of a flow sensor at the airway (e.g., D-Lite), for example, the leak may be caused by a deflated cuff on the endotracheal tube, or a tube that has become displaced. When a laryngeal mask airway (LMA) is being used, a closed loop indicates that the LMA is well seated as there is no leak around the cuff. This is useful, particularly during spontaneous ventilation with pressure support.

In another example (from the author's experience), during a head and neck surgery during which only exhaled tidal volumes were being monitored on the machine's spirometer, it was noted that although the ventilator was set to deliver a 600-mL tidal volume, the exhaled tidal volume was only 400 mL. A spirometry sensor was placed between the Y-piece of the circle system and the tracheal tube connector. The flow-volume loop obtained was closed, and the inspired tidal volume was also 400 mL. This indicated that either the ventilator was not functioning correctly, or more likely, that there was a leak between the ventilator and the breathing system. The leak was found to be the result of a cut that had been accidentally made when the circle system tubing had been placed into a tube tree. The tubing was replaced, and tidal volume was restored to 600 mL.

PEEP and optimizing compliance

Compliance is not a fixed number; rather, it varies with FRC.[16] Ideally, the lung volume at the beginning of inspiration (FRC) should be such that compliance is on the steep part of the compliance-versus-FRC curve for that patient. Application of PEEP during positive-pressure ventilation causes an increase in FRC. If baseline volume-pressure and flow-volume loops have been saved, application of PEEP will result in the origin of the volume-pressure loop being shifted to the right, and an inspired volume that is less than expired volume for the single breath immediately following application of PEEP. The volume difference represents the increase in FRC (Figure 15.20). The volume-pressure loop can be used to titrate PEEP to an optimal compliance, either by looking at the displayed numeric value or by comparing subsequent volume-pressure loops with baseline and noting the slope. PEEP is titrated to maximize compliance. Compared with baseline, PEEP will decrease the expiratory flow rate, making the expiratory part of the loop flatter.

Volumetric capnography and oxygraphy

The ability to integrate instantaneous carbon dioxide concentration and gas flow breath by breath makes possible the continuous measurement of timed carbon dioxide production (VCO_2). The plot of exhaled carbon dioxide concentration against exhaled volume is called the *volumetric capnogram*, from which the quantity of carbon dioxide exhaled per breath can be computed. Monitors that have this feature average the values over time and display a reading of VCO_2 in mL/min.[17,18]

Similarly, the integration of oxygen concentration and gas flow signals permits computation of minute oxygen consumption, as well as the respiratory exchange ratio (VCO_2/VO_2).[7–9]

Complications

As with other monitoring devices and technology, complications may be caused by pure device failure or by vulnerable monitoring devices,[19] but more commonly they are the results of use(r) error. Some flow sensors require zeroing/calibration at the beginning of the day's cases or at other times.[20] Water accumulating in monitoring tubing may cause spurious readings of flow and volume. Flow sensors are commonly concealed within the workstation; therefore, breakage may not be obvious as the source of a breathing circuit leak.[21]

Contemporary monitoring systems are very reliable and integrated with sophisticated prioritized alarm systems. It is essential that the caregiver understand how to set appropriate alarm limits and audible alarm volumes so that critical incidents do not go undetected, and adverse outcomes can be averted.

Credentialing

No special credentialing is required to use the pressure, volume, and flow monitoring described in this chapter. However, the new electronic anesthesia workstations are more complex and less intuitive than traditional anesthesia machines. Adequate in-servicing of all those who will use these monitors is essential so they may be used safely and with confidence. In this regard, the Anesthesia Patient Safety Foundation has sponsored a technology training initiative aimed at improving formal training and assessment before using any advanced medical device. Anesthesia caregivers must know how to set appropriate alarm limits on their monitors, how to set an alarm volume that will be audible in the procedural environment, how to recognize the alarm, and to have an appropriate response to the alarm situation.[22]

A number of reports describe critical incidents and/or adverse outcomes associated with failure to use breathing system monitoring appropriately. A review of the first 2000 incidents reported to the Australian Incident Monitoring Study found 317 incidents that involved problems with ventilation.[23] The major portion (47%) were disconnections; 61 percent of these were detected by a monitor. Monitor detection was by a low circuit pressure alarm in 37 percent, but this alarm failed to warn of nonventilation in 12 incidents (in 6 because it was not switched on and in 6 because of a failure to detect the disconnection).

Practice Parameters

The ASA standards for basic anesthestic monitoring (approved by the ASA House of Delegates on October 21, 1986, and last amended on October 20, 2010)[24] include the following statements that pertain to pressure and volume monitoring:

STANDARD II

During all anesthetics, the patient's oxygenation, ventilation, circulation and temperature shall be continually evaluated.

VENTILATION
OBJECTIVE

To ensure adequate ventilation of the patient during all anesthetics.

METHODS

I) Every patient receiving general anesthesia shall have the adequacy of ventilation continually evaluated. Qualitative clinical signs such as chest excursion, observation of the reservoir breathing bag and auscultation of breath sounds are useful. Continual monitoring for the presence of expired carbon dioxide shall be performed unless invalidated by the nature of the patient, procedure or equipment. Quantitative monitoring of the volume of expired gas is strongly encouraged.*

3) When ventilation is controlled by a mechanical ventilator, there shall be in continuous use a device that is capable of detecting disconnection of components of the breathing system.

The device must give an audible signal when its alarm threshold is exceeded.

[Note that "continual" is defined as "repeated regularly and frequently in steady rapid succession," whereas "continuous" means "prolonged without any interruption at any time."

* Under extenuating circumstances, the responsible anesthesiologist may waive the requirements marked with an asterisk (*); it is recommended that when this is done, it should be so stated (including the reasons) in a note in the patient's medical record.

The monitoring equipment needed to meet these standards is now part of every anesthesia delivery system. All contemporary workstations include spirometry (for exhaled volume, and in many, also inhaled volume), and all include pressure monitoring and alarms. Despite all the integrated monitoring, it may still be possible to not recognize failure to ventilate. There may be occasions, such as during median sternotomy or cardiopulmonary bypass, when the surgical procedure requires that ventilation be temporarily interrupted. During this time, the ventilation monitors may also be disabled, and there are reports of failure to reinstitute ventilation once sternotomy has been completed, or when coming off cardiopulmonary bypass. Centers that perform cardiopulmonary bypass have weaning protocols that include reinstitution of ventilation and ventilatory monitoring. After brief periods of apnea, there have been cases of failure to resume ventilation leading to a critical incident. It is therefore essential that critical alarms be silenced for brief amounts of time only (<2 min).

In 1997, the ASA Closed Claims Project reported on claims involving anesthesia delivery equipment. At that time there were 72 such claims in the database, 76 percent of which resulted in death or severe neurological injury.[25] In 78 percent of the 72 claims, the reviewers considered that the use or better use of monitoring could have prevented an adverse outcome. There have been enormous improvements in the technology whereby pressure, volume, and flow are monitored. The intelligent use of these monitors with their associated alarms has the potential to significantly improve patient safety.

Acknowledgment

The author is grateful to Dr. Daniel Raemer for reviewing this chapter and for his valuable contributions.

References

1. Cobbold RSC. Displacement, force and motion transducers. In *Transducers for Biomedical Measurements: Principles and Applications*. New York: John Wiley & Sons, 1974, p. 120.
2. Wright BM. A respiratory anemometer. *J Physiol (Lond)* 1955;**127**:25P.
3. Nunn JF, Ezi-Ashi TI. The accuracy of the respirometer and ventigrator. *Br J Anaesth* 1962;**34**:422–32.
4. Fleisch A. Der pneumotachometer. *Arch Ges Physiol* 1925;**209**:713–22.
5. Sykes MK, Vickers MD, Hull CJ. Measurement of gas flow and volume. In *Principles of Clinical Measurement*. Oxford: Blackwell Scientific, 1981, p. 198.
6. Tham R, Oberle M. How do flow sensors work? *APSF Newsletter* 2008;**23**:10–12.
7. Barnard JP, Sleigh JW. Breath-by-breath analysis of oxygen uptake using the Datex Ultima. *Br J Anaesth* 1995;**74**:155–8.
8. Takala J, Meriläinen P. *Handbook of Indirect Calorimetry and Gas Exchange*. Helsinki: Datex-Ohmeda 876710–01, 2001; p. 30.
9. Takala J. Appliguide. Clinical application guide of gas exchange and indirect calorimetry. Helsinki: Datex-Ohmeda 895143–1, 2000.
10. Raphael DT, Weller RS, Doran DJ. *Anesth Analg* 1988;**67**:876–83.
11. Scheller MS, Jones BR, Benumof JL: Influence of fresh gas flow and I:E ratio on tidal volume and PaCO2 in ventilated patients. *J Cardiothorac Anesth* 1989;**3**:564.
12. Bardoczky GI, D'Hollander A. Continuous monitoring of the flow-volume loops and compliance during anesthesia. *J Clin Monit* 1992;**8**:251–2.
13. Bardoczky GI, Defrancquen P, Engelman E, Capello M. Continuous monitoring of pulmonary mechanics with the sidestream spirometer during lung transplantation. *J Cardiothoracic Vasc Anes* 1992;**6**:731–4.
14. Bardoczky GI, Levarlet M, Engelman E, Defrancquen P. Continuous spirometry for detection of double-lumen endobronchial tube displacement. *Br J Anaesth* 1993;**70**:499–502.
15. Bardoczky GI, Engelman E, D'Hollander A. Continuous spirometry: an aid to monitoring ventilation during operation. *Br J Anaesth* 1993;**71**:747–51.
16. Lumb AB. Elastic forces and lung volumes. In *Nunn's Applied Respiratory Physiology*, 5th ed. Woburn, MA: Butterworth Heinemann, 2000, p. 47.
17. Lucangelo U, Gullo A, Bernabe F, Blanch L. Capnographic measures: volumetric capnography. In Gravenstein JS, Jaffe MB, Paulus DA, eds. *Capnography: Clinical Aspects*, New York: Cambridge University Press, 2004, pp. 313–9.
18. Jaffe MB, Orr J. Combining flow and carbon dioxide. In Gravenstein JS, Jaffe MB, Paulus DA, eds. *Capnography: Clinical Aspects*, New York: Cambridge University Press, 2004, pp. 423–6.
19. Bader SO, Doshi KK, Grunwald G. A novel leak from an unfamiliar component. *Anesth Analg* 2006;**102**:975–6.
20. Aisys Carestation. User's reference manual, part 1 of 2. Madison,WI: GE, Datex-Ohmeda, 2005; Section 5–9.
21. Patil V, Mackenzie IM. Hidden gas leak on a Datex-Ohmeda Aestiva/5 anesthetic machine. *Anesth Analg* 2007;**104**:234–5.
22. Olympio MA. Formal training and assessment before using advanced medical devices in the OR. *APSF Newsletter* 2007;**22**:63–65.
23. Russell WJ, Webb RK, Van der Walt JH, Runciman WB. The Australian Incident Monitoring Study. Problems with ventilation: an analysis of 2000 incident reports. *AIC* 1993;**21**:617–20.
24. American Society of Anesthesiologists. *Standards for Basic Anesthetic Monitoring*. http://www.asahq.org/publicationsAndServices/standards/02.pdf.
25. Caplan RA, Vistica MF, Posner KL, Cheney FW. Adverse anesthetic outcomes arising from gas delivery equipment: A closed claims analysis. *Anesthesiology* 1997;**87**:741–8.

Chapter 16

Pulse oximetry

Tuula S. O. Kurki and James B. Eisenkraft

Introduction

Oxygen moves down a partial pressure gradient from the environment, through the respiratory tract and lungs, arterial blood, and capillaries, to the mitochondria in cells, where it is used. The steps in this process are known as the *oxygen cascade*.[1] The monitoring of oxygenation is essential to the safe practice of anesthesiology and is valuable in many other clinical and non-clinical situations. Monitoring of the inspired (and exhaled) oxygen concentrations has been described in Chapter 14. *Oximetry* is defined as the measurement of the saturation of the hemoglobin in the blood with oxygen. Pulse oximetry is the measurement of the percentage saturation of hemoglobin with oxygen in the arterial blood, noninvasively and continuously.

Oxygen is transported in the circulation in two forms: some is physically dissolved in plasma, but most is chemically bound to hemoglobin (Hb) as oxyhemoglobin (HbO$_2$). The percentage of hemoglobin that is bound with oxygen is termed the *percentage saturation of hemoglobin*, or sometimes *percent oxygen saturation*. The relationship between oxygen hemoglobin saturation and plasma PO$_2$ is sigmoid in shape and is called the *oxygen–hemoglobin dissociation curve*. The P50 is the PO$_2$ at which the hemoglobin is 50 percent saturated with oxygen. For normal adult hemoglobin the P50 is about 27 mmHg. An increase in P50 results in a rightward-shifting of the curve, and vice versa. Several factors affect the relationship between PaO$_2$ and saturation. An increase in body temperature, acidemia, 2,3-DPG, and carbon dioxide content will increase P50.

Although normal hemoglobins combine with oxygen, there are some forms of hemoglobin, called *dyshemoglobins*, that do not. The most important ones are carboxyhemoglobin (COHb) and methemoglobin (metHb). This leads to two definitions of hemoglobin saturation:

Functional saturation (SaO$_2$%) is the amount of oxyhemoglobin divided by the total amount of hemoglobin that is capable of carrying oxygen:

$$SaO_2\% = HbO_2/(HbO_2 + DHb) \times 100,$$

where DHb is the quantity of deoxygenated hemoglobin present.

Fractional saturation (HbO$_2$%) is the amount of oxyhemoglobin divided by the *total* amount of hemoglobin present (which includes dyshemoglobins):

$$HbO_2\% = HbO_2/(HbO_2 + DHb + COHb + metHb).$$

When the quantity of dyshemoglobins is small, SaO$_2$ and HbO$_2$ are essentially the same.

Oxygen transport (oxygen flux) is the total amount of oxygen transported to the tissues per minute. It is determined by arterial oxygen tension (PaO$_2$), arterial hemoglobin oxygen saturation, Hb concentration, and cardiac output.

Let us consider normal oxygen carriage by 100 mL (1 dL) of blood with a hemoglobin concentration of 15 g/dL, no dyshemoglobins present, and PaO$_2$ of 100 mmHg.

The quantity of oxygen carried (CaO$_2$; arterial oxygen content) is:

$$[Hb\,concn. \times 1.34 \times SaO_2\%] + [PaO_2 \times 0.003]$$

or

$$[15 \times 1.34 \times 100\%] + [100 \times 0.003]$$
$$= [20.1 + 0.3] = 20.4 \text{ mL oxygen/dL of blood.}$$

$$Oxygen\ flux = CaO_2 \times cardiac\ output\ (L/min).$$

The measurement of arterial hemoglobin oxygen saturation requires that an arterial blood sample be drawn and analyzed in a laboratory co-oximeter (or hemoximeter). This is essentially a spectrophotometer than uses six or more wavelengths of light to measure DHb, HbO$_2$, COHb, metHb, and total Hb concentration. Using these data, it can display a saturation value expressed as SaO$_2$ or HbO$_2$%. Alternatively, the PO$_2$ of the arterial sample can be measured in a blood gas analyzer, and a *calculated* saturation derived from the PaO$_2$ via the hemoglobin–oxygen dissociation curve. The *calculated* saturation will be erroneous and possibly misleading in the presence of significant amounts of dyshemoglobins or dyes.

Methods to measure arterial hemoglobin–oxygen saturation have evolved considerably over the past 200 years. The fascinating history of oximetry and the discovery of pulse oximetry are the subject of a number of excellent reviews.[2,3] J. R. Squire, working in London in 1940, was the first to realize that the differences in transmission of red and infrared light before and after expelling the blood from the web of the hand with a pressure cuff was a function of saturation.[4] The development of oximetry was stimulated during World War II in an effort to warn military pilots of dangerous hypoxia. In 1942, Millikan developed a lightweight red and infrared ear oximeter, for which he coined the word "oximeter."[5]

In 1972 Takuo Aoyagi, an electrical engineer at the Nihon Kohden company in Tokyo, was interested in measuring cardiac output noninvasively by the dye dilution method, using a commercially available ear oximeter. He balanced the red and infrared signals to cancel the pulse noise that prevented measuring the dye washout accurately and discovered that changes of oxygen saturation voided his pulse cancellation. Aoyagi then realized that these pulsatile changes could be used to compute saturation from the ratio of ratios of pulsatile changes in the red and infrared regions of the electromagnetic spectrum. His ideas, equations and instrument were adapted, improved, and successfully marketed by Minolta in about 1978, stimulating other companies to further improve and market pulse oximeters worldwide in the mid-1980s.[3]

Technical concepts

The pulse oximeter uses a combination of two technologies: spectrophotometry, whereby the saturation of hemoglobin with oxygen is estimated; and optical plethysmography, which focuses the measurement on pulsatile arterial blood.

Spectrophotometry

The color of blood is a function of the hemoglobin oxygen saturation. As hemoglobin becomes deoxygenated, it becomes less permeable to red light, and its color changes gradually to blue. The color change is the result of changes in the optical properties of the heme moiety in hemoglobin. Pulse oximetry estimates the hemoglobin oxygen saturation in blood by determining the "blueness" of the arterial blood between a light source and a photodetector.[6] The spectrophotometric method depends on an approximate Lambert–Beer relationship, which states that there is a logarithmic dependence between the transmissivity (T) of light at a given wavelength (λ) through a substance, and the product of the absorption coefficient (β_λ) of the substance at that wavelength, the distance that the light travels through the material (i.e. the path length, l), and the concentration (c) of absorbing species in the material. Transmissivity, T, is the intensity of light emerging from the medium (I_{out}), divided by the intensity of the incident light (I_{in}):

$$T = I_{out}/I_{in} = e^{-\beta\lambda l.c}$$

For liquids transmissivity, T, is expressed as absorbance of light, A, where

$$A = -\log_{10} I_{out}/I_{in}$$

Absorbance of light, A, is therefore a function of concentration, c.

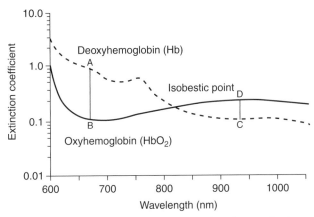

Figure 16.1. Absorbance versus radiation wavelength curves for deoxygenated and oxygenated hemoglobin. Line A–B shows that as hemoglobin becomes more oxygenated, absorbance at 660 nm decreases. Line C–D shows that as hemoglobin becomes more oxygenated, absorbance at 940 nm increases.

If more than one absorber is present (e.g. oxyhemoglobin and deoxygenated hemoglobin), the total absorbance is the sum of their individual absorbances.

Figure 16.1 shows the absorbance spectra for oxygenated and deoxygenated hemoglobins. The plots show absorbance of light (extinction coefficient) on the y-axis, against wavelength of incident light on the x-axis. To distinguish between the concentration of two absorbers, oxyhemoglobin and deoxyhemoglobin, it is necessary to measure absorption at two wavelengths. The two basic wavelengths that the pulse oximeter uses are one near infrared (940 nm) and the other near red (660 nm). Figure 16.1 shows that at wavelength 660 nm, as hemoglobin becomes more oxygenated (going from point A to point B), absorbance of light decreases. At wavelength 940 nm, as hemoglobin becomes more oxygenated (going from point C to point D), absorbance of light increases. These changes are shown in Figure 16.2a (absorbance vs saturation at 660 nm) and Figure 16.2b (absorbance vs saturation at 940 nm). Dividing the relationship in Figure 16.2a by that in Figure 16.2b, one obtains a plot of saturation on the y-axis against the ratio of absorbance at 660 nm to that at 940 nm on the x-axis (Figure 16.3). This is essentially a linear relationship and forms the basis for the calibration algorithm of the two-wavelength pulse oximeter. In other words, if one can measure the ratio of absorbance of light at 660 nm to that at 940 nm in arterial blood, this ratio can be used to estimate the arterial hemoglobin oxygen saturation.

The pulse oximeter sensor probe (finger clip or ear clip) incorporates a light source that consists of two light-emitting diodes (LEDs): one that emits light in the red region at a wavelength of 660 nm, and the other, infrared light at 940 nm. A photodetector is located on the other side of the clip to measure the intensity of light that is transmitted through the sensor site (usually a fingertip). The two LEDs cycle on and off between 2000 and 3000 times per second, with only one on at a time, and a third point in the cycle when both are off, so the photodetector can adjust for ambient light.

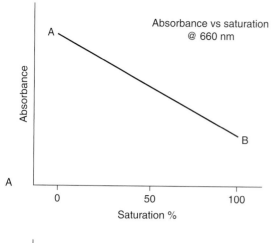

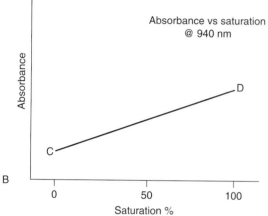

Figure 16.2. Plot of absorbance versus saturation at (a) 660 nm and (b) 940 nm. Points A, B, C, and D are as in Figure 16.1.

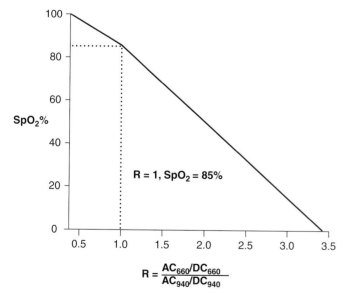

$$R = \frac{AC_{660}/DC_{660}}{AC_{940}/DC_{940}}$$

Figure 16.3. Example of the calibration algorithm of a two-wavelength pulse oximeter. The pulse oximeter saturation reading (SpO$_2$) is based on the ratio of pulse-added absorbances at 660 and 940 nm. When the ratio is high, SpO$_2$ is low, and vice versa. A ratio of 1 corresponds to an SpO$_2$ of about 85%.

Optical plethysmography

At the pulse oximeter sensor site (fingertip), during each arterial pulsation the site expands in volume as arterial blood enters during systole, and then contracts as the blood leaves during diastole. As a result, the path length of light through the fingertip increases and decreases cyclically with each pulsation, and is "seen" by the photodetector as pulsatile changes in absorbance at the two wavelengths of light, 660 nm and 940 nm.

Light absorbance in tissue can be considered to be due to two components: a nonpulsatile component caused by nonpulsatile blood and tissue (i.e., bone, skin, muscle) pigmentation that produces a (non-pulsatile) direct current (DC), and a pulsatile component caused by pulsation of the artery, which produces an alternating current (AC; Figure 16.4). During systole, light absorption is increased at both wavelengths, and these *pulse-added absorbances* are therefore caused by hemoglobin in the arterial blood. The ratio of pulse-added absorbances AC660/AC940 nm (Figures 16.2 and 16.3) is made independent of the intensity of the incident light by calculating the *ratio of ratios*, R, where R = [(AC 660/DC 660) / (AC 940/DC 940)]. In Figure 16.3, it can be seen that when R is large, saturation is low, when R is small, saturation is high, and that R = 1 corresponds to a saturation of approximately 85 percent.

Despite the theoretical relationship between hemoglobin saturation and R, pulse oximeters must be calibrated empirically to relate the pulse oximeter saturation reading, designated SpO$_2$, to R. The empiric calibration curves of pulse oximeters are created by exposing healthy adult human volunteers to gas mixtures of decreasing FIO$_2$, and therefore of desaturation. When in a steady state, an arterial blood sample is drawn for measurement of saturation in a laboratory hemoximeter (considered the gold standard). The hemoximeter readings are used with the simultaneously recorded values of R, to plot the points needed to create the empiric calibration algorithm. The algorithms are also tested in human subjects in oximetry laboratories before the devices receive FDA approval and are commercially released for market. Pulse oximeters therefore do not require user calibration. The accuracy at low saturations (<70%) and under conditions of poor peripheral perfusion has been shown to vary among different pulse oximeters.[7,8] In the range of SpO$_2$ values 100 percent to 70 percent, the standard deviation (SD) of the SpO$_2$ reading is specified by the manufacturers as ± 2 percent, when compared with the laboratory hemoximeter oxyhemoglobin concentrations.[7–10]

Assuming that for any given hemoximeter reading of saturation, the SpO$_2$ reading has a normal distribution, then if the SpO$_2$ is 96 percent, there is a 68 percent likelihood that the true saturation is between 94 percent and 98 percent (i.e. ± 1 SD), and a 95 percent likelihood that it is between 92 percent and 100 percent (i.e. ± 2 SD).

The pulse oximeter does not actually *measure* saturation; rather, it measures an R value and uses this to *predict*, via a look-up table in the software, what the laboratory hemoximeter saturation reading would be if a simultaneously obtained

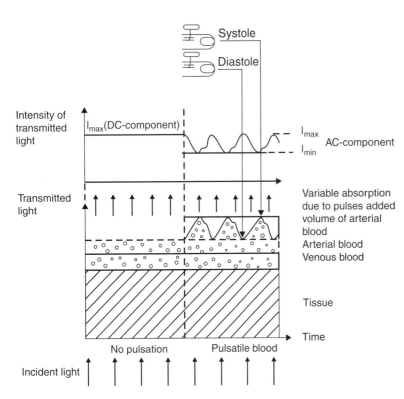

Figure 16.4. Absorption of radiation as it passes through a fingertip. Pulse-added absorption is due to arterial blood pulsations. Incident light passes through fixed or constant absorbers, including skin; bone; blood in veins, assumed to be nonpulsatile; and blood in arteries at end-diastole, also assumed to be nonpulsatile. The pulse-added component is assumed to be due to arterial blood and is responsible for the AC signal. The nonpulsatile component is responsible for the DC signal. Permission given by General Electric Company.

arterial sample were analyzed. The accuracy of the prediction will depend on how closely the characteristics of the patient being monitored resemble those of the human volunteers from whose data the algorithm was created.

When creating the empiric calibration algorithms, pulse oximeter manufacturers had to make a decision whether to use the hemoximeter value for *fractional* saturation or for *functional* saturation. Can this make any difference? Assume that an arterial sample analyzed in the laboratory hemoximeter gives the following readings:

$$DHb = 0, HbO_2 = 96\%, COHb = 2\%, \text{ and metHb} = 2\%.$$
$$\text{Functional saturation } (SaO_2) = 96/(96 + 0) = 100\%.$$
$$\text{Fractional saturation } (HbO_2\%) = 96/(96 + 2 + 2) = 96\%.$$

Most manufacturers chose to use functional saturation in creating their algorithms. Regardless of whether $HbO_2\%$ or $SaO_2\%$ was used, it is important to remember that the two wavelength pulse oximeter measures neither fractional nor functional saturation.

One of the major problems of the older pulse oximeters was failure or spurious readings during patient movement or in the presence of a low signal (as a result of low pulse amplitude). Motion artifact may be caused by movement of the probe on the patient, causing erratic changes in path length of light. More recently, it has been recognized that it is mainly the result of venous pulsations.[11,12] Recall that in the preceding description of optical plethysmography, it was assumed that the venous blood did not pulsate and was a fixed absorber of light, contributing to the DC signal. The newest-generation

pulse oximeters incorporate special algorithms to overcome the effects of motion (motion resistant) and have improved signal-to-noise ratios, allowing more accurate operation during periods of low perfusion.[13] However, if no pulse is detectable, the pulse oximeter will fail.[9] Failure modes have been the subject of much discussion, as some pulse oximeters give no SpO_2 reading and a warning, whereas others may display a spurious reading.

Another limitation of conventional two-wavelength pulse oximeters is that they give spurious readings in the presence of dyshemoglobins. This is because with only two wavelengths of light, they can solve for only two unknowns, DHb and HbO_2. This is analogous to solving simultaneous equations; that is, one needs at least as many equations as unknowns to solve for each unknown.

Carboxyhemoglobin

In dogs given CO in 100 percent oxygen to breathe, increasing amounts of COHb caused the SpO_2 reading to decrease from 100 percent down to the low 90s (Figure 16.5).[14,15] In this situation, the two-wavelength pulse oximeter SpO_2 overreads the fractional saturation, and underreads the functional saturation (which is 100% when breathing an $FIO_2 = 1$).

Methemoglobinemia

When methemoglobinemia was induced in dogs breathing 100 percent oxygen, the greater the concentration of methemoglobin, the more the SpO_2 reading tended toward 85 percent (Figure 16.6).[16] This is an example of the "R = 1,

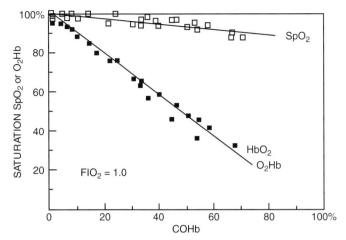

Figure 16.5. Plot of SpO_2 and HbO_2 against COHb in dogs breathing FIO_2 of 1. All the hemoglobin that can carry oxygen is fully saturated (as $FIO_2 = 1$); therefore, functional saturation is 100%. The HbO_2 line is the fractional saturation of hemoglobin, as all the hemoglobin that is not COHb is HbO_2. From Barker SJ, Tremper KK. The effect of carbon monoxide inhalation on pulse oximetry and transcutaneous PO2. *Anesthesiology* 1987;66:677–679, with permission.

$SpO_2 = 85\%$" phenomenon. Reference to the absorbance spectrum for methemoglobin shows that the absorbances at 660 nm and 940 nm are similar (Figure 16.7). The greater the metHb%, the more will the ratio of pulse-added absorbances (R) be driven toward 1, and therefore SpO_2 toward 85 percent. There are

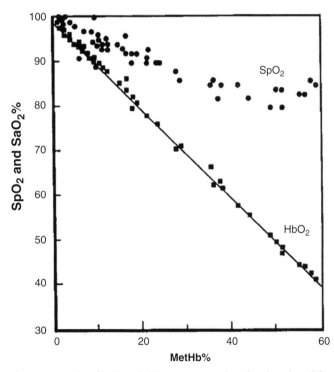

Figure 16.6. Plot of SpO_2 and HbO_2 against metHb in dogs breathing FIO_2 of 1. All the hemoglobin that can carry oxygen is fully saturated (as $FIO_2 = 1$); therefore, functional saturation is 100%. The HbO_2 line is the fractional saturation of hemoglobin, as all the hemoglobin that is not metHb is HbO_2. As the percentage of metHb increases, the SpO_2 tends toward 85%. From Barker SJ, Tremper KK, Hyatt J. Effects of methemoglobinemia on pulse oximetry and mixed venous oximetry. *Anesthesiology* 1989;70:112–7, with permission.

numerous case reports of spurious SpO_2 readings caused by methemogobin.[17–19]

Multiple-wavelength pulse oximeters

Recently, the limitations of the conventional two-wavelength pulse oximeter in the presence of COHb and metHb have been addressed by building multiple-wavelength pulse oximeters. The more wavelengths that are used, the greater the number of absorbers that can be measured. The Masimo Corporation (Irvine, CA) invented Masimo Rainbow SET Pulse CO-Oximetry in 2005 – the first-and-only upgradable technology platform allowing noninvasive and continuous monitoring of multiple blood constituents that previously required invasive procedures, including total hemoglobin (SpHb), oxygen content (SpOC), carboxyhemoglobin (SpCO), methemoglobin (SpMet), and Pleth Variability Index (PVI), in addition to SpO_2, pulse rate, and perfusion index (PI) (Figure 16.8). Masimo's Rainbow Series of Pulse CO-Oximeters are the first commercial devices to provide noninvasive and continuous monitoring of hemoglobin concentration. FDA-cleared in 2008, noninvasive hemoglobin is being used in numerous hospitals throughout the United States and abroad, where it is reportedly making a positive impact on patient care, and widespread clinical evaluations are underway.

Reflectance pulse oximetry

Most pulse oximeters use transmission spectrophotometry as the basic method for detecting absorbances of the red and infrared light as they pass through the probe site. There is another type of pulse oximetry, called *reflectance pulse oximetry*, that requires use of probes designed to measure the absorbance of reflected (rather than transmitted) red and infrared light. The sensors can be conveniently placed on the patient's forehead. The reflectance method is especially suitable for burn patients and in other situations in which an extremity is not available for transmission sensor placement. It is also useful in patients who have peripheral vasoconstriction when transmission finger probes cannot be used because of a lack of the plethysmographic signal and low-flow situation. For example, Nellcor (Pleasanton, CA), recommends placement of its OxiMax reflectance sensor on the forehead, just above the eyebrow, centering it with the iris. The blood supply of the skin of the lower forehead just above the eyebrows is from the supraorbital artery, a branch of the internal carotid artery, and therefore is well maintained. In addition, the area shows less vasoconstrictor response to cold or other stimuli, compared with other peripheral sites.[20,21]

The main problem with reflectance oximetry is that the pulsatile component is small compared with the transmissive component (1/10 of the transmissive component). In addition, forehead pulse oximetry may provide spuriously low readings owing to transmitted venous pulsations.[22,23] This is particularly marked when the patient is in a head-down position. A potential solution to the problem of venous pulsations is use of an elastic headband that applies 10 to 20 mmHg pressure to the

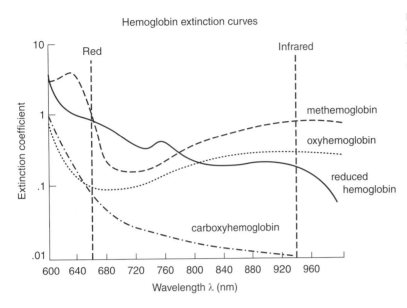

Hemoglobin extinction curves

Figure 16.7. Plot of absorbance vs wavelength for deoxygenated hemoglobin, HbO$_2$, COHb, and metHb. For metHb, the absorbances at 660 and 940 nm are essentially the same; therefore, R = 1, and SpO$_2$ reads 85%. From Tremper KK, Barker SJ. Pulse oximetry. *Anesthesiology* 1989;70:98–108, with permission.

forehead probe, to apply a pressure greater than venous pressure.[24]

Parameters monitored

The pulse oximeter displays SpO$_2$, which is an estimate of arterial hemoglobin oxygen saturation. It can be measured at different sites: from the fingertip, the palm, the ear, the nose, the tongue, or the toe, using specially designed sensors or probes. These probes are designed for transmission and detection of transmitted red and infrared light. Sensors are also available that use the reflectance method, and can be attached to the forehead (Nellcor, Masimo).

Pulse oximeters can measure the pulse rate at the sensor site. Pulse rate is not always identical with the heart rate as monitored on ECG, depending on whether there are extra supraventricular or ventricular beats that do not generate a peripheral pulse waveform. Some pulse oximeters display signal strength or signal-to-noise ratio by a series of ascending light bars (laddergram) (Nellcor; Pleasanton, CA). Some pulse oximeters display an actual plethysmographic waveform and calculate a modulation percentage (GE) or PI (GE, Masimo). These provide information about the condition of the peripheral circulation. If there is vasodilatation, the signal is strong, PI values are high, and modulation percentage is on a large scale

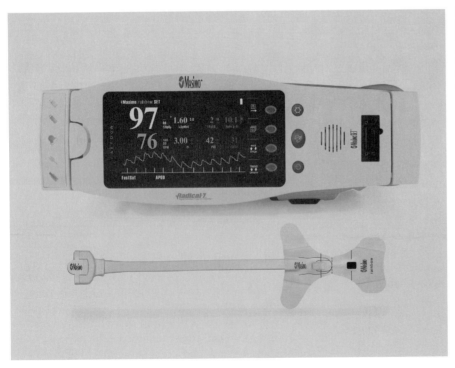

Figure 16.8. The Masimo Radical-7 (Masimo Rainbow SET Pulse CO-Oximeter) is a 3-in-1 (bedside, handheld, transport) pulse CO-oximeter featuring Masimo Rainbow SET for noninvasive and continuous measurement of hemoglobin, oxygen content, carboxyhemoglobin, methemoglobin, Pleth Variability Index, oxyhemoglobin, perfusion index, pulse rate, and, most recently, acoustic respiration rate. By permission from Masimo Corp., Irvine, CA.

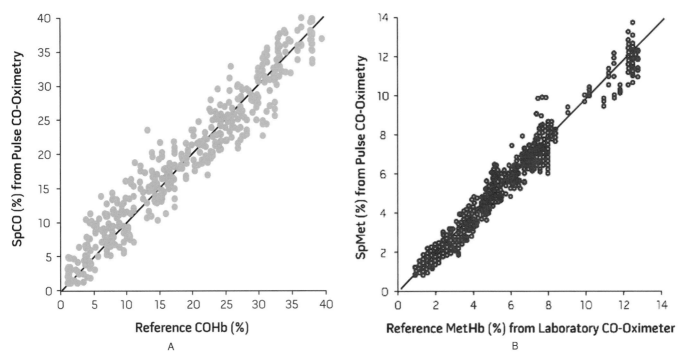

Figure 16.9. A: Plot of SpCO (Masimo Pulse CO-Oximeter measurement of COHb), against COHb, as measured from a blood sample analyzed in a laboratory hemoximeter. B: Plot of SpMet (Masimo Pulse CO-Oximeter measurement of metHb), against metHb, as measured from a blood sample analyzed in a laboratory hemoximeter. From Masimo Corp., Irvine, CA, with permission.

(up to 20%–50%). If there is vasoconstriction, the plethysmographic pulse wave amplitude is small, PI is small, and modulation percentage is small.

Some pulse oximeters offer a plethysmographic variability index (PVI) (Masimo; Irvine, CA).[25] In hypovolemic patients, one can observe fluctuations in the plethysmographic amplitude during the respiratory cycle owing to changes in the balance between intrathoracic pressure and intravascular blood volume; in hypovolemic patients, the PVI will increase. Some pulse oximeters offer a so-called slow pleth recording, whereby the user can observe the fluctuations of plethysmographic amplitude during the respiratory cycle on the display (GE). The plethysmographic amplitude information can be used to evaluate the volume status or vasodilation/vasoconstriction status of a patient. In the intensive care unit, the pulse volume amplitude information can be used as a dynamic parameter to assess the volume status, for example, of a septic patient.[26–29]

Newer models of pulse oximeters (Masimo Rainbow SET) can measure COHb (SpCO) and metHb (SpMet) concentrations by using eight wavelengths of light (Figure 16.9).[30–32] Total Hb (SpHb) can be measured with the Masimo pulse oximeter Rainbow SET which uses 12 wavelengths of light (600–940 nm).[21] This is the first noninvasive continuous Hb measurement device to become available.[33] There are now reports of its use by clinicians (Figure 16.10) and widespread clinical evaluations are ongoing.

Pulse oximeters are valuable in the early detection of hypoxemia, especially because the human eye can be poor at detecting this condition. The low SpO_2 alarm is usually set at 94 percent as a default, but the value set should be considered on an individual basis. For example, during head and neck surgery under MAC, administration of oxygen by nasal cannula or face mask has resulted in fires and burns. It is now recommended that supplemental oxygen be provided only if necessary, and

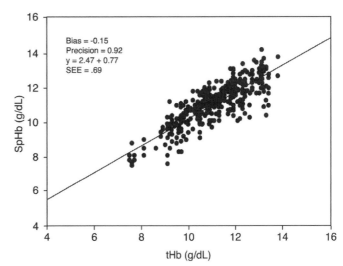

Figure 16.10. A scatterplot of 165 reference hemoglobin values as determined by laboratory CO-Oximetry (tHb) and 335 simultaneous noninvasive hemoglobin values (SpHb) collected from 20 subjects undergoing hemodilution. The average difference (bias) between SpHb and tHb was −0.15 g/dL, 1 SD of the difference (precision) was 0.92 g/dL, and the average root-mean-square difference was 0.94 g/dL. From Macknet. The accuracy of noninvasive and continuous total hemoglobin measurement by pulse CO-oximetry in human subjects Undergoing Hemodilution. *Anesth Analg* 2010; 111:1424–6, with permission

that a lower SpO_2 may often be acceptable. For many patients, maintaining an SpO_2 of 90 percent ($PaO_2 = 60$ mmHg) may be adequate.[34]

Although pulse oximeters monitor the R value beat to beat, the SpO_2 is not displayed beat-to-beat because of potential artifacts and rapidly changing values. Instead, the SpO_2 displayed is the average of the many values measured over a brief time period, or epoch. This is often 10 to 15 seconds, although in some pulse oximeters the epoch duration can be changed by the user. The advantage of a longer epoch is that there is less artifact; the disadvantage is that if saturation is decreasing, there is increased delay in triggering a low SpO_2 alarm. The pulse oximeter probe site can also affect the time to recognition of hypoxemia.[35,36]

Pulse oximeters cannot be used as a monitor of extreme hyperoxia, because of the shape of the hemoglobin–oxygen dissociation curve. When the PO_2 is greater than 140 mmHg, hemoglobin oxygen saturation and SpO_2 are 100 percent. At higher PaO_2s, the SpO_2 will still read 100 percent. In neonates and premature newborn babies, the SpO_2 high alarm can be adjusted to lower values (e.g. 87%–93%) to prevent too high an oxygen concentration, which may cause damage to the eyes (retrolental fibroplasia), resulting in impaired vision or even permanent blindness of the neonate.[37]

Pulse oximeters have been used as perfusion monitors, and have helped to ensure proper positioning of patients on the operating room table. Hovagim and associates reported eight cases in which the use of pulse oximetry alerted the anesthesiologist to a patient's improper positioning.[38] Pulse oximeters have also been used to monitor therapy to maintain patency of a ductus arteriosus. In the latter case, one pulse oximeter probe is placed on the right arm (preductal), and one on a lower extremity (postductal). As long as the ductus remains patent, the preductal SpO_2 is greater than the postductal SpO_2. When the ductus closes, the SpO_2s become similar.[39] Pulse oximetry has also been shown to decrease the frequency of arterial blood gas sampling in the ICU.[40]

Evidence of utility

In 1986, the American Society of Anesthesiologists (ASA) adopted the Standards for Basic Intra-Operative Monitoring, based on the Harvard standards published earlier that year. These standards encouraged the use of pulse oximetry and capnography.[41] Despite the lack of any prospective, double-blind controlled study that establishes (to commonly accepted levels of statistical significance) that pulse oximetry improves outcome, in 1990, pulse oximetry monitoring essentially became one of the ASA standards for basic anesthetic monitoring.[42] Prior to this time, the use of pulse oximetry had become a de facto standard of care in American anesthesia because there was a widely held belief among anesthesia providers that pulse oximetry was a good thing, and the vast majority of anesthetics involved use of pulse oximetry.[43] A number of studies have shown that the clinical use of

pulse oximetry actually decreased the number and severity of episodes of hypoxemia.[44,45] It is therefore reasonable to believe that use of pulse oximetry represents an improvement in the quality of care and in patient safety.

In 1989 and 1990, the ASA Closed Claims Study reported that there had been a significant decrease in mortality related to hypoxemia since pulse oximetry became a mandatory minimum monitoring standard.[46] From an analysis of 1175 claims, the authors concluded that the combination of pulse oximetry and capnography "could be expected" to help prevent anesthetic-related morbidity and mortality. The ASA Closed Claims Study also reported that 57 percent of anesthesia-related deaths were preventable by the use of pulse oximetry and capnography. With the use of such monitoring in more than one million anesthetics, the anesthesia-related arrests decreased from 0.13/10,000 to 0.04/10,000 anesthetics.[46]

In 1993, Moller and colleagues reported the results of the first large prospective randomized multicenter clinical trial on perioperative pulse oximetry monitoring.[47,48] In five Danish hospitals, by random assignment, monitoring did or did not include pulse oximetry for patients age 18 years or older, scheduled for elective or emergency operations, or for regional or general anesthesia, except during cardiac or neurosurgical procedures. Of the 20,802 patients studied, 10,312 were assigned to the oximetry group and 10,490 to the control group. During anesthesia and in the postanesthesia care unit (PACU), significantly more patients in the oximetry group had at least one respiratory event than those in the control group in both the OR and PACU. This was the result of a 19-fold increase in the incidence of diagnosed hypoxemia in the oximetry group compared with the control group, in both the OR and PACU. Equal numbers of in-hospital deaths were reported in the two groups. Questionnaires completed by the anesthesiologists at the five institutions revealed that 18 percent had experienced a situation in which use of a pulse oximeter helped to avoid a serious event or complication, and that 80 percent felt more secure when they used a pulse oximeter. The study also demonstrated a significant decrease in the rate of myocardial ischemia with pulse oximetry use. Although monitoring prompted a number of changes in patient care, a reduction in overall rate of postoperative complications was not observed. In this study, pulse oximetry did not affect the overall outcome of anesthesia.[47,48]

In 2006, Cheney and coworkers reported on trends in anesthesia-related death and brain damage based on the 6894 closed anesthesia malpractice claims in the ASA Closed Claims Project database.[49] Trends in the proportion of claims for death or permanent brain damage between 1975 and 2000 were analyzed. The authors concluded that the significant decrease in the proportion of claims for death or permanent brain damage from 1975 through 2000 seemed to be unrelated to a marked increase in the proportion of claims in which pulse oximetry and end-tidal carbon dioxide monitoring were used. Following the introduction and use of these monitors, there was a significant reduction in the proportion of respiratory damaging events and an increase in the proportion of cardiovascular damaging events responsible for death or permanent brain damage. Therefore, it is difficult to show the efficacy and benefits of its use in clinical outcome.

A systematic review by Pedersen and colleagues investigated outcome in 21,733 patients and included four studies for the analysis.[50] Results indicated that hypoxemia was reduced in the pulse oximetry group, both in the operating room and in the recovery room. In the recovery room, the incidence of hypoxemia was 1.5 to three times less in the pulse oximetry group. There was no difference in cognitive function between the groups. No statistically significant differences were detected between the groups in complications, mortality, or hospital stay.[50]

Robbertze and coworkers[51] reported that a higher proportion of patients in non-OR anesthesia claims underwent monitored anesthesia care (58% vs 6%, $P < 0.001$). Inadequate oxygenation/ventilation was the most common specific damaging event in non-OR anesthesia claims (33% vs 2% in operating room claims, $P < 0.001$). The proportion of deaths was increased in non-OR anesthesia claims (54% vs 24%, $P = 0.003$). Non-OR anesthesia claims were more often judged as having substandard care ($P = 0.003$) and being preventable by better monitoring ($P = 0.007$). The researchers concluded that non-OR anesthesia claims had a higher severity of injury and more substandard care than OR claims. Inadequate oxygenation/ventilation was the most common mechanism of injury. Maintenance of minimum monitoring standards and airway management training is required for staff involved in patient sedation.[51]

Evidence for a beneficial effect of pulse oximetry in the postoperative care of cardiac surgical patients was studied by Bierman and associates in a sample of 35 cardiac surgical patients.[52] They concluded that pulse oximetry improves patient safety through the detection of clinically unapparent episodes of desaturation and can allow a reduction in the number of blood gas analyses used without adverse effects to the patient.

In summary, use of pulse oximetry has become the standard of care despite any data showing a statistically significant improvement in outcome associated with its use. Use of pulse oximetry is one of the ASA minimum standards for basic anesthetic monitoring in the operating room,[53] PACU,[54] ICU,[55] non-OR locations,[56] office-based anesthesia locations,[57] and ambulatory facilities.[58] The recent evidence of a Cochrane review[59] shows that no statistically significant differences were detected between the groups in complications or mortality or hospital stay. Hypoxemia events were reduced 1.5- to threefold in the PACU. The earlier reports from the ASA Closed Claims studies have suggested benefits to pulse oximetry use, along with a significant decrease in mortality related to hypoxemia in different environments.[53,55]

Complications

As with any monitoring device, complications can be caused by pure failure of the equipment, but are more often the result of use(r) error, which includes misinterpretation of data and failure to recognize spurious readings. When used in patients with low perfusion states or during motion, the pulse oximeter may display erroneous readings that may, in turn, lead to inappropriate changes in oxygen therapy. Pulse oximeters can detect only hypoxemia. If the patient is hyperoxic, the SpO2 reads 100 percent and the pulse oximeter cannot provide warning of the hyperoxia.

Pressure on the sensor, especially under conditions of low perfusion, can cause damage to the skin, ischemia, and even skin blisters.[60,61] There are also reports of burns on fingers or toes (in children).[62] The taped-on sensors should not be taped too tightly; this will prevent extra compression and tissue ischemia. During long procedures, the sensors and underlying skin should be evaluated every two hours. Shelley and colleagues noted that use of their setup in a subsequent study of forehead reflectance pulse oximetry resulted in a burn on the forehead of one of their research subjects.[28] This occurred with the probe secured by a Tegaderm dressing and without application of external pressure. When a forehead sensor is used, the skin at the site must be checked at regular intervals.

Dyshemoglobins will cause the two-wavelength pulse oximeter to display spurious readings.[14–17] In the presence of COHb, the SpO2 overreads the fractional saturation (HbO2%).[14] Similar overestimation of HbO2% may occur if there is significant metHb in the blood.[16] At the level of 35 percent metHb in the blood, a two-wavelength pulse oximeter will read an SpO2 of 84 percent to 86 percent, and the values do not decrease even if metHb levels increase. Thus, if there is any suspicion of COHb (burn victim, smoke inhalation) or metHb poisoning (e.g. after benzocaine treatment),[63] an arterial blood sample should be drawn and a laboratory co-oximetry analysis performed. The new multiwavelength pulse oximeters (Masimo Rainbow SET) are able to measure COHb and metHb concentrations (Figure 16.9).[18,30,31]

Mild anemia does not affect pulse oximetry readings under normal circumstances. If the hemoglobin concentration is very low (Hct <15%), then the pulse oximeter may fail, mainly because of low perfusion at the probe site.[64,65]

Fetal hemoglobin (HbF) will not cause significant inaccuracy in pulse oximetry because it involves amino acid changes only in the globin chains.[66,67] Spurious readings are associated with changes in the heme moiety of hemoglobin.

Venous pulsations at the sensor site can cause spuriously low readings of SpO2 because the pulse oximeter is unable to distinguish arterial from venous blood pulsations. When there is a continuous column of blood between the right heart and the forehead sensor site (i.e. jugular vein valve absent), venous pulsations can be transmitted from the chest.[68] Spuriously low SpO2 readings are therefore most likely to occur during positive-pressure ventilation, in the head-down (Trendelenburg) position, and when venous drainage from the neck is impeded. The SpO2 underreading can be significant, depending on the venous pulse pressure and the distensibility of the venous system at the probe site. Barker describes one case (anterior neck surgery) in which the forehead reflectance pulse oximeter (Nellcor Max-Fast) read an SpO_2 of 60 percent to 70 percent for the entire case, while an earlobe sensor and arterial blood gas analysis indicated saturation percentages in the mid-90s.[22]

Skin pigmentation has been reported to cause inaccurate SpO_2 readings at low oxygen saturations, especially if the skin is very dark.[69] Some nail polishes and artificial nails will affect the accuracy of the pulse oximetry. Dark colors, particularly blue and green, cause spuriously low SpO_2 readings.[70,71]

Intravenously administered dyes (methylene blue, indigo carmine, indocyanine green) cause spuriously low SpO_2 readings,[72-75] Methylene blue has its major spectral absorbance peak at 668 nm, which is close to the wavelength at which pulse oximeters read the red absorbance for deoxygenated hemoglobin. The effect may last 10 to 60 minutes with a dose of 2 to 5 mg/kg of methylene blue, and 1 to 15 minutes for indocyanine green at a dose of 0.5 to 2 mg/kg.

Clinical motion is one of the most common causes of inaccuracy in SpO_2 if the patient is awake and moving the extremities, or is shivering.[76,77] Most contemporary pulse oximeters incorporate motion-resistant algorithms that will diminish these effects on the SpO_2 readings.

A low perfusion state is one of the most challenging problems, especially in the ICU and PACU. If the extremities (fingers, toes, ears) are hypoperfused, peripheral blood flow is minimal, and skin is cold, then the pulse oximeter may be unable to detect an adequate plethysmographic wave and therefore may be unable to follow the changes in absorbances during the cardiac cycle.

Palve and Vuori studied the lowest values of pulse pressure (dPP) and peripheral temperature (Tp) associated with reliable readings from three different early pulse oximeters, along with the ability of the pulse oximeters to work immediately before and after total cardiopulmonary bypass (CPB).[78] In their study, the lowest mean dPP with a reliable O_2 saturation reading was 13 mmHg and the lowest mean Tp was 23.6°C. The dPP needed for a reliable reading before total CPB did not differ significantly from that needed after total CPB. No significant differences in performance were found among the three oximeters during this study.

Irita and associates[79] compared the performance of a newer pulse oximeter (Masimo SET) with that of a conventional (Nihon Kohden AY-900P) pulse oximeter during hypothermic CPB with nonpulsatile flow. The newer device displayed accurate SpO_2 significantly more frequently and for longer than a conventional oximeter. The authors concluded that the more recently developed pulse oximeters seem to perform better during hypoperfusion.

Use of electrocautery can induce "noise" in the pulse oximetry waveform and interfere with measurement of SpO_2.[80] Intense ambient light – for example, in the operating room under the surgical lamps – can cause spuriously high readings.[81] It is therefore generally recommended that the sensor and sensor site be covered to avoid interference by ambient light.

Use of a conventional pulse oximeter device with a normal sensor within the magnetic field of an MRI can cause burning or melting of the cable on the skin and burns of the sensor site.[82-84] The monitor will also move in the magnetic field. Specially designed pulse oximeters, which use a fiberoptic cable to transmit light to and from the MRI-compatible sensors, are now available for use in the MRI suite. In addition, the monitor itself must be isolated from the magnetic field.

The failure rate of pulse oximetry has been the subject of several studies.[85-86] Recognition that there is a failure rate is important clinically, as well as medicolegally, because its use is considered the standard of care.[80] Moller and coworkers,[47] reviewing handkept anesthesia records, reported a total failure rate of the oximetry in 10,802 patients of 2.5 percent, but the failure rate increased to 7.2 percent in patients who were ASA physical status 4. Freund and colleagues[86] reviewed the handkept records of 11,046 cases studied at four University of Washington Hospitals, and reported an overall failure rate of 1.24 percent, but 4.24 percent at the Veterans Hospital, where ASA physical status tended to be greater.

Reich and coworkers[85] studied predictors of pulse oximetry data failure by reviewing 9203 electronic medical records, and reported a failure rate of 9.18 percent. The independent preoperative predictors of pulse oximetry data failure were ASA physical status 3, 4, or 5 and orthopedic, vascular, or cardiac surgery. Intraoperative hypothermia, hypotension, hypertension, and duration of procedure were also independent risk factors for pulse oximetry data failure. These authors concluded that pulse oximetry data failure rates based on review of computerized records were markedly greater than those previously reported with handkept records. Physical status, type of surgery, and intraoperative variables were risk factors for pulse oximetry data failure. They also recommended that regulations and expectations regarding pulse oximetry monitoring should reflect the limitations of the technology.

Credentialing

Pulse oximeters are user-friendly, the sensors are easy to apply, and no credentialing is required. However, users should receive in-service training for correct application of sensors. Some recommend that LEDs in the finger probes be applied to the surface of the fingernail and the photodetector on the palmar side of the fingertip. If, however, the patient is wearing nail polish that might interfere with the accuracy of the SpO_2 reading, then the probe can be rotated through 90 degrees on the fingertip so the nail is no longer in the path of the emitted light.[87] Some sensors, especially those used in neonates, need special attention before application on a newborn. Disposable adhesive sensors can be used on the finger, palm, sole, or toe. Clip-on probes are used on the ear, or sometimes on the nose.

Misapplication of a sensor can cause pulse oximetry failure or spurious readings. Thus, if a finger probe is applied such that some of the emitted light passes tangential to, rather than through, the fingertip to reach the photodetector, similar amounts of light at 660 and 940 nm reach the detector. This leads to a spuriously low SpO$_2$ reading because of an "R = 1, SpO$_2$ = 85%" situation, sometimes called the *penumbra effect*.[88] In-servicing is important when forehead sensors are used for reflectance pulse oximetry. The elastic headband used to apply pressure to the probe site must not be too tight; otherwise, pressure injury or a burn may result. Use of pulse oximetry in the MRI suite also warrants specific in-service training.

Practice parameters

The intraoperative and postoperative use of pulse oximetry for patient monitoring is considered to be the standard of care. The evolution of pulse oximetry in ASA standards has been eloquently described by Eichhorn.[43] The ASA standards for basic anesthetic monitoring (last amended October 2010)[42] standard II, Oxygenation, 2, state:

Blood oxygenation: During all anesthetics, a quantitative method of assessing oxygenation such as pulse oximetry shall be employed.* When the pulse oximeter is utilized, the variable pitch pulse tone and the low threshold alarm shall be audible to the anesthesiologist or the anesthesia care team personnel.* Adequate illumination and exposure of the patient are necessary to assess color.*"

["† Note that "continual" is defined as "repeated regularly and frequently in steady rapid succession" whereas "continuous" means "prolonged without any interruption at any time." Under extenuating circumstances, the responsible anesthesiologist may waive the requirements marked with an asterisk (*); it is recommended that when this is done, it should be so stated (including the reasons) in a note in the patient's medical record.]

The ASA standards for postanesthesia care state:[53]

STANDARD IV

THE PATIENT'S CONDITION SHALL BE EVALUATED CONTINUALLY IN THE PACU.

1. The patient shall be observed and monitored by methods appropriate to the patient's medical condition. Particular attention should be given to monitoring oxygenation, ventilation, circulation, level of consciousness and temperature. During recovery from all anesthetics, a quantitative method of assessing oxygenation such as pulse oximetry shall be employed in the initial phase of recovery.* This is not intended for application during the recovery of the obstetrical patient in whom regional anesthesia was used for labor and vaginal delivery.

The astute reader will note that the ASA standards directly quoted here require "a quantitative method of assessing oxygenation," but do not require pulse oximetry specifically. The standards as written, therefore, will not have to be rewritten (and reapproved) if and when alternative or superior technologies become available.

Many states, including New York and New Jersey, have written similar monitoring of oxygenation requirements into the state health regulations. For example, the New York regulation

(405.13. Anesthesia Services. 2.[iii][d] states that "monitoring the patient's oxygenation shall be continuously monitored to ensure adequate oxygen concentration in the inspired gas and the blood through the use of a pulse oximeter or superior equipment."[89]

Pulse oximetry is included in the international standards for the safe practice of anaesthesia, 2008[90] and in ambulatory anesthesia.[58] Monitoring of SpO$_2$ is the standard of care in PACUs, non-OR anesthetizing locations such as catheterization/angiography laboratories, MRI units, radiology and endoscopy suites, office-based anesthesia, during transport of critically ill patients, in the emergency department, and during ambulance transport.[53–58] Preoperative evaluation clinics, sleep laboratories, pulmonary function laboratories, and spirometry and exercise laboratories also use SpO$_2$ monitoring.

Pulse oximeters are widely available to clinicians and to the general public, and used in many nonmedical locations (Figure 16.11). In malls, markets, and airplanes, pulse oximeters have been used as a spot-check device in emergency situations to determine whether a patient is hypoxemic and to rapidly obtain pulse rate information. In CPR situations SpO$_2$, pulse rate, and plethysmographic amplitude values help to determine the efficacy of CPR (i.e. if there is pulsatile flow in the peripheral extremities). Small portable pulse oximeters are used by mountain climbers, pilots, and divers to prevent and detect hypoxemia.

The plethysmographic pulse wave and the changes in plethysmographic amplitude are among new areas of research interest. Evaluation of the stage of hypovolemia and the effects of volume loading on the plethysmographic pulse volume amplitude changes during respiratory cycle can be used as a measure of hypovolemia and responsiveness to volume loading.[91,92] The plethysmogram can also be used for the assessment of arterial patency and arterial occlusion (Allen test). In

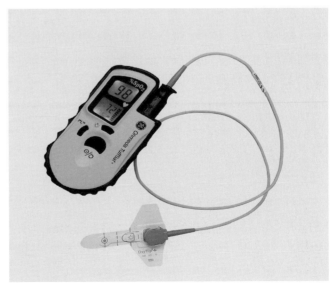

Figure 16.11. Hand-held pulse oximeter (Tuffsat, GE). Permission given by General Electric Company.

the future, one may see many new parameters derived from plethysmographic waveforms obtained from various sites.[93,94]

In the preanesthesia assessment clinic, a multiwavelength pulse oximeter is especially useful in the evaluation of patients who are scheduled for surgery. The ability to noninvasively measure SpO_2, $HbO_2\%$, COHB, metHb, total hemoglobin, pulse rate, and perfusion indices constitutes a major advance in perioperative patient care. Pulse oximetry is widely accepted for clinical (and outside-hospital) use.

Since its discovery and introduction into widespread clinical (and nonclinical) uses, there have been significant advances in the science of pulse oximetry, the most recent being the ability to monitor hemoglobin continuously and noninvasively. The future development of this monitoring modality presents many exciting possibilities.[31,95,96,97]

References

1. Lumb AB. Oxygen. In *Nunn's Applied Respiratory Physiology*, 5th ed. Woburn, MA: Butterworth-Heinemann, 2000, pp. 249–305.

2. Severinghaus JW. Historical development of oxygenation monitoring. In Payne JP, Severinghaus JW, eds. *Pulse Oximetry*, Berlin: Springer, 1986, pp. 1–18.

3. Severinghaus JW, Aoyagi T. Discovery of pulse oximetry. *Anesth Analg* 2007;**105**:S1–4.

4. Squire JR. Instrument for measuring quantity of blood and its degree of oxygenation in the web of the hand. *Clin Sci* 1940;**4**: 331–9.

5. Millikan GA. The oximeter: an instrument for measuring continuously oxygen saturation of arterial blood in man. *Rev Sci Instrum* 1942;**13**:434–44.

6. Pologe JA. Pulse oximetry: technical aspects. *Int Anesthesiol Clin* 1987;**25**:137–53.

7. Severinghaus JW, Naifeh KH. Accuracy of response of six pulse oximeters to profound hypoxia. *Anesthesiology* 1987;**67**:551–8.

8. Severinghaus JW, Naifeh KH, Koh SO. Errors in 14 pulse oximeters during profound hypoxia. *J Clin Monit* 1989;**5**:72–81.

9. Severinghaus JW, Spellman MJ Jr. Pulse oximeter failure thresholds in hypotension and vasoconstriction. *Anesthesiology* 1990;**73**:532–7.

10. Severinghaus JW, Kelleher JF. Recent developments in pulse oximetry. *Anesthesiology* 1992;**76**:1018–38.

11. Barker SJ, Shah NK. Effects of motion on performance of pulse oximeters in volunteers. *Anesthesiology* 1996;**85**:774–81.

12. Goldman JM, Petterson MT, Kopotic RJ, Barker SJ. Masimo signal extraction pulse oximetry. *J Clin Monit Comput* 2000;**16**:475–83.

13. Barker SJ. Motion resistant pulse oximetry: a comparison of new and old models. *Anesth Analg* 2002;**95**:967–72.

14. Barker SJ, Tremper KK. The effect of carbon monoxide inhalation on pulse oximetry and transcutaneous PO_2. *Anesthesiology* 1987;**66**:677–679.

15. Vegfors M, Lennmarken C. Carboxyhaemoglobinaemia and pulse oximetry. *Br J Anaesth* 1991;**66**:625–6.

16. Barker SJ, Tremper KK, Hyatt J. Effects of methemoglobinemia on pulse oximetry and mixed venous oximetry. *Anesthesiology* 1989;**70**:112–7.

17. Eisenkraft JB. Pulse oximeter desaturation due to methemoglobinemia. *Anesthesiology*. 1988;**68**:279–82.

18. Annabi EH, Barker SJ. Severe methemoglobinemia detected by pulse oximetry. *Anesth Analg* 2009;**108**:898–9.

19. Varon AJ. Methemoglobinemia and pulse oximetry. *Crit Care Med* 1992;**20**:1363–4.

20. Eisenkraft JB. Forehead pulse oximetry: friend and foe. *Anesthesiology* 2006;**105**:1075–7.

21. Cortinez LI, MacLeod DB, Wright D, et al. Assessment of vasoactivity at different sites using oximeter's plethysmograph. *Anesthesiology* 2003;**99**:A-560.

22. Barker SJ. Problems with forehead reflectance pulse oximetry. *Respir Care* 2006;**51**:715–6.

23. Shelley KH, Tamai D, Jablonka D, et al. The effect of venous pulsation on the forehead pulse oximeter wave form as a possible source of error in SpO2 calculation, *Anesth Analg* 2005;**100**: 743–7.

24. Agashe GS, Coakley J, Mannheimer PD. Forehead pulse oximetry: headband use helps alleviate false low readings likely related to venous pulsation artifact. *Anesthesiology* 2006;**105**:1111–6.

25. Cannesson M, Delannoy B, Morand A, et al. Does the pleth variability index indicate the respiratory-induced variation in the plethysmogram and arterial pressure waveforms? *Anesth Analg* 2008;**106**: 1189–94.

26. Feissel M, Teboul JL, Merlani P, Badie J, Faller JP, Bendjelid K. Plethysmography dynamic indices predict fluid responsiveness in septic ventilated patients. *Intensive Care Med* 2007;**33**:993–9.

27. Bendjelid K. The pulse oximetry plethysmographic curve revisited. *Curr Opin Crit Care*. 2008;**14**:348–53.

28. Shelley KH. Photo-plethysmograpy: beyond the calculation of arterial oxygen saturation and heart rate. *Anesth Analg* 2007;**105**: S31–36.

29. Reisner A, Shaltis PA, McCombie D, et al. Utility of the photoplethysmogram in circulatory monitoring. *Anesthesiology* 2008;**108**:950–8.

30. Barker, SJ, Curry J, Redford D, Morgan S. Measurement of carboxyhemoglobin and methemoglobin by pulse oximetry: A human volunteer study. *Anesthesiology* 2006;**105**:892–7

31. Barker SG, Badal JJ. The measurement of dyshemoglobins and total hemoglobin by pulse oximetry. *Current Opinion in Anesthesiology* 2008;**21**:805–10.

32. Feiner JR, Bickler PE, Mannheimer PD. Accuracy of methemoglobin detection by pulse co-oximetry during hypoxia. *Anesth Analg* 2010;**111**:143–8.

33. Macknet MR, Allard M, Applegate RL, Rook J. The accuracy of noninvasive and continuous total hemoglobin measurement by pulse co-oximetry in human subjects undergoing hemodilution. *Anesth Analg* 2010;**111**: 1424–6.

34. American Society of Anesthesiologists Task Force on Operating Room Fires, Caplan RA, Barker SJ, Connis RT, et al. *Anesthesiology* 2008;**108**:786–801.

35. Dimich I, Singh PP, Adell A, Hendler M, Sonnenklar N, Jhaveri M. Evaluation of oxygen saturation monitoring by pulse oximetry in neonates in the delivery system. *Can J Anesth* 1991;**38**:985–8.

36. Sugino S, Kanaya N, Mizuuchi M, et al. Forehead is as sensitive as finger pulse oximetry during general anesthesia. *Can J Anesth* 2004;**51**:432–6.

37. Wallace DK. Oxygen saturation levels and retinopathy of prematurity – are we on target? *J AAPOS* 2006;**10**:382–3.

38. Hovagim A, Backus WW, Manecke G, et al. Pulse oximetry and patient positioning. *Anesthesiology* 1989;**71**:454–6.

39. Toth B, Becker A, Seelbach-Goebel B. Oxygen saturation in healthy newborn infants immediately after birth measured by pulse oximetry. *Arch Gynecol Obstet* 2002;**266**:105–7.

40. Durbin CG, Rostow SK. More reliable oximetry reduces the frequency of arterial blood gas analyses and hastens weaning after

cardiac surgery: a prospective, randomized trial of the clinical impact of a new technology. *Crit Care Med* 2002;**30**:1735–40.

41. Eichhorn JH, Cooper JB, Cullen DJ, et al. Standards for patient monitoring during anesthesia at Harvard Medical School. *JAMA* 1986;**256**:1017–20.

42. American Society of Anesthesiologists. Standards of the American Society of Anesthesiologists: Standards for Basic Anesthetic Monitoring. Available at http://www.asahq.org/publicationsAndServices/standards/02.pdf.

43. Eichhorn JH. Pulse oximetry as a standard of practice in anesthesia. *Anesthesiology* 1993;**78**:423–5.

44. Moller JT, Jensen PF, Johannessen, Espersen K. Hypoxemia is reduced by pulse oximetry monitoring in the operation theater and in the recovery room. *Br J Anaesth* 1992;**68**:146–50.

45. Cote CJ, Goldstein EA, Cote MA, Hoaglin DC, Ryan JF. A single blind study of pulse oximetry in children. *Anesthesiology* 1988;**68**:184–8.

46. Caplan RA, Posner KL, Ward RJ, Cheney FW. Adverse respiratory events in anesthesia: a closed claims analysis. *Anesthesiology* 1990;**72**:828–33.

47. Moller JT, Pedersen T, Rasmussen LS, et al. Randomized evaluation of pulse oximetry in 20,802 patients: I. *Anesthesiology* 1993;**78**:436–44.

48. Moller JT, Johannessen NW, Espersen K, et al. Randomized evaluation of pulse oximetry in 20,802 patients: II. *Anesthesiology* 1993;**78**:445–53.

49. Cheney FW, Posner KL, Lee LA, Caplan RA, Domino KB. Trends in anesthesia-related death and brain damage: a closed claims analysis. *Anesthesiology* 2006;**105**:1081–6.

50. Pedersen T, Moller AM, Dyrlund Pedersen B. Pulse oximetry for perioperative monitoring: Systematic review of randomized, controlled trials. *Anesth Analg* 2003;**96**:426–31.

51. Robbertze R, Posner KL, Domino KB. Closed claims review of anesthesia for procedures outside the operating room. *Curr Opin Anesthesiol* 2006;**19**:436–42.

52. Bierman MI, Stein KL, Snyder JV. Pulse oximetry in the postoperative care of cardiac surgical patients. A randomized controlled trial. *Chest* 1992;**102**:1367–70.

53. *Standards fo Basic Anesthetic Monitoring* Park Ridge, IL: American Society of Anesthesiologists, 1986, and last amended October 20, 2010, http://www.asahq.org/Standards/02.html.

54. *Standards for Postanesthesia Care* (last amended October 19, 1994). Park Ridge, IL: American Society of Anesthesiologists, 2001, http://www.asahq.org/Standards/02.html

55. Guidelines Committee, American College of Critical Care Medicine, Society of Critical Care Medicine and the Transfer Guidelines Task Force. Guidelines for the transfer of critically ill patients. *Am J Crit Care* 1993;**2**:189–95.

56. *Guidelines for Non-Operating Room Anesthetizing Locations* (Approved by House of Delegates, October 19, 1994). Park Ridge, IL: American Society of Anesthesiologists, 2001.

57. *Guidelines for Office-Based Anesthesia* (approved by House of Delegates, October 13, 1999). Park Ridge, IL: American Society of Anesthesiologists, 2001.

58. *Guidelines for Ambulatory Anesthesia and Surgery* (last amended October 21, 1998). Park Ridge, IL: American Society of Anesthesiologists, 2001, http://www.asahq.org/Standards/02.html.

59. Pedersen T, Dyrlund Pedersen B, Moller AM. Pulse oximetry for perioperative monitoring. *Cochrane Database Syst Rev* 2003;**3**.

60. Sloan TB. Finger injury by an oxygen saturation monitor probe. *Anesthesiology* 1988;**68**:936–8.

61. Berge KH, Lainier WL, Scanlon PD. Ischemic digital skin necrosis: a complication of the reusable Nellcor pulse oximeter probe. *Anesth Analg* 1988;**67**:712–3.

62. Miyasaka K, Ohata JO. Burn, erosion and "sun" tan with the use of pulse oximetry in infants. *Anesthesiology* 1987;**67**:1008–9.

63. Ash-Bernal R, Wise R, Wright SM. Acquired methemoglobinemia: A retrospective series of 138 cases at two teaching hospitals. *Medicine* (Baltimore) 2004;**83**:265–73.

64. Severinghaus JW, Koh SO. Effect of anemia on pulse oximeter accuracy at low saturation. *J Clin Monit* 1990;**6**:85–88.

65. Lee S, Tremper KK, Barker SJ. Effects of anemia on pulse oximetry and continuous mixed venous hemoglobin saturation monitoring in dogs. *Anesthesiology* 1991;**75**:118–22.

66. Rajadurai VS, Walker AM, Yu VY, Oates A. Effect of fetal haemoglobin on the accuracy of pulse oximetry in preterm infants. *J Paediatr Child Health* 1992;**28**:43–6.

67. Arikan GM, Haeusler MC, Haas J, Scholz H. Does the hemoglobin concentration in fetal blood interfere with the accuracy of fetal reflection pulse oximetry? *Fetal Diagn Therap* 1998;**13**:236–40.

68. Sami HM, Kleinman BS, Lonchyna VA. Central venous pulsations associated with a falsely low oxygen saturation measured by pulse oximetry. *J Clin Monit* 1991;**7**:309–12.

69. Feiner J, Severinghaus JW, Bickler PE. Dark skin decreases the accuracy of pulse oximetrers at low oxygen saturation: The effects of pulse oximeter probe type and gender. *Anesth Analg* 2007;**105**:S18–23.

70. Ralston AC, Webb RK, Runciman WB. Potential errors in pulse oximetry. III: effects of interferences, dyes, dyshaemoglobins, and other pigments. *Anaesthesia.* 1991;**46**:291–5.

71. Cote CJ, Goldstein EA, Fuchsman WH, Hoaglin DC. The effect of nail polish on pulse oximetry. *Anesth Analg* 1988;**67**:683–6.

72. Sidi A, Paulus DA, Rush W, et al. Methylene blue and indocyanine green artifactually lower pulse oximetry readings of oxygen saturation. Studies in dogs. *J Clin Monit* 1987;**3**:249–56.

73. Yusim Y, Livingstone D, Sidi A. Blue dyes, blue people: the systemic effects of blue dyes when administered via different routes. *J Clin Anesth* 2007;**19**:315–21.

74. Scheller MS, Unger RJ, Kelner MJ. Effects of intravenously administered dyes on pulse oximetry readings. *Anesthesiology* 1986;**65**:550–2.

75. Gorman ES, Shnider MR. Effect of methylene blue on the absorbance of solutions of haemoglobin. *Br J Anaesth.* 1988;**60**:439–44.

76. Barker SJ, Shah NK. The effects of motion on the performance of pulse oximeters in volunteers. *Anesthesiology* 1997;**86**:101–8.

77. Petterson MT, Begnoche VL, Graybeal JM. The effect of motion on pulse oximetry and its clinical significance. *Anesth Analg* 2007:**105**:S78–84.

78. Palve H, Vuori A. Minimum pulse pressure and peripheral temperature needed for pulse oximetry during cardiac surgery with cardiopulmonary bypass. *J Thorac Cardiovasc Anesth* 1991;**5**:327–30.

79. Irita K, Kai Y, Akiyoshi K, et al. Performance evaluation of a new pulse oximeter during mild hypothermic cardiopulmonary bypass. *Anesth Analg* 2003;**96**:11–4.

80. Block FE, Detko GJ. Minimizing interference and false alarms from electrocautery in the Nellcor N-100 pulse oximeter. *J Clin Monit* 1986;**2**:203–5.

81. Hanowell L, Eisele JH, Downs D. Ambient light affects pulse oximeters. *Anesthesiology* 1987;**67**:864–5.

82. Jorgensen NH, Messick JM, Gray J, Nugent M, Berquist TH. ASA monitoring standards and magnetic resonance imaging. *Anesth Analg* 1994;**79**:1141–7.

83. Salvo I, Colombo S, Capocasa T, Torri G. Pulse oximetry in MRI units. *J Clin Anesth* 1990;**2**:65–6.

84. Bashein G, Syrory G. Burns associated with pulse oximetry during magnetic resonance imaging. *Anesthesiology* 1991;**75**:382–3.

85. Reich DL, Timcenko A, Bodian CA, et al. Predictors of pulse oximetry data failure. *Anesthesiology* 1996;**84**:859–64.

86. Freund PR, Overand PT, Cooper J. A prospective study of intraoperative pulse oximetry failure. *J Clin Monit* 1991;**7**: 253–8.

87. White PF, Boyle WA. Nail polish and oximetry. *Anesth Analg* 1989;**68**:546–7.

88. Kelleher JH, Ruff RH. The penumbra effect: vasomotion-dependent pulse oximeter artifact due to probe malposition. *Anesthesiology* 1989;**71**:787–91.

89. New York State Laws and Regulations. http://www.health.state.ny.us/nysdoh/phforum/nycrr10.htm.

90. 2008 International Standards for a Safe Practice of Anaesthesia. An update of the Standards developed by the International Task Force on Anaesthesia by the World Federation of Societies of Anaesthesiologists 13 June 1992. http://www.isaweb.in/forms/ansafprac.pdf.

91. Shelley KH. Photoplethysmography: beyond the calculation of arterial oxygen saturation and heart rate. *Anesth Analg* 2007;**105**:S31–36.

92. Reisner A, Shaltis PA, Mc Combie D, Asada H. Utility of the photoplethysmogram in circulatory monitoring. *Anesthesiology* 2008;**108**:950–8.

93. Awad AA, Haddadin AS, Tantawy H, et al. The relationship between the photoplethysmographic waveform and systemic vascular resistance. *J Clin Monit Comput* 2007;**21**:365–72.

94. Phillips JP, Kyriacou PA, Jones DP, Shelley KH, Langford RM. Pulse oximetry and photoplethysmographic waveform analysis of the esophagus and bowel. *Curr Opin Anaesthesiol* 2008;**21**: 779–83.

95. Feissel M, Teboul JL, Merlani P, Badie J, Faller JP, Bendjelid K. Plethysmography dynamic indices predict fluid responsiveness in septic ventilated patients. *Intensive Care Med* 2007;**33**: 993–9.

96. Pizov R, Eden A, Bystritski D, Kalina E, Tamir A, Gelman S. Arterial and plethysmographic waveform analysis in anesthetized patients with hypovolemia. *Anesthesiology* 2010;**113**:89–91.

97. McGrath SP, Ryan KL, Wendelken SM, Rickards CA, Convertino VA. Pulse oximeter plethysmographic waveform changes in awake, spontaneously breathing, hypovolemic volunteers. *Anesth Analg* 2011;**112**:368–74.

Neurologic intraoperative electrophysiologic monitoring

Michael L. McGarvey and Albert T. Cheung

Introduction

Surgical operations have the potential to cause intraoperative neurologic injury by vascular compromise or direct injury to nerves and other central nervous system structures (Table 17.1). Intraoperative neurologic injuries causing permanent disability are considered major surgical complications and contribute to both surgical mortality and long-term morbidity. Because the severity of intraoperative neurologic injuries correlates highly with postoperative outcomes and the potential for rehabilitation, any technique that may lessen, reverse, or even prevent neurologic injury is considered valuable.

Strategies to avoid, prevent, and enable early intervention for treatment of intraoperative neurologic injuries require techniques to detect impending neurologic injury in anesthetized patients. Neurologic intraoperative electrophysiologic monitoring (NIOM) provides a means for early identification of impending or ongoing intraoperative neurologic injuries, thus permitting a chance to intervene before the injury becomes permanent or to initiate therapy at the time of injury to lessen the extent of damage (Table 17.2). Changes to a patient's neurologic electrophysiologic baselines during the procedure alert the operative team that a potential injury may be occurring. The goal of NIOM is to detect dysfunction resulting from ischemia, mass effect, stretch, heat, or direct injury in real time before it causes permanent neurologic injury Monitoring may also be useful in identifying and preserving neurologic structures during a procedure when they are at risk (mapping).

In extraoperative testing of evoked potentials, individual neurophysiologic laboratories establish their standard normal values for patients. This is not the case in the operating room, in which physiologic effects of anesthesia, temperature, and environment have a significant effect on neurophysiologic testing. In the operating room, patients serve as their own baseline, and it is changes in this baseline that serve as a warning. In this setting, changes in anesthetic and temperature during an operation may have a significant impact on neurophysiologic testing; this must be taken into account when interpreting these tests.

Furthermore, the operating room is a very hostile environment when trying to monitor the electrical impulses of the human body. Electrical interference from 60 Hz noise, electrocautery, electrical drills, microscopes, and other equipment used during operations often create artifacts that make

Table 17.1. Operations and associated neurologic injuries

Operation	Injuries
Carotid endarterectomy	Stroke
Cerebral aneurysm	Stroke
Brain tumor	Stroke, brain injury
Acoustic neuroma	Nerve injury
ENT resections	Nerve injury
Scoliosis	Spinal cord ischemia, spinal cord injury
Thoracic aorta	Stroke, encephalopathy
Cardiac operations	Stroke, encephalopathy
Thoracoabdominal aorta	Stroke, spinal cord ischemia
Thoracic endovascular aortic repair	Stroke, spinal cord ischemia

monitoring difficult. Additional technical difficulties encountered in the intraoperative setting include liquid saturation of equipment, disconnected wires, equipment malfunction, and limited access to the patient. Considering these challenges, successful intraoperative monitoring requires experienced technicians and neurophysiologists who are accustomed to working closely with the anesthesia and surgical teams. Testing and certification in the United States for intraoperative monitoring

Table 17.2. Neurologic intraoperative electophysiologic monitoring techniques

Technique	Utility
Electroencephalography (EEG)	Detection of brain ischemia
	Detection of seizure activity
	Assessment of brain metabolic activity
Somatosensory evoked potential (SSEP)	Detection of stroke
	Sensory nerve ischemia
	Sensory nerve injury
	Spinal cord injury
	Spinal cord ischemia
Motor-evoked potential (MEP)	Motor nerve ischemia
	Motor nerve injury
	Spinal cord injury
	Spinal cord ischemia
Brainstem auditory evoked potential (BAEP)	Injury to auditory pathway
	Injury to eighth cranial nerve
Visual-evoked potential (VEP)	Integrity of visual pathway
	Injury to occipital lobes
	Injury to optic nerve
Nerve integrity monitor (NIM)	Injury to peripheral nerves
Electomyelogram (EMG)	Injury to peripheral nerves
Nerve conduction study (NCS)	Injury to peripheral nerves

technicians is through the American Board of Registration of Electroencephalographic and Evoked Potential Technologists (http://abret.org). For professional neurophysiologists, certification is available through the American Clinical Neurophysiology Society (https://www.acns.org) and the American Society of Neurophysiologic Monitoring (http://www.asnm.org).

There are several challenges to establishing the efficacy of NIOM. The first is that there have been no blinded or randomized trials to support the efficacy of NIOM in humans. Unfortunately, there will likely never be a substantial trial to test the efficacy of NIOM.[1] The reason behind the lack of high-level evidence is that monitoring has become well-established and accepted as the standard of care in many clinical practices. Moreover, the risk-to-benefit ratio for NIOM is favorable because employing NIOM is a very low-risk procedure compared with the risks associated with the operation. The consensus in the surgical community is that monitoring is useful and there would be ethical and medicolegal dilemmas in withholding monitoring in patients who are at potential risk of neurologic injury. Thus, motivation to perform randomized controlled trials to test the effectiveness of NIOM does not exist.

A second limitation of evidence to support the efficacy of NIOM is that if NIOM were effective in preventing an intraoperative neurologic injury, it is difficult to establish a direct relationship between significant intraoperative NIOM changes with neurologic injury if the neurologic injury were avoided. For example, if employing NIOM detects an impending injury that alerts the intraoperative team to avoid or effectively reverse the injury, the benefit of NIOM can never be verified because a neurologic examination cannot be performed in the anesthetized patient during operation and the patient will exhibit a normal neurologic examination after the operation.

Finally, acute intraoperative neurologic injuries are relatively uncommon and often heterogeneous, and a large number of patients would need to be studied to test the effectiveness of NIOM. For these reasons, the clinical utility of NIOM relies on experimental evidence, animal studies, case series with comparisons to historical controls, and expert consensus. Additional support for the clinical utility of NIOM is based on studies and clinical experience assessing the sensitivity and specificity of NIOM for detecting intraoperative injuries by demonstrating that monitoring can detect injury in cases in which injury has occurred (true positives), monitoring showing that no injury occurred (true negatives), the false-negative rate (injury occurred but not detected), and the false-positive rate (injury was predicted by NIOM at the end of a procedure but injury did not occur). Multimodality monitoring can also be performed to compare the ability of different NIOM techniques to predict injury within the same patient.

Neurologic electrophysiologic techniques

Various portions of the nervous system can be monitored by using several NIOM techniques. The specific neurologic tissues at risk, as well as the type of potential injury, vary with different surgical procedures. Specific techniques include electroencephalography (EEG), evoked potentials including somatotosensory evoked potentials (SSEP), brainstem auditory evoked potentials (BAEP), visual evoked potentials (VEP), electromyography (EMG), nerve conduction studies (NCSs), and transcortical electrical motor evoked potentials (TcMEPs).

Electroencephalography

EEG is a measure of spontaneous electrical brain activity recorded from electrodes placed in standard patterns on a patient's scalp or directly on the cortex with sterile electrode strips or grids. Although there is controversy regarding which montages and the number of electrodes that are optimal when recording the EEG from the scalp, the standard 10/20 system of electrode placement is typically used.[2] The differences in activity between individual electrodes is amplified and then recorded as continuous wavelets, which have different frequencies and amplitudes. These data can be displayed as a raw EEG (Figure 17.1) on a display in a series of channels or broken down into its basic components of frequency and amplitude and displayed as a spectral analysis. A change in a patient's background EEG activity from baseline during a procedure may indicate ischemia of the cerebral cortex, either focally or through a generalized loss of activity over the entire cortex (Figure 17.2). A greater than 50 percent attenuation of non-delta EEG activity or an increase in delta activity greater than 1 Hz is generally considered a significant change within two minutes of an intervention that may produce cerebral ischemia (Figures 17.2 and 17.3).[3,4] At many centers, EEG is routinely used intraoperatively during carotid endarterectomy (CEA), cerebral aneurysm and arteriovenous malformation surgery, or in other procedures that place the cortex at risk.[1,5-7]

One of the most common uses of NIOM is EEG during CEA and other intracranial vascular procedures, when the brain is at risk for ischemic injury as a result of hypoperfusion. Although commonly used to monitor CEAs, few data exist to support its use, including a lack of randomized trials. Intraoperative stroke is rare, occurring in approximately 2 percent to 3 percent of CEAs, with a large proportion of these strokes caused by embolism.[5-7] Despite the lack of data from randomized trials, it is clear that a small proportion of these strokes is the result of hypoperfusion, and it is known from both animal studies and human blood flow studies that loss of EEG activity reflects reduction of blood flow in the brain.[8,9] In a large series of 1152 CEAs, a persistent significant change on intraoperative EEG (12 cases) had 100 percent predictive value for an intraoperative neurologic complication.[6] A critical point during CEA is clamping of the carotid artery to perform the endarterectomy. If ischemia is detected during clamping of the carotid artery, increasing the blood pressure with vasopressor therapy or placement of a carotid shunt may be used to alleviate the ischemia. Significant EEG changes can occur in up to 25 percent of cases during carotid clamping; however, strokes do not occur in a majority of these cases, even without shunting.[3,6,9,10]

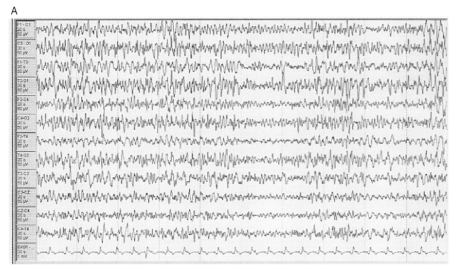

Figure 17.1. Effect of clamping the left internal carotid artery during a left carotid endarterectomy. This EEG was recorded with double-distance electrodes at a paper speed of 2 seconds/epoch. (A) Baseline EEG recorded prior to incision following induction. (B) Demonstration of the effect of clamping the left carotid artery with decrease of EEG amplitude greater than 50% and onset of delta activity greater than 1 Hz in the left hemispheric electrodes (even-numbered electrodes). The surgeon was informed of this change, a right carotid shunt was placed, and the EEG returned to baseline.

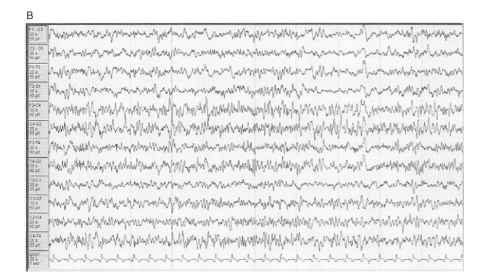

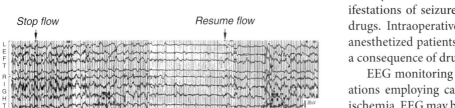

Figure 17.2. Global cerebral hypoperfusion was detected by intraoperative EEG manifested as bilateral slowing and decreased amplitude of the continuous EEG during a brief episode of normothermic (36°C) circulatory arrest in a patient undergoing repair of a proximal descending thoracic aortic aneurysm. Normal EEG activity resumed after restoration of normal circulatory function. Systemic blood flow was interrupted (stop flow) and restored (resume flow) at the times indicated by the arrows. Global cerebral hypoxia (without hypoperfusion) will also produce EEG slowing, but the changes are more gradual compared to acute malperfusion. LEFT = EEG recordings from left cortex; RIGHT = EEG recordings from right cortex.

Intraoperative EEG monitoring can also detect seizure activity in anesthetized patients in whom the neurologic manifestations of seizure are masked by neuromuscular blocking drugs. Intraoperative seizures may occur in patients at risk, anesthetized patients being treated for status epilepticus, or as a consequence of drug-induced seizure activity (Figure 17.4).

EEG monitoring may also be used in cardiovascular operations employing cardiopulmonary bypass to detect cerebral ischemia. EEG may be very useful in detecting cerebral malperfusion in these cases, particularly in aortic dissection repairs, when cannulation of the false lumen can cause malperfusion of the aortic arch branch vessels on initiation of cardiopulmonary bypass. In a review of 97 patients undergoing Type A aortic dissections repairs using EEG monitoring, 6 patients underwent immediate therapeutic interventions based on changes detected by EEG monitoring.[11] Cerebral malperfusion can be quickly detected by intraoperative EEG, permitting time for intervention (Figure 17.2).

A. Before release

B. After release

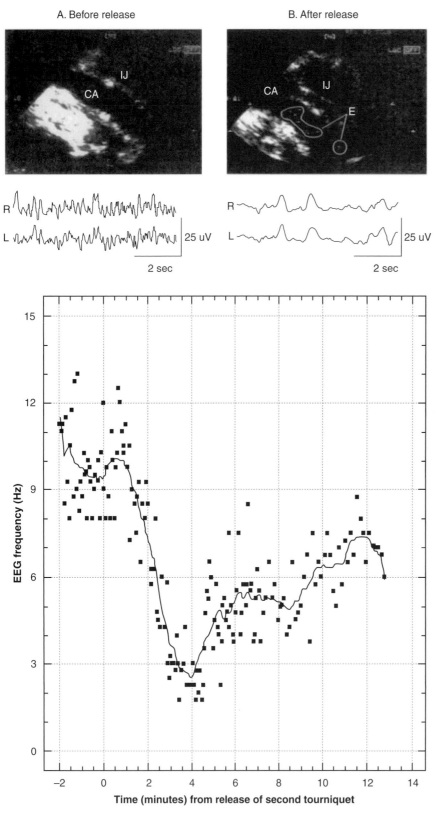

Figure 17.3. Paradoxical cerebral arterial embolism detected by intraoperative EEG and carotid duplex imaging in a patient undergoing bilateral knee replacement. During the operation, sequential release of lower extremity tourniquets was associated with venous thromboemboli that traversed a patent foramen ovale, causing paradoxical embolization to the brain. Top panel displays representative ultrasound images of the right carotid artery (top) and right (R) and left (L) prefrontal-to-frontal (Fp1-F3) EEG waveforms (below) obtained shortly before (A) and after (B) release of the second lower extremity tourniquet. Multiple intravascular emboli (E) were observed in the carotid artery (CA) but not in the internal jugular vein (IJ). Release of the second tourniquet was also associated with marked bilateral slowing and reduction of fast EEG activity within 80 seconds of detection of emboli in the carotid artery (lower panel). Diffuse bilateral EEG slowing caused by the paradoxical embolism to the brain was associated with a fatal neurologic injury. From Weiss, SJ, Cheung, AT, Stecker, MM et al, Fatal paradoxical cerebral embolization during bilateral knee arthroplasty. *Anesthesiology*, 1996, 84 (3) .

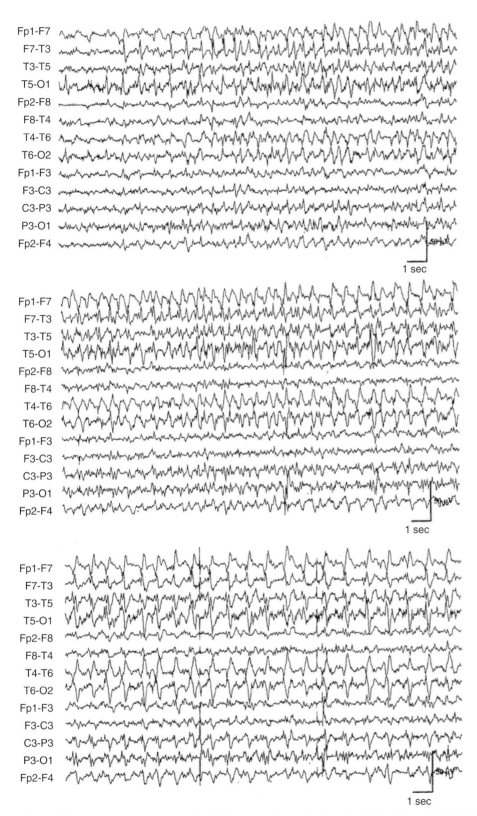

Figure 17.4. Intraoperative recording of the EEG in an anesthetized patient who had an intraoperative seizure in response to the rapid intravascular injection of lidocaine. Serial EEG tracings show the appearance of period complexes over the left hemisphere that evolved in frequency and location over time consistent with seizure activity. EEG seizure patterns include generalized spike and wave activity, repetitive rapid spiking that change in frequency and location over 20 to 300 seconds, or focal or generalized buildup of fast activity that evolves over time into generalized spike discharges. Modified from Cheung AT et al. *Anesthesiology* 2001;94:1143–7.

Anesthetic agents that produce unconsciousness have the potential to attenuate EEG amplitude and frequencies. Barbiturates, propofol, and etomidate cause dose-dependent slowing of the EEG and may suppress it altogether when administered as an intravenous bolus. Inhaled anesthetic agents suppress EEG activity in a dose-dependent fashion, with isoflurane producing burst suppression at an end-tidal concentration of 1.75 vol%. Opioid narcotic analgesics at doses typically administered for general anesthesia have very little effect on the EEG. For these reasons, when EEG monitoring is required during general anesthesia, a balanced anesthetic technique is employed using a sedative hypnotic in low doses, narcotic analgesics, neuromuscular blocking agents, and an inhaled anesthetic at a constant concentration of 0.5 MAC. Marking the EEG in the event of bolus sedative hypnotic administration or when the inhaled anesthetic concentration is changed will help to distinguish EEG changes caused by general anesthetics from changes as a consequence of neurologic injury.

Hypothermia produces dose-dependent slowing of the EEG. The predictable actions of hypothermia on EEG activity have made EEG a useful monitor to determine the adequacy of deliberate hypothermia for suppression of brain metabolic activity. In cardiac and neurosurgical procedures requiring temporary circulatory arrest, the onset of electrocortical silence on the EEG during deliberate hypothermia can be used to optimize conditions for deep hypothermic circulatory arrest. Studies have shown that periodic complexes appear on the EEG at an average nasopharyngeal temperature of 29.6°C, burst suppression appears at an average temperature of 24.4°C, and electrocortical silence appears at an average temperature of 17.8°C (Figure 17.5).[12] Because brain temperature cannot be measured directly, EEG changes can be used as a physiologic surrogate to assess the metabolic activity of the brain during progressive levels of deliberate hypothermia. When EEG was employed to manage patients undergoing deep hypothermic circulatory arrest, it was found that electrocortical silence occurred over a range of nasopharyngeal temperatures among patients and that the only absolute predictors of electrocortical silence were a nasopharygeal temperature of 12.5°C or at least 50 minutes of cooling on cardiopulmonary bypass (Figure 17.6).

Somatosensory evoked potentials

Evoked potentials are measures of nervous system electrical activity resulting from a specific stimulus that is applied to the patient. Electrodes record responses to repetitive stimuli as averaged wavelets at different locations in the nervous system as this evoked activity propagates along its course.

SSEPs are produced by repetitive electrical stimulation of a peripheral nerve while recording averaged potentials as they travel through afferent sensory system. SSEP waveforms are recorded from the peripheral nerves, spinal cord, brainstem, and primary somatosensory cortex (Figure 17.7). The recording of waveforms at sequential locations along the complete afferent sensory system allows for localization of dysfunction during procedures. This dysfunction could be caused by ischemia, mass effect, or local injury. Stimulation and recording parameters for intraoperative SSEPs have been established.[13,14] SSEPs recorded from stimulation of the median nerve (alternatively, the ulnar nerve) at the wrist are used intraoperatively during carotid endarterectomy and intracranial surgery for anterior circulation vascular lesions.[15,16] SSEPs recorded from stimulation of the posterior tibial nerve at the ankle (alternatively, from the common peroneal nerve at the popliteal fossa) in the leg are used during intracranial surgeries involving vascular lesions in the posterior cerebral circulation.[17] Monitoring both upper and lower extremity SSEPs during procedures that place the spinal cord at risk may be useful in procedures to treat scoliosis, spinal tumors, or descending aortic repairs. SSEPs from the sensory nerves of arms and legs have been used to ensure their integrity during peripheral nerve surgery.

The accepted criterion for significant SSEP change, suggesting a potential injury, is a decrease of spinal or cortical amplitudes by 50 percent or an increase in latency by 10 percent from baseline that is reproducible on two subsequent trials.[18] One potential shortcoming of SSEP monitoring, particularly in procedures that place the spinal cord at risk, is that SSEP impulses travel in the dorsal columns of the spinal cord; thus motor pathways are not technically monitored by this modality. SSEP changes may at best reflect injury to the anterior motor tracts during monitoring

Use of SSEP to identify early spinal cord injury has become widespread. The risk of spinal injury varies with different surgeries, but has reported to occur in 1 percent to 2 percent of scoliosis repairs. Significant changes in SSEP have been predictive of injury in several small case series in complex cervical and thoracic spine procedures, but false positives and false negative do occur.[19–24] The risk for injury in cases involving intramedullary spinal lesions, such as tumors, has been reported to be up to 65.4 percent.[25,26] Permanent loss of SSEP signals in descending aortic repairs indicating spinal ischemia has accurately predicted paraplegia (Figure 17.8). Furthermore, good outcomes have been reported in small case series when spinal SSEP changes are reversed with maneuvers that improve spinal perfusion.[27–31] There is a direct correlation to the time of loss of SSEP (40–60 minutes) and the incidence of paraplegia.[32]

Upper extremity SSEP monitoring has been used for monitoring during CEA. A benefit of using SSEP over EEG in CEA is that SSEP allows for monitoring of subcortical structures, although EEG does provide neurophysiologic information for a much larger area of cortex.

The utility of SSEP monitoring during intracranial aneurysm repair has also been studied. In repairs of intracranial aneurysm, temporary occlusion of a proximal vessel such as the carotid may be necessary to increase the safety of aneurysm clip placement. During these periods, monitoring with SSEP may enable longer periods of temporary ischemia, identification of inadequate collateral flow, or malpositioning of aneurysm clips.[17,33]

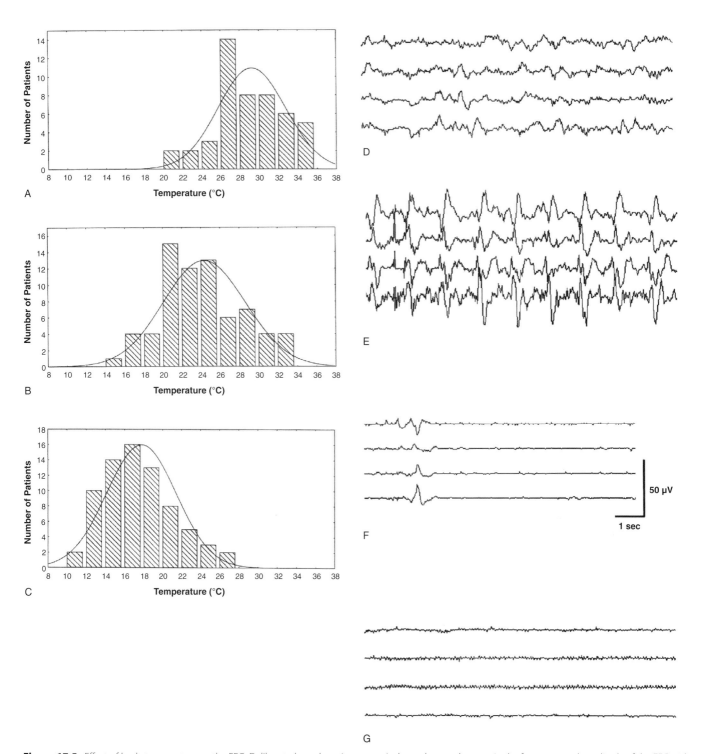

Figure 17.5. Effect of body temperature on the EEG. Deliberate hypothermia progressively produces a decrease in the frequency and amplitude of the EEG with eventual electrocortical silence (ECS) or disappearance of the EEG. The left panel shows the distribution of nasopharyngeal temperatures at which periodic complexes appear (A), burst suppression appears (B), and ECS appears (C). The right panel shows the typical appearance of the EEG at normothermia (D), progressing to periodic complexes (E), burst suppression (F), and ECS (G) as temperature decreases during cooling to deep hypothermia on cardiopulmonary bypass. Data from ref. 12.

Another standard for SSEP monitoring is for localization and mapping of the sensory–motor cortex during resections of tumors and vascular lesions near the motor cortex.[34] Identification of the motor cortex may allow it to be spared in these types of procedures. In this technique, SSEPs are recorded from strips or grids placed directly over the exposed cortex. The recording of a median nerve SSEP by this technique will reveal the largest amplitude N-20 wave over the somatosensory cortex in

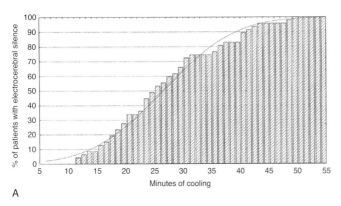
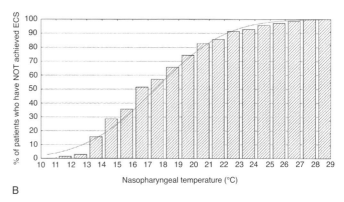

Figure 17.6. Variability in the duration of cooling on cardiopulmonary bypass (A) and nasopharyngeal temperature (B) necessary to achieve ESC with deep hypothermia. At least 50 minutes of cooling or a nasopharyngeal temperature of 12.5°C is necessary to ensure ECS in at least 95% of patients. Data from ref. 12.

a referential montage and a phase reversal of the cortical SSEP in a bipolar montage, thus identifying the location of the central sulcus and motor cortex.

Intraoperative monitoring of SSEP has also been used to detect acute intraoperative stroke. SSEP changes indicating hemispheric stroke are acute unilateral decrease or loss of cortical SSEP with preservation of peripheral nerve and spinal SSEP (Figures 17.9 and 17.10). Intraoperative SSEP monitoring has contributed to the elucidation of mechanisms for thromboembolic stroke during open cardiac operations and thoracic endovascular aortic repairs.[35–37]

General anesthetic agents may interfere with intraoperative SSEP monitoring by increasing SSEP latency and decreasing SSEP amplitude.[38] Inhaled volatile anesthetics cause dose-dependent changes in SSEP latency and amplitude. Combining nitrous oxide with inhaled volatile anesthetics produces an additive effect on the SSEP. In general, although some attenuation of SSEP signals occurs, satisfactory intraoperative monitoring of SSEP can be accomplished with a balanced anesthetic technique at 0.5 MAC concentrations of inhaled anesthetics. Maintaining a constant end-tidal concentration of the inhaled

anesthetic is important to minimize anesthetic-induced alterations of SSEP signals. Intravenous bolus administration of barbiturates and propofol will also increase SSEP latency and decrease SSEP amplitude, with the greatest effect on cortical SSEPs. However, SSEP monitoring can be accomplished during general anesthesia with a continuous infusion of propofol at a dose in the range of 25 mcg/kg/min to 50 mcg/kg/min if the dose is kept constant.

Unlike barbiturates, etomidate and ketamine increase transiently cortical SSEP potentials after intravenous administration. Benzodiazepines have only mild depressant effects on the SSEP, whereas opioid analgesics have no effects, making these agents useful as part of a balanced anesthetic regimen for intraoperative SSEP monitoring. Neuromuscular blocking drugs do not affect the SSEP but improve conditions for intraoperative monitoring by suppressing artifacts caused by muscle contractions in response to the electrical stimulation. Regional nerve blocks or central neural axial blocks with local anesthetic agents will abolish SSEP arising from the affected limbs.

Hypothermia causes marked predictable changes in the SSEP, as it does in the EEG. Progressive levels of hypothermia

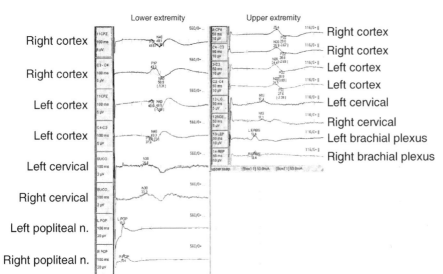

Figure 17.7. Normal appearance of somatosensory evoked potentials (SSEPs) originating from electrical stimulation of anterior tibial nerves in the lower extremities (left panel) and the median nerves in the upper extremities (right panel). Electrical stimulation of the anterior tibial nerve at the ankle generates SSEPs recorded from in the ipsilateral popliteal nerve, ipsilateral cervical spinal cord, and contralateral brain cortex. Electrical stimulation of the median nerve at the wrist generates SSEPs recorded from in the ipsilateral brachial plexus, ipsilateral cervical spinal cord, and contralateral brain cortex. SSEP latency is the duration of time between stimulus and the measured SSEP peak in milliseconds. SSEP amplitude is the peak-to-peak height of the SSEP in microvolts. The presence, latency, and amplitude of SSEP signals are used to assess the integrity of the sensory pathway from the peripheral nerve to the sensory cortex.

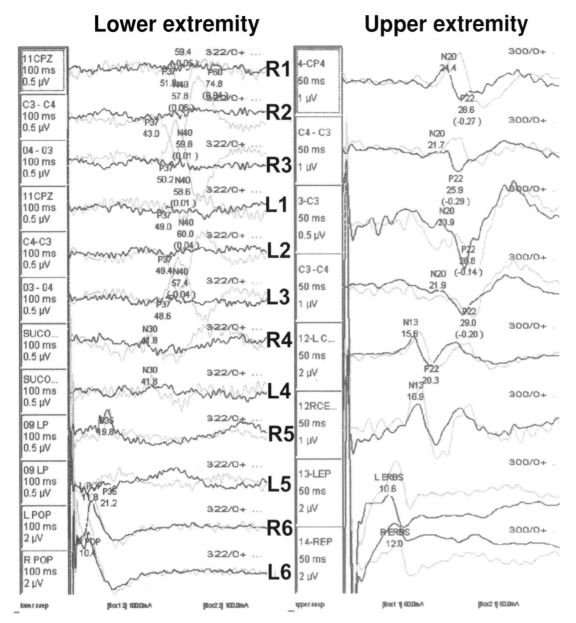

Figure 17.8. Intraoperative somatosensory evoked potential (SSEP) monitoring used to detect spinal cord ischemia in a patient undergoing repair of a thoracoabdominal aortic aneurysm with partial left heart bypass. SSEPs from lower extremity stimulation at the anterior tibial nerve (left panel) were compared with SSEPs from the upper extremity stimulation at the median nerve (right panel). Disappearance of SSEP signals from the right (R) and left (L) lower extremities recorded at the cortex (R1, R2, R3, L1, L2, L3) and spine (R4, L4) with preservation of SSEP signals from the lumbar plexus (R5, L5) and popliteal nerves (R6, L6) indicated the acute onset of spinal cord ischemia. Upper-extremity SSEP signals were maintained during the episode. The light gray tracings were the baseline SSEP signals used for comparison.

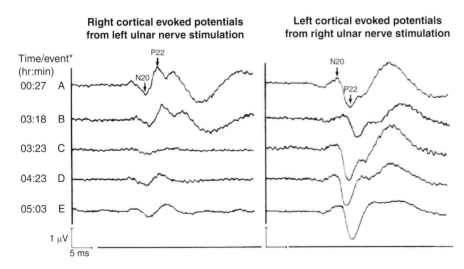

Figure 17.9. Acute intraoperative thromboembolic stroke detected by somatosensory evoked potential (SSEP) monitoring in a patient undergoing mitral valve replacement. Representative cortical N20–P22 SSEPs from right ulnar nerve stimulation (right) and left ulnar nerve stimulation (left) obtained at five elapsed times after the start of operation (time 0). The acute unilateral loss in amplitude of the right cortical N20–P22 SEP from left ulnar nerve stimulation at an elapsed time of 03:23 (h:min) indicated an acute thromboembolic stroke in the territory of the right cerebral hemisphere that occurred shortly after removal of the ascending aortic cross-clamp and the initiation of left ventricular ejection at 03:21. The acute cortical stroke was manifested by an acute unilateral decrease in the cortical N20–P22 SSEP without changes in the right or left Erb's point, N13, and N18 SSEPs. Modified from ref. 37.

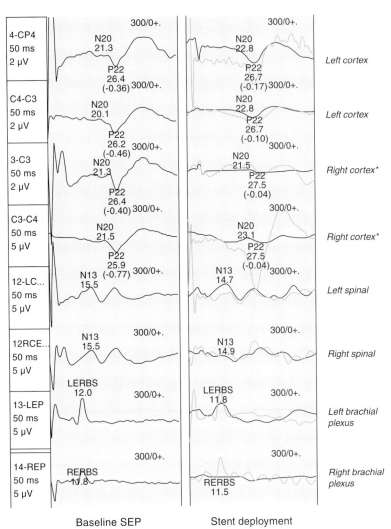

4-CP4 50 ms 2 µV	300/0+. N20 21.3 P22 26.4 (-0.36)
C4-C3 50 ms 2 µV	N20 20.1 P22 26.2 (-0.46)
3-C3 50 ms 2 µV	N20 21.3 P22 26.4 (-0.40)
C3-C4 50 ms 5 µV	N20 21.5 P22 25.9 (-0.77)
12-LC... 50 ms 5 µV	N13 15.5
12RCE... 50 ms 5 µV	N13 15.5
13-LEP 50 ms 5 µV	LERBS 12.0
14-REP 50 ms 5 µV	RERBS 11.8

Baseline SEP   Stent deployment

Right panel labels:
N20 22.8, P22 26.7 (-0.17) — Left cortex
N20 22.8, P22 26.7 (-0.10) — Left cortex
N20 21.5, P22 27.5 (-0.04) — Right cortex*
N20 23.1, P22 27.5 (-0.04) — Right cortex*
N13 14.7 — Left spinal
N13 14.9 — Right spinal
LERBS 11.8 — Left brachial plexus
RERBS 11.5 — Right brachial plexus

Figure 17.10. Intraoperative detection of an acute right cortical thromboembolic stroke during endovascular stent graft repair of a thoracic aortic aneurysm. Acute loss of SSEP amplitude in the right brain cortical SSEPs arising from left median nerve stimulation (right panel) in comparison to baseline (left panel) was consistent with a right hemispheric stroke caused by dislodgment and embolism of vulnerable atheromatous plaque during wire instrumentation of the aortic arch. Postoperatively, neurologic examination revealed left hemiplegia, and computed tomographic (CT) scan of the head revealed an embolic infarct in the territory of the right middle cerebral artery.

prolong SSEP latency, decrease SSEP amplitude, and eventually abolish SSEP signals. The N20–P22 cortical SSEP signal disappeared at a mean nasopharyngeal temperature of 21.4°C and the N13 SSEP disappeared at a mean nasopharyngeal temperature of 28.6°C in a group of cardiac surgical patients undergoing SSEP monitoring during deep hypothermic circulatory arrest for thoracic aortic operations (Figure 17.11).

Transcranial motor-evoked potentials

TcMEPs are performed by delivering electrical current to the motor cortex from electrodes on the scalp and recording either TcMEP waveforms (D and I waves) from epidural electrodes near the spine itself or recording myogenic evoked potentials from muscles in the upper and lower extremities (Figure 17.12). Motor-evoked potentials may also be recorded by direct electrical stimulation of the motor cortex following craniotomy (as a means of functional mapping of the motor cortex) or via transcortical magnetic stimulation. TcMEP provides a real-time assessment of the descending motor pathway from the cortex to muscle during procedures that place the corticospinal

tracks at risk. TcMEP is being used increasingly in advanced neurosurgical, aortic, and orthopedic centers for monitoring motor pathways of the brain and spinal cord during procedures. TcMEP appears to have a superior temporal resolution for detection of ischemia compared with SSEP (less than 5 minutes vs 30 minutes). This is likely because TcMEP measures the functional integrity of spinal gray matter, which is very sensitive to ischemia, in addition to the functional integrity of spinal motor myelinated tracts.

One downside to TcMEP measurements is that there are no precise criteria in the literature to define a critical change in the TcMEP waveform indicating that injury is occurring. Studies have used different thresholds for a reduction in compound muscle action potential (CMAP) amplitude (25% vs 50% vs 80%) or different stimulation threshold changes (the amount of stimulation current it takes to generate the CMAP) to signify a critical change.[39,40]

The ability to perform TcMEP is also limited by its sensitivity to anesthetics, paralytic agents, and temperature. The use of paralytic agents is discouraged and, if used at all, should be extremely limited and kept constant (at less than 40%

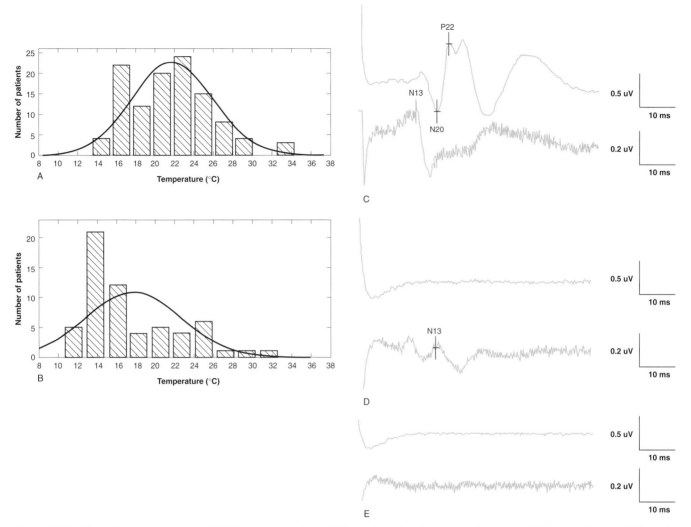

Figure 17.11. Effect of body temperature on SSEP latency and amplitude. Deliberate hypothermia progressively increases SSEP latency, decreases SSEP amplitude, and eventually causes the disappearance of SSEPs. The left panel shows the distribution of nasopharyngeal temperatures at which the N20–P22 (A) and N13 (B) SSEP disappear. The right panel shows the typical appearance of the N20–P22 and N13 SSEPs at normothermia (C), disappearance of the N20–P22 SSEP and prolongation of the latency of the N13 SSEP at moderate hypothermia (D), and disappearance of both N20–P22 and N13 SSEP at deep hypothermic conditions (E). Data from ref.12.

neuromuscular blockade) so that changes in TcMEP can be interpreted accurately. This also means that patients may be subjected to a higher risk of injury from spontaneous movements or stimulation during their procedures.

Another limitation of TcMEP monitoring is that TcMEPs are often difficult to obtain from the leg. It is unclear whether technical limitations in the instruments and equipment used to monitor TcMEP or preexisting injuries in patients are the cause of inability to elicit lower extremity TcMEP signals in some patients.[39-43] Complications directly associated with monitoring are of greater concern during TcMEP monitoring than with other NIOM modalities. The stimulus intensity required to generate the TcMEP response may, in rare instances, cause seizures or tongue lacerations.[41,44,45] Finally, establishing the efficacy of TcMEP has been limited because of the lack of approved equipment and experience in performing this technique.

The optimal approach to detect intraoperative spinal cord ischemia or injury during high-risk procedures is controversial, and it is unclear whether SSEP or TcMEP is superior for this purpose. Intraoperative monitoring of spinal cord function is useful in orthopedic procedures involving structural or vascular lesions, as well as repairs of the descending aorta, which put the spinal cord at risk of ischemia (Table 17.1).[46,47] SSEP monitoring has been the traditional standard for intraoperative monitoring of the spinal cord, and it has been employed in routine clinical practice for spinal procedures since the 1980s.[1] However, SSEP, in theory, monitors only the sensory white matter tracts of the spinal cord, and the posterior columns in particular. It is controversial whether SSEP is sufficiently sensitive for detecting injury to the corticospinal tracts in the cord, regions that are specifically susceptible to ischemia during these procedures. Although multiple studies have reported improved outcomes with SSEP monitoring

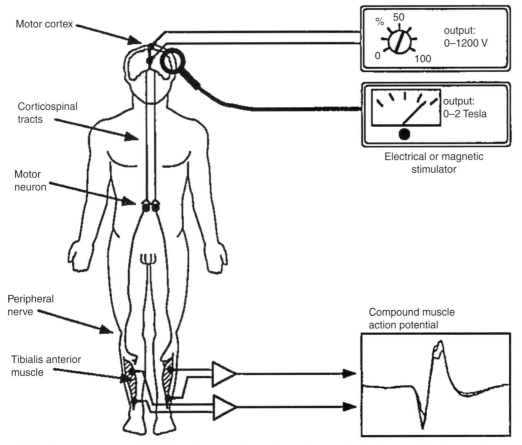

Figure 17.12. Motor-evoked potential (MEP) monitoring is performed by applying an electrical or magnetic stimulus to the scalp over the motor cortex. Nerve action potentials travel from the motor cortex along the corticospinal tracts to activate alpha-motor neurons in the anterior horn of the spinal cord. The subsequent nerve action potentials travel along peripheral nerves to the motor end-plate, generating a compound muscle action potential that can be recorded from electrodes over the muscle.

during aortic and spine surgery,[28,29,48,49] other studies suggest that TcMEP monitoring had increased sensitivity for predicting motor injury.[39,42,43,50–52]

Several series have been performed in which TcMEP and SSEP were monitored simultaneously during the same procedure (Table 17.3). This is a rare instance in which head-to-head comparisons have been performed between two monitoring techniques. In these comparisons, TcMEP appeared to be more sensitive and detected the onset and recovery of spinal cord ischemia earlier than SSEP, permitting intraoperative interventions such as the reimplantation of intercostal arteries into the thoracoabdominal aortic graft for the prevention of spinal cord ischemia associated with thoracoabdominal aortic aneurysm repair (Figure 17.13).[4,39,53] In these studies, anesthesia was tailored to optimize TcMEP monitoring. The limited use of paralytic agents increased the difficulty of SSEP monitoring because of interference from motor artifacts generated by eliciting TcMEP signals. At present, there is no definitive evidence to support the superiority of either SSEP or TcMEP monitoring in procedures that place the spinal cord at risk.[41,44,55] The technical challenges of performing and interpreting TcMEP must be weighed against the decreased sensitivity of SSEP, and suc-

cessful monitoring with either technique depends greatly on the institutional expertise and experience.

Intraoperative monitoring of TcMEP is challenging because general anesthetic agents are potent suppressants of TcMEP signals, and neuromuscular blocking drugs interfere with the generation of the compound muscle action potential (Table 17.4). Under conditions of general anesthesia, changes or alterations in TcMEP signals resulting from changes in anesthetic concentrations or actions must be distinguished from changes caused by injury or ischemia as a consequence of the operation. Inhaled volatile anesthetic agents at clinically effective concentrations suppress both cortical activation and the activation of spinal motor neurons in the anterior horn. If inhaled volatile anesthetics are used when monitoring TcMEP, they must be administered in very low concentrations, such as 0.2 to 0.5 MAC for isoflurane or less than 50 percent for nitrous oxide. Barbiturates and propofol also cause dose-dependent depression of TcMEP signals and may cause transient, long-lasting depression, or even obliteration, of signals after acute bolus intravenous administration. However, the short duration of action of propofol, and the ability to titrate its actions when administered as a continuous intravenous infusion, have allowed this

Table 17.3. Studies comparing intraoperative somatosensory evoked potential monitoring (SSEP) with transcranial motor evoked potential monitoring (TcMEP)

Study, Year (type of surgery: cervical/thoracic spine,[1] TAAA[2])	Number of patients	Number of subjects with significant intraoperative SSEP/TCMEP changes			Number of subjects with persistent significant changes who awoke with motor deficit (additional false-negatives bold, false-positives in italics)				Sensitivity of having a significant change and having a motor deficit (%)		Specificity of having a significant change and having a motor deficit (%)	
		Both SSEP/TcMEP	TcMEP alone	SSEP alone	Total	Both SSEP/TCMEP	TCMEP alone	SSEP alone	TcMEP	SSEP	TcMEP	SSEP
Pelosi, 2002[1]	104	7	7	0	3	1	2(**1**)(*1*)	1(**2**)	67	33	99	100
Hilibranbrand, 2004[1]	427	4	8	0	2	1	2	1(**1**)	100	50	100	100
	118	5	37	0	5	1(*4*)	4(**1**)(*14*)	1(**4**)	80	20	89	100
Weinzierl, 2007[1]	69	6	12	2	10	2(**1**)(*1*)	8(**2**)(*1*)	2(**8**)(2)	80	20	98	96
Meylaerts, 1999[2]	38	5	13	11	0	0	0	0(*15*)	N/A	N/A	71	100
Total	756	27	77	13	20	5(**1**)(*5*)	16(**4**)(*16*)	5(**16**)(*17*)	80	24	96	98

211

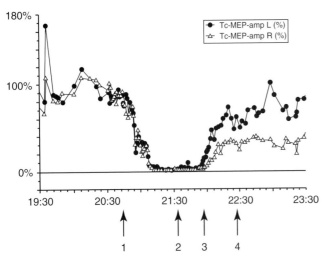

Figure 17.13. Changes in motor-evoked potential (MEP) amplitudes recorded from the right (TcMEP-amp R) and left (TcMEP-amp L) tibialis anterior muscle as a percentage of the baseline amplitude over time during the course of a thoracoabdominal aortic aneurysm repair. The designated intraoperative events were (1) aorta cross-clamped at T5 and L1 levels, (2) proximal aorta anastomosed to a Dacron vascular graft, (3) Dacron vascular graft anastomosed to the distal aorta, and (4) recovery of spinal cord function. Medical surgical interventions prompted by the decrease in MEP during operation at each time point were (1) vasopressor therapy and increase in partial left heart bypass flow rate to increase the proximal and distal aortic pressures and (2) reattachment of T8–9 intercostal arteries. Modified from Jacobs MJ et al. *J Vasc Surg* 1999;**29**:48–59.

agent to be used successfully at concentrations ranging from 25 mcg/kg/min to 100 mcg/kg/min for anesthetic maintenance when monitoring TcMEP. At the higher propofol infusion rates, multipulse stimulation techniques can be applied to improve TcMEP amplitude. Intravenous bolus doses of benzodiazepines will also cause suppression of TcMEP but are less potent depressants of TcMEP than the barbiturates and propofol.

In contrast to barbiturates and propofol, the intravenous anesthetics ketamine and etomidate have very little effect on TcMEP. However, side effects limit the total dose and duration of ketamine and etomidate that can be administered for a surgical procedure. Ketamine may cause emergence delirium, and etomidate causes dose-dependent adrenal cortical suppression. Nevertheless, ketamine and etomidate are useful anes-

Table 17.4. Anesthetic agents in order of potency on suppression of transcranial motor-evoked potentials

1. Fentanyl, sufentanil or remifentanil: continuous infusion
2. Etomidate[1]: 10–30 mcg/kg/min*
3. Ketamine[2]: 1–4 mg/kg/hr (postoperative delirium)*
4. Propofol: ≤ 50–100 mcg/kg/min*
5. Midazolam: 0.1 mg/kg/hr*
6. Nitrous oxide ≤ 50%
7. Volatile anesthetics (e.g. isoflurane: none or ≤0.2%–0.5%)

* Bolus dosing of these agents can cause transient, long-lasting depression or obliteration of MEP or SEP responses.
[1] Etomidate causes dose-dependent adrenocortical depression.
[2] Ketamine may cause postoperative delirium.

thetic adjuncts when necessary for TcMEP monitoring. Opioid narcotics have no, or only minimal, effects on TcMEP, so they are important anesthetic adjuncts. Fentanyl, sufentanil, or remifentanil administered as continuous intravenous infusions are commonly used as part of the anesthetic regimen when monitoring intraoperative TcMEP.

Neuromuscular blocking drugs attenuate TcMEP by blocking nerve transmission at the neuromuscular junction, decreasing the amplitude of the compound muscle action potential. An optimal condition for TcMEP monitoring requires the complete avoidance of neuromuscular blocking agents; that is not always possible, however, because muscle relaxation and prevention of patient movement are often necessary for operation and cannot be achieved with narcotic analgesics and the doses of general anesthetics used for TcMEP monitoring. For this reason, short- or intermediate-acting neuromuscular blocking agents, such as atracurium, cisatracurium, or vecuronium, can be administered as continuous intravenous infusions with the dose titrated to maintain a constant EMG response or single muscle twitch amplitude. Typically, partial neuromuscular blockade at a single muscle twitch height of 20 percent to 50 percent of baseline permits TcMEP monitoring under satisfactory operative conditions.

The technical challenges of monitoring TcMEP during general anesthesia require coordination between the monitoring team and the anesthesiologist. No single anesthetic regimen has been developed to suit all operations in which TcMEP monitoring is required. Several anesthetic regimens have been described. For TcMEP monitoring to detect spinal cord ischemia in patients undergoing thoracoabdominal aortic aneurysm repair, general anesthesia was induced using fentanyl 10 mcg/kg, thiopental 2–5 mg/kg, and atracurium 0.5 mg/kg. General anesthesia was then maintained using intravenous infusions of fentanyl 15 mcg/kg/hr, scopolamine 8 mcg/kg/hr, and atracurium 0.2 mcg/kg/min titrated to maintain compound muscle action potential at 20 percent of baseline by measuring thenar CMAP every two minutes through stimulation of the median nerve. The amplitudes of recorded TcMEP were then corrected for the level of neuromuscular blockade.[54]

Another anesthetic regimen described for monitoring TcMEP in patients undergoing neurosurgical operations was continuous intravenous infusion of propofol 10 mg/kg/hr and remifentanil 0.25 mcg/kg/min. With this anesthetic regimen, no muscle relaxants were administered, except for cisatracurium 0.15 mg/kg intravenously to facilitate tracheal intubation at induction.[39] Other anesthetic regimens that have been described include the use of diazepam 0.1–0.15 mg/kg by mouth as a preanesthetic medication, and etomidate 0.3–0.4 mg/kg or thiopental 3.5–4.0 mg/kg for induction. Anesthesia was maintained with fentanyl 3–5 mcg/kg, midazolam 0.03–0.07 mg/kg, and nitrous oxide 70 percent in oxygen.[56] Successful monitoring of TcMEP for neurosurgical and orthopedic procedures has also been reported using low-dose inhaled isoflurane at 0.25%–1.0% or halothane at 0.25%–0.5% to maintain general anesthesia.[56] (The references to the use of halothane,

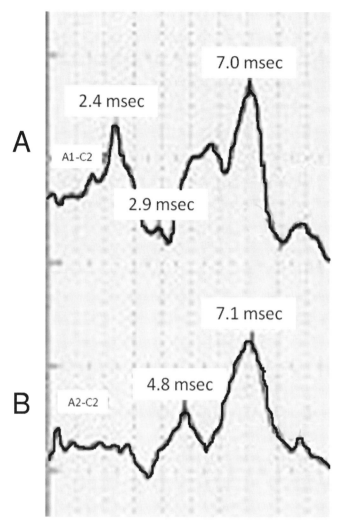

Figure 17.14. A baseline intraoperative BAEP recorded after stimulation of the left ear during a left acoustic neuroma resection (clicks delivered at 130dB to ipsalateral ear with white noise delivered to contralateral ear). (A) Ipsilateral recording at the left ear electrode demonstrating wave I at 2.4 ms, wave II at 3.9 ms, wave III at 4.8 ms, and a wave IV–V complex at 7 ms. (B) Contralateral recording from right ear. Note the absence of wave I from this ear, demonstrating that the distal components are bilateral, whereas wave I is only ipsalateral. Loss of amplitude or increased latency in any of the components may serve as a warning of injury, whereas persistence of wave V throughout the procedure correlates to preservation of hearing postoperatively.

scopolamine, and atracurium are included for completeness, and not as a recommendation for use in current anesthesia practice for patients receiving TcMEP monitoring.)

Brainstem auditory evoked potentials

BAEPs are wavelets generated by the auditory nerve and brainstem in response to repetitive clicks delivered to the ear. Typically, five wavelets are recorded from electrodes placed near the ear, with the first recorded wavelet representing the response from peripheral cochlear nerve, whereas the next four wavelets are generated from ascending structures in the brainstem. Changes in latency and amplitude of these five waves are used to assess the integrity of the auditory pathway during procedures that put them at risk (Figure 17.14).[57] BAEPs are commonly used in posterior fossa neurosurgical procedures, such as acoustic neuroma resections, which place the eighth nerve at risk from either ischemia or stretch injury. BAEP may also be useful in identifying and preventing injury in procedures such as tumor resections or arteriovenous malformation (AVM) repairs, which place the brainstem itself at risk because of ischemia or mass effect. BAEP monitoring may be used to monitor surgical procedures involving the brainstem and posterior fossa that place the eighth nerve and the auditory pathway at risk.[58–61] General anesthetics, including inhaled anesthetics and intravenous anesthetics, have little effect on BAERs.

Visual-evoked potentials

Visual-evoked potentials (VEPs) are wavelets generated by the occipital cortex in response to visual stimuli (typically, flashing lights delivered with LED goggles in the operative setting). VEPs are recorded from electrodes overlying the occipital cortex and provide information about the integrity of the visual pathway during procedures. VEPs have been have been monitored during neurosurgical procedures involving mass and vascular lesions near the optic nerve and chiasm. The evidence supporting VEP monitoring is sparse, in part because of difficulty in obtaining signals in the operating room.[62–65] Inhaled and intravenous anesthetics cause a dose-dependent decrease in VEP amplitude and increase in VEP latency.

Electromyography and nerve conduction studies

EMG and NCS can be performed on both peripheral and cranial nerves to assess their integrity and to localize these nerves by recording CMAPs from the muscles they supply. Monitoring is performed by placing pins or electrodes in muscles and then identifying the nerve supplying the muscle by stimulating it during the procedure (mapping). NCS can also be performed by determining whether a specific length of nerve will conduct electrical activity between a stimulating and recording electrode. If a nerve does not conduct the signal, this may indicate that it has been significantly injured along its course. Peripheral nerves are at risk of crush, stretch, ligation, ischemic, and hyperthermic injury during many surgical procedures as a result of malpositioning, electrocautery, or direct injury.

Monitoring is also performed by observing spontaneous activity from the muscle, which may indicate that a nerve supplying it is suffering unexpected injury. Cranial motor nerves are often monitored in this fashion. Cranial nerve VII is often monitored during posterior fossa procedures, when it is at high risk of injury, and during parotid gland procedures or other ENT procedures involving the face, ear, or sinuses. All peripheral nerves in the extremities and trunk can similarly be monitored. Monitoring of peripheral nerves can aid in localizing and protecting nervous tissue during nerve repairs or during tumor resections. Cranial nerve monitoring is employed in operations of the posterior fossa and brainstem.[66,67] There are no large published studies evaluating the utility of EMG or NCS for monitoring other cranial or peripheral nerves.

Performing EMG or NCS in anesthetized patients requires the avoidance of neuromuscular blocking drugs. If neuromuscular blocking drugs are required for tracheal intubation for the induction of general anesthesia, short-acting neuromuscular blocking agents can be chosen. Full recovery from the neuromuscular blocking drug can be verified with the use of a nerve stimulator prior to performing EMG or NCS.

Areas of uncertainty and multimodality monitoring

Although there is a legitimate concern regarding the unproven benefit of NIOM because of the lack of randomized trials, there are several situations in which monitoring appears to have an established utility. Specifically, the improved outcomes reported in large case series support the continued use of EEG in CEA, SSEP in spinal surgery, BAEP in posterior fossa procedures, and EMG in procedures placing the facial nerve at risk. There are a several areas in which the evidence has either not supported the use of monitoring or in which further clinical research needs to be performed to demonstrate a clear benefit prior to recommending that these techniques become the standard of care in clinical practice. These techniques include VEP monitoring, SSEP and BAEP monitoring in procedures placing the brainstem at risk, EEG in neurosurgical vascular procedures, SSEP in CEA, and EMG in cases placing peripheral and cranial nerves, other than the seventh nerve, at risk.

There is early evidence supporting the use of TcMEP in complex cervical and thoracic spinal procedures and descending thoracic aortic procedures. It appears that TcMEP may be more sensitive than SSEP in detecting and predicting motor deficits in patients undergoing procedures that place their spinal cords at risk of motor deficits. This benefit must now be weighed against the potential risks of using TcMEP prior to its becoming the standard over SSEP for monitoring these procedures. The risks include potential skin injury, anesthetic restrictions, cost, false-positive rate, and the need for increased professional oversight. Further clinical research in the use of TcMEP is necessary to establish this promising technique. The exception at this time may be a clear benefit of the use of TcMEP in the treatment of intramedullary spinal cord tumors.

The difficulty of assessing the benefit of intraoperative monitoring techniques in isolation raises the question of whether using multiple electrophysiologic techniques or nonelectrical techniques during high-risk procedures adds any benefit. Adding multiple techniques during one procedure may aid in identifying injury but also may add confusion when the modalities do not correlate, as well as adding cost. A benefit of dual monitoring, however, is that if one modality fails for technical reasons, the other modality is still available.

Guidelines

In 1990, the Therapeutics and Technology Subcommittee of the American Academy of Neurology (AAN) determined that the following techniques were useful and noninvestigational: EEG and SSEPs as adjuncts in CEA and brain surgeries in which cerebral blood flow was compromised, SSEP monitoring performed in procedures involving ischemia or mechanical trauma to the spine, and BAEP and cranial nerve monitoring in surgeries performed in the region of the brainstem or ear.[1] There have been no further recommendations from the AAN regarding NIOM.

Summary and authors' recommendations

The following suggestions have been derived from the review of the available data concerning NIOM. These recommendations serve as a guide only and are based on the authors' interpretation of the available data, should take into account the individual institutional expertise and experience, and are not meant to replace clinical judgment. There should be judicious use of neurophysiologic monitoring. It should be reserved for surgical cases in which the nervous system is at significant risk. When neurologic injury is very likely, neurophysiologic monitoring should be employed whenever feasible, as outlined below.

1. Although it is relatively rare, neurologic injury as a result of hypoperfusion may occur during carotid endarterectomy. EEG can identify this complication and appears to improve outcomes by indicating when carotid shunting is necessary. The available data support its use over other modalities at this time, although a randomized trial comparing modalities such as TCD, SSEP, stump pressure, and nonselective shunting is needed. EEG's use in other procedures in which the cerebral cortex is at risk may be beneficial, but there is a lack of data to support it.

2. SSEPs are useful in identifying ischemia in the brain during complex neurosurgical vascular procedures, injury to the spinal cord in complex cervical and thoracic spinal procedures, and ischemia in descending thoracic aortic repairs. It is unclear whether SSEP or TcMEP is superior for detecting potential injury in the spinal cord, given the current data available. This is deserving of further study. It is the authors' recommendation based on this review that SSEP be used during all complex cervical and thoracic spine and descending aortic procedures that place the spinal cord at significant risk of injury.

3. At this time, TcMEP should be considered as a useful adjunct in monitoring the spinal cord during procedures placing it at risk of injury, but more clinical data are required to determine whether TcMEP should be considered a standard. The authors recommend that SSEP should also be monitored in all cases in which TcMEP is employed. A randomized controlled trial comparing TcMEP and SSEP spinal monitoring may be possible from an ethical standpoint and should be considered.

4. BAEP monitoring is useful in identifying injury and improving outcomes during neurosurgical procedures involving the posterior fossa that place the eighth cranial nerve at risk, and the authors recommend its use. The recommendation is strongest in cases of acoustic neuroma

resection in which the tumor is less than 2 cm in diameter. It is unclear whether BAEP and SSEP monitoring is useful during procedures that place the brainstem at risk, but given the potential benefit of monitoring, the authors recommend its use while more outcome data are collected.

5. Monitoring of the seventh cranial nerve in operations performed in the region of the brainstem or ear using spontaneous EMG and mapping with direct simulation of the seventh cranial nerves has been associated with improved outcomes, and the authors recommend its use. Whether there is a benefit from monitoring of other cranial nerves or peripheral nerves during procedures that place them at risk is unclear, but the authors recommend monitoring whenever feasible while further outcome data are collected.

6. It is unclear whether VEP monitoring can adequately identify injury to the visual pathways and improve outcomes in surgical procedures placing them at risk. The authors recommend that at present, VEP use should likely be limited to research protocols.

References

1. Assessment: intraoperative neurophysiology. Report of the Therapeutics and Technology Assessment Subcommittee of the American Academy of Neurology. *Neurology* 1990;**40**:1644–6.

2. Laman DM, Van Der Reijden CS, Wieneke GH, van Duijn H, van Huffelen AC. EEG evidence for shunt requirement during carotid endarterectomy: optimal EEG derivations with respect to frequency bands and anesthetic regimen. *J Clin Neurophysiol* 2001;**18**:353–63.

3. Blume WT, Ferguson GG, McNeill DK. Significance of EEG changes at carotid endarterectomy. *Stroke* 1986;**17**:891–7.

4. Laman DM, Wieneke GH, van Duijn H, Veldhuizen RJ, van Huffelen AC. QEEG changes during carotid clamping in carotid endarterectomy: spectral edge frequency parameters and relative band power parameters. *J Clin Neurophysiol* 2005;**22**:244–52.

5. Sundt TM Jr, Sharbrough FW, Anderson RE, Michenfelder JD. Cerebral blood flow measurements and electroencephalograms during carotid endarterectomy. *J Neurosurg* 1974;**41**:310–20.

6. Sundt TM Jr, Sharbrough FW, Piepgras DG, Kearns TP, Messick JM Jr, O'Fallon WM. Correlation of cerebral blood flow and electroencephalographic changes during carotid endarterectomy: with results of surgery and hemodynamics of cerebral ischemia. *Mayo Clin Proc* 1981;**56**:533–43.

7. Sharbrough FW, Messick JM **Jr**, Sundt TM Jr. Correlation of continuous electroencephalograms with cerebral blood flow measurements during carotid endarterectomy. *Stroke* 1973;**4**:674–83.

8. Algotsson L, Messeter K, Rehncrona S, Skeidsvoll H, Ryding E. Cerebral hemodynamic changes and electroencephalography during carotid endarterectomy. *J Clin Anesth* 1990;**2**:143–51.

9. Zampella E, Morawetz RB, McDowell HA, et al. The importance of cerebral ischemia during carotid endarterectomy. *Neurosurgery* 1991;**29**:727–30; discussion 730–1.

10. Redekop G, Ferguson G. Correlation of contralateral stenosis and intraoperative electroencephalogram change with risk of stroke during carotid endarterectomy. *Neurosurgery* 1992;**30**:191–4.

11. Bavaria JE, Brinster DR, Gorman RC, Woo YJ, Gleason T, Pochettino A. Advances in the treatment of acute type A dissection: an integrated approach. *Ann Thorac Surg* 2002;**74**:S1848–52; discussion S1857–63.

12. Stecker MM, Cheung AT, Pochettino A, et al. Deep hypothermic circulatory arrest: I. Effects of cooling on electroencephalogram and evoked potentials. *Ann Thorac Surg* 2001;**71**:14–21.

13. Guideline 9D: Guidelines on short-latency somatosensory evoked potentials. *J Clin Neurophysiol* 2006;**23**:168–79.

14. Cruccu G, Aminoff MJ, Curio G, et al. Recommendations for the clinical use of somatosensory-evoked potentials. *Clin Neurophysiol* 2008;**119**:1705–19.

15. Schramm J, Koht A, Schmidt G, Pechstein U, Taniguchi M, Fahlbusch R. Surgical and electrophysiological observations during clipping of 134 aneurysms with evoked potential monitoring. *Neurosurgery* 1990;**26**:61–70.

16. Buchthal A, Belopavlovic M. Somatosensory evoked potentials in cerebral aneurysm surgery. *Eur J Anaesthesiol* 1992;**9**:493–7.

17. Lopez JR, Chang SD, Steinberg GK. The use of electrophysiological monitoring in the intraoperative management of intracranial aneurysms. *J Neurol Neurosurg Psychiatry* 1999;**66**:189–96.

18. Burke D, Nuwer MR, Daube J, et al. Intraoperative monitoring. The International Federation of Clinical Neurophysiology. *Electroencephalogr Clin Neurophysiol Suppl* 1999;**52**:133–48.

19. Luders H, Lesser RP, Hahn J, et al. Basal temporal language area demonstrated by electrical stimulation. *Neurology* 1986;**36**:505–10.

20. Minahan RE, Sepkuty JP, Lesser RP, Sponseller PD, Kostuik JP. Anterior spinal cord injury with preserved neurogenic 'motor' evoked potentials. *Clin Neurophysiol* 2001;**112**:1442–50.

21. More RC, Nuwer MR, Dawson EG. Cortical evoked potential monitoring during spinal surgery: sensitivity, specificity, reliability, and criteria for alarm. *J Spinal Disord* 1988;**1**:75–80.

22. Mostegl A, Bauer R, Eichenauer M. Intraoperative somatosensory potential monitoring. A clinical analysis of 127 surgical procedures. *Spine* 1988;**13**:396–400.

23. Szalay EA, Carollo JJ, Roach JW. Sensitivity of spinal cord monitoring to intraoperative events. *J Pediatr Orthop* 1986;**6**:437–41.

24. Jones SJ, Edgar MA, Ransford AO, Thomas NP. A system for the electrophysiological monitoring of the spinal cord during operations for scoliosis. *J Bone Joint Surg Br* 1983;**65**:134–9.

25. Constantini S, Miller DC, Allen JC, Rorke LB, Freed D, Epstein FJ. Radical excision of intramedullary spinal cord tumors: surgical morbidity and long-term follow-up evaluation in 164 children and young adults. *J Neurosurg* 2000;**93**:183–93.

26. Cristante L, Herrmann HD. Surgical management of intramedullary spinal cord tumors: functional outcome and sources of morbidity. *Neurosurgery* 1994;**35**:69–74.

27. Galla JD, Ergin MA, Lansman SL, et al. Use of somatosensory evoked potentials for thoracic and thoracoabdominal aortic resections. *Ann Thorac Surg* 1999;**67**:1947–52; discussion 1953–8.

28. Grabitz K, Sandmann W, Stuhmeier K, et al. The risk of ischemic spinal cord injury in patients undergoing graft replacement for thoracoabdominal aortic aneurysms. *J Vasc Surg* 1996;**23**: 230–40.

29. Griepp RB, Ergin MA, Galla JD, et al. Looking for the artery of Adamkiewicz: a quest to minimize paraplegia after operations for aneurysms of the descending thoracic and thoracoabdominal aorta. *J Thorac Cardiovasc Surg* 1996;**112**:1202–13; discussion 1213–5.

30. Laschinger JC, Cunningham JN, Jr., Nathan IM, Knopp EA, Cooper MM, Spencer FC. Experimental and clinical assessment of the adequacy of partial bypass in maintenance of spinal cord blood flow during operations on the thoracic aorta. *Ann Thorac Surg* 1983;**36**:417–26.

31. Robertazzi RR, Cunningham JN **Jr**. Monitoring of somatosensory evoked potentials: a primer on the intraoperative detection of spinal cord ischemia during aortic reconstructive surgery. *Semin Thorac Cardiovasc Surg* 1998;**10**:11–7.

32. Sloan TB, Jameson LC. Electrophysiologic monitoring during surgery to repair the thoraco-abdominal aorta. *J Clin Neurophysiol* 2007;**24**:316–27.

33. Mizoi K, Yoshimoto T. Intraoperative monitoring of the somatosensory evoked potentials and cerebral blood flow during aneurysm surgery – safety evaluation for temporary vascular occlusion. *Neurol Med Chir (Tokyo)* 1991;**31**:318–25.

34. Legatt AD, Kader A. Topography of the initial cortical component of the median nerve somatosensory evoked potential. Relationship to central sulcus anatomy. *J Clin Neurophysiol* 2000;**17**:321–5.

35. Gutsche JT, Cheung AT, McGarvey ML, et al. Risk factors for perioperative stroke after thoracic endovascular aortic repair. *Ann Thorac Surg* 2007;**84**:1195–200; discussion 1200.

36. Stecker MM, Cheung AT, Patterson T, et al. Detection of stroke during cardiac operations with somatosensory evoked responses. *J Thorac Cardiovasc Surg* 1996;**112**:962–72.

37. Cheung AT, Savino JS, Weiss SJ, et al. Detection of acute embolic stroke during mitral valve replacement using somatosensory evoked potential monitoring. *Anesthesiology* 1995;**83**:208–10.

38. Banoub M, Tetzlaff JE, Schubert A. Pharmacologic and physiologic influences affecting sensory evoked potentials: implications for perioperative monitoring. *Anesthesiology* 2003;**99**:716–37.

39. Weinzierl MR, Reinacher P, Gilsbach JM, Rohde V. Combined motor and somatosensory evoked potentials for intraoperative monitoring: intra- and postoperative data in a series of 69 operations. *Neurosurg Rev* 2007;**30**:109–16; discussion 116.

40. Langeloo DD, Lelivelt A, Louis Journee H, Slappendel R, de Kleuver M. Transcranial electrical motor-evoked potential monitoring during surgery for spinal deformity: a study of 145 patients. *Spine* 2003;**28**:1043–50.

41. Legatt AD. Current practice of motor evoked potential monitoring: results of a survey. *J Clin Neurophysiol* 2002;**19**:454–60.

42. Hilibrand AS, Schwartz DM, Sethuraman V, Vaccaro AR, Albert TJ. Comparison of transcranial electric motor and somatosensory evoked potential monitoring during cervical spine surgery. *J Bone Joint Surg Am* 2004;**86**-A:1248–53.

43. Pelosi L, Lamb J, Grevitt M, Mehdian SM, Webb JK, Blumhardt LD. Combined monitoring of motor and somatosensory evoked potentials in orthopaedic spinal surgery. *Clin Neurophysiol* 2002;**113**:1082–91.

44. MacDonald DB. Safety of intraoperative transcranial electrical stimulation motor evoked potential monitoring. *J Clin Neurophysiol* 2002;**19**:416–29.

45. Macdonald DB. Intraoperative motor evoked potential monitoring: overview and update. *J Clin Monit Comput* 2006;**20**:347–77.

46. McGarvey ML, Cheung AT, Szeto W, Messe SR. Management of neurologic complications of thoracic aortic surgery. *J Clin Neurophysiol* 2007;**24**:336–43.

47. McGarvey ML, Mullen MT, Woo EY, et al. The treatment of spinal cord ischemia following thoracic endovascular aortic repair. *Neurocrit Care* 2007;**6**:35–9.

48. Dawson EG, Sherman JE, Kanim LE, Nuwer MR. Spinal cord monitoring. Results of the Scoliosis Research Society and the European Spinal Deformity Society survey. *Spine* 1991;**16**:S361–4.

49. Schepens MA, Boezeman EH, Hamerlijnck RP, ter Beek H, Vermeulen FE. Somatosensory evoked potentials during exclusion and reperfusion of critical aortic segments in thoracoabdominal aortic aneurysm surgery. *J Cardiovasc Surg* 1994;**9**:692–702.

50. Costa P, Bruno A, Bonzanino M, et al. Somatosensory- and motor-evoked potential monitoring during spine and spinal cord surgery. *Spinal Cord* 2007;**45**:86–91.

51. Meylaerts SA, Jacobs MJ, van Iterson V, De Haan P, Kalkman CJ. Comparison of transcranial motor evoked potentials and somatosensory evoked potentials during thoracoabdominal aortic aneurysm repair. *Ann Surg* 1999;**230**:742–9.

52. van Dongen EP, Schepens MA, Morshuis WJ, et al. Thoracic and thoracoabdominal aortic aneurysm repair: use of evoked potential monitoring in 118 patients. *J Vasc Surg* 2001;**34**:1035–40.

53. Dong CC, MacDonald DB, Janusz MT. Intraoperative spinal cord monitoring during descending thoracic and thoracoabdominal aneurysm surgery. *Ann Thorac Surg* 2002;**74**:S1873–6; discussion S1892–8.

54. Shine TS, Harrison BA, De Ruyter ML, et al. Motor and somatosensory evoked potentials: their role in predicting spinal cord ischemia in patients undergoing thoracoabdominal aortic aneurysm repair with regional lumbar epidural cooling. *Anesthesiology* 2008;**108**:580–7.

55. Legatt AD. Ellen R. Grass Lecture: Motor evoked potential monitoring. *Am J Electroneurodiagnostic Technol* 2004;**44**:223–43.

56. Adams DC, Emerson RG, Heyer EJ, et al. Monitoring of intraoperative motor-evoked potentials under conditions of controlled neuromuscular blockade. *Anesth Analg* 1993;**77**:913–8.

57. Manninen PH, Patterson S, Lam AM, Gelb AW, Nantau WE. Evoked potential monitoring during posterior fossa aneurysm surgery: a comparison of two modalities. *Can J Anaesth* 1994;**41**:92–7.

58. Nadol JB, Jr., Chiong CM, Ojemann RG, et al. Preservation of hearing and facial nerve function in resection of acoustic neuroma. *Laryngoscope* 1992;**102**:1153–8.

59. Radtke RA, Erwin CW, Wilkins RH. Intraoperative brainstem auditory evoked potentials: significant decrease in postoperative morbidity. *Neurology* 1989;**39**:187–91.

60. James ML, Husain AM. Brainstem auditory evoked potential monitoring: when is change in wave V significant? *Neurology* 2005;**65**:1551–5.

61. Harper CM, Harner SG, Slavit DH, et al. Effect of BAEP monitoring on hearing preservation during acoustic neuroma resection. *Neurology* 1992;**42**:1551–3.

62. Cedzich C, Schramm J, Mengedoht CF, Fahlbusch R. Factors that limit the use of flash visual evoked potentials for surgical monitoring. *Electroencephalogr Clin Neurophysiol* 1988;**71**:142–5.

63. Sasaki T, Ichikawa T, Sakuma J, et al. Intraoperative monitoring of visual evoked potentials. *Masui* 2006;**55**:302–13.

64. Chacko AG, Babu KS, Chandy MJ. Value of visual evoked potential monitoring during trans-sphenoidal pituitary surgery. *Br J Neurosurg* 1996;**10**:275–8.

65. Herzon GD, Zealear DL. Intraoperative monitoring of the visual evoked potential during endoscopic sinus surgery. *Otolaryngol Head Neck Surg* 1994;**111**:575–9.

66. Niparko JK, Kileny PR, Kemink JL, Lee HM, Graham MD. Neurophysiologic intraoperative monitoring: II. Facial nerve function. *Am J Otol* 1989;**10**:55–61.

67. Terrell JE, Kileny PR, Yian C, et al. Clinical outcome of continuous facial nerve monitoring during primary parotidectomy. *Arch Otolaryngol Head Neck Surg* 1997;**123**: 1081–7.

Chapter 18

Level of consciousness monitoring

Marc J. Bloom

Technical concepts

Origin of EEG

Most of the monitors available today for monitoring level of consciousness during anesthesia (a.k.a. anesthesia effect or brain function monitors) use electroencephalography (EEG) as the fundamental signal. The EEG is a voltage measured on the surface of the scalp. This electrical signal is sometimes mistakenly believed to originate from the propagation of action potentials through axons of the central nervous system. However, although action potentials represent an electrical signal of nearly 100 millivolts, the field of this electrical signal is almost entirely contained within a few diameters of the axon and cannot be measured by electrodes on the scalp. Instead, the source of this electrical signal is actually from the depolarization of the cell body and dendritic tree caused by the release of neurotransmitters at the synapse. Even this electrical field from a single neuron is too weak to be measured at the scalp surface. EEG can be measured because nerve cells do not fire completely independently. There is an overriding inhibitory influence that keeps neurons from firing until an appropriate input arrives. When an incoming afferent volley arrives, it tends to cause a group of cells within an area to all depolarize in near-synchrony. This temporal and spatial summation allows for an electrical field of high enough strength to be measured on the surface of the scalp.

To facilitate use, all the currently available monitors use a set of adhesive electrodes. This limits placement of the electrodes to areas without hair; therefore, all the devices have been calibrated for frontal EEG obtained from the forehead.

Parameter extraction

Although it has been recognized for at least 30 years that there were recognizable and measurable changes in the EEG caused by deepening of anesthetic levels, a reliable monotonic measure defied description for many years. Initial attempts at describing EEG slowing using measures such as median frequency were only weakly correlated with clinically observed anesthetic effects. It was also observed that high frequencies would drop out as anesthetic level was deepened; attempts to measure this effect, such as the spectral edge frequency, were pursued early on as a measure of anesthetic effect. Again, those measures

initially looked promising, but correlation was not high enough to be clinically useful.

Discriminant functions

Instead of trying to predetermine which parameter might best describe aesthetic effects on EEG, a new approach was taken. Many derived parameters from EEG were fed into a statistical package, and a discriminant function was derived. The earliest – and, thus far, most commercially successful – of these efforts is that of the bispectral index (BIS) from Aspect Medical Inc. (Norwood, MA; Figure 18.1). Even this product was initially limited in its success, because anesthetic depth was difficult to define. Although minimum alveolar concentration (MAC) worked fairly well for defining the potency of inhaled anesthetics, after parenteral drugs were introduced into the anesthetic regime, the components of anesthesia became separable. The initial attempts to use BIS as a predictor of movement in response to skin incision met with limited and disappointing results.

Anesthesia, as practiced today, has at least four separable components: a sedative/hypnotic component, an analgesic component, an autonomic component, and an amnesic component. Later versions of the BIS discriminant function focused solely on the sedative component and succeeded with a remarkably high correlation with the clinically assessed state.

Parameters monitored

Bispectral index

To derive their indices, all the devices on the market today have followed a similar process. Initially, patients or volunteers were subjected to carefully controlled levels of sedation. In the ideal case, these levels are defined behaviorally. At each level of sedation, from wide awake through completely unresponsive, samples of EEG were taken. The discriminant function was then optimized to produce the highest performance of correct classification of new samples of EEG.

In the case of BIS, the details of the components of the discriminant function and the process of computing the index are laid out in a review by Rampil.[1] Along with a ratio of beta frequency power at light levels of sedation, and a measure of EEG suppression at deepest levels of sedation, BIS includes a

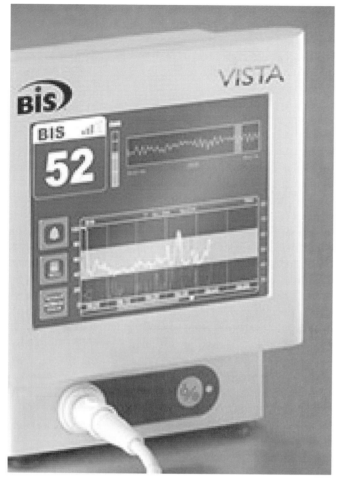

Figure 18.1. Vista BIS Monitor, Aspect Medical Systems. Image used by permission from Nellcor Puritan Bennett LLC, Boulder, CO, doing business as Covidien.

What is a bispectrum?

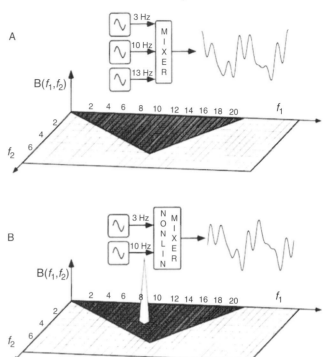

Figure 18.2. Schematic description of a bispectrum. (A) Three independent waves mixed together showing no bispectral interaction. (B) Two waves mixed together producing an interaction component in the bispectrum. Image used by permission from Nellcor Puritan Bennett LLC, Boulder, CO, doing business as Covidien.

component derived from the bispectrum of the EEG. The bispectrum is a measure of the relative synchrony or phase-locking of frequencies in the EEG (see Figures 18.2 and 18.3)

The result of this calculation produced an index with performance results that were clinically relevant. Table 18.1 shows a comparison of the correlation coefficients for a various levels of sedation for BIS and drug concentration.[2] Of note in Table 18.1 is the strong correlation between these values and behavior when using propofol as the sedative. The correlation coefficient with this value is even higher than that of actually measuring the blood level. This says that even for identical blood levels, people have different degrees of sedation. Also of note is the high correlation between both BIS and end-tidal potent agent concentration. The high correlation between exhaled gas concentration and behavior is the reason why potent agent anesthetics are still a mainstay of modern anesthetic practice. Correlation is nearly as high with the benzodiazepines. However, for alfentanil and all of the rest of the fentanyl family, there is no correlation between either the blood level or BIS and level of consciousness.

The statistically derived indices, such as BIS, are often difficult to understand because they have no physiologic correlate.

BIS represents the probability that a patient will respond to a command, but not the probability that the patient will remember being asked to follow the command (see Figure 18.4). If the BIS value is above 80, it is highly likely that the patient will follow a command, but if the BIS value is below 60, is highly unlikely that the patient will follow a command. The curves for each class of drugs nearly overlie each other, indicating that the

BIS calculation

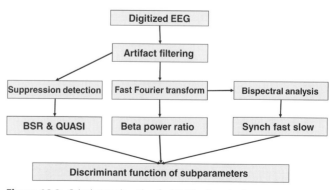

Figure 18.3. Calculation algorithm for BIS. The three basic components are burst suppression, beta power ratio, and the ratio of bicoherence up to 47 Hz, divided by the bicoherence from 40 to 47 Hz. Image used by permission from Nellcor Puritan Bennett LLC, Boulder, CO, doing business as Covidien.

Table 18.1. Correlations coefficients of bispectral index and drug concentration parameters with sedation

Drug (n)	Bispectral index	Target concentration	Actual concentration	Log concentration
Propofol (399)	0.88 *	−0.81	−0.78	−0.77
Isoflurane (70)	0.85	−0.89	−0.89	−0.85
Midazolam (50)	0.76	−0.77	−0.75	−0.65
Alfentanil (50)	0.44 *	−0.17	−0.25	−0.24

* $p < 0.05$ versus target concentration.

index is nearly drug-independent with respect to determination of the level of consciousness.[2]

A secondary result of the validation trials on BIS has spawned considerable controversy. Although the discriminant function was optimized to classify levels of consciousness, in all cases, the ability to remember was lost at a higher index value than a loss of consciousness. Therefore, it was concluded, and later demonstrated, that using a BIS monitor decreased the risk of intraoperative explicit recall.[3]

Entropy

Because EEG is known to be a nonlinear signal, another processing technique that has been applied to the analysis of EEG is entropy analysis. Entropy describes the irregularity, complexity, or unpredictability of a signal. Although measures of entropy could be made directly on the raw EEG signal, the current monitor on the market, the GE Entropy module (GE Healthcare Clinical Systems, Wauwatosa, WI) uses a measure of the entropy of the Fourier transform of the EEG.[4] The raw EEG is acquired from a frontal EEG electrode strip very similar to that of the BIS monitor. The power spectrum is derived from the raw EEG, and a Shannon function is applied to the power spectrum, as shown in Figure 18.5.[5]

Two values are computed. State entropy is computed over the frequency range up to 32 Hz, and response entropy is computed to a higher frequency of 47 Hz. Higher portions of

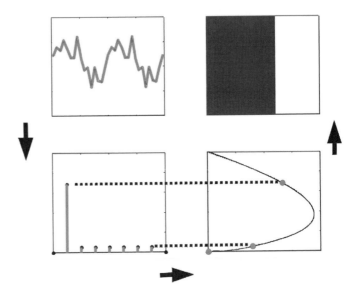

Figure 18.5. The conversion process for deriving an entropy value. The power spectrum is derived from the raw EEG, and a Shannon function is then applied to the power spectrum. Used with permission from ref. 5.

the response entropy spectrum are dominated by the EMG signal, but this is computed over a shorter time span, giving it a quicker response when the patient's state suddenly changes. Raw entropy values are converted to a scale from 0 to 100, using a spline curve as shown in Figure 18.6.[5]

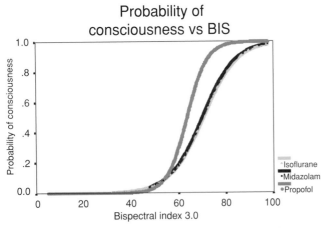

Probability of consciousness vs BIS

Isoflurane
Midazolam
Propofol

Figure 18.4. The cumulative probability of following a command given a particular BIS. (Modified from ref. 2, with permission.) Image used by permission from Nellcor Puritan Bennett LLC, Boulder, CO, doing business as Covidien.

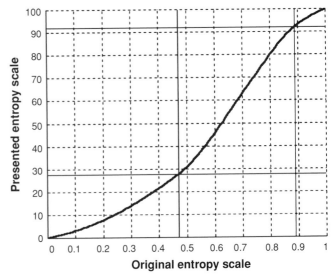

Figure 18.6. The rescaling function to produce the clinical entropy index. Used with permission from ref. 5.

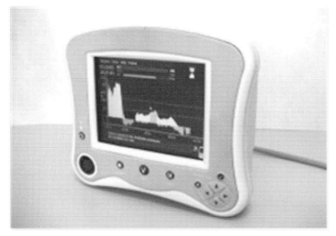

Figure 18.7. The Hospira SEDLine Device. Image use with permission.

Patient state index

The Patient State Index (PSI; Figure 18.7), originally developed by Physiometrics and now marketed by Hospira (Lake Forest, IL), is also a discriminant function derived from quantitative measures of the EEG. After a series of filters and tests for artifacts, the power spectrum of the EEG is computed and divided into sub-bands, including delta, theta, alpha, beta, and gamma, along with total power. The original configuration of the electrodes sampled the EEG from both the frontal and parietal regions and then derived features for the discriminant function.[6] The original features included

- Absolute power gradient between frontal and vertex regions in gamma
- Absolute power changes between frontal and central regions in beta
- Absolute power changes between frontal and parietal regions in alpha
- Total spectral power in the frontal region
- Mean frequency of the total spectrum in the frontal region
- Absolute power in delta at the vertex
- Posterior relative power in slow delta

Using a set of normative data, each of the features is transformed to a standardized Z-score relative to its distribution in a reference state and then expressed as a probability of deviation from that state. Two additional algorithms are used to detect arousal and burst suppression.[7]

Newer versions of devices computing PSI have eliminated the posterior electrodes. Therefore, it is unclear how the original feature set, which included regional comparisons, has been modified in the current systems.

SNAP index

Another algorithm known as the *SNAP* index was recently reintroduced by Stryker (Kalamazoo, MI). The *SNAP* index distinguishes itself from other algorithms by incorporating higher-frequency signals, from 80 to 420 Hz. It is not clear from published studies which proportion of this higher-frequency signal represents EMG versus EEG signals. The details of the computation of the *SNAP* index have been shown only as vague box diagrams in publications thus far.[8] Direct comparisons of the BIS index and the *SNAP* index show at least a 15-point bias between the two indices, and a standard deviation of at least 25 points, indicating that the two computations are neither directly comparable nor interchangeable (i.e. neither is accepted as a gold standard – see Chapter 3).

Narcotrend index

The Narcotrend monitor (MonitorTechnik, Bad Bramstedt, Germany),[9] developed in Hannover, Germany, computes an index from a similarly developed discriminant function. The parameters of the function are derived from amplitude measures and autoregressive coefficients, as well as coefficients from fast Fourier transformation and spectral coefficients. In this case, the discriminant function was optimized to classify EEG segments according to the original classical stages of anesthesia, as described by Guedel. However, the index was later transformed into a scale from 0 to 100, similar to those of other monitors. Once again, direct comparison with indices such as the BIS have shown significant correlation but have also indicated that the indices are not interchangeable.

Evidence of utility

The most important question in the development of these monitors is whether they in fact make a difference in the performance and outcome in anesthetic delivery. Few true outcome studies have been published.

Bispectral index

Utility trial

The most notable of these was a study of the utility of the BIS by Gan et al.[10] This randomized prospective study was designed to test for improvement in overall anesthetic management, and the ability to lower the effective minimum dose. Patients were randomized to receive either standard anesthetic care or standard care supplemented with a BIS monitor. Propofol was used as the primary hypnotic agent (Figure.18.8).

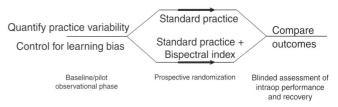

Figure 18.8. The design of the Bispectral Index Clinical Utility trial.

The results demonstrated a 13 percent to 23 percent decrease in propofol use, a 35 percent to 40 percent faster time to wakeup and extubation, and a 16 percent faster eligibility for postanesthesia care unit (PACU) discharge. Twice as many patients were rated as eligible for discharge on admission to PACU, and the BIS-monitored patients had better nursing assessments overall. There was no difference between the groups in untoward intraoperative events.

B-Aware trial

A more controversial outcome (i.e. decreasing the risk of intraoperative awareness) has been the subject of several studies. The B-Aware trial[11] was a prospective randomized double-blind multicenter study of higher-risk patients. Higher risk was defined as patients undergoing cardiac trauma, airway surgery, or cesarean section, and these patients were randomized to receive either standard practice anesthesia or BIS-guided anesthesia delivery.

Awareness incidence was determined by interviewers and a research committee that did not know who had been BIS monitored (double-blind). The study was conducted independently from Aspect Medical, but partial funding and equipment were provided. A total of 2503 patients were enrolled in the study. The incidence of confirmed awareness was 0.17 percent in the BIS group, and 0.91 percent in the routine care group ($p = 0.022$).

Cochrane Review

In 2007, in an extensive review of the published literature, twenty studies with 4056 participants were evaluated to assess whether use of a BIS monitor reduced anesthetic use, recovery time, recall awareness, and cost.[12] They included only randomized controlled trials comparing BIS with standard clinical practice in titrating anesthetic agents. The results were that BIS-guided anesthesia reduced the requirements for propofol by 1.3 mg/kg/hr, and for volatile agents by 0.17 MAC. Recovery times to eye opening, response to command, extubation, and orientation were all significantly shortened by BIS. BIS also shortened the duration of PACU stay but did not reduce the time to discharge to home. The authors' conclusions were that anesthesia guided by BIS within the recommended range (40 to 60) was associated with improved anesthetic delivery and postoperative recovery from relatively deep anesthesia. In addition, BIS-guided anesthesia had a significant association with reduced incidence of intraoperative recall in surgical patients at high risk of awareness.

Avidan study

Further controversy arose over these results in 2008, when a study was published in the *New England Journal of Medicine* by Avidan and colleagues.[13] This study of 2000 patients randomly assigned to either BIS-targeted anesthesia or end-tidal anesthetic gas (ETAG) targeted anesthesia found two patients in each group with unintended intraoperative awareness. The authors concluded that the results did not reproduce previous studies that reported a lower incidence of anesthesia awareness with BIS monitoring, and that the use of BIS was not associated with reduced administration of volatile anesthetic agent. They stated that anesthesia awareness occurred even when BIS values and the ETAG concentrations were within the target ranges.

Part of the controversy has arisen from the fact that in both the BIS-guided cases of awareness, there were significant gaps in the recorded BIS values during the period when the awareness may have occurred. Similarly, in both the ETAG-guided cases, the anesthetic concentration fell below the 0.7 MAC minimum value in the period when awareness may have occurred. What this study does seem to show is that maintaining a minimum of the end-tidal concentration of at least 0.7 MAC may be as effective as BIS monitoring in reducing the risk of intraoperative awareness. Questions still remain about the necessary sample size to validate the conclusions of the study, and a larger follow on study is in progress.[14-18]

Entropy

Studies of efficacy and utility are far fewer for Entropy. Two studies published by Vanluchene and colleagues[19,20] demonstrated similar prediction probability performance (Pk) and comparable sensitivity and specificity to the BIS. A study in 2005 by Vakkuri and associates[21] compared anesthesia guided by Entropy to that of conventional practice for consumption of anesthetic agents and recovery times. Using a total intravenous anesthesia (TIVA) regimen, propofol consumption was significantly decreased in the Entropy group, whereas hemodynamic and other adverse changes were no different between the groups. Improvements in outcome measures such as decreased awareness from light anesthesia, or decreased mortality from deep anesthesia, have not been demonstrated with Entropy devices.

Patient state index

Similar studies on PSI[6] have demonstrated a reduction in propofol consumption and faster emergence and recovery without an increase in adverse events. Again, improvements in outcome measures such as decreased awareness from light anesthesia, or decreased mortality from deep anesthesia, have not been demonstrated.

Narcotrend index

Studies by Kreuer,[22] Rundshagen,[23] and Schmidt[24,25] have compared the Narcotrend monitor with BIS monitoring and standard practice. When compared with standard practice, patients with either monitor needed significantly less propofol, opened their eyes earlier, and were extubated sooner. None of these studies[22-25] addressed the question of whether Narcotrend monitoring could effectively reduce the risk of intraoperative awareness.

Complications

When one is using an anesthetic effect monitor, an important question is, "What harm might it cause?" Perhaps the most common complication of the use of such monitors is the risk of overdosing an anesthetic because of an elevated index caused by artifacts. There are no studies published on the incidence of overdose caused by the misinterpretation of such indices, however.

Another risk in the use of these monitors stems from the fact that there is some time lag between a change in the physiologic state and a change in the computed index. The delay can be on the order of tens of seconds; therefore, a patient may react before an index gives any warning.[26] These indices are all retrospective and not predictive. It remains the job of the clinician to use all the available monitors and other information to anticipate a patient's response.

Although there are occasional reports of skin damage from the application of EEG electrodes, there are no published studies on the incidence of such complications. It is clear that additional caution is warranted in situations in which any additional pressure might be applied to the electrodes, such as patients in the prone position.

Credentialing

Little formal education is available for the application and use of monitors of anesthetic depth. Occasional lectures and mini-workshops are offered at some conferences, but most clinicians learn to use these monitors by trial and error. Some companies provide clinical specialists who provide onsite training to clinicians who buy a specific product.

Practice parameters

There are various reasons for choosing to use an anesthetic effect monitor. The most prominent reason, perhaps owing to its notoriety, is for reduction of the risk of awareness. As indicated earlier, studies by Myles[11] and Ekman[27] showed a reduction in the incidence of awareness, but studies such as that of Avidan[12] indicate that the exact circumstances that require anesthetic effect monitoring are not yet clearly defined. However, studies with various monitors[6,22,28–31] have shown a consistent ability to reduce anesthetic requirements and consumption. This fact, coupled with the finding that excessive doses of anesthetics were associated with increased mortality,[32,33] suggests that the value of anesthetic effect monitoring is not just in reducing the incidence awareness but also in preventing overdosage, to use an optimal level of anesthesia.

There are other likely benefits to using anesthetic effect monitors, such as faster emergence[10] and earlier recovery,[10,34,35] as well as a decrease in postoperative nausea and vomiting (PONV).[17,18] These secondary benefits help to optimize clinical care and increase patient satisfaction (see Figure 18.9).

Although these benefits might suggest that anesthetic effect monitoring should become a standard of care, an American Society of Anesthesiology Task Force examined the available

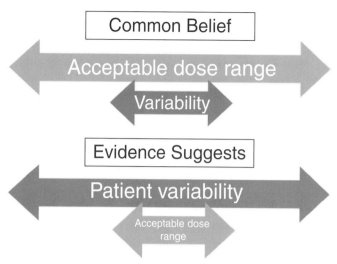

Figure 18.9. Although it is generally believed that interpatient variability is much less than the clinically acceptable dose range, evidence is growing that interpatient variability is much greater than expected, and that the extremes of the clinical dosing range produce undesirable effects, making it difficult to predetermine the optimal anesthetic dose for a particular patient.

literature and generated a practice advisory for brain function monitoring in 2006.[36] The task force did not find sufficient evidence at the time to recommend routine use of such monitors solely for the reduction of intraoperative awareness. It did recommend, however, that in patients with specific risk factors, the decision to use brain function monitors should be made on a case-by-case basis.

The risk factors included

1. A history of substance use or abuse
2. A previous episode of intraoperative awareness
3. A history of, or anticipated, difficult intubation
4. Patients on high doses of opioids
5. ASA physical status 4 or 5
6. Patients with limited hemodynamic reserve
7. Cardiac surgery
8. Cesarean section
9. Airway surgery
10. Trauma surgery
11. Emergency surgery
12. Use of neuromuscular blockers
13. Planned use of nitrous–opioid anesthesia

Reasons that level of consciousness/anesthesia effect/brain function monitoring has not become part of routine practice include the fact that reliability of such monitors is hard to measure because there is no gold standard against which to compare these measurements. Similarly, reproducibility is hard to assess, given that studies have shown that the various indices are not interchangeable and cannot be readily compared.[37–41]

Another significant impediment to widespread adoption is the costs involved in such monitoring – approximated at $17.50 per patient. If we assume an awareness incidence of 0.18 percent,[27] then preventing one case of intraoperative awareness, with a monitor assumed to be 80 percent effective, the number needed to treat is 694, and the cost is approximately $12,000. However, if we assume the incidence in a high-risk population to be about 0.91 percent,[11] then the number needed to treat is reduced to 137, at a cost of about $2400. These costs may be partly recovered by the reduced consumption of drugs, faster emergence from anesthesia, and reduced PACU times. Other potential cost savings, such as reduced incidence of PONV and lower liability from unintended awareness and consequent posttraumatic stress disorder, are difficult or impossible to quantify.

In summary, although brain function monitors appear to correlate directly with anesthetic effects on the level of consciousness and may assist with preventing both underdosage with possible unintended awareness and overdosage with the potential risk of adverse outcomes, they have not yet become a part of standard anesthetic care.

Although these monitors may offer qualitative improvements in a patient's anesthetic experience and improved resource utilization, it remains the individual anesthesia provider's decision whether to use such technology. The American Society of Anesthesiologists Practice Advisory may help practitioners decide on the circumstances under which these monitors may be of greatest potential benefit.

References

1. Rampil IJ. A primer for EEG signal processing in anesthesia [see comments]. *Anesthesiology* 1998;**89**(4)9:80–1002.
2. Glass PS, et al. Bispectral analysis measures sedation and memory effects of propofol, midazolam, isoflurane, and alfentanil in healthy volunteers. *Anesthesiology* 1997;**86**(4):836–47.
3. Myles PS. Prevention of awareness during anaesthesia. *Best Pract Res Clin Anaesthesiol* 2007;**21**(3):345–55.
4. Bein B. Entropy. *Best Pract Res Clin Anaesthesiol* 2006;**20**(1):101–9.
5. Viertio-Oja H, et al. Description of the entropy algorithm as applied in the Datex-Ohmeda S/5 Entropy Module. *Acta Anaesthesiologica Scandinavica* 2004;**48**(2):154–61.
6. Drover DR, et al. Patient State Index: titration of delivery and recovery from propofol, alfentanil, and nitrous oxide anesthesia. *Anesthesiology* 2002;**97**(1):82–9.
7. Drover D, et al. Patient State Index. *Best Pract Res Clin Anaesthesiol* 2006;**20**(1):121–8.
8. Wong CA, et al. A comparison of the SNAP II and BIS XP indices during sevoflurane and nitrous oxide anaesthesia at 1 and 1.5 MAC and at awakening. *Br J Anaesth* 2006;**97**(2):181–6.
9. Kreuer S, et al. The Narcotrend monitor. *Best Pract Res Clin Anaesthesiol* 2006;**20**(1):111–9.
10. Gan TJ, et al. Bispectral index monitoring allows faster emergence and improved recovery from propofol, alfentanil, and nitrous oxide anesthesia. BIS Utility Study Group. *Anesthesiology* 1997;**87**(4):808–15.
11. Myles PS, et al. Bispectral index monitoring to prevent awareness during anaesthesia: the B-Aware randomised controlled trial [see comment]. *Lancet* 2004;**363**(9423):1757–63.
12. Punjasawadwong Y, Boonjeungmonkol N, Phongchiewboon A. Bispectral index for improving anaesthetic delivery and postoperative recovery. *Cochrane Database of Systematic Reviews* 2007(4):CD003843.
13. Avidan MS, et al. Anesthesia awareness and the bispectral index [see comment]. *N Engl J Med* 2008;**358**(11):1097–108.
14. Wong J, et al. Titration of isoflurane using BIS index improves early recovery of elderly patients undergoing orthopedic surgeries. *Can J Anaesth* 2002;**49**(1):13–8.
15. White PF, Song D. Bispectral index monitoring and fast tracking after ambulatory surgery: an unexpected finding? [comment]. *Anesthesiology* 2004;**100**(1):194–5; author reply 195–6.
16. Liu SS. Effects of bispectral index monitoring on ambulatory anesthesia: a meta-analysis of randomized controlled trials and a cost analysis. *Anesthesiology* 2004;**101**(2):311–5.
17. Luginbuhl M, et al. Different benefit of bispectral index (BIS) in desflurane and propofol anesthesia. *Acta Anaesthesiologica Scandinavica* 2003;**47**(2):165–73.
18. Nelskyla KA, et al. Sevoflurane titration using bispectral index decreases postoperative vomiting in phase II recovery after ambulatory surgery [see comment]. *Anesth Analg* 2001;**93**(5):1165–9.
19. Vanluchene ALG, et al. Spectral entropy measurement of patient responsiveness during propofol and remifentanil. A comparison with the bispectral index. *Br J Anaesth* 2004;**93**(5):645–54.
20. Vanluchene ALG, et al. Spectral entropy as an electroencephalographic measure of anesthetic drug effect: a comparison with bispectral index and processed midlatency auditory evoked response. *Anesthesiology* 2004;**101**(1):34–42.
21. Vakkuri A, et al. Time-frequency balanced spectral entropy as a measure of anesthetic drug effect in central nervous system during sevoflurane, propofol, and thiopental anesthesia. *Acta Anaesthesiol Scand* 2004;**48**(2):145–53.
22. Kreuer S, et al. Narcotrend monitoring allows faster emergence and a reduction of drug consumption in propofol-remifentanil anesthesia [see comment]. *Anesthesiology* 2003;**99**(1):34–41.
23. Rundshagen I, et al. Narcotrend-assisted propofol/remifentanil anaesthesia vs clinical practice: does it make a difference? [see comment]. *Br J Anaesth* 2007;**99**(5):686–93.
24. Schmidt GN, et al. Narcotrend and bispectral index monitor are superior to classic electroencephalographic parameters for the assessment of anesthetic states during propofol-remifentanil anesthesia. *Anesthesiology* 2003;**99**(5):1072–7.
25. Schmidt GN, et al. Comparative evaluation of Narcotrend, bispectral index, and classical electroencephalographic variables during induction, maintenance, and emergence of a propofol/remifentanil anesthesia. *Anesth Analg* 2004;**98**(5):1346–53.
26. Pilge S, et al. Time delay of index calculation: analysis of cerebral state, bispectral, and Narcotrend indices. *Anesthesiology* 2006;**104**(3):488–94.
27. Ekman A, et al. Reduction in the incidence of awareness using BIS monitoring. *Acta Anaesthesiol Scand* 2004;**48**(1):20–6.
28. Basar H, et al. Effect of bispectral index monitoring on sevoflurane consumption. *Eur J Anaesthesiol* 2003;**20**(5):396–400.
29. Yli-Hankala A, et al. EEG bispectral index monitoring in sevoflurane or propofol anaesthesia: analysis of direct costs and immediate recovery. *Acta Anaesthesiol Scand* 1999;**43**(5):545–9.
30. Recart A, et al. The effect of cerebral monitoring on recovery after general anesthesia: a comparison of the auditory evoked

potential and bispectral index devices with standard clinical practice. *Anesth Analg* 2003;**97**(6):1667–74.

31. Vakkuri A, et al. Sevoflurane requirement for laparoscopic tubal ligation: an electroencephalographic bispectral study. *Eur J Anaesthesiol* 1999;**16**(5):279–83.

32. Monk TG, et al. Anesthetic management and one-year mortality after noncardiac surgery [see comment]. *Anesth Analg* 2005;**100**(1):4–10.

33. Lindholm M-L, et al. Mortality within 2 years after surgery in relation to low intraoperative bispectral index values and preexisting malignant disease. *Anesth Analg* 2009;**108**(2):508–12.

34. White PF, et al. Does the use of electroencephalographic bispectral index or auditory evoked potential index monitoring facilitate recovery after desflurane anesthesia in the ambulatory setting? *Anesthesiology* 2004;**100**(4):811–7.

35. White PF. Use of cerebral monitoring during anaesthesia: effect on recovery profile. *Best Pract Res Clin Anaesthesiol* 2006;**20**(1):181–9.

36. American Society of Anesthesiologists. Practice Advisory for Intraoperative Awareness and Brain Function Monitoring. *Anesthesiology* 2006;**104**(4):847–64.

37. Schneider G, et al. EEG-based indices of anaesthesia: correlation between bispectral index and patient state index? *Eur J Anaesthesiol* 2004;**21**(1):6–12.

38. Kreuer S, et al. Comparison of BIS and AAI as measures of anaesthetic drug effect during desflurane-remifentanil anaesthesia [see comment]. *Acta Anaesthesiol Scand* 2004;**48**(9):1168–73.

39. Kreuer S, et al. Comparability of Narcotrend index and bispectral index during propofol anaesthesia. *Br J Anaesth* 2004;**93**(2):235–40.

40. Kreuer S, et al. A-line, bispectral index, and estimated effect-site concentrations: a prediction of clinical end-points of anesthesia. *Anesth Analg* 2006;**102**(4):1141–6.

41. Wong CA, et al. A comparison of the SNAP II and BIS XP indices during sevoflurane and nitrous oxide anaesthesia at 1 and 1.5 MAC and at awakening. *Br J Anaesth* 2006;**97**(2):181–6.

Chapter 19

Transcranial Doppler

Dean B. Andropoulos

Introduction

Transcranial Doppler (TCD) ultrasound is a sensitive, real-time monitor of cerebral blood flow velocity and emboli that has been used for neurologic monitoring during adult open cardiac surgery, vascular surgery, intracranial aneurysm surgery, and congenital heart surgery. This chapter will review the technical concepts of TCD, parameters monitored and clinical uses of intraoperative TCD, evidence of utility for TCD, use to improve neurological outcomes, risks and complications of TCD, and finally, training and certification for TCD.

Technical considerations for transcranial Doppler ultrasound

Currently available instruments use pulsed-wave ultrasound of 2 MHz frequency with a power of 100 mW, which is range-gated with a sample volume length of up to 15 mm. As in cardiac Doppler examination, TCD measures cerebral blood flow velocity (CBFV), not absolute cerebral blood flow. Several transducer probes are available, ranging from very small disc probes suitable for infants and children, to larger, heavier disk probes with holders that attach to fixation devices for adolescents and adults (Figure 19.1). Microvascular probes are also available for the assessment of cerebral hemodynamics during cerebral aneurysm surgery.[1,2] These small probes have a diameter of 1.5 mm or less and use frequencies of 16 or 20 MHz. The probes are placed on the vessel of interest by the neurosurgeon using either a malleable wand or a rigid suction cannula. Intraoperative TCD monitoring usually requires fixation of the ultrasonic probe with a specialized holder to prevent probe movement, avoid compression of cranial or facial tissues, and permit the surgeon to have access to cranial or neck regions (Figures 19.2–19.5). These TCD and microvascular probes are small in size and their design must incorporate shielding from radiofrequency artifact from electrosurgical units.

High-pass filtering of TCD signals is necessary to minimize vessel wall motion artifact. During surgery, extremely low CBFV signals are often encountered, especially during cardiopulmonary bypass with deep hypothermia. Filter settings as low as 50 Hz may be required to visualize these low CBFVs. TCD devices used during cardiac surgery must have appropriate filter settings to accurately monitor low flow states;

sometimes, the filter needs to be turned off completely in circumstances of very low CBFV.

Cerebral blood flow velocity measurement

As discussed in Chapter 12, erythrocytes moving toward or away from the ultrasonic transducer are insonated; the

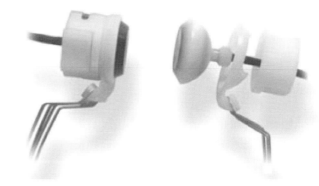

Figure 19.1. 2-MHz probes for intraoperative monitoring, capable of attachment to several external fixation devices. Courtesy of Compumedics DWL Doppler, Compumedics Ltd, www. dwl.de/.

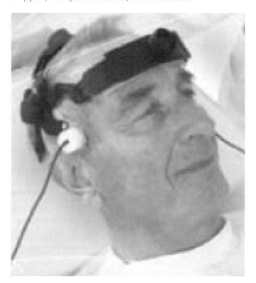

Figure 19.2. Padded adjustable Doppler probe holder, with probe secured over temporal window. Courtesy of Compumedics DWL Doppler, Compumedics Ltd, www. dwl.de/.

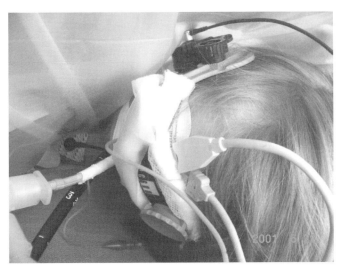

Figure 19.3. Padded probe fixation device in a child with probe secured over the temporal window.

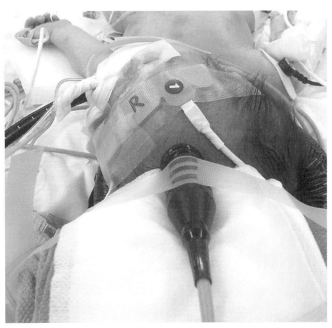

Figure 19.5. Alternative monitoring site with hand-held probe secured over anterior fontanelle in a neonate, with sample volume directed at right middle cerebral artery–anterior cerebral artery junction.

difference in frequency between the transmitted ultrasound and its reflected waves (echoes) enables the calculation of erythrocyte velocity using the Doppler equation. Because of laminar flow, these echoes create a family of distinct frequencies, and spectral analysis permits presentation of the blood flow velocity as a function of time through the sample volume. The signal power of each velocity component is determined and is displayed as a color- or gray-scaled spectral profile. Through fast Fourier transformation (FFT), the spectral analyzer automatically calculates CBFV parameters such as peak systolic, end-diastolic, and intensity-weighted mean CBFVs (cm/sec), as well as pulsatility indices (PIs), which describe the downstream resistance. The PI is equal to the peak velocity minus the end-diastolic velocity, divided by the mean velocity (Figure 19.6). The information can be stored digitally and analyzed offline at a later time. As with cardiac ultrasound, the advantage of pulsed-wave Doppler ultrasound is that a precise sample volume can

be selected, which insonates only the arteries of interest, without contamination from other sources. The peak CBFV can be trended easily because of a favorable signal-to-noise ratio; however, during surgery with bypass and nonpulsatile flow, mean CBFV will be the only velocity parameter displayed. The direction of blood flow should be clearly labeled; the usual convention is to have flow toward the transducer displayed above the zero velocity baseline, and flows away from the transducer below the baseline.

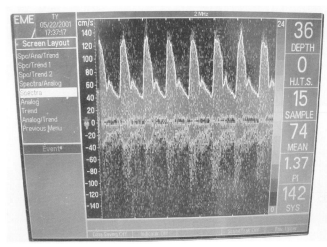

Figure 19.6. Transcranial Doppler cerebral blood flow velocity (CBFV) spectrum in an adult patient. Depth is depth of sample volume in mm, HITS is the high-intensity transient signal (embolus) counter, sample is width of sample volume in mm, mean is mean CBFV in cm/sec, PI is pulsatility index, equal to the peak velocity minus the end-diastolic velocity, divided by the mean velocity. Sys is systolic CBFV.

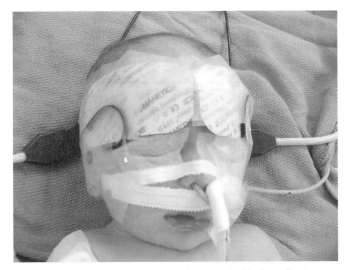

Figure 19.4. Neonatal/pediatric disk probe secured with clear adhesive dressing over temporal window.

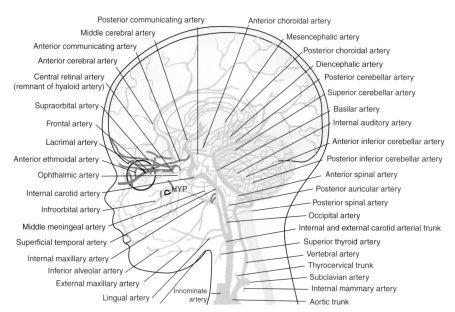

Figure 19.7. Transcranial Doppler anatomy in an infant. The usual sample volume for intraoperative monitoring is the junction of the middle and anterior cerebral arteries. Reproduced with permission from ref. 7.

TCD measurements reflect the CBFV in the insonated vessel in cm/sec, which is not synonymous with cerebral blood flow in cm^3/sec. Flow velocity is a function of pressure gradient across the cerebral vascular bed, cerebral vascular resistance to flow, and diameter of the vessel being insonated. If a vessel becomes narrowed in the region of insonation, the CBFV through the vessel will increase, although total blood flow decreases. In normal patients, cerebral autoregulation is intact, so small decreases or increases in blood pressure cause compensatory vasodilation and vasoconstriction in the peripheral arterioles to maintain the total cerebral blood flow constant.

CBFV depends on the diameter of the blood vessel, whereas cerebral blood flow depends on cerebral vascular resistance, which changes in response to changes in CO_2, temperature, cerebral perfusion pressure, and pump flow. Thus, CBFV often correlates well with cerebral blood flow in the individual patient, particularly at deep hypothermia, when autoregulation is lost and the caliber of the blood vessels is unchanged. However, the clinician must always be mindful and estimate the state of the patient's cerebral vascular resistance to translate TCD into meaningful information for clinical decision making.

Interpretation of CBFV changes occurring during surgery or critical care is heavily influenced by the patient's underlying pathology and the use of anesthetics and other vasoactive agents. Chronic hypertension, diabetes mellitus, cerebral atherosclerosis, and nicotine use may diminish or abolish cerebral pressure autoregulation,[3] making both flow and flow velocity dependent on systemic arterial pressure. Cerebral pressure flow autoregulation is also blunted at moderate hypothermia and abolished at deep hypothermia during cardiopulmonary bypass (CPB).[4] These patients may also lack cerebral arterial reactivity to changes in PaCO$_2$. With these progressive disorders, changes in blood flow may not be reflected in trends in the same direction as CBFV. In addition, with unilateral

or asymmetric carotid stenosis or previous cerebral infarction, vascular reactivity in the two hemispheres may differ.[5] In such cases, unilateral insonation may result in a misperception about brain tissue at risk. This is also a significant issue in patients with intracranial vascular disease. Knowledge of the status of the patient's intracranial vasculature preoperatively may be helpful in guiding intraoperative monitoring.

The most consistent and reproducible technique for clinical use in patients of all ages is to monitor the middle cerebral artery (MCA) through the temporal window, which can usually be found just above the zygoma and just anterior to the tragus of the ear (Figures 19.2–19.4).[6] Several transducer probes are available, ranging from very small disk probes suitable for infants and children, to larger, heavier probes for adolescents and adults. The depth of the sample volume and angle of insonation are adjusted until the bifurcation of the MCA and the anterior cerebral artery (ACA) are detected, ideally at a zero degree angle of insonation, which yields the most accurate CBFV information, just as in cardiac ultrasound (Figure 19.7). Correct position and sample volume adjustment are heralded by a maximal antegrade signal (positive deflection, toward the transducer) from the MCA, accompanied by retrograde flow as the ACA is insonated (negative deflection, away from the transducer). This spectrum should be the same or very similar velocity and waveform as the MCA flow (Figure 19.8). The same location should be monitored for an individual patient.

Insonation at the MCA–ACA bifurcation also offers the advantage of minimizing interpatient variability. In addition, the MCA supplies the largest volume of tissue of any of the basal cerebral arteries.[7] After obtaining an optimal signal, the probe must be secured, usually by adhesive tape or clear adhesive dressing for the small disk probe, or by adjustments to a padded head ring, or adhesive disk in larger patients. Care must be taken with the padded head ring to thoroughly pad

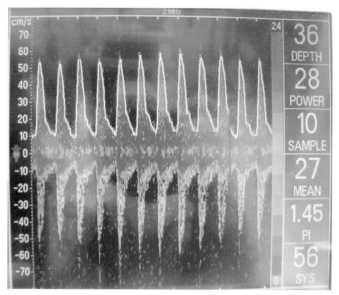

Figure 19.8. Sample volume near the junction of the middle cerebral artery (positive deflection, toward the transducer) and anterior cerebral artery (negative deflection, away from the transducer) in an infant.

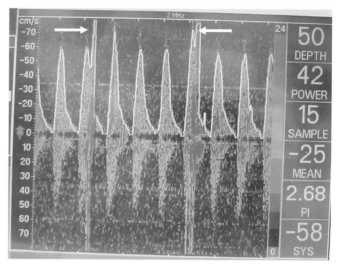

Figure 19.9. High-intensity transient signals (HITS). Note two deep signals with a velocity well above the systolic velocity in an infant before cardiopulmonary bypass (arrows).

all pressure points and to pay particular care to the orbits. For smaller patients, securing the probe by wrapping the head with an elastic bandage is discouraged because pressure sores may develop under the area of the transducer. Also, adjustment to the probe position is often necessary during the case, so access to the transducer is important. In infants, an alternative site for monitoring is through the anterior fontanelle, using a hand-held pencil-type probe, placing the probe over the lateral edge of the fontanelle, and aiming caudally, at a larger depth than for the temporal window, at the internal carotid artery (Figure 19.5)

The depth of measurement and normal flow velocities for the MCA for infants, children, and adults are listed in Table 19.1. These normal velocities were determined in patients without cerebrovascular or cardiovascular disease. In addition to the problems in adults with cerebrovascular disease noted earlier, congenital cardiac defects producing large diastolic runoffs,

such as a large patent ductus arteriosus, will have an effect on diastolic blood flow to the brain. These normal velocities were obtained in awake children and adults under perfect examination conditions. Hemodynamic instability, less-than-optimal probe positioning, and general anesthesia may reduce these velocities in clinical practice. Often the clinician must accept a stable baseline for the individual patient and use it as the basis for comparison, rather than expect a perfect signal. Typically, the skull attenuates about 80 percent of the ultrasonic energy prior cerebral vessel insonation.[8] Because of temporal bone hyperostosis related to age, sex, and race, inadequate temporal ultrasonic windows occur in a significant subpopulation of patients.[9,10] Identification of this situation prior to surgery often enables the sonographer to use an alternative insonation site (i.e. foramenal or submandibular).

Cerebral emboli detection and counting

Cerebral emboli are very common during open-heart surgery in adults and children. Emboli are easily detected by TCD, although artifacts, such as electrocautery and physical contact with the ultrasound transducer, may be observed (Figure 19.9).[11] True emboli have characteristic audio and visual signals and are designated as high-intensity transient signals (HITS) that can actually be counted by the TCD software. The filtering criteria must be set to exclude artifacts, and the HITS counter can be a gauge of the number of emboli detected in the artery being monitored.

Uses of transcranial Doppler monitoring in the intraoperative setting

TCD has widespread application in a number of clinical settings in the operating room, including assessment of intracranial hemodynamics, circle of Willis anatomy and function, ischemic

Table 19.1. Normal transcranial Doppler values for infants, children, and adults; temporal window

Age	Depth	Mean velocity (cm/sec)	Peak systolic velocity (cm/sec)	End-diastolic velocity (cm/sec)
0–3 mo	25	24–42 ± 10	46–75 ± 15	12–24 ± 8
3–12 mo	30	74 ± 14	114 ± 20	46 ± 9
1–3 yr	35–45	85 ± 10	124 ± 10	65 ± 11
3–6 yr	40–45	94 ± 10	147 ± 17	65 ± 9
6–10 yr	45–50	97 ± 9	143 ± 13	72 ± 9
10–18 yr	45–50	81 ± 11	129 ± 17	60 ± 8
>18 yr	30–65	62 ± 12	100 ± 20	45 ± 15

Normal transcranial Doppler parameters in infants, children, and adults. Values were obtained in awake, normal patients without cardio- or cerebral vascular pathology, breathing room air. For adults, a mean velocity >80–100 cm/sec may signify significant stenosis or hyperemia.
Reproduced with permission from refs. 6 and 54.

threshold and CBFV monitoring during carotid endarterectomy, intracranial aneurysm repair, CPB, detection of cerebral emboli, and use in congenital heart surgery.

Assessment of intracranial hemodynamics

The specific objectives of intraoperative TCD monitoring need to be understood and discussed with the surgical team preoperatively. Again, TCD measures CBFV, and the use of CBFV measurements as an estimate of cerebral blood flow is neither appropriate nor recommended. In contrast, continuous CBFV recordings from a single insonation site can provide reliable and clinically valuable trend information. TCD monitoring can identify changes in flow direction or detect sudden dramatic CBFV change (i.e. relative hypo- or hyperperfusion). Change in the ratio of velocities at peak systole and end-diastole or PIs also can be used to estimate cerebral vascular resistance (i.e. venous obstruction or intracranial hypertension).[12] In certain clinical situations, each of these pieces of information, which are often unobtainable by other means, may prevent a neurologic injury.[13] Interpretation of sudden cerebral hemodynamic changes requires the anesthesiologist to pay attention to maneuvers by the surgeon or perfusionist that can cause these changes. Thus, in the surgical environment, the anesthesiologist should have immediate visual access to the surgical field to facilitate rapid integration of surgical information.

Circle of Willis function

Circle of Willis CBFV measurements are based on established criteria including cranial window, sample volume depth and extension, spatial relationships of probe angle to intracranial vessels, relative flow velocity, and response of oscillation maneuvers.[9,14] The most proximal segment of the middle cerebral artery (M1) is the most frequently used for TCD monitoring applications because it carries up to 40 percent of the hemispheric blood flow. This segment generally has the highest peak and intensity-weighted mean CBFV of any intracranial vessel, although there is a large variation (i.e. 35–90 cm/sec) in the awake adult patient.[15] Correct identification of this segment is especially important when assessing collateral flow during carotid occlusion. With carotid occlusion, the TCD signal from the ipsilateral internal carotid artery disappears, but with normal intact circle of Willis function, CBFV is maintained in the ipsilateral MCA segment. Typically, the MCA can be insonated at a depth of 50 mm in adults and can be traced back to the bifurcation to the carotid artery as the depth increases. With bifurcation of the MCA into the ACA, flow direction is toward the transducer in the MCA and away from the transducer for the ACA.

Carotid endarterectomy and the ischemic threshold

An absolute CBFV threshold for ischemia has not been established, and so common practice relies on changes relative to the patient's baseline to determine risk of ischemia.

In unanesthetized patients, clinical signs of cerebral hypoperfusion appear with reductions in middle cerebral artery flow velocity of greater than 60 percent.[16] During carotid endarterectomy, an exponential relationship between carotid clamp-related decreases in middle cerebral artery mean CBFV and carotid artery stump pressure has been described. The CBFV fell to undetectable levels at a stump pressure of 15 mmHg.[17] The authors concluded that TCD "provided an excellent indicator as to the necessity of shunting." An additional study found that patients with stump pressures below 30 mmHg had significantly lower CBFV than those with higher pressures.[18]

A multicenter retrospective study of carotid endarterectomy patients suggested that severe ischemia (i.e. high probability of new neurological deficit) was associated with a greater than 85 percent reduction in CBFV, and moderate ischemia represented a 60 percent to 85 percent decrease.[19,20] Jorgensen and colleagues found that during carotid endarterectomy under general anesthesia with combined TCD, cerebral blood flow, and EEG monitoring, a greater than 60 percent decrease in mean CBFV below the preocclusion reference resulted in flow of approximately 20 mL/100 g/min and pathologic EEG suppression.[21] Spencer[22] suggested that CBFV reductions of greater than 70 percent persisting for more than 5 minutes signified cerebral ischemia in need of immediate corrective action. In the absence of definitive criteria for the ischemic threshold, a 70 percent reduction in mean CBFV appears to be a reasonable temporary guide.[23] However, some patients have adequate leptomeningeal collateral flow, and EEG activity occasionally may remain unchanged in the presence of a severely decreased or absent MCA CBFV spectrum.

Intracranial aneurysm repair

Occlusion of an intracranial artery is often necessary for catheter or surgical treatment of a giant cerebral aneurysm, and testing the integrity of the circle of Willis and collateral arterial supply is important to plan the approach. TCD monitoring during manual[24] or intravascular balloon[25] carotid artery occlusion can identify the lack of adequate alternative arterial supply to the hemisphere of interest. The appearance of neurologic sequelae correlated with the magnitude of the *relative* CBFV decrease from individualized preocclusion reference, but not with the *absolute* CBFV. In these studies, neurologic signs of transient focal deficit consistently occurred with CBFV decreases greater than 65 percent.

Cardiopulmonary bypass

TCD has been used to continuously assess changes in cerebral hemodynamics during CPB. TCD indicates CBF presence and direction and is able to detect an evolving ischemic process arising from a malpositioned bypass cannula or inadvertent occlusion of the great vessels (Figure 19.10). During surgical repair of the aortic arch, TCD documents CBF direction during attempts at selective antegrade or retrograde cerebral perfusion in both

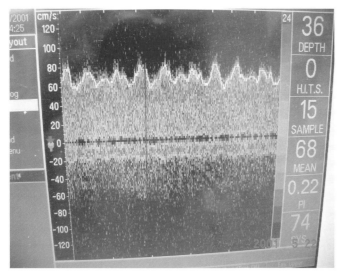

Figure 19.10. Transcranial Doppler signal during cardiopulmonary bypass in an adult patient. Note minimal pulsatility. Sudden decrease or cessation of flow, as may be seen with aortic cannula malposition, is rapidly detected.

adults and children (Figure 19.11). Because peak CBFV changes in large basal cerebral arteries are usually related to peak CBF changes, TCD may aid in the determination of safe upper and lower limits for pump flow and perfusion pressure. In addition, end-diastolic CBFV change is inversely related to change in cerebrovascular resistance. A sudden increase in resistance during cardiopulmonary bypass may indicate impaired venous return, possibly caused by a malpositioned or partially occluded venous cannula. Persistence of the pattern following termination of bypass may suggest developing cerebral edema and the need for its treatment.

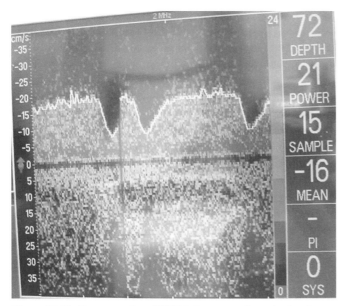

Figure 19.11. Documentation of CBFV during antegrade cerebral perfusion in a neonate. The very low flow rate is indicated by variation in CBFV in parallel with the roller head rate of rotation by the CPB pump.

Two different approaches have been used in adult patients for TCD ischemia detection during CPB. The first is simply a modification of the relative ischemia criteria used for non-CPB surgery, based on the view that larger decreases in CBFV are needed to reliably identify hypoperfusion with extracorporeal circulatory support. In a retrospective study of coronary artery bypass patients, Edmonds[26] defined cerebral ischemia as a mean CBFV decline of 80 percent below the preincision baseline. Decreases of this magnitude occurred in 13 percent of the cases and were associated with EEG suppression and/or cerebral oxygen desaturation. Nearly all the decreases were correctable by increasing mean arterial pressure, cardiopulmonary bypass pump outflow, or arterial CO_2 tension. The 3 percent neurologic deficit incidence in this patient cohort was half that of a historical control group that received no neuromonitoring.

The other approach to TCD monitoring during CPB is qualitative, with goals of maintaining a measurable CBFV spectral signal and verifying that the flow direction is as expected,[27] to prevent the infrequent but devastating injury that may be associated with cannula malposition or other technical errors with the conduct of CPB. This approach seems especially well suited for procedures that involve multimodality neuromonitoring and the use of deep hypothermic circulatory arrest with selective cerebral perfusion. The effectiveness of the qualitative method has been described for both adult[28,29] and pediatric[30] cardiac surgery.

TCD has been used extensively in pediatric cardiac surgical research to examine cerebral physiology in response to cardiopulmonary bypass, hypothermia, low-flow bypass, regional low-flow perfusion to the brain, and circulatory arrest. Hillier and associates[31] used TCD to study cerebrovascular hemodynamics during hypothermic bypass with deep hypothermic circulatory arrest (DHCA) in 10 infants. Cerebral blood flow velocity did not return to baseline levels after DHCA. Calculated cerebral vascular resistance (mean arterial pressure – central venous pressure/CBFV) was increased immediately after DHCA and remained so until the end of bypass. The observed decrease in CBFV during cooling was thought to be the result of decreased metabolic demand by the brain and thus less blood flow, although α-stat strategy was used. This could be explained by relative cerebral vasoconstriction during cooling in smaller arterioles downstream to the MCA and ACA, as these large arteries do not change their caliber in response to changes in $PaCO_2$.[32] TCD of the MCA through the temporal window was used to describe the cerebral pressure–flow velocity relationship during hypothermic bypass in 25 neonates and infants less than nine months old. CBFV was examined over a wide range of cerebral perfusion pressure varying from 6 to 90 mm Hg, at three temperatures – normothermia (36–37°C), moderate hypothermia (23–25°C), and profound hypothermia (14–20°C). Cerebral pressure flow autoregulation was preserved at normothermia, partially affected at moderate hypothermia, and totally lost at profound hypothermia, results that agree with previous research done using xenon to quantitate cerebral blood flow.[4]

TCD has also been used to determine the threshold of detectable cerebral perfusion during low-flow cardiopulmonary bypass. Zimmerman and coworkers[33] studied 28 neonates undergoing the arterial switch operation with α-stat pH management. At 14°C to 15°C the pump flow was sequentially reduced to 0 mL/kg/min. All patients had detectable cerebral blood flow down to 20 mL/kg/min, whereas 1 had no perfusion at 20 mL/kg/min, and 8 had none at 10 mL/kg/min, leading the authors to conclude that 30 mL/kg/min was the minimum acceptable flow in this population. Finally, Andropoulos and associates[34] used TCD of the MCA to determine the level of bypass flow necessary during regional low-flow perfusion for neonatal aortic arch reconstruction (Figure 19.11) They studied 34 neonates undergoing the Norwood operation or aortic arch advancement and established a baseline mean CBFV under hypothermic full flow bypass (17–22°C, 150 mL/kg/min) using pH stat management. During these conditions, the mean CBFV was 22 cm/sec. The researchers then used TCD to determine how much bypass flow was necessary to match this value, finding that a mean of 63 mL/kg/min was necessary. Interestingly, this necessary level of bypass flow did not correlate with mean arterial pressure in the radial artery or cerebral saturation measured by near-infrared spectroscopy (NIRS). The necessary flow as determined by TCD varied widely, leading the authors to conclude that TCD was a valuable monitor to ensure adequate but not excessive cerebral blood flow during this complicated technique.

Detection and quantification of cerebral emboli

TCD is very sensitive to the presence of emboli, regardless of their size or composition.[35] Detection of embolization provided by TCD can improve surgical and perfusion technique[26] and facilitate correction of technical problems such as an air leak.[36] Echogenic substances with acoustic impedance greater than that of erythrocytes have been referred to as microemboli, microbubbles, particulate emboli, formed-element emboli, and Doppler microembolic signals (MES),[37] whereas the term *high-intensity transient signals* (HITS) appears currently to be the most widely used.[38]

The basic features of Doppler embolic signals were initially defined by Spencer and colleages.[17] Subsequently, an international consensus committee[39] characterized the basic ultrasonic criteria of particulate (i.e. formed-element) HITS:

1. Transient, with a duration <300 ms;
2. Duration dependent on passage time through the sample volume;
3. High-intensity, with an amplitude >3 dB above background flow signal;
4. Unidirectional; and
5. Acoustically resemble "snaps, tonal chirps, or moans."

Gavrilescu and associates[40] compared the ultrasonic signatures of particulate HITS to those presumably representing uncoated bubbles. Distinguishing characteristics of the latter were their bidirectionality and higher intensities (>25 dB above background). In contrast, acoustic artifacts, although also bidirectional, are predominantly of low frequency (<400 Hz). They may arise from movement of the probe or probe cable, electrical interference, and patient actions such as coughing, swallowing, talking, and facial movement. Recent development of multifrequency and multigated Doppler instruments has led to claims of improved sensitivity and specificity of emboli detection. For example, Brucher and Russell[41] reported 99 percent correct classification of gaseous and particulate emboli using an in vitro test system. However, the US Food and Drug Administration has yet to clear for clinical use ultrasonographs equipped with this technology, and in clinical practice it is difficult to distinguish differences between solid and gaseous emboli using standard commercially available TCD systems.

An important limitation of the current generation of emboli measurement systems is the inability of the automated features of the system to detect the most ominous situation, a massive gaseous embolization called an embolic *shower* or *curtain*. Because all current emboli detection algorithms focus on the discrete nature of individual transient embolic events, sustained high-intensity signals are unrecognized; the anesthesiologist needs to be vigilant to recognize these events.

HITS may be detected in as many as 60 percent of carotid endarterectomies.[42] In this setting, the emboliform ultrasonic signals will be primarily of particulate origin, either thrombus or atheroma. These emboli appear to be responsible for approximately half the cerebrovascular complications associated with this procedure.[22] Payne and colleagues[43] found that in the first hours after endarterectomy, neurologic injury often accompanied HITS formation at a rate exceeding two per minute. Aggressive thrombolysis subsequently eliminated both HITS and the neurologic complications.

HITS composition during cardiac surgery is less certain because of the frequent unintentional introduction of air into the cerebral circulation during cardiopulmonary bypass and the production of cavitation bubbles by mechanical prosthetic devices. Some studies have implicated HITS in the etiology of both neurologic injury and cognitive decline after cardiac surgery,[16,44] whereas others have not.[45] Although some investigators have found the severity of the injury or decline to be related to aggregate HITS,[44,46] others found no relationship.[47,48] No study has proposed a critical HITS injury threshold. There is retrospective evidence that HITS reduction is associated with a decreased incidence of cerebral injury.[49] Despite the association of aggregate HITS in some studies with neurocognitive injury, however, the relative impact of particulate and gaseous emboli is unclear.

Outcome studies using transcranial Doppler

The majority of outcome studies assessing the use of TCD have focused on the association between the number of detected microemboli and later cognitive dysfunction or brain injury. In a review of the occurrence and clinical impact of microembolic signals during cardiac surgery, Dittrich and Ringelstein[50] reviewed more than 50 studies in more than 1500 patients with TCD microemboli during or after coronary artery bypass graft (CABG), valve surgery, left ventricular assist device (LVAD) placement, and catheter interventions. Prevalence of HITS in these studies ranged from 0 to 100 percent of patients, with most studies having a prevalence of 40 percent to 80 percent, and number of HITS from one to several hundred per patient, with most experiencing <20 HITS. There were a few studies demonstrating a difference in number of HITS in those patients with postoperative neurocognitive dysfunction or thromboembolic events, but the great majority of studies could detect no association. The authors' conclusions were that the number of HITS can provide clues to successfully modify surgical interventions, but TCD detection of HITS is not an accepted surrogate parameter for the prediction or prevention of neuronal damage with cognitive decline. They cited the limitations of different monitoring devices, protocols, and monitoring time period as hampering the interpretation of the results of these trials. There is still no reliable method to distinguish between gaseous and solid emboli, and there are no large prospective, randomized trials with long-term neurological outcome studies to determine the utility of HITS detection by TCD.

In a recent systematic review of 14 cardiac surgery articles, 5 carotid endarterectomy articles, and 2 orthopedic surgery articles after screening for adequate study design and methods, Martin and associates[51] determined that HITS occurred during nearly all cardiac surgical procedures. Off-pump CABG was associated with significantly fewer HITS (i.e. 30 or less off pump vs several hundred with CPB). In both orthopedic surgery (range 0–40 HITS) and carotid endarterectomy (range 0–700 HITS), many patients had HITS; the numbers were lower than with cardiac surgery with CPB (0–5260 HITS). The authors concluded that no consistent association between HITS and neurocognitive outcome could be determined, and that the studies were limited by differences in monitoring techniques, and in timing and type of neurocognitive tests.

In a careful study of HITS in pediatric cardiac surgery of 25 patients, O'Brien and associates[11] noted that all patients had HITS (range 2–2664), 42 percent of all emboli occurred within three minutes of the release of the aortic crossclamp, and there was no difference in the number of HITS for patients with and without obligate intracardiac shunting. The number of HITS was not associated with gross neurologic deficits postoperatively (Figure 19.12).

In retrospective reviews of adult and pediatric cardiac surgery cases with CPB, Edmonds and co-workers[26,52] determined that a multimodality neurologic monitoring strategy for including NIRS, processed EEG, and TCD reduced acute postoperative neurological changes (25% to 6% in children, 6% to 3% in adults). However, TCD abnormalities were involved in only 5 percent to 10 percent of these patients, and often the other modalities, such as NIRS, were abnormal during abnormal TCD conditions as well. Taken together, there is insufficient evidence from the few randomized, prospective, controlled studies (or other study designs) performed that TCD monitoring will improve acute or longer-term neurologic outcomes.

In addition to limited evidence of utility for routine use in intraoperative monitoring, TCD is difficult to perform for long periods by the anesthesiologist, because of the frequent adjustments to the probe that are often necessary to maintain an optimal signal. There is a significant learning curve for placement of the probe and fixation devices. These practical considerations make this technique difficult to implement in multiple operating rooms simultaneously. A monitoring technician can be used; however, this staffing may not be reimbursible by third-party payors, making TCD monitoring by a separate person besides the anesthesiologist financially unsustainable in many settings.

Complications of transcranial Doppler ultrasound

Prolonged high-intensity ultrasound has potential risks to patients primarily from overheating of tissues in the path of the ultrasound energy.[53] The highest energy absorption coefficients occur in bone. Because all the energy studies have been performed in vitro, the potential intracranial cooling effect associated with tissue perfusion is unknown. The maximum output of 100 mW/cm^2 recommended by the American Institute of Ultrasound in Medicine has been adopted by all manufacturers of TCD devices cleared for use by the US Food and Drug Administration, which should be well below any threshold for significant heating. The effects of continuous long-term exposure, such as that which may occur in the surgical/critical care environments, are not fully understood. Therefore, the acoustic power and pulse amplitude should be kept to a minimum commensurate with the production of waveforms that can be accurately measured. This is particularly important with transorbital insonation, which is not recommended for intraoperative or continuous critical care monitoring. Pressure sores or pressure injury to scalp, forehead, or orbits are possible if probes and fixation devices are applied too tightly, without adequate padding, or improperly, without checking for impingement on vital structures.

Sources of TCD artifact that give erroneous signals and could result in inappropriate interventions include radiofrequency interference from electrosurgical units from the immediate or neighboring operating rooms; inadequate probe fixation, resulting in ambiguous, obscured, or evanescent CBFV spectra; or mechanical contact of the probe by surgical instruments. No monitoring at all is preferable to potentially misleading information.

Education, credentialing, and certification in transcranial Doppler ultrasound

There is currently no credentialing by any professional anesthesiology or critical care organization. The American Society of Neurophysiologic Monitoring (ASNM, www.ASNM.org)

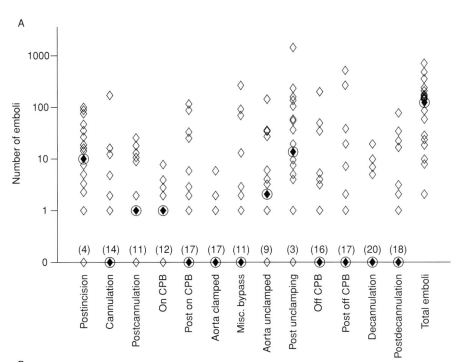

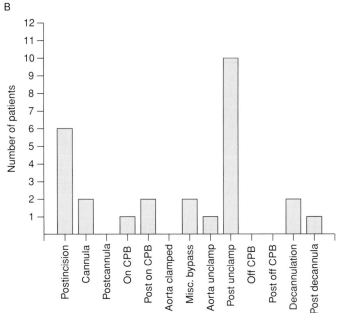

Figure 19.12 (a) Number of emboli detected during 13 phases of cardiac surgery with bypass in 25 pediatric patients. Each symbol denotes one patient. Numbers in parentheses are numbers of patients experiencing no emboli at each phase. The circled solid diamond symbol indicates median number of emboli at each time period. (b) The time interval associated with the greatest number of emboli in each of 25 patients. The greatest number of emboli were apparent either after skin incision or >3 min after the aortic clamp was released. Reproduced with permission from ref. 11.

recommends certification by the American Board of Neurophysiologic Monitoring (ABNM), or its equivalent, as a measure of professional level qualification in multimodality neuromonitoring. Criteria for ABNM certification include[1] an advanced degree – master's, Ph.D., M.D., or D.O.;[2] documented clinical experience, with the requirement of at least 300 monitored cases over a minimum of three years;[3] surgeon attestations regarding monitoring experience;[4] the passing of two examinations, one written and the other oral. These examinations focus on electrophysiological techniques, and neither covers TCD monitoring in any detail nor certifies competence in the production or interpretation of ultrasonic waveforms.

Training for physician proficiency in interpretation of cerebrovascular ultrasound studies, with particular emphasis on applied principles of ultrasound physics, fluid dynamics, and various aspects of TCD examination, is offered by the American Society of Neuroimaging (ASN; www.asnweb.org). Nevertheless, certification of technical sonographic expertise in TCD evaluation of intracranial vessels is currently not available in the United States. At the beginning of 2006, the ASN board of directors approved creation of the first national examination to assess a technologist's ability to apply knowledge, concepts, and principles of neurovascular ultrasound that constitute the basis of safe and effective patient care. It is designed to measure the candidate's application of medical knowledge and understanding of biomedical and clinical sciences that are considered to be essential for the unsupervised performance of neurovascular ultrasound.

Practice parameters for transcranial Doppler ultrasound

Currently there are no practice parameters establishing recommendations to use TCD for intraoperative monitoring, nor can it be considered the standard of care for any type of surgical procedure. The ASNM and ASN state, "On the basis of current clinical literature and scientific evidence, TCD monitoring is an established monitoring modality for the: 1) assessment of cerebral vasomotor reactivity and autoregulation; 2) documentation of the circle of Willis functional status; 3) identification of relative cerebral hypo- and hyperperfusion; 4) detection of cerebral emboli (Class II and III evidence, Type B recommendation)."[55]

Conclusions

TCD has been an important research tool for cardiac and vascular surgery and may have utility for specialized CPB techniques, such as antegrade or retrograde cerebral perfusion, in both adult and pediatric patients. In addition, TCD will detect intraoperative cerebral emboli. However, lack of outcome benefit, and the technical difficulties with obtaining and maintaining a valid TCD signal in the intraoperative setting limit its utility for routine use by the anesthesiologist.

References

1. Bailes JE, Lokesh ST, Fukushima T, et al. Intraoperative microvascular Doppler sonography in aneurysm surgery. *Neurosurgery* 1997;**40**:965–72.
2. Edmonds HL, Isley MR, Sloan T, et al. American Society of Neurophysiologic Monitoring (ASNM) and American Society of Neuroimaging (ASN) Joint Guidelines for Transcranial Doppler (TCD) Ultrasonic Monitoring. www.ASNM.org, January 25, 2009.
3. Muller M, Schimrigk K. Vasomotor reactivity and pattern of collateral blood flow in severe occlusive carotid artery disease. *Stroke* 1996;**27**;296–99.
4. Greeley WJ, Ungerleider RM, Kern FH, et al. Effects of cardiopulmonary bypass on cerebral blood flow in neonates, infants, and children. *Circulation* 1989;**80**:I209–15.
5. Eames PJ, Blake MJ, Dawson SL, et al. Dynamic cerebral autoregulation and beat to beat blood pressure control are impaired in acute ischaemic stroke. *J Neurol Neurosurg Psychiatry* 2002;**72**:467–72.
6. Fischer AQ, Truemper EJ. Applications in the neonate and child. In Babikian VL, Wechsler LR (eds.). *Transcranial Doppler Ultrasonography*, 2nd ed. Oxford: Butterworth-Heineman, 1993, pp. 355–75.
7. Truemper EJ, Fischer AQ. Cerebrovascular developmental anatomy and physiology in the infant and child. In Babikian VL, Wechsler LR (eds.). *Transcranial Doppler Ultrasonography*, 2nd ed. Oxford: Butterworth-Heineman, 1993, pp. 281–320.
8. Grolimund, P. Transmission of ultrasound through the temporal bone. In Aaslid R (ed.), *Transcranial Doppler Sonography*. New York: Springer-Verlag, 1986, pp. 10–21.
9. Saver JL, Feldman F. Basic transcranial Doppler examination: technique and anatomy. In Babikian VL, Wechsler LR (eds.). *Transcranial Doppler Ultrasonography*. St. Louis: Mosby, 1993, pp. 11–28.
10. Bass A, Krupski WC, Schneider PA, et al. Intraoperative transcranial Doppler: limitations of the method. *Vasc Surg* 1989;**10**;549–53.
11. O'Brien JJ, Butterworth J, Hammon JW, et al. Cerebral emboli during cardiac surgery in children. *Anesthesiology* 1997;**87**:1063–9.
12. Hassler W. Steinmetz H, Gawlowski J. Transcranial Doppler ultrasonography in raised intracranial pressure and in intracranial circulatory arrest. *J Neurosurg* 1988;**68**:745–50.
13. Guerra WK, Gaab MR, Dietz H, et al. Surgical decompression for traumatic brain swelling: indications and results. *J Neurosurg* 1999;**90**:187–96.
14. Fujioika K, Douville CM. Anatomy and free-hand examination techniques. In Newell DW, Aaslid R (eds.). *Transcranial Doppler*. New York: Raven Press, 1992, pp. 9–31.
15. Adams RJ, Nichols FT, Hess DC. Normal values and physiological variables. In Newell DW, Aaslid R (eds.). *Transcranial Doppler*. New York: Raven Press, 1992, pp. 41–48.
16. Edmonds HL, Pollock SB, Thomas MH. Transcranial Doppler guides emboli reduction during myocardial revascularization. *Stroke* 1998;**29**:2237.
17. Spencer MP, Thomas GI, Moehring MA. Relation between middle cerebral artery blood flow-velocity and sump pressure during carotid endarterectomy. *Stroke* 1992;**23**:1439–45.
18. Kalra M, al-Khaffaf H, Farell A, et al. Comparison of measurement of stump pressure and transcranial measurement of flow-velocity in the middle cerebral artery in carotid surgery. *Ann Vasc Surg* 1994;**8**:225–31.
19. Halsey J. Risks and benefits of shunting in carotid endarterectomy. The International Transcranial Doppler Collaborators. *Stroke* 1992;**23**:1583–7.
20. Halsey J. Monitoring blood flow velocity in the middle cerebral artery during carotid endarterectomy. In Babikian VL, Wechsler LR (eds.). *Transcranial Doppler Ultrasonography*. St. Louis: Mosby, 1993, pp. 216–21.
21. Jorgensen LG. Transcranial Doppler ultrasound for cerebral perfusion. *Acta Physiologica Scand* 1995;**625** [supplement]: 1–44.
22. Spencer MP. Transcranial Doppler monitoring and causes of stroke from carotid endarterectomy. *Stroke* 1997;28;685–91.
23. Babikian VL, Cantelmo NL, Wijman CA. Neurovascular monitoring during carotid endarterectomy. In Babikian VL, Wechsler LR (eds.), *Transcranial Doppler Ultrasonography,* 2nd ed. Boston: Butterworth-Heinemann, 1999, pp. 231–45.
24. Giller CA Mathews D, Walker B, et al. Prediction of tolerance to carotid artery occlusion using transcranial Doppler ultrasound. *J Neurosurg* 1994;**81**:15–19.
25. Schneweis S, Urbach H, Solymosi L, et al. Preoperative risk assessment for carotid occlusion by transcranial Doppler ultrasound. *J Neurol Neurosurg Psychiatry* 1997;**62**:485–9.
26. Edmonds HL. Protective effect of neuromonitoring during cardiac surgery. *Ann NY Acad Sci* 2005;**1053**:12–19.
27. Edmonds HL, Rodriguez RA, Audenaert SM, et al. The role of neuromonitoring in cardiovascular surgery. *J Cardiothorac Vasc Anesth* 1996;**10**:15–23.

28. Ganzel BL, Edmonds HL, Pank JR, et al. Neurophysiological monitoring to assure delivery of retrograde cerebral perfusion. *J Thorac Cardiovasc Surg* 1997;**113**:748–57.

29. Estrera AL, Garami Z, Millar CC, et al. Determination of cerebral blood flow dynamics during retrograde cerebral perfusion using power M-mode transcranial Doppler. *Ann Thorac Surg* 2003;**76**:704–9.

30. Andropoulos DB, Stayer SA, Diaz LK, et al. Neurological monitoring for congenital heart surgery. *Anesth Analg* 2004;**99**:1365–75.

31. Hillier SC, Burrows FA, Bissonnette B, Taylor RH. Cerebral hemodynamics in neonates and infants undergoing cardiopulmonary bypass and profound hypothermic circulatory arrest: assessment by transcranial Doppler sonography. *Anesth Analg* 1991;**72**:723–8.

32. Huber P, Handa J. Effect of contrast material, hypercapnia, hyperventilation, hypertonic glucose and papaverine on the diameter of the cerebral arteries: Angiographic determination in man. *Invest Radiol* 1967;**2**:17–32.

33. Zimmerman AA, Burrows FA, Jonas RA, Hickey PR. The limits of detectable cerebral perfusion by transcranial Doppler sonography in neonates undergoing deep hypothermic low-flow cardiopulmonary bypass. *J Thorac Cardiovasc Surg* 1997;**114**:594–600.

34. Andropoulos DB, Stayer SA, McKenzie ED, Fraser CD Jr. Novel cerebral physiologic monitoring to guide low-flow cerebral perfusion during neonatal aortic arch reconstruction. *J Thorac Cardiovasc Surg* 2003;**125**:491–9.

35. Mullges W, Berg D, Babin-Ebell J et al. Cerebral microembolus generation in different extracorporeal circulation systems. *Cerebrovasc Dis* 1999;**9**:265–9.

36. Yeh TJ, Austin EH III, Sehic A, Edmonds HL Jr. Role of neuromonitoring in the detection and correction of cerebral air embolism. *J Thorac Cardiovasc Surg* 2003;**126**:589–91.

37. Spencer MP. Detection of embolism with Doppler ultrasound: a review. *Echocardiography* 1996;**13**:519–27.

38. Hennerici MG. High intensity transcranial signals (HITS): a questionable "jackpot" for the prediction of stroke risk. *J Heart Valve Dis* 1994;**3**:124–5.

39. Consensus Committee, 9th International Cerebral Hemodynamics Symposium. Basic identification criteria for Doppler microembolic signals. *Stroke* 1995;**26**:1123.

40. Gavrilescu T, Babikian VL, Cantelmo NL, et al. Cerebral microembolism during carotid endarterectomy. *Am J Surg* 1995;**170**:159–64.

41. Brucher R, Russell D. Automatic online embolus detection and artifact rejection with the first multi-frequency transcranial Doppler. *Stroke* 2002;**33**:1969–74.

42. Jansen C, Vriens EM, Eikelboom BC, et al. Carotid endarterectomy with transcranial Doppler and electroencephalographic monitoring: a prospective study in 130 operations. *Stroke* 1993;**24**:665–9.

43. Payne DA, Jones CI, Hayes PD, et al. Beneficial effects of clopidogrel combined with aspirin in reducing cerebral emboli in patients undergoing carotid endarterectomy. *Circulation* 2004;**109**:1476–81.

44. Stump DA, Kon NA, Rogers AT, et al. Emboli and neuropsychological outcome following cardiopulmonary bypass. *Echocardiography* 1996;**13**:555–8.

45. Georgiadis D, Kaps M, Berg J, et al. Transcranial Doppler detection of microemboli in prosthetic heart valve patients: dependency upon valve type. *Eur J Cardiothorac Surg* 1996;**10**:253–7.

46. Clark RE, Brillman J, Davis DA, et al. Microemboli during coronary artery bypass grafting: genesis and effect on outcome. *J Thorac Cardiovasc Surg* 1995;**109**:249–58.

47. Lund C, Hol PK, Lundblad R, et al. Comparison of cerebral embolization during off-pump and on-pump coronary artery bypass surgery. *Ann Thorac Surg* 2003;**76**:765–70.

48. Ferrari J, Baumgartner H, Tentschert S, et al. Cerebral microembolism during transcatheter closure of patent foramen ovale. *J. Neurol* 2004;**251**:825–9.

49. Kaposzta Z, Martin JF, Markus HS. Switching off embolization from symptomatic carotid plaque using S-nitrosoglutathione. *Circulation* 2002;**105**:1480–4.

50. Dittrich R, Ringelstein B. Occurrence and clinical impact of microembolic signals during or after cardiosurgical procedures. *Stroke* 2008;**39**:503–11.

51. Martin KK, Wigginton JB, Babikian VL, et al. Intraoperative cerebral high-intensity transient signals and postoperative cognitive function: a systematic review. *Am J Surg* 2009;**197**:55–63.

52. Austin EH III, Edmonds HL Jr, Auden SM. Benefit of neurophysiologic monitoring for pediatric cardiac surgery. *J Thorac Cardiovasc Surg* 1997;**114**:707–17.

53. Nyborg WL. Optimization of exposure conditions for medical ultrasound. *Ultrasound Med Biol* 1985;**11**:245–60.

54. Lao A, Sharma VK, Katz ML, Alexandrov AV. Diagnostic criteria for transcranial doppler ultrasound. In McGahan JP, Goldberg BB (eds.). *Diagnostic Ultrasound*, 2nd ed. New York: Informa Healthcare, 2008, pp. 543–5.

55. Edmonds HL Jr, Isley MR, Sloan TB, Alexandrov AV, Razumovsky AY. American Society of Neurophysiologic Monitoring and American Society of Neuroimaging Joint Guidelines for Transcranial Doppler Ultrasonic Monitoring. *J Neuroimaging*. 2010 Mar 17. [Epub ahead of print].

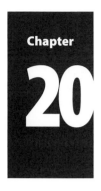

Multimodality monitoring in critically ill neurologic patients

Jennifer A. Frontera

Introduction

Multimodality monitoring is the integration of biochemical, metabolic, clinical, and radiographic variables into an evaluation of physiology that allows for real-time diagnosis and goal-directed therapy of critically ill neurologic patients. The neurologic exam is one of the most important elements in guiding treatment of patients with brain or spinal cord injury, but comatose or sedated patients pose special challenges in management because detecting changes in brain function is limited in these populations. Multimodality monitoring allows evaluation of brain tissue function and viability. Traditional methods of physiologic monitoring entail measurement of blood pressure, heart rate, cardiac filling pressures, and temperature, whereas multimodality monitoring also monitors parameters such as intracranial pressure, brain oxygen tension, brain metabolism and interstitial metabolites, cerebral blood flow, and electrophysiology. Electrophysiologic monitoring includes electroencephalography (EEG) and evoked potential monitoring. Continuous, quantitative, real-time assessments of brain function allow for proactive and individualized goal-directed management.

Monitoring technologies

Intracranial pressure and compliance monitoring

In adults, the cranium is a rigid vault that contains the brain parenchyma (80% by volume), cerebrospinal fluid (CSF; 10% by volume), and blood (10% by volume). CSF is produced at a rate of 20 mL/hr (500 mL/day), and approximately 150 mL of CSF bathe the entire neuroaxis. Factors that contribute to elevated intracranial pressure include masses (tumor, hematoma, air, abscess), hydrocephalus (either obstructive or the result of overproduction, such as from a choroid plexus papilloma), parenchymal edema (vasogenic, hydrostatic/transmural, cytotoxic, or hypoosmotic), and abnormal blood flow (caused by either increased cerebral blood flow secondary to autoregulatory failure or abnormal egress of venous outflow because of sinus obstruction).

To understand how cerebral blood flow (CBF) is related to intracranial pressure (ICP), it is important to understand the concept of cerebral autoregulation. The brain is able to maintain CBF over a wide range of systemic blood pressures by regulating the caliber of small arterioles (Figure 20.1). At high mean arterial pressures (MAPs), arterioles vasoconstrict; conversely, at low MAPs, they vasodilate. When MAP becomes higher than the capacity for the brain to compensate, arterioles passively vasodilate and cerebral blood volume (CBV) increases, leading to an increase in ICP (autoregulation breakthrough zone). When MAP becomes pathologically low, the arterioles are maximally vasodilated, CBV is increased, and consequently ICP increases (vasodilatory cascade zone). This is the reason that cerebral perfusion pressure (CPP) is typically maintained at ≥ 60 mmHg when managing elevated ICP. Lundberg A plateau ICP waves (described later) develop in the vasodilatory cascade zone and can be aborted by increasing MAP.

Under normal conditions, compensation for increased intracranial volume occurs, including egress of CSF, and venous blood results in a relatively constant ICP as the intracranial volume expands. At a critical intracranial volume, these compensation mechanisms become exhausted and ICP increases exponentially. This concept is known as the *Monroe–Kelly doctrine* (Figure 20.2). The intracranial compliance (Δ volume/Δ pressure), which is initially high, can decrease suddenly and cause an elevated ICP with small volume changes. The concept of compliance is crucial, because certain populations have greater compliance than others. Monitoring absolute ICP values can be problematic in patients who are on the edge of their compliance curve. These patients may have "normal" ICP values but may be at risk for dramatic ICP spikes with straining (Valsalva maneuvers), sneezing, or small increases in intracranial volume. In fact, herniation with "normal" ICP values is well described.[1,2] In one study, only 25 percent of patients with large strokes who herniated had an elevated ICP at the time of decompensation.[3] Compliance can be estimated in patients who have an external ventricular drain by draining a specific volume of CSF and looking at the change in ICP (using the formula for compliance = Δ volume/Δ pressure).

The cranial vault consists of different compartments, each of which can have a different pressure. When pressure gradients exist between compartments, shift and herniation can occur, even if the absolute pressures in any given compartment are within the normal range (up to 20 mmHg or 25 cmH$_2$O). When the basal cisterns are compressed, ICP gradients can increase

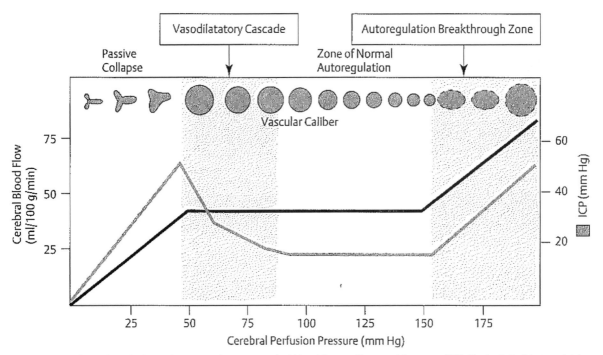

Figure 20.1. Effects of cerebral vascular autoregulation on cerebral blood flow and intracranial pressure (ICP). The brain is able to maintain cerebral blood flow over a wide range of systemic blood pressures by regulating the caliber of small arterioles. Reproduced from Seder, D, Mayer, SA and Frontera, JA, Management of elevated intracranial pressure. In *Decision Making in Neurocritical Care*, 2009; with permission from Thieme Publishers.

dramatically; when there is more than 3 mm of shift, ICP gradients are present.

Although there is no level 1 evidence demonstrating the benefit of ICP monitoring, it has been shown in a small traumatic brain injury (TBI) series to reduce mortality.[4] A large, randomized study demonstrating improved outcomes with ICP monitoring in TBI patients would require 700 patients at an estimated cost of $5 million to detect a 10 percent mortality difference.[5] The only way to diagnose elevated ICP reliably is to measure it directly.

Indications for ICP monitoring include patients with intracranial pathology who have a poor neurologic exam with

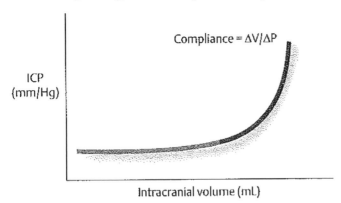

Figure 20.2. Normal compensation for increased intracranial volume maintains relatively constant intracranial pressure (ICP) as the intracranial volume expands. At a critical intracranial volume, compensation mechanisms are exhausted and ICP increases exponentially. This concept is known as the *Monroe–Kelly doctrine*. Reproduced with kind permission from Springer Science+Business Media from Rose, JC, Optimizing blood pressure in neurological emergencies, *Neurocritcal Care* 1:3;2004.

suspected elevated ICP, patients with symptomatic hydrocephalus who will benefit from CSF diversion via an external ventricular drain, patients with head trauma who have a Glasgow Coma Scale (GCS) $\leq$ 8 and an abnormal head CT, or a GCS $\leq$ 8 with a normal head CT and two of the following: systolic blood pressure <90 mmHg, posturing, or age >40 years.[6]

Although ICP can be measured by simply performing manometry during lumbar puncture, this procedure may not be safe in patients with ventricular obstruction or shift and does not provide a continuous measure of ICP.

The gold standard for intracranial pressure monitoring is the external ventricular drain (EVD). This device can be placed at the bedside and is typically inserted by a neurosurgeon or neurointensivist at Kocher's point anteriorly, which lies at the perpendicular intersection of the midpupillary line posteriorly and the superiorly directed line between the midpoint of the external auditory meatus and lateral canthus. In an average patient, the site of insertion lies 10 cm from the nasion posteriorly (or 1 cm anterior to the coronal suture) and 3 cm lateral to the midline. The catheter is typically inserted 6 to 8 cm in depth from the outer table of the skull, targeting the third ventricle. The benefits of Kocher's point include avoidance of the sagittal sinus, lateral bridging veins, and eloquent areas of the brain, such as the motor strip.[7]

An EVD allows for both global measurement of ICP and treatment of elevated ICP via CSF drainage. There is a 5 percent to 20 percent infection rate with EVDs and a 2 percent hemorrhage rate with placement in noncoagulopathic patients. When the drain is open an ICP value can be transduced,

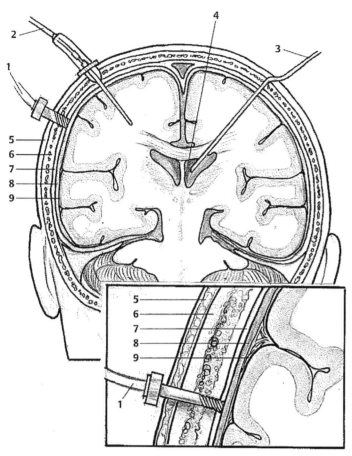

Figure 20.3. Different types of intracranial pressure monitors. Intracranial pressure may be monitored in the ventricles, parenchyma, or the subdural space. Reproduced from *Decision Making in Neurocritical Care*, JA Frontera, ed., chapter 15, page 204; with permission from Thieme Publishers.

1. Subdural bolt
2. Intraparenchymal monitor
3. External ventricular drain
4. Lateral ventricle
5. Skin
6. Skull
7. Dura
8. Subdural space
   (this is a potential space)
9. Arachnoid layer

but this is not an accurate measurement of ICP; to correctly measure ICP, the drain should be closed and a triphasic waveform should be present on the monitor. Specialized EVDs that allow for drainage with concurrent continuous ICP monitoring are available. Such EVDs contain a fiberoptic transducer at the tip and combine technology available in parenchymal ICP monitors with drainage capacity (Integra Neurosciences; Plainsboro, NJ), but they are more expensive than a standard EVD and their caliber is larger, which may increase placement-related bleeding risk.

Inaccuracies in ICP measurement can occur when the EVD has not been properly zeroed, when the foramen of the ventricular catheter or the tubing becomes clogged (with blood, air, CSF protein, choroid plexus, etc.), or when there is kinking in the tubing (which can occur with tunneling after insertion). Flushing of ventriculostomy tubing to restore patency of the EVD should always be performed in a sterile fashion with a minimum volume of normal saline. Similarly, tapping of shunt tubing should be minimized and performed only using sterile technique. Always check that the ICP transducer is at the level of the foramen of Monroe. Transducers that are lower than this level will give falsely elevated ICP values.

Intraparenchymal monitors (Camino, Integra Neurosciences; Plainsboro, NJ; Figure 20.3) are placed via a bolt or tunneled through a craniotomy defect into the white matter of the parenchyma. These monitors have the advantage of a low bleeding and infection risk but do undergo some drift in values, and ICP readings may fluctuate by 3 mmHg. Multiple intraparenchymal monitors may be placed to measure ICP gradients, and/or a monitor may be placed specifically in a penumbral area, giving a regional ICP value. Multilumen bolts allow for placement of several multimodality monitors through the same burrhole (i.e. brain oxygen monitoring, brain temperature, parenchymal ICP monitoring, and microdialysis catheters can be placed through one multilumen bolt). Given the low bleeding risk, parenchymal monitors are favored in patients with coagulopathies who require ICP monitoring, such as patients with fulminant liver failure. Similarly, in patients with small ventricles for whom EVD placement may be difficult, as in patients with severe cerebral edema, parenchymal ICP monitoring may be favored.

Epidural and subarachnoid/subdural monitors are used infrequently because of unreliable ICP measurements. Pros and cons of these devices are delineated in Table 20.1.

Table 20.1. Characteristics of intracranial pressure monitoring systems

Type of Monitor	Pro	Con
Intraventricular	Gold standard, more global ICP measurement, allows for diagnosis and treatment	Highest infection rate (5–20%), risk of hemorrhage (2%)
Intraparenchymal	Infection and hemorrhage rate low (1%), easy to place	Measure regional ICP, cannot recalibrate after placement, drift (readings may vary by 3 mmHg)
Subarachnoid/ subdural	Infection and hemorrhage rate low	Unreliable measurements, not often used
Epidural	Low risk of hemorrhage compared with intraventricular and intraparenchymal monitors, occasional use with coagulopathic liver patients	Unreliable measurements

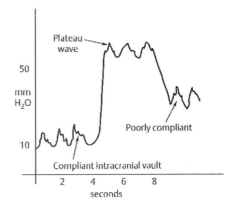

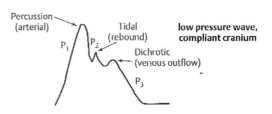

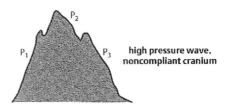

Figure 20.4. The intracranial pressure waveform is composed of a P1 arterial percussion wave, a P2 tidal rebound wave, and a P3 dichrotic venous outflow wave. Normal intracranial compliance and poor compliance result in different waveform patterns. Reproduced from Seder, D, Mayer, SA and Frontera, JA, Management of elevated intracranial pressure. In *Decision Making in Neurocritical Care*, 2009; with permission from Thieme Medical Publishers.

Typically, antibiotics (such as a second-generation cephalosporin) are administered prior to insertion or removal of an ICP monitoring device, when there is maximal risk of brain or CSF contamination. Whether to administer antibiotics for the duration of the time the monitor is in place is a matter of controversy. Although in the past, routine ventriculostomy exchanges were performed after five days, this is no longer recommended.

For all monitors, transducers should be placed at the level of the foramen of Monroe (tragus of the ear). Similarly, to accurately calculate CPP (CPP = MAP − ICP), arterial pressure transducers should also be placed at the level of the foramen of Monroe (Figure 20.3).

The ICP waveform is comprised of a P1 arterial percussion wave, a P2 tidal rebound wave, and a P3 dichrotic venous outflow wave (Figure 20.4). Patients with poor intracranial compliance have a prominent P2 wave and a large systolic-to-diastolic gradient (pulse pressure). Lundberg A waves are plateau waves of elevated intracranial pressures of up to 50 to 100 mmHg, lasting 5 to 20 minutes. These plateau waves are thought to be related to a vasodilatory cascade that occurs when cerebral perfusion pressure is abnormally low. Treatment entails improving cerebral perfusion pressure by improving mean arterial pressure. Lundberg B waves represent ICP spikes of shorter duration (usually minutes) that are related to variations in the respiratory cycle. Lundberg C waves are of uncertain significance and represent elevated ICP waves related to the cardiac cycle.

Noninvasive estimates of ICP include transcranial Doppler pulsatility index, intraocular pressure/tonometry, and tympanic membrane displacement, all of which are poor substitutes for direct measurement of ICP and have not been directly validated. Radiographic imaging such as CT and MRI can give clues to elevated ICP (shift, edema, hydrocephalus, etc.) but can be normal even when the ICP is elevated. For example, in a prospective study of 753 TBI patients, 10 percent to 15 percent of patients with a normal head CT developed elevated ICP.[18]

Transcranial Doppler ultrasound

Transcranial Doppler ultrasound (TCD) is a bedside, noninvasive ultrasound technique that entails Doppler of medium-sized intracranial and extracranial blood vessels. Standard TCD provides only Doppler information; newer modalities, such as transcranial color Doppler (TCCD), provide ultrasound and Doppler information, but are technically harder to perform. TCD can give an estimate of CBF assuming that the insonated vessel caliber does not change during the time of insonation. According to Ohm's law:

CBF = CPP/CVR where CBF is cerebral blood flow, CPP is cerebral perfusion pressure, and CVR is cerebrovascular resistance.

CVR = (length × resistivity) / cross-sectional area.

TCD is most commonly used in subarachnoid hemorrhage (SAH) patients to monitor for vasospasm (Type A, level I–II

Table 20.2. Sensitivity and specificity of transcranial Doppler for detecting angiographic or symptomatic cerebral vasospasm

| Vessel | Angiographic vasospasm[19] | | Symptomatic vasospasm[20] | |
	Sensitivity	Specificity	Sensitivity	Specificity
ICA	25–30	83–91	80	77
MCA	39–94	70–100	64	78
ACA	13–71	65–100	45	84
Vertebral artery	44–100	82–88	–	–
Basilar artery	77–100	42–79	–	–
PCA	48–60	78–87	–	–

ICA = internal carotid artery; MCA = middle cerebral artery; ACA = anterior cerebral artery; PCA = posterior cerebral artery.

evidence per the American Academy of Neurology). The sensitivity and specificity of TCD for detecting angiographic or symptomatic spasm are delineated in Table 20.2.

The varying sensitivities and specificities depend on the mean flow velocity (MFV) cutpoint used to predict either symptomatic or angiographic vasospasm. In a study of 101 SAH patients, the positive predictive value for angiographic vasospasm for a MFV >200 cm/sec was 87 percent, whereas the negative predictive value for a MFV <120 cm/s was 94 percent.[21] Likelihood ratios for intermittent values were less useful. Unfortunately, in this study 57 percent of the subjects had MFV between 120 and 200 cm/sec, making TCD an unreliable predictor of angiographic spasm. Similarly, when predicting symptomatic vasospasm using a MFV cutpoint of 120 cm/sec, TCD had an overall 39 percent positive predictive value and 90 percent negative predictive value.[20]

Lindegaard ratios[22] are designed to correct TCD values for hyperemia that may be caused by increased cardiac output (resulting from sepsis, pressors, anemia, etc.) and are calculated as MCA MFV/ ICA MFV. Lindegaard ratios have been shown to improve the positive predictive value of TCD for symptomatic vasospasm.[23] Currently, most physicians will follow daily TCD values in subarachnoid hemorrhage patients as part of a multimodality regimen including the clinical exam and imaging studies to monitor patients for clinically relevant vasospasm. We do not use TCD as a surrogate for diagnosing vasospasm.

TCD can also be used to estimate autoregulation. Induced blood pressure changes and dynamic cerebral autoregulation correlating systemic arterial blood pressure and intracranial mean flow velocities can estimate autoregulation. If MFV varies directly with systemic blood pressure, there is a loss of autoregulation. Chemical autoregulation can be estimated using a CO_2 or acetazolamide challenge. If autoregulation is intact, there should be a 2 percent change in MFV per change in CO_2 in response to CO_2 inhalation. Abnormalities in dynamic cerebral autoregulation and CO_2 reactivity have been demonstrated in patients with SAH and vasospasm.[24-26]

TCD can be used as a confirmatory test for brain death. As ICP elevates, the pulse pressure in the brain increases, as reflected by an increase in pulsatility index. When the ICP becomes critically high, intracranial circulatory arrest occurs.

This is demonstrated on TCD by isolated or reverberating systolic flow with no diastolic outflow. To confirm brain death, isolated systolic flow must be demonstrated in the anterior circulation bilaterally and in the posterior circulation. TCD cannot be performed in roughly 10 percent of the population because of differences in skull thickness. The sensitivity of TCD for brain death confirmation is 91 percent to 100 percent, with 97 percent to 100 percent specificity.[19]

Continuous EEG

Continuous electroencephalography (cEEG) is one of the only ways to continuously monitor neuronal function. In the ICU setting, EEG is critical for detecting subtle or nonconvulsive seizures. Up to 35 percent of neurocritical care patients suffer nonconvulsive seizures, and 75 percent of these patients are in nonconvulsive status epilepticus.[27,28] In a medical ICU setting, 8 percent of patients without a primary neurological diagnosis were found to have nonconvulsive seizures when monitored with cEEG.[29] Nonconvulsive seizures and status epilepticus are associated with morbidity and mortality.[29,30] Early detection of seizures is crucial because delayed treatment increases mortality substantially. Mortality is 36 percent if treatment is begun after 30 minutes of nonconvulsive status epilepticus, as compared with 75 percent if treatment is delayed by more than 24 hours.[31]

Patients with unexplained coma, fluctuating mental status, uncharacterized spells such as posturing, twitching, gaze deviation, or agitation, or heart rate and blood pressure lability are candidates for cEEG monitoring. EEG is also used to titrate seizure therapy to burst suppression (typically one burst every 4–6 seconds) and can be used to confirm brain death (criteria include >2 microvolt sensitivity, 1–30 Hz, a minimum of 8 electrodes 10 cm apart, an impedance between 100 and 10,000 Ω, and 30 minutes of flatline recording). EEG can also be useful for prognostication. Alpha coma and burst suppression after cardiac arrest augur a poor prognosis, whereas sleep architecture, a normal anterior-to-posterior gradient, and reactivity to stimulation indicate a favorable prognosis.

EEG data can be compressed for evaluation of long epochs of monitoring using compressed spectral array (CSA), density spectral array, and bandwidth power trends. CSA provides easy

Table 20.3. Established criteria for normality in brain tissue oxygen tension and brain temperature monitoring

	Normal	Abnormal
Brain tissue oxygen tension (PbO2)	20 mmHg in white matter 35–40 mmHg in gray matter	<15 mmHg indicates hypoxia <10 mmHg indicates ischemia
Brain temperature	Correlates with body temperature, can be 1°C higher than core temperature	<36.8°C or >37.2°C considered abnormal

recognition of state changes, trends, and left/right asymmetries but can be misleading in the ICU because artifacts are often of high amplitude. CSA does not detect individual epileptiform discharges and should always be used in conjunction with the raw EEG waveforms.

Brain oxygen monitoring

Brain tissue oxygen partial pressure (PbO_2) monitoring can be performed by placing a probe either through a bolt or tunneled through a craniotomy defect. The Licox probe (Integra Neurosciences; Plainsboro, NJ), which is the only commercially available probe in the United States, uses a polarographic Clark microelectrode. The Licox is typically placed through a double or triple lumen bolt along with other components of multimodality monitoring, such as a parenchymal ICP monitor, brain tissue temperature monitor, and a microdialysis probe (discussed later). The bolt is usually placed in a penumbral zone of tissue at risk, targeting the white matter. Initial values can be misleading; thus, probes are typically allowed to stabilize for at least one to two hours before PbO_2 values are considered valid. Unfortunately, the Licox is not MRI-compatible. The PbO_2 value is an averaged partial pressure measurement of capillary and interstitial brain oxygen content over an area of 17 mm^2. Normal values for PbO_2 are listed in Table 20.3.

In order to understand what PbO_2 values represent, it is important to review the metabolism of oxygen. To summarize

Oxygen delivery to the brain can be represented by

$$DO_2 = CBF \times CaO_2,$$

where DO_2 is oxygen delivery and CaO_2 is the arterial oxygen content.

Oxygen consumption by the brain can be represented by

$$VO_2 = CBF \times (CaO_2 - CvO_2),$$

where VO_2 is oxygen consumption and CvO_2 is the venous content.

$$CaO_2 = (1.34 \times \text{hemoglobin concentration} \times SaO_2)$$
$$+ (0.003 \times PaO_2),$$

where SaO_2 is the arterial oxyhemoglobin saturation and PaO_2 is the arterial oxygen tension.

Oxygen extracted by the brain can be represented by

$$OEF = (CaO_2 - CvO_2)/CaO2,$$

where OEF is oxygen extraction fraction.

Oxygen metabolized by the brain (cerebral metabolic rate of oxygen, $CRMO_2$) can be represented by

$$CMRO_2 = VO_2 + CIO_2,$$

where CIO_2 is the amount of oxygen accumulated in brain tissue. Under normal conditions CIO_2 is negligible such that

$$CMRO_2 \approx VO_2 \text{ or}$$
$$CMRO_2 = CBF \times (CaO_2 - CvO_2).$$

Because $OEF = (CaO_2 - CvO_2)/CaO_2$, substituting in $CMRO_2$ can be expressed as

$$CMRO_2 = CBF \times OEF \times CaO_2,$$

where OEF is oxygen extraction fraction.

Several studies have linked changes in PbO_2 to changes in CBF and PaO_2.[35-37] Animal studies have shown a relationship between PbO_2 and MAP that resembles an autoregulatory curve (Figure 20.1), suggesting that PbO_2 is affected by factors that regulate CBF.[35] Others have shown that PbO_2 is closely tied to measures of CPP.[38-41]

Although pressure autoregulation suggests a relationship between CBF and CPP or MAP, it is important to understand that other factors affect cerebral autoregulation. Chemoregulation means that CBF varies based on CO_2/pH levels and, to some extent, on O_2 tissue levels. Metabolic autoregulation occurs such that CBF is coupled to the brain's metabolic demands. Because CO_2 is a byproduct of metabolism, chemoregulation and metabolic autoregulation are closely related. Similarly, there are neural inputs that control CBF. In one model, astrocytes are able to trigger vasodilation by activating astrocytic metabotropic glutamate receptors, triggering an astrocytic calcium wave. As the calcium wave invades an astrocytic endplate, Ca^{2+} stimulates phospholipase A2 to produce arachidonic acid (AA). The AA is metabolized by cyclooxygenase (COX)-1 into a vasodilating prostaglandin (PG).[42] Again, neural autoregulation and metabolic autoregulation are closely tied, because more metabolically active brain tissue will trigger neural vasodilation. When metabolism and CBF are coupled, the inactive or anesthetized brain will have a low CBF and, consequently, a low PbO_2. Hence, low PbO_2 may not necessarily be abnormal and conversely, very high PbO_2 may represent hyperemia when there is uncoupling.

In an elegant study of TBI patients, a multivariate analysis was conducted to determine the relationship among PbO_2 and CBF, CaO_2, CvO_2, OEF, DO_2, $CMRO_2$, and $CBF \times (PaO_2 - PvO_2)$, which approximates the diffusion of oxygen per unit time across the blood–brain barrier, as derived earlier. This study found that only $CBF \times (PaO_2 - PvO_2)$ was significantly correlated to PbO_2, indicating that PbO_2 largely represents the amount of dissolved oxygen content in the brain.[43]

Understanding what PbO_2 represents is crucial to modifying therapy. PbO_2 serves largely as a monitor of either low CBF (which is related to cerebral perfusion pressure by the equation CBF = CPP/CVR) or low arterial oxygen tensions. Because CPP = MAP – ICP, modifying arterial blood pressure or treating elevated ICP can improve CBF and improve PbO_2. In the past, clinicians have treated low PbO_2 values by increasing FiO_2 and, hence, improving arterial oxygen tension. Because arterial oxygen content depends on hemoglobin concentration and the amount of oxygen dissolved in the blood (CaO_2 = [1.34 × Hg concentration × SaO_2] + PaO_2 × [0.003]), improvements in PbO_2 values can be made by transfusion and increasing FiO_2. However, given the oxygen saturation curve, increasing FiO_2 to supraphysiologic levels may only increase the partial pressure of brain oxygen, resulting in a minimal improvement in the delivery of O_2 to the tissues. One study found that increasing FiO_2 led to a 40 percent reduction in microdialysis lactate levels in 12 TBI patients, suggesting less tissue ischemia with improved PbO_2 values after an FiO_2 intervention.[44] Alternatively, another study found that increasing FiO_2 had no impact on lactate/pyruvate ratios in a group of TBI patients.[45] Because lactate/pyruvate ratios are more reliable that the lactate or pyruvate ratio alone, the first study is limited by not examining the ratio. A small study examined PET values of $CMRO_2$ and CBF before and after a one-hour 100% FiO_2 challenge.[46] Although there was a significant change in PaO_2 and a small change in CaO_2, there were no significant changes in MAP, CBF, or $CMRO_2$. The authors concluded that use of 100 percent FiO_2 is not justified for acute TBI. FiO_2 challenges, however, can be used for brief periods (20–30 minutes) to ascertain that the PbO_2 probe is functioning.

Although PbO_2 does not represent oxygen consumption, oxygen extraction fraction or oxygen delivery, abnormal PbO_2 values have been linked to poor functional and cognitive outcomes in critically ill neurologic patients.[47–50] Mortality after TBI was increased in patients with prolonged periods of PbO_2 <8–10 mmHg[51–53] and PbO_2 was identified as the most powerful predictor of outcome after TBI in a multivariate model including GCS, ICP, cerebral perfusion pressure (CPP), and microdialysis values.[54] Prolonged brain tissue hypoxia has been associated with significantly worse outcomes in patients with subarachnoid hemorrhage.[55] PbO_2 monitoring has also been used in clinical practice to monitor for vasospasm after subarachnoid hemorrhage[56,57] and to monitor induced hypothermia for ICP control after TBI.[58]

Only one study has demonstrated that PbO_2-guided therapy improves outcome. In a study of TBI patients with a GCS <8, 28 patients were treated with goal-directed therapy aimed at maintaining an ICP <20 mmHg and PbO_2 >25 mmHg and were compared with 25 historical controls who received traditional treatment aimed at maintaining an ICP <20 mmHg and a CPP >60 mmHg. To maintain a PbO_2 >25 mmHg, adjustments could be made to CPP, FiO_2, seizure control, ICP management (including hemicraniectomy), or transfusion to a

Table 20.4. Established criteria for normality in cerebral microdialysis monitoring

Microdialysis

Normal	Glucose >2 mmol/L
	Glutamate <15 mmol/L
	Lactate/pyruvate 15–25 mmol/L
Abnormal	Glucose <2 mmol/L
	Glutamate >15 mmol/L
	Lactate/pyruvate >25–40 mmol/L

hemoglobin >10 mg/dL. The mean ICP and CPP was similar in both groups. Patients who underwent ICP and PbO_2 goal-directed therapy had a mortality rate of 25 percent, compared with 44 percent in the historical control group ($P < 0.05$); however, there was no significant difference in discharge disposition between the two groups. Limitations of this study include the fact that historical controls were used. The group with PbO_2-directed therapy also underwent decompressive hemicraniectomy for ICP control, whereas the control group did not, and this may have affected the outcome. Finally, because many interventions were used sequentially to improve PbO_2, it is difficult to identify the most salient ways to respond to reduced PbO_2 values.

Microdialysis

Although the brain constitutes only 2 percent of the average person's body weight, it consumes 20 percent of the body's O_2 and receives 20 percent of cardiac output. Microdialysis can measure products of metabolism by sampling interstitial metabolites such as glucose, lactate, pyruvate, glutamate, and glycerol. The only commercially available probe is the CMA 600 (CMA Microdialysis; Stockholm, Sweden). The microdialysis probe is a 0.62-mm semipermeable membrane catheter perfused with artificial CSF at a flow rate of 0.3 μL/min. The probe is inserted through a bolt or tunneled through a craniotomy and is typically placed in a penumbral zone. The catheter samples an area of 2 to 3 mm^2 of brain tissue and allows for diffusion of molecules <10,000 to 20,000 Daltons in size. The relative recovery of metabolites depends on perfusion flow, probe membrane surface, interstitial volume fraction, interstitial diffusion characteristics, temperature, and turnover of diffusable substances.[59] Microdialysis samples are typically evaluated every 10 to 60 minutes and analyzed by enzyme spectrophotometry or high-performance liquid chromatography.[60–62] Hemorrhage or gliosis around the probe can lead to unreliable microdialysis results. Normal microdialysis values are listed in Table 20.4.

To understand the meaning of microdialysis values, it is important to review the glycolysis pathway (Figure 20.5). In conditions of ischemia, glucose is decreased, lactate is increased, pyruvate is decreased (hence, the lactate/pyruvate or L/P ratio is increased), and glutamate levels are increased. Decreased microdialysis glucose levels can be the result of decreased systemic supply, decreased perfusion, or increased

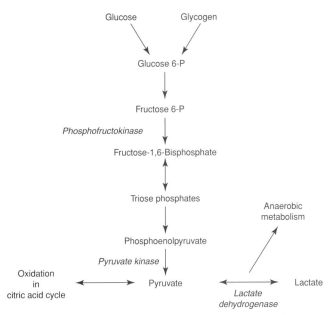

Figure 20.5. The glycolysis pathway is illustrated. Cerebral microdialysis may be used to monitor for elevations in lactate, lactate:pyruvate ratio, or glutamate, which are typically indicative of anaerobic metabolism, ischemia, or mitochondrial dysfunction.

Table 20.5.	Issues concerning intracranial probe placement for oxygen tension and cerebral microdialysis monitoring
Pros	**Cons**
Continuous parametric measurement of averaged capillary and interstitial oxygen pressure or frequent (hourly) measures of metabolic function	Probe placement is crucial to success; if a probe is located in infarcted tissue or hematoma, information is not useful
Can study changes in metabolism or oxygenation in response to therapeutic interventions (such as blood pressure management, transfusion, changes in FiO_2)	Samples only 2–3 mm around the probe and gives regional values
Can give insight into penumbral tissue viability and identify tissue at risk before injury becomes permanent	Invasive and labor-intensive
	No well-constructed studies demonstrating that PbO_2 or microdialysis-guided treatment improve outcome

cellular uptake and utilization. Conversely, increased microdialysis glucose levels can be caused by hyperemia, increased systemic glucose values, or decreased cellular glucose utilization. Decreased utilization may be a normal response to decreased metabolic activity or may be the result of a mitochondrial abnormality that precludes utilization. Elevations in lactate, L/P, or glutamate are typically indicative of anaerobic metabolism, ischemia, or mitochondrial dysfunction. Using the L/P ratio is considered more reliable than following lactate levels alone. Elevated levels of glycerol indicate destruction of cell membranes, which is usually caused by energy failure. Other metabolites, such as adenosine, urea, amino acids, nitrite, and nitrates, can be measured but are not FDA-approved at this time.[63] Concomitant use of PbO_2 or other direct measures of CBF can clarify the interpretation of microdialysis values. Reduced glucose values in the context of elevated L/P, elevated glutamate, reduced PbO_2, and reduced CBF indicate ischemia, for example. Abnormal microdialysis values have been correlated with abnormal PbO_2, jugular venous saturation, ICP, hypoxia, CBF, and OEF.[60,61,64-70]

There have been no randomized trials or outcome studies of microdialysis-guided therapy to demonstrate the utility of microdialysis in management. However, several studies have shown that changes in microdialysis values are predictive of poor outcome. Elevated L/P and glutamate predicted death or severe disability one year after SAH, after controlling for age and admission neurologic status.[75] In TBI patients, persistently low glucose levels and elevated lactate/glucose levels have been related to poor outcome and increased mortality.[64,70] In addition to cerebral metabolites, microdialysis can be used to measure brain parenchymal drug levels or to deliver therapeutic

agents regionally.[85-88] Microdialysis has been recommended by a consensus panel for use in patients with severe TBI who require ICP/CPP monitoring.[60] The pros and cons of microdialysis and brain oxygen monitoring are listed in Table 20.5.

Jugular venous oxygen saturation

Jugular venous bulb sampling can provide an estimate of global cerebral oxygen delivery. Typically, a pediatric central venous catheter with a fiberoptic tip to allow for continuous oxygen saturation measurement is inserted in a retrograde fashion into the dominant jugular vein. The tip of the catheter should be located at the level of the first or second vertebral body to prevent contamination with venous blood from the external jugular vein. The catheter requires calibration every 8 to 12 hours to ensure accuracy.[89,90] If the continuously measured $SjvO_2$ varies by more than 4 percent from the venous oxygen saturation measured on a jugular bulb blood sample, the catheter should be recalibrated. In addition to venous oxygen saturation values, blood sampling from the jugular bulb catheter can be performed to measure PvO_2. Given the hemoglobin concentration, venous oxygen can be calculated by the equation below:

$CvO_2 = (1.34 \times$ hemoglobin concentration $\times SjvO_2) + (0.003 \times PvO_2)$, where $SjvO_2$ is the jugular venous oxyhemoglobin saturation and PvO_2 is the venous oxygen tension. Cerebral oxygen metabolism can be estimated by

$$CMRO_2 = CBF \times (CaO_2 - CvO_2), \text{ and similarly,}$$
$$OEF = (CaO_2 - CvO_2)/CaO_2.$$

The arteriovenous difference in oxygen supply is known as $AVDO_2$ and can be expressed as

$$AVDO_2 = (CaO_2 - CvO_2) \text{ and}$$
$$AVDO_2 = CMRO_2/CBF.$$

If the brain's oxygen metabolism is constant, $AVDO_2$ is inversely proportional to CBF. A normal $SjvO_2$ ranges from 60 percent to 80 percent. Lower $SjvO_2$ indicates low CBF, ischemia, or elevated metabolic rate, such as that which can occur with fever or seizures. Elevated $SjvO_2$ (>80%) may represent hyperemia (abnormally elevated CBF), metabolic suppression, poor oxygen unloading, or an inability to utilize delivered O_2 (mitochondrial injury or massive infarction). $SjvO_2$ represents global changes in oxygen utilization; therefore, smaller regional changes can be missed. $SjvO_2$ can be misleading in cases in which the hemoglobin or arterial oxygen levels fluctuate or when large areas of the brain are infarcted (leading to elevated $SjvO_2$ levels).

Jugular bulb desaturation events have been associated with poor outcome after TBI.[91-93] In a study of 353 TBI patients, CPP plus $SjvO_2$-directed management, compared with CPP-directed therapy in historical controls, produced significantly better outcomes at six months.[94] In a randomized trial of ICP- versus CBF-directed therapy, there was a significant decrease in the number of $SjvO_2$ desaturation events in the CBF group, but there was no difference in clinical outcome.[95] Jugular bulb saturation monitoring has also been used during neurosurgical procedures[96] and in the treatment of SAH.[97]

Cerebral blood flow

Cerebral blood flow is related to MAP, ICP, and brain metabolism and is maintained by pressure, chemical, and neural autoregulation, as described earlier. The gold standard for estimating CBF is performed using the Kety–Schmidt technique, in which the concentration of a freely diffusible indicator is directly measured in arterial and jugular venous blood samples and in the cerebral tissue.[98] Normal and abnormal CBF values are listed in Table 20.4. Continuous measurement of CBF can be performed using thermal diffusion flowmetry. Using this method, thermal conductivity is measured between two probes after one is heated 1 to 2 fC (Bowman CBF monitor; Hemedex Inc., Cambridge, MA). Continuous CBF monitoring correlates with CBF measurements performed using xenon CT. Limitations of catheter CBF monitoring include that only a small portion of tissue is monitored and artifacts may arise because of probe placement. Imaging modalities used to estimate CBF include O-15 PET (which also provides $CMRO_2$ and OEF), xenon CT (requiring inhalation of nonradioactive xenon with subsequent CT imaging), SPECT (which requires isotope administration prior to imaging and has limited spacial resolution), CT perfusion (which provides a quantitative measurement of CBF, CBV, and mean transit time), and MR perfusion (which provides qualitative measurements requiring comparison across hemispheres).

Conclusions

Multimodality monitoring allows physicians to augment the clinical exam with direct measures of brain physiology. The data can be managed using computer-assisted graphical analysis and real-time analysis to manage patients in an individualized goal-directed fashion. It is the goal of modern neurocritical care to identify physiologic and metabolic risk factors early to intervene and to mitigate secondary injury.

References

1. Mayer SA, Coplin WM, Raps EC. Cerebral edema, intracranial pressure, and herniation syndromes. *J Stroke Cerebrovasc Dis* 1999;**8**:183–191.
2. Pratt RW, Mayer SA. Normal pressure "herniation." *Neurocrit Care* 2005;**2**:172–175.
3. Frank JI. Large hemispheric infarction, deterioration, and intracranial pressure. *Neurology* 1995;**45**:1286–1290.
4. Lane PL, Skoretz TG, Doig G, Girotti MJ. Intracranial pressure monitoring and outcomes after traumatic brain injury. *Can J Surg* 2000;**43**:442–448.
5. Murray GD, Butcher I, McHugh GS, et al. Multivariable prognostic analysis in traumatic brain injury: results from the impact study. *J Neurotrauma* 2007;**24**:329–337.
6. Brain Trauma Foundation. Guidelines for the management of severe traumatic brain injury. *J Neurotrauma* 2007;24 Suppl 1:S1–106.
7. Connolly ES. *Fundamentals of Operative Techniques in Neurosurgery*. New York, Thieme, 2002.
8. Bota DP, Lefranc F, Vilallobos HR, Brimioulle S, Vincent JL. Ventriculostomy-related infections in critically ill patients: a 6-year experience. *J Neurosurg* 2005;**103**:468–472.
9. Dettenkofer M, Ebner W, Els T, et al. Surveillance of nosocomial infections in a neurology intensive care unit. *J Neurol* 2001;**248**:959–964.
10. Dettenkofer M, Ebner W, Hans FJ, et al. Nosocomial infections in a neurosurgery intensive care unit. *Acta Neurochir (Wien)* 1999;**141**:1303–1308.
11. Frontera JA, Fernandez A, Schmidt JM, et al. Impact of nosocomial infectious complications after subarachnoid hemorrhage. *Neurosurgery* 2008;**62**:80–87; discussion 87.
12. Zolldann D, Thiex R, Hafner H, Waitschies B, Lutticken R, Lemmen SW. Periodic surveillance of nosocomial infections in a neurosurgery intensive care unit. *Infection* 2005;**33**:115–121.
13. Holloway KL, Barnes T, Choi S, et al. Ventriculostomy infections: the effect of monitoring duration and catheter exchange in 584 patients. *J Neurosurg* 1996;**85**:419–424.
14. Park P, Garton HJ, Kocan MJ, Thompson BG. Risk of infection with prolonged ventricular catheterization. *Neurosurgery* 2004;**55**:594–599; discussion 599–601.
15. Wong GK, Poon WS, Wai S, Yu LM, Lyon D, Lam JM. Failure of regular external ventricular drain exchange to reduce cerebrospinal fluid infection: result of a randomised controlled trial. *J Neurol Neurosurg Psychiatry* 2002;**73**:759–761.
16. Alleyne CH, Jr., Hassan M, Zabramski JM. The efficacy and cost of prophylactic and periprocedural antibiotics in patients with external ventricular drains. *Neurosurgery* 2000;**47**:1124–1127; discussion 1127–1129.
17. Poon WS, Ng S, Wai S. CSF antibiotic prophylaxis for neurosurgical patients with ventriculostomy: a randomised study. *Acta Neurochir Suppl* 1998;**71**:146–148.
18. Eisenberg HM, Gary HE Jr, Aldrich EF, et al. Initial CT findings in 753 patients with severe head injury. A report from the NIH Traumatic Coma Data Bank. *J Neurosurg* 1990;**73**:688–698.
19. Sloan MA, Alexandrov AV, Tegeler CH, et al. Assessment: transcranial Doppler ultrasonography: report of the Therapeutics

and Technology Assessment Subcommittee of the American Academy of Neurology. *Neurology* 2004;**62**:1468–1481.

20. Suarez JI, Qureshi AI, Yahia AB, et al. Symptomatic vasospasm diagnosis after subarachnoid hemorrhage: Evaluation of transcranial Doppler ultrasound and cerebral angiography as related to compromised vascular distribution. *Crit Care Med* 2002;**30**:1348–1355.

21. Vora YY, Suarez-Almazor M, Steinke DE, Martin ML, Findlay JM. Role of transcranial Doppler monitoring in the diagnosis of cerebral vasospasm after subarachnoid hemorrhage. *Neurosurgery* 1999;**44**:1237–1247; discussion 1247–1248.

22. Lindegaard KF, Nornes H, Bakke SJ, Sorteberg W, Nakstad P. Cerebral vasospasm after subarachnoid haemorrhage investigated by means of transcranial Doppler ultrasound. *Acta Neurochir Suppl (Wien)* 1988;**42**:81–84.

23. Naval NS, Thomas CE, Urrutia VC. Relative changes in flow velocities in vasospasm after subarachnoid hemorrhage: a transcranial Doppler study. *Neurocrit Care* 2005;**2**:133–140.

24. Frontera JA, Rundek T, Schmidt JM, et al. Cerebrovascular reactivity and vasospasm after subarachnoid hemorrhage: a pilot study. *Neurology* 2006;**66**:727–729.

25. Lang EW, Diehl RR, Mehdorn HM. Cerebral autoregulation testing after aneurysmal subarachnoid hemorrhage: The phase relationship between arterial blood pressure and cerebral blood flow velocity. *Crit Care Med* 2001;**29**:158–163.

26. Soehle M, Czosnyka M, Pickard JD, Kirkpatrick PJ. Continuous assessment of cerebral autoregulation in subarachnoid hemorrhage. *Anesth Analg* 2004;**98**:1133–1139.

27. Claassen J, Mayer SA, Kowalski RG, Emerson RG, Hirsch LJ. Detection of electrographic seizures with continuous EEG monitoring in critically ill patients. *Neurology* 2004;**62**:1743–1748.

28. Jordan KG. Neurophysiologic monitoring in the neuroscience intensive care unit. *Neurol Clin* 1995;**13**:579–626.

29. Towne AR, Waterhouse EJ, Boggs JG, et al. Prevalence of nonconvulsive status epilepticus in comatose patients. *Neurology* 2000;**54**:340–345.

30. Jaitly R, Sgro JA, Towne AR, Ko D, DeLorenzo RJ. Prognostic value of EEG monitoring after status epilepticus: A prospective adult study. *J Clin Neurophysiol* 1997;**14**:326–334.

31. Young GB, Jordan KG, Doig GS. An assessment of nonconvulsive seizures in the intensive care unit using continuous EEG monitoring: An investigation of variables associated with mortality. *Neurology* 1996;**47**:83–89.

32. Claassen J, Mayer SA, Hirsch LJ. Continuous EEG monitoring in patients with subarachnoid hemorrhage. *J Clin Neurophysiol* 2005;**22**:92–98.

33. Vespa PM, Boscardin WJ, Hovda DA, et al. Early and persistent impaired percent alpha variability on continuous electroencephalography monitoring as predictive of poor outcome after traumatic brain injury. *J Neurosurg* 2002;**97**:84–92.

34. Vespa PM, Nuwer MR, Juhasz C, et al. Early detection of vasospasm after acute subarachnoid hemorrhage using continuous EEG ICU monitoring. *Electroencephalogr Clin Neurophysiol* 1997;**103**:607–615.

35. Hemphill JC 3rd, Knudson MM, Derugin N, Morabito D, Manley GT. Carbon dioxide reactivity and pressure autoregulation of brain tissue oxygen. *Neurosurgery* 2001;**48**:377–383; discussion 383–384.

36. Rosenthal G, Hemphill JC, Sorani M, et al. The role of lung function in brain tissue oxygenation following traumatic brain injury. *J Neurosurg* 2008;**108**:59–65

37. Scheufler KM, Rohrborn HJ, Zentner J. Does tissue oxygen-tension reliably reflect cerebral oxygen delivery and consumption? *Anesth Analg* 2002;**95**:1042–1048.

38. Filippi R, Reisch R, Mauer D, Perneczky A. Brain tissue PO2 related to SjvO2, ICP, and CPP in severe brain injury. *Neurosurg Rev* 2000;**23**:94–97.

39. Haitsma IK, Maas AI. Advanced monitoring in the intensive care unit: brain tissue oxygen tension. *Curr Opin Crit Care* 2002;**8**:115–120.

40. Johnston AJ, Steiner LA, Coles JP, et al. Effect of cerebral perfusion pressure augmentation on regional oxygenation and metabolism after head injury. *Crit Care Med* 2005;**33**:189–195; discussion 255–257.

41. Rose JC, Neill TA, Hemphill JC 3rd. Continuous monitoring of the microcirculation in neurocritical care: an update on brain tissue oxygenation. *Curr Opin Crit Care* 2006;**12**:97–102.

42. Takano T, Tian GF, Peng W, et al. Astrocyte-mediated control of cerebral blood flow. *Nat Neurosci* 2006;**9**:260–267.

43. Rosenthal G, Hemphill JC **3rd**, Sorani M, et al. Brain tissue oxygen tension is more indicative of oxygen diffusion than oxygen delivery and metabolism in patients with traumatic brain injury. *Crit Care Med* 2008;**36**:1917–1924.

44. Menzel M, Doppenberg EM, Zauner A, Soukup J, Reinert MM, Bullock R. Increased inspired oxygen concentration as a factor in improved brain tissue oxygenation and tissue lactate levels after severe human head injury. *J Neurosurg* 1999;**91**:1–10.

45. Magnoni S, Ghisoni L, Locatelli M, et al. Lack of improvement in cerebral metabolism after hyperoxia in severe head injury: A microdialysis study. *J Neurosurg* 2003;**98**:952–958.

46. Diringer MN, Aiyagari V, Zazulia AR, Videen TO, Powers WJ. Effect of hyperoxia on cerebral metabolic rate for oxygen measured using positron emission tomography in patients with acute severe head injury. *J Neurosurg* 2007;**106**:526–529.

47. Stiefel MF, Spiotta A, Gracias VH, et al. Reduced mortality rate in patients with severe traumatic brain injury treated with brain tissue oxygen monitoring. *J Neurosurg* 2005;**103**:805–811.

48. Meixensberger J, Jaeger M, Vath A, Dings J, Kunze E, Roosen K. Brain tissue oxygen guided treatment supplementing ICP/CPP therapy after traumatic brain injury. *J Neurol Neurosurg Psychiatry* 2003;**74**:760–764.

49. Meixensberger J, Renner C, Simanowski R, Schmidtke A, Dings J, Roosen K. Influence of cerebral oxygenation following severe head injury on neuropsychological testing. *Neurol Res* 2004;**26**:414–417.

50. Van Den Brink WA, van Santbrink H, Steyerberg EW, et al. Brain oxygen tension in severe head injury. *Neurosurgery* 2000;**46**:868–876; discussion 876–878.

51. Bardt TF, Unterberg AW, Hartl R, Kiening KL, Schneider GH, Lanksch WR. Monitoring of brain tissue PO2 in traumatic brain injury: effect of cerebral hypoxia on outcome. *Acta Neurochir Suppl* 1998;**71**:153–156.

52. Bardt TF, Unterberg AW, Kiening KL, Schneider GH, Lanksch WR. Multimodal cerebral monitoring in comatose head-injured patients. *Acta Neurochir (Wien)* 1998;**140**:357–365.

53. Valadka AB, Gopinath SP, Contant CF, Uzura M, Robertson CS. Relationship of brain tissue PO2 to outcome after severe head injury. *Crit Care Med* 1998;**26**:1576–1581.

54. Zauner A, Doppenberg EM, Woodward JJ, Choi SC, Young HF, Bullock R. Continuous monitoring of cerebral substrate delivery and clearance: initial experience in 24 patients with severe acute brain injuries. *Neurosurgery* 1997;**41**:1082–1091; discussion 1091–1093.

55. Kett-White R, Hutchinson PJ, Al-Rawi PG, Gupta AK, Pickard JD, Kirkpatrick PJ. Adverse cerebral events detected after subarachnoid hemorrhage using brain oxygen and microdialysis probes. *Neurosurgery* 2002;**50**:1213–1221; discussion 1221–1222.

56. Charbel FT, Du X, Hoffman WE, Ausman JI. Brain tissue PO(2), PCO(2), and pH during cerebral vasospasm. *Surg Neurol* 2000;**54**:432–437; discussion 438.

57. Vath A, Kunze E, Roosen K, Meixensberger J. Therapeutic aspects of brain tissue PO2 monitoring after subarachnoid hemorrhage. *Acta Neurochir Suppl* 2002;**81**:307–309.

58. Gupta AK, Al-Rawi PG, Hutchinson PJ, Kirkpatrick PJ. Effect of hypothermia on brain tissue oxygenation in patients with severe head injury. *Br J Anaesth* 2002;**88**:188–192.

59. Benveniste H. Brain microdialysis. *J Neurochem* 1989;**52**:1667–1679.

60. Bellander BM, Cantais E, Enblad P, et al. Consensus meeting on microdialysis in neurointensive care. *Intensive Care Med* 2004;**30**:2166–2169.

61. Johnston AJ, Gupta AK. Advanced monitoring in the neurology intensive care unit: Microdialysis. *Curr Opin Crit Care* 2002;**8**:121–127.

62. Wartenberg KE, Schmidt JM, Mayer SA. Multimodality monitoring in neurocritical care. *Crit Care Clin* 2007;**23**:507–538.

63. Sarrafzadeh AS, Kiening KL, Unterberg AW. Neuromonitoring: brain oxygenation and microdialysis. *Curr Neurol Neurosci Rep* 2003;**3**:517–523.

64. Goodman JC, Valadka AB, Gopinath SP, Uzura M, Robertson CS. Extracellular lactate and glucose alterations in the brain after head injury measured by microdialysis. *Crit Care Med* 1999;**27**:1965–1973.

65. Sarrafzadeh AS, Sakowitz OW, Callsen TA, Lanksch WR, Unterberg AW. Detection of secondary insults by brain tissue PO2 and bedside microdialysis in severe head injury. *Acta Neurochir Suppl* 2002;**81**:319–321.

66. Carter LP, Weinand ME, Oommen KJ. Cerebral blood flow (CBF) monitoring in intensive care by thermal diffusion. *Acta Neurochir Suppl (Wien)* 1993;**59**:43–46.

67. Dunn IF, Ellegala DB, Fox JF, Kim DH. Principles of cerebral oxygenation and blood flow in the neurological critical care unit. *Neurocrit Care* 2006;**4**:77–82.

68. Gopinath SP, Valadka AB, Goodman JC, Robertson CS. Extracellular glutamate and aspartate in head-injured patients. *Acta Neurochir Suppl* 2000;**76**:437–438.

69. Reinert M, Khaldi A, Zauner A, Doppenberg E, Choi S, Bullock R. High extracellular potassium and its correlates after severe head injury: Relationship to high intracranial pressure. *Neurosurg Focus* 2000;**8**:e10

70. Vespa PM, McArthur D, O'Phelan K, et al. Persistently low extracellular glucose correlates with poor outcome 6 months after human traumatic brain injury despite a lack of increased lactate: a microdialysis study. *J Cereb Blood Flow Metab* 2003;**23**: 865–877.

71. Nilsson OG, Brandt L, Ungerstedt U, Saveland H. Bedside detection of brain ischemia using intracerebral microdialysis: Subarachnoid hemorrhage and delayed ischemic deterioration. *Neurosurgery* 1999;**45**:1176–1184; discussion 1184–1185.

72. Persson L, Valtysson J, Enblad P, Warme PE, Cesarini K, Lewen A, Hillered L. Neurochemical monitoring using intracerebral microdialysis in patients with subarachnoid hemorrhage. *J Neurosurg* 1996;**84**:606–616.

73. Sarrafzadeh AS, Sakowitz OW, Kiening KL, Benndorf G, Lanksch WR, Unterberg AW. Bedside microdialysis: a tool to monitor cerebral metabolism in subarachnoid hemorrhage patients? *Crit Care Med* 2002;**30**:1062–1070.

74. Unterberg AW, Sakowitz OW, Sarrafzadeh AS, Benndorf G, Lanksch WR. Role of bedside microdialysis in the diagnosis of cerebral vasospasm following aneurysmal subarachnoid hemorrhage. *J Neurosurg* 2001;**94**:740–749.

75. Sarrafzadeh A, Haux D, Kuchler I, Lanksch WR, Unterberg AW. Poor-grade aneurysmal subarachnoid hemorrhage: relationship of cerebral metabolism to outcome. *J Neurosurg* 2004;**100**:400–406.

76. Miller CM, Vespa PM, McArthur DL, Hirt D, Etchepare M. Frameless stereotactic aspiration and thrombolysis of deep intracerebral hemorrhage is associated with reduced levels of extracellular cerebral glutamate and unchanged lactate pyruvate ratios. *Neurocrit Care* 2007;**6**:22–29.

77. Berger C, Sakowitz OW, Kiening KL, Schwab S. Neurochemical monitoring of glycerol therapy in patients with ischemic brain edema. *Stroke* 2005;**36**:e4–6.

78. Berger C, Schabitz WR, Georgiadis D, Steiner T, Aschoff A, Schwab S. Effects of hypothermia on excitatory amino acids and metabolism in stroke patients: a microdialysis study. *Stroke* 2002;**33**:519–524.

79. Dohmen C, Bosche B, Graf R, et al. Identification and clinical impact of impaired cerebrovascular autoregulation in patients with malignant middle cerebral artery infarction. *Stroke* 2007;**38**:56–61.

80. Schneweis S, Grond M, Staub F, et al. Predictive value of neurochemical monitoring in large middle cerebral artery infarction. *Stroke* 2001;**32**:1863–1867.

81. Bachli H, Langemann H, Mendelowitsch A, Alessandri B, Landolt H, Gratzl O. Microdialytic monitoring during cerebrovascular surgery. *Neurol Res* 1996;**18**:370–376.

82. Hutchinson PJ, Al-Rawi PG, O'Connell MT, Gupta AK, Pickard JD, Kirkpatrick PJ. Biochemical changes related to hypoxia during cerebral aneurysm surgery: combined microdialysis and tissue oxygen monitoring: case report. *Neurosurgery* 2000;**46**: 201–205; discussion 205–206.

83. Mendelowitsch A, Sekhar LN, Wright DC, et al. An increase in extracellular glutamate is a sensitive method of detecting ischaemic neuronal damage during cranial base and cerebrovascular surgery. An in vivo microdialysis study. *Acta Neurochir (Wien)* 1998;**140**:349–355; discussion 356.

84. Xu W, Mellergard P, Ungerstedt U, Nordstrom CH. Local changes in cerebral energy metabolism due to brain retraction during routine neurosurgical procedures. *Acta Neurochir (Wien)* 2002;**144**:679–683.

85. Bouw R, Ederoth P, Lundberg J, Ungerstedt U, Nordstrom CH, Hammarlund-Udenaes M. Increased blood-brain barrier permeability of morphine in a patient with severe brain lesions as determined by microdialysis. *Acta Anaesthesiol Scand* 2001;**45**:390–392.

86. Joukhadar C, Derendorf H, Muller M. Microdialysis. A novel tool for clinical studies of anti-infective agents. *Eur J Clin Pharmacol* 2001;**57**:211–219.

87. Mindermann T, Zimmerli W, Gratzl O. Rifampin concentrations in various compartments of the human brain: a novel method for determining drug levels in the cerebral extracellular space. *Antimicrob Agents Chemother* 1998;**42**:2626–2629.

88. Tisdall M, Russo S, Sen J, et al. Free phenytoin concentration measurement in brain extracellular fluid: A pilot study. *Br J Neurosurg* 2006;**20**:285–289.

89. Goetting MG, Preston G. Jugular bulb catheterization: experience with 123 patients. *Crit Care Med* 1990;**18**:1220–1223.

90. Gopinath SP, Valadka AB, Uzura M, Robertson CS. Comparison of jugular venous oxygen saturation and brain tissue PO_2 as monitors of cerebral ischemia after head injury. *Crit Care Med* 1999;**27**:2337–2345.

91. Cormio M, Valadka AB, Robertson CS. Elevated jugular venous oxygen saturation after severe head injury. *J Neurosurg* 1999;**90**:9–15.

92. Gopinath SP, Robertson CS, Contant CF, et al. Jugular venous desaturation and outcome after head injury. *J Neurol Neurosurg Psychiatry* 1994;**57**:717–723.

93. Macmillan CS, Andrews PJ, Easton VJ. Increased jugular bulb saturation is associated with poor outcome in traumatic brain injury. *J Neurol Neurosurg Psychiatry* 2001;**70**:101–104.

94. Cruz J. The first decade of continuous monitoring of jugular bulb oxyhemoglobin saturation: management strategies and clinical outcome. *Crit Care Med* 1998;**26**:344–351.

95. Robertson CS, Valadka AB, Hannay HJ, et al. Prevention of secondary ischemic insults after severe head injury. *Crit Care Med* 1999;**27**:2086–2095.

96. Gunn HC, Matta BF, Lam AM, Mayberg TS. Accuracy of continuous jugular bulb venous oximetry during intracranial surgery. *J Neurosurg Anesthesiol* 1995;**7**:174–177.

97. Chieregato A, Targa L, Zatelli R. Limitations of jugular bulb oxyhemoglobin saturation without intracranial pressure monitoring in subarachnoid hemorrhage. *J Neurosurg Anesthesiol* 1996;**8**:21–25.

98. Kety SS, Schmidt CF. The determination of cerebral blood flow in man by the use of nitrous oxide in low concentrations. *Am J Physiol* 1945;**143**:53–66.

Near-infrared spectroscopy

Dean B. Andropoulos

Introduction

Near-infrared spectroscopy (NIRS) is used to measure both cerebral and somatic oxyhemoglobin saturation. Since its now-classic description in 1977 by Jobsis,[1] this technology has been the subject of more than 1000 publications. Because of its non-invasive, compact, portable nature, and potential to measure tissue oxygenation in the brain and other organ systems during surgery and critical illness, it is gaining more widespread clinical use. This chapter examines the technical aspects of NIRS, parameters measured and clinical uses in adult and pediatric cardiac and noncardiac surgery and critical care, evidence for effectiveness in improving clinical outcomes, and pitfalls and complications of NIRS usage.

Technical concepts of near-infrared spectroscopy

NIRS is a noninvasive optical technique used to monitor brain tissue oxygenation. Most devices use two to four wavelengths of infrared light at 700 to 1000 nm, where oxygenated and deoxygenated hemoglobin have distinct absorption spectra.[2–4] Commercially available devices measure the concentration of oxy- and deoxyhemoglobin, using variants of the Beer–Lambert equation: $\log (I/I_0) = \varepsilon_\lambda L C$, where I_0 is the intensity of light before passing through the tissue, I is the intensity of light after passing through the tissue, and the I/I_0 ratio is absorption. Absorption of the near-infrared light depends on the optical path length (L), the concentration of the chromophore in that path (C), and the molar absorptivity of the chromophore at the specific wavelength used (ε_λ).

Cerebral oximetry assumes that 75 percent of the cerebral blood volume in the light path is venous, and 25 percent is arterial. This 75:25 ratio is derived from theoretical anatomical models. Watzman and colleagues attempted to verify this index in children with congenital heart disease by measuring jugular venous bulb saturation ($SjvO_2$) and arterial saturation, and comparing it with cerebral saturation measured with frequency-domain NIRS.[5] The actual ratio in patients varied widely, but averaged 85:15.

In the various models of cerebral oximeters currently on the market, the sensor electrode is placed on the forehead (Figure 21.1A) below the hairline. A light-emitting diode (LED) or laser emits infrared light, which passes through a banana-shaped tissue volume in the frontal cerebral cortex, to two or three detectors placed 3 to 5 cm from the emitter. The screen displays regional cerebral oxygen saturation (rSO_2), and trend over time (Figures 21.1B, C). By using different sensing optodes and multiple wavelengths, extracranial and intracranial hemoglobin absorption can be separated. Deep arcs of light travel across the skin and skull but do not penetrate the cerebral cortex. Deep arcs of light cross the skin, skull, dura, and cortex (Figure 21.2). Subtracting the two absorptions measured, the shallow from the deep, leaves absorption that is due to intracerebral chromophores; this processing renders the cerebral specificity of the oximeter (Figure 21.3). However, the accuracy of NIRS is confounded by the light scattering, which alters the optical path length; the available commercial clinical devices solve this problem differently. The depth of light penetration is 2 to 4 cm.

Three cerebral oximeters are currently widely commercially available: the INVOS 5100, NIRO-200, and FORE-SIGHT. Of the three, the Somanetics INVOS 5100 system (Somanetics Inc., Troy, MI) is in most common use. It has disposable probes, including an adult probe for patients over 40 kg, as well as a pediatric probe designed for patients 4 to 40 kg, which uses a different algorithm that takes into account the thinner skull and extracranial tissues compared with those of the adult.[6] More recently, a neonatal probe has become available that is easier to apply, as it conforms well to the smaller forehead shape. It uses two wavelenghs, 730 and 810 nm; has one LED and two detectors, spaced at 3 cm and 4 cm apart from the emitter; and uses spatially resolved spectroscopy (Figure 21.4). The distinct absorption coefficients of oxy- and deoxyhemoglobin permit measurement of the relative signals from these compounds in the light path. The INVOS device reports oxyhemoglobin/total hemoglobin (oxy- + deoxyhemoglobin) × 100, as the measured regional cerebral oxygen saturation (rSO_2), in percentage. The rSO_2 is reported as a percentage on a scale from 15% to 95%. A subtraction algorithm, based on probe size, removes most of the transmitted shallow (3 cm detector) signal, leaving more than 85 percent of the remaining signal derived from the brain frontal cortex. This device is US Food and Drug Administration (FDA) approved for use in children and adults as a trend-only monitor. It is compact, noninvasive,

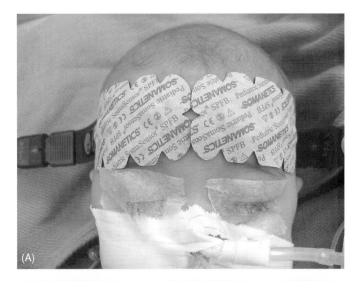

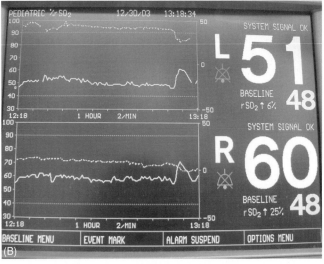

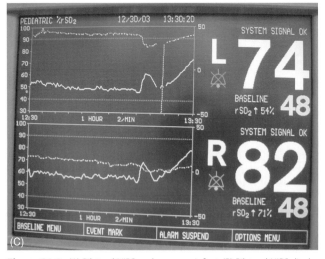

Figure 21.1. (A) Bilateral NIRS probes on an infant. (B) Bilateral NIRS display in a neonate with hypoplastic left heart syndrome in the prebypass period. The bilateral baseline rSO2 of 48% has been recorded; the device displays the current rSO2, the baseline values, and the relative change from baseline values, updated every 4 seconds. (C) NIRS display on bypass in same patient as (B), during cooling with pH stat blood gas management, demonstrating the expected significant increase in rSO2 bilaterally.

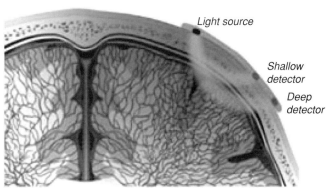

Figure 21.2. Deep arcs of light cross skin, skull, dura, and cortex to measure cerebral rSO2. Courtesy of Somanetics Corporation.

and requires little warmup. A signal strength indicator displays adequacy of detected signal. The device does not depend on pulsatility as a pulse oximeter does and operates at all temperatures. Cerebral blood volume index (Crbvi) can also be calculated, representing the total hemoglobin in the light path, which may be used as an estimate of cerebral blood volume; however, this is an FDA-approved application only for research purposes, but not for clinical use.

The NIRO-200 (Hamamatsu Photonics; Hamamatsu, Japan) uses three wavelengths of near-infrared light (775, 810, and 850 nm) emitted by a laser diode and detected by a photodiode. It uses spatially resolved spectrophotometry; the three wavelengths allow better determination of light path length according to the Beer–Lambert law, which allows calculation of absolute concentrations of oxygenated and total hemoglobin. The NIRO-200 reports a tissue oxygenation index (TOI) as well as hemoglobin indices, including changes in total hemoglobin and in oxy- and deoxyhemoglobin. The probes are not disposable, but are attached with a disposable probe holder. This device may potentially be more accurate than the INVOS system because of the increased number of wavelengths of light; however, it is not FDA-approved for use in the United States.

A more recent FDA-approved device is the FORE-SIGHT monitor (Casmed; Branford, CT). This device uses four wavelengths of light: 690, 778, 800, and 850 nm. The purpose of the additional wavelengths is to better discriminate non-hemoglobin sources of infrared absorption, which may lead to a more accurate calculation of oxygenated and total hemoglobin concentrations.[7] The FORE-SIGHT monitor reports the percentage of oxygenated hemoglobin to total hemoglobin as cerebral tissue oxygen saturation (SCTO2), and is marketed as an absolute cerebral tissue oxygen saturation. Currently available probes are disposable, and are appropriate only for patients from 2.5 to 8 kg, and >40 kg.

Comparison between these commercial devices reveals differences in measured values owing to the different numbers of wavelengths and subtraction algorithms, thus making direct data comparisons difficult.[3] However, regardless of the device used, it is important to remember that all devices measure combined arterial and venous blood oxygen saturation and cannot

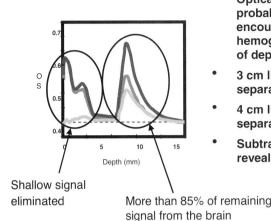

- Optical sampling density (OSD) or probability that a photon will encounter a molecule of hemoglobin plotted as a function of depth from surface

- 3 cm light-source to detector separation distance (medium gray)

- 4 cm light-source to detector separation distance added (dark gray)

- Subtracting the 3 cm from the 4 cm reveals final signal rSO_2 (light gray)

Shallow signal eliminated

More than 85% of remaining signal from the brain

Figure 21.3. Subtraction algorithm for Somanetics 5100A NIRS device. This algorithm differs for the adult probe vs the pediatric probe, accounting for the thicker scalp, skull, and meninges of the adult. Courtesy of Somanetics Corporation.

be assumed to be identical to $SjvO_2$. Maneuvers to increase arterial oxygen saturation, such as increasing FiO_2, will increase cerebral oxygenation as measured by these devices, but the $SjvO_2$ may remain unchanged. The FORE-SIGHT device is still relatively new, and comparison data with the INVOS are not available. However, the FORE-SIGHT monitor may predict a more accurate value for the true brain saturation compared with the INVOS monitor, which will make between patient comparisons easier.

In an attempt to validate the noninvasive measurement of cerebral oxygen saturation in children with congenital heart disease, $SjvO_2$ and rSO_2 were compared. In 40 infants and children undergoing congenital heart surgery or cardiac catheterization, the correlation for paired measurements was inconclusive except for infants less than one year of age.[8] In 30 patients undergoing cardiac catheterization, an improved correlation $r = 0.93$ was found, and there was a linear correlation between changes in arterial CO_2 and cerebral saturation.[9]

Somatic near-infrared oximetry

Using the same principles of unique light absorption spectra of hemoglobin species, NIRS has also been used to measure tissue

oxygenation in skeletal muscle – quadriceps, forearm, or thenar eminence muscle in adults and children.[10] In addition, a probe placed over the flank at the T10–L2 level will measure tissue saturation in skeletal muscle, and in small infants, renal oxygenation, owing to the small light penetrance distance needed in these small patients.[11] Finally, mesenteric saturation has also been measured in infants with a probe placed in the midline between the umbilicus and the symphysis pubis.[12]

Parameters monitored with near-infrared spectroscopy

To simplify terminology, the term rSO_2, for regional oxygen saturation, will be used for the remainder of this chapter, regardless of the device used. Cerebral rSO_2 measurements are an estimate of venous-weighted oxyhemoglobin saturation in the sample volume illuminated by the light path – the frontal cerebral cortex, in most situations. rSO_2 can be altered by any of the factors that affect the cerebral oxygen supply–demand ratio and are especially affected by the unique features of the cerebral circulation, including cerebral autoregulation and alterations in cerebral blood flow according to $PaCO_2$. Any factor that decreases cerebral oxygen consumption will generally increase rSO_2, and any factor that increases oxygen delivery to the brain will also generally increase rSO_2. Table 21.1 lists some of the common alterable clinical factors that can be used to change rSO_2. Because cerebral rSO_2 is influenced by arterial oxygenation, improving this parameter will often increase rSO_2, even if $SjvO_2$ is little altered.

To optimize the utility of NIRS monitoring during the perioperative period, an accurate concept of normal baseline values and a threshold for cerebral injury and for intervention are important to understand. Using the INVOS system, baseline cerebral rSO_2 in 1000 adult cardiac surgery patients before anesthesia, breathing room air, was $67 \pm 10\%$, slightly lower than young adult healthy volunteers at $71 \pm 6\%$.[13] If bilateral forehead probes were used, the mean and median left–right differences were both 0%, and 5 percent of patients had an

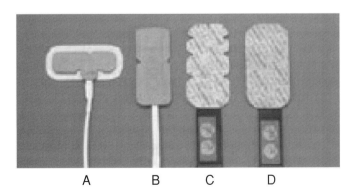

Figure 21.4. Different NIRS probes for neonate cerebral 1–4 kg (A), neonatal somatic 1–4 kg (B), pediatric cerebral/somatic (4–40 kg) (C), adult >40 kg (D). Courtesy of Somanetics Corporation.

Table 21.1. Factors increasing rSO$_2$

Factors decreasing CMRO$_2$ and generally increasing rSO$_2$

Hypothermia

Increasing sedation, anesthesia, analgesia with GABAergic agents, opioids, dexmedetomidine

Treating seizures

Factors increasing oxygen delivery to brain and generally increasing rSO$_2$

Increasing PaCO$_2$

Increasing hemoglobin

Increasing cardiac output

Increasing FiO$_2$ or other ventilatory maneuvers to increase SpO$_2$

Increasing mean arterial pressure (outside limits of autoregulation, i.e. hypotension)

Increasing CPB flow rate

Increasing CPP

Minimizing cerebral venous pressure to increase CPP, i.e. obstructed venous bypass cannula

interhemispheric difference of >10%. In addition, 5.4 percent of the values were less than 50%, 1.6 percent less than 40%, and 1.5 percent were greater than 85%. Thus, a normal baseline range of 50% to 85%, and left–right interhemispheric difference of less than 10%, can be expected for these patients. A threshold for hypoxic injury, and thus for intervention, is difficult to precisely define; however, in two studies of 104 patients undergoing awake carotid endarterectomy with regional anesthesia and cerebral oximetry monitoring, patients who developed neurologic symptoms with carotid clamping had an average 20 percent *relative* decline in rSO$_2$, versus only 9 percent in asymptomatic patients.[14,15]

For pediatric patients undergoing congenital heart surgery, baseline rSO$_2$ varies with cardiac lesion.[4] The baseline cerebral saturation is about 70 percent in acyanotic patients without large left-to-right intracardiac shunts, breathing room air. On room air, rSO$_2$ for cyanotic patients, or acyanotic patients with large left-to-right intracardiac shunts, is usually 40% to 60%; hypoplastic left heart syndrome (HLHS) patients receiving <21% FiO$_2$ preoperatively have lower rSO$_2$, averaging 53%, versus those receiving FiO$_2$ 0.21 and 3% inspired CO$_2$, where rSO$_2$ averages 68%.[16]

Taking into account the adult carotid surgery data cited previously, as well as pediatric cardiac surgery outcome data (discussed later), some practitioners would consider a relative decline from a baseline of 20 percent or more (e.g. from a baseline of 60% to a nadir of 48%) cause for intervention. The software on most oximeters will continuously calculate this relative difference from baseline. Other practitioners would use an absolute value of rSO$_2$ of 50% as cause for intervention.

Cerebral oximetry reflects a balance between oxygen delivery and oxygen consumption by the brain (CMrO$_2$). The cerebral oxygen content will therefore be affected both by the arterial saturation of hemoglobin and by the hemoglobin concentration. There then must exist a cerebral saturation value, or ischemic threshold, below which brain injury is likely because of oxygen deprivation, as demand outstrips supply. In a neonatal piglet study using frequency domain NIRS, Kurth and col-

leagues showed that cerebral lactate levels rose at rSO$_2$ values of 44% or lower; major EEG changes occurred when the cerebral saturation declined to 37%, with reductions in cerebral ATP levels when oximetry readings were 33% or lower.[17] This concept was confirmed in another neonatal piglet model using hypoxic gas mixtures for 30 minutes at normothermia, demonstrating that rSO$_2$ > 40% did not change EEG or brain pathology obtained 72 hours later; rSO$_2$ 30% to 40% produced no EEG changes, but at 72 hours there were ischemic neuronal changes in the hippocampus, and mitochondrial injury occurred. At rSO$_2$ < 30%, there was circulatory failure, EEG amplitude decreased, and there was vacuolization of neurons and severe mitochondrial injury.[18] Finally, in a similar piglet model, the hypoxic–ischemic cerebral saturation-time threshold for brain injury found that rSO$_2$ of 35% for two hours or more produced brain injury.[19] In general, most pediatric clinical studies use either 20 percent below established baseline or an oximetry reading of 45% to 50% for the threshold for treatment based on evidence of new MRI lesions or clinical exam that brain injury is more likely to develop under these circumstances.[20,21]

In the absence of absolute criteria for intervention to prevent neurologic injury (discussed later, under Outcomes), each anesthesiologist must take into account the unique pathophysiology of each patient and the monitoring system used, and decide on criteria for intervention, much like all the other physiologic variables measured for surgery and critical care.

Clinical data in adult cardiac surgery

The significant incidence of neurocognitive dysfunction, stroke, seizures, and other adverse neurological effects after cardiac surgery with cardiopulmonary bypass (CPB) have led to the appealing concept that monitoring cerebral oxygen saturation and preventing prolonged decreases in cerebral oxygenation could reduce adverse outcomes. Figure 21.5 represents a typical clinical scenario for bilateral cerebral NIRS monitoring in an adult patient undergoing complex aortic arch surgery. Common periods for risk of cerebral desaturation include hemodynamic instability/low cardiac output in the prebypass period, institution of CPB with hemodilution, hypocarbia accompanying alpha stat blood gas management and cooling of the patient, periods of low-flow bypass or circulatory arrest, warming on bypass with low hematocrit, and postbypass period with low cardiac output, anemia, or arrhythmias.

In addition, NIRS is capable of detecting sudden cerebral desaturation from cannulation problems or malposition. Jannelle and associates described a case of a 75-year-old patient undergoing repair of a DeBakey type 1 aortic dissection with deep hypothermia.[22] After 40 minutes of CPB, during replacement of the aortic valve, profound right hemispheric desaturation occurred despite a nasopharyngeal temperature of 18°C and an isoelectric electroencephalogram. After deep hypothermic circulatory arrest (DHCA) was instituted, the aorta was opened and the dissection was noted to extend into the right

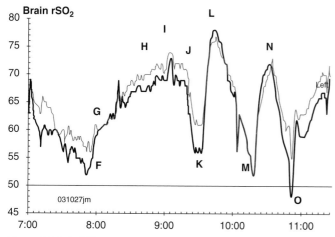

Figure 21.5. Left (thinner gray) and right (thicker black) lines demonstrate rSO₂ changes in an adult undergoing complex aortic arch reconstruction. The horizontal line signifies 20% relative decline from awake baseline. F illustrates rSO₂ decrease owing to moderate hypocapnia; G is response to decreasing minute ventilation and increasing PaCO₂; H is institution of cardiopulmonary bypass; I is cooling with pH stat management; J is the onset of a period of retrograde cerebral perfusion at deep hypothermia; K is restoration of full flow bypass; L is the onset of rewarming; M is at full rewarming, propofol administered to increase depth of anesthesia; N is separation from bypass with hypotension; O is administration of intravascular volume and phenylephrine. Reproduced with permission from ref. (13).

common carotid artery. Retrograde cerebral perfusion was instituted, the rSO₂ improved, and the patient was discharged home without apparent deficits (Figure 21.6).

NIRS can be used to monitor the brain during antegrade or retrograde cerebral perfusion for aortic surgery. Orihashi and colleagues reported a series of 59 patients undergoing aortic arch surgery with antegrade selective cerebral perfusion.[23] Sixteen patients developed an acute neurological syndrome, including seizures, coma, and hemiparesis; new cerebral

infarction was documented in six of these patients. Despite aortic cross-clamp time, selective cerebral perfusion (SCP) time, and DHCA times being equal in patients with and without injury, rSO₂ time below both 55% (67 vs 11 minutes) and 60% (141 vs 50 minutes) was significantly longer in patients with an acute neurologic injury. The same group documented selective cerebral perfusion catheter malposition in two cases, heralded by sudden decrease in rSO₂, confirmed by transesophageal echocardiography.[24]

NIRS has also been used for novel procedures such as aortic endovascular stent grafting. Santo and coworkers[25] describe a 26-year-old male who suffered a traumatic aortic tear. During the stenting, recurrent left-sided rSO₂ decreases from 60% to 75% down to 40% to 60% guided the surgical perfusion strategy, and persistent low left-sided rSO₂ directed the surgeon to remove a nearly occlusive thrombus from the left common carotid artery segment of the graft. The patient recovered well with only a mild right arm paresis.

Clinical data in pediatric cardiac surgery

Changes in cerebral oxygenation have been characterized during cardiopulmonary bypass in children with or without deep hypothermic circulatory arrest (Figure 21.7).[26] rSO₂ predictably decreases during DHCA to a nadir approximately 60 percent to 70 percent below baseline values obtained prebypass;[26] the nadir is reached at about 40 minutes, after which there is no further decrease. At this point, it appears that the brain does not continue the uptake of oxygen; interestingly, this time period appears to correlate with clinical and experimental studies suggesting that 40 to 45 minutes is the limit for safe duration for circulatory arrest.[27,28] The DHCA initiation at higher temperature results in a faster fall in rSO₂, reaching the

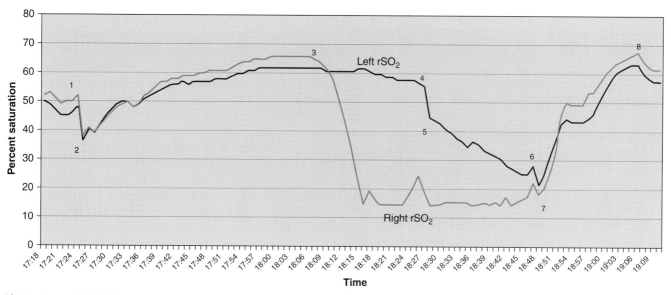

Figure 21.6. Cerebral rSO₂ values during cardiopulmonary bypass in an adult with extension of aortic dissection during emergency repair. 1 = Begin cardiopulmonary bypass; 2 = begin cooling; 3 = sudden right hemispheric desaturation; 4 = begin deep hypothermic circulatory arrest; 5 = begin retrograde cerebral perfusion; 6 = begin deep hypothermic circulatory arrest; 7 = begin anterograde cerebral perfusion; 8 = begin rewarming. Reproduced with permission from ref. (22).

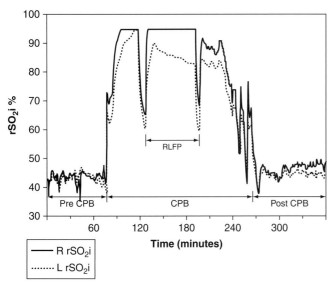

Figure 21.7. Typical changes in regional cerebral oxygen saturation (rSO$_2$) during cardiac surgery in a neonate with hypoplastic left heart syndrome undergoing Norwood stage I palliation, with cardiopulmonary bypass, regional cerebral low-flow perfusion (RLFP), and deep hypothermic circulatory arrest. Note the precipitous decline at minute 115 with onset of DHCA for atrial septectomy, and again at minute 185 for replacement of aortic cannula.

Table 21.2. Treatment algorithm for low cerebral oxygen saturation (rSO$_2$)[45]

1. Establish baseline rSO$_2$ on FiO$_2$ 0.21, PaCO$_2$ 40 mmHg, stable baseline hemodynamics, awake before induction of anesthesia, or prebypass if possible
2. Treat decreased rSO$_2$ of >20% relative value below baseline, or <50% absolute value
3. Pre/post bypass (in order of ease/rapidity to institute):
   a. Increase FiO$_2$
   b. Increase PaCO$_2$
   c. Increase cardiac output/O$_2$ delivery with volume infusions, inotropic support, vasodilators, etc.
   d. Increase depth of anesthesia
   e. Decrease temperature
   f. Increase hemoglobin
4. During CPB:
   a. Increase CPB flow and/or mean arterial pressure
   b. Increase PaCO$_2$
   c. Increase FiO$_2$
   d. Decrease temperature
   e. Increase hemoglobin
   f. Check aortic and venous cannula positioning
   g. Check for aortic dissection

Source: Ref. 45.

nadir sooner.[29] Reperfusion immediately results in an increase in rSO$_2$ levels, seen at full bypass flow before DHCA.

The question often arises whether bilateral cerebral hemisphere NIRS monitoring is necessary. In a study of 20 patients undergoing anterograde cerebral perfusion (ACP) via the right innominate artery, half the patients had a left–right difference of greater than 10 percent.[30] In 60 neonates undergoing surgery with conventional bypass, only 10 percent had a difference of more than than 10 percent between left and right sides at baseline; this difference persisted in only one patient.[31] Based on these data, bilateral monitoring is probably necessary only when special CPB techniques are used for aortic arch reconstruction, or when anatomical variants, such as bilateral superior vena cavae or abnormalities of the brachiocephalic vessels, are present.

Treatment of low rSO$_2$

Whether during adult or pediatric cardiac surgery with CPB, the general approach to treating low rSO$_2$ is similar and involves increasing oxygen delivery to the brain or decreasing oxygen consumption. One approach to treatment is displayed in Table 21.2.

Clinical data in noncardiac surgery and critical care

Cerebral oximetry has also been used for carotid endarterectomy monitoring. Moritz and associates studied 75 patients undergoing awake carotid endarterectomy under regional anesthesia, and compared the ability of NIRS, transcranial Doppler (TCD) of the middle cerebral artery, carotid stump pressure, and somatosensory evoked potentials to detect neurological deterioration, which occurred in 12 of the 75 patients.[32] A

20 percent relative reduction in rSO$_2$ from baseline had a 83 percent sensitivity and 83 percent specificity to detect a neurological event. NIRS, TCD, and stump pressures all performed well, and were equivalent at detecting ischemic events (area under the receiver operating curve 0.905, 0.973, and 0.925, respectively), whereas somaotosensory evoked potentials performed poorly (AUC 0.749). However, 21 percent of patients had technical difficulties with the TCD signal, and this method was deemed impractical by the authors.

NIRS has also been found to be useful for monitoring during cerebral aneurysm embolization. In a study of 32 adults undergoing this procedure under general anesthesia, angiographically confirmed vasospasm of the anterior circulation was reliably accompanied by a decrease in rSO$_2$.[33] The greater the decrease in rSO$_2$, the more severe the vasospasm. With a baseline mean of 73%, a decrease to 68% was observed for mild vasospasm (25% narrowing), 66% for moderate vasospasm (50% narrowing), and 52% for severe (75% narrowing) vasospasm.

In critical care medicine, cerebral NIRS has been used to monitor the adequacy of cerebral oxygen delivery and as a surrogate marker for the adequacy of global oxygen delivery in patients after cardiac surgery, and patients on extracorporeal membrane oxygenation (ECMO) or ventricular assist devices.[7,34] Changes in rSO$_2$ have a close correlation with changes in mixed venous saturation (SvO$_2$) in both single- and two-ventricle patients after congenital cardiac surgery.[35,36]

Clinical uses of somatic NIRS in adult and pediatric surgery and critical care

NIRS can be used to measure tissue oxygenation during surgery and critical illness; because of its noninvasive, continuous nature, it has intuitive appeal in conditions in which low cardiac output and other causes of shock would benefit from such continuous monitoring. In a study of 26 adult trauma patients, a tissue $rSO_2 < 70\%$ within the first hour of admission, measured at the thenar eminence, predicted the need for blood transfusion, with a specificity of 78 percent, sensitivity of 88 percent, positive predictive value of 64 percent, and negative predictive value of 93 percent.[37] Conventional measures on admission, such as blood pressure, heart rate, admission hemoglobin, lactate, and base deficit, could not reliably predict the need for transfusion during the hospital stay.

In another study of 383 adult trauma patients, a thenar eminence rSO_2 value of $< 75\%$ during the 24 hours after admission predicted multiple organ dysfunction syndrome in the 50 patients who developed it.[38] The sensitivity was 78 percent, specificity 39 percent, positive predictive value 18 percent, negative predictive value 91 percent. The low positive predictive value signifies the high false-positive rate. A maximum calculated base deficit of –6 mEq/L performed similarly to the tissue NIRS value.

NIRS also may have value in predicting surgical site infections. In a study of 59 adult patients, tissue rSO_2 was measured at the forearm and surgical wound site preoperatively, and at 12, 24, and 48 hours postoperatively.[39] In the 17 patients who developed a surgical site infection, mean rSO_2 at 12 hours was 42%, versus 58% in those who did not ($p = 0.005$). When a cutoff of wound $rSO_2 < 53\%$ was used, this value had a sensitivity of 71 percent and a specificity of 73 percent to predict wound infection.

Somatic NIRS using a probe placed on the flank at T10–L2 was studied in a series of neonates after during and single ventricle surgical palliation by Hoffman and coworkers.[11] In nine neonates undergoing CPB with regional cerebral perfusion (RCP), mean cerebral rSO_2 prebypass was 65% and somatic rSO_2 59%, and during RCP cerebral rSO_2 was 81% versus somatic rSO_2 41%, signifying relative tissue hypoxia because of lack of perfusion to subdiaphragmatic organs during this technique. After CPB, cerebral rSO_2 decreased to 53%, but somatic rSO_2 increased to 76%.[11] In 79 postoperative neonates undergoing Norwood Stage I palliation for hypoplastic left heart syndrome, a cerebral–somatic rSO_2 difference of less than 10 percent significantly increased the risk for biochemical shock, mortality, or other complications (Figure 21.8). Mean somatic $rSO_2 < 70\%$ was associated with a significantly increased risk of prolonged ICU stay, shock, and other complications.

Somatic NIRS has also been used to measure mesenteric rSO_2 in neonates and infants after cardiac surgery, with a probe placed on the abdomen between the umbilicus and symphysis pubis. In a study of 20 patients, Kaufman and colleagues[41] compared mesenteric NIRS and flank NIRS at T10–L2 with gastric pH measured by tonometry and lactate values. In 122 simultaneous measurements made in the first 48 hours after surgery, mesenteric rSO_2 correlated significantly with gastric pH ($r = 0.79$), serum lactate ($r = 0.77$), and SvO_2 ($r = 0.89$). These correlations were all better than those using flank NIRS. The authors concluded that mesenteric NIRS is a sensitive monitor

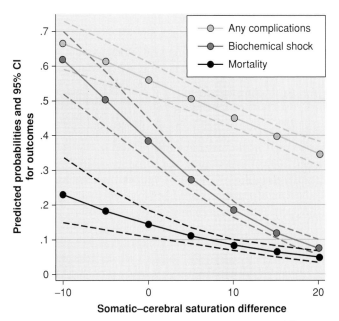

Figure 21.8. Relationship between somatic rSO_2–cerebral rSO_2 difference, and the incidence of complications in 79 patients in the 48 hours after Norwood stage I palliation for hypoplastic left heart syndrome. Reproduced with permission from ref. (40).

of splanchnic tissue oxygenation and may have utility at managing these patients and improving outcomes.

These studies lend credence to the idea that NIRS-directed targeted interventions could be used to improve oxygen delivery to tissues and organs and potentially improve outcomes from surgery, anesthesia, and critical illness. To date, there is a lack of such published studies, but the noninvasive continuous nature of NIRS monitoring should make such studies more likely to be performed.

Outcome studies of near-infrared spectroscopy
Association of low cerebral saturation with adverse neurologic outcome

There is evidence from adult cardiac surgery studies that low intraoperative cerebral rSO_2 is associated with postoperative neurocognitive dysfunction. In a study of 41 adults undergoing cardiac surgery with CPB, Nollert and colleagues found that three of the four patients with new postoperative changes on psychometric testing had significant periods of low rSO_2.[42]

In a study of 101 adult patients undergoing cardiac surgery with bypass, Yao and associates[43] determined that time spent at $rSO_2 < 40\%$ was associated with abnormalities on postoperative neuropsychologic testing. Patients with more than 10 minutes at $rSO_2 < 40\%$ had a 32 percent to 42 percent incidence of abnormalities on two separate tests, versus 10 percent to 13 percent for those who had less than 10 minutes at $rSO_2 < 40\%$ Goldman and coworkers[44] compared permanent stroke incidence in 1245 consecutive adult patients undergoing cardiac surgery with bypass without NIRS monitoring with 1034 subsequent patients who underwent NIRS monitoring with a treatment protocol to optimize cerebral oxygenation. The permanent stroke rate was 2.5 percent in the unmonitored group versus 0.97 percent in the monitored group ($p = 0.044$).

In an important – and, to date, the only – prospective, randomized, controlled study of NIRS monitoring versus no NIRS monitoring for adult cardiac surgery, Murkin and colleagues[45] studied 200 patients undergoing coronary artery bypass graft (CABG), randomized to either intraoperative rSO_2 monitoring with active intervention or blinded rSO_2 monitoring. Baseline values were obtained preinduction with patients breathing oxygen via nasal cannula. For the intervention group, the goal was to keep rSO_2 above 75 percent of the baseline value – that is, if the baseline rSO_2 were 70%, the goal was to keep rSO_2 above 53%. Mild hypothermia of $32°C$ to $35°C$ with alpha stat management was used on CPB. If rSO_2 was below 75 percent of baseline, a prioritized intervention protocol was instituted, including checking for head and facial plethora and adjusting head position or venous cannula; increasing $PaCO_2$ to 40 mmHg or more whether on or off CPB; increasing mean arterial pressure to greater than 60 mmHg, if low, with phenylephrine; decreasing jugular venous pressure to less than 10 mmHg if elevated; increasing CPB flow or cardiac output; increasing hematocrit if below 20 percent; increasing FiO_2; or administering propofol to increase depth of anesthesia. Primary outcome was a composite of postoperative complications as defined by the Society of Thoracic Surgeons, and included new Q wave myocardial infarction; clinical stroke confirmed by CT scan; prolonged ventilation of more than 24 and 48 hours; dialysis-dependent renal failure; reoperation or reexploration for bleeding; arrthymia requiring treatment; wound infection; readmission; or death. Fewer patients in the monitoring and intervention group experienced major organ morbidity or mortality as defined above: three patients versus 11 patients ($p = 0.048$) (Figure 21.9). Additionally, severe cerebral desaturation, defined as rSO_2 less than 70 percent of baseline for more than 150 minutes intraoperatively, was seen in no monitor/intervention patient, versus being seen in six blinded control patients ($p = 0.014$). This properly designed study presents the best argument to date that NIRS monitoring with an active intervention protocol can improve outcomes for adult cardiac surgery.

There is increasing evidence from pediatric cardiac surgery studies that prolonged low NIRS values are associated with adverse short-term neurologic outcomes. Dent and fellow researchers studied 15 neonates undergoing the Norwood operation who underwent preoperative, intraoperative, and postoperative rSO_2 monitoring.[20] A prolonged low rSO_2 (>180 minutes with $rSO_2 \leq 45\%$) was associated with a higher risk of new ischemic lesions on postoperative MRI when compared to the presurgical study, with a sensitivity of 82 percent, specificity of 75 percent, positive predictive value of 90 percent, and negative predictive value of 60 percent. Therefore, both the extent of decreased cerebral saturation (ischemic threshold) and the time

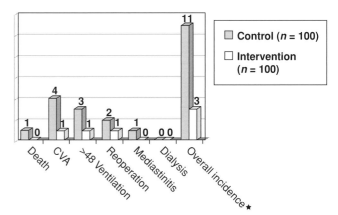

Figure 21.9. Incidence of 30-day major organ morbidity and mortality in 200 adult patients undergoing coronary artery bypass grafting *$p = 0.048$. Control group had NIRS monitoring for data collection only, with monitor values not available to the anesthesiologist. Intervention group had NIRS monitoring with data available to anesthesiologist, and active intervention protocol. Reproduced with permission from ref. (45).

spent below this ischemic threshold are important in predicting the development of new postoperative brain injury by MRI.

There is additional clinical evidence suggesting that low cerebral saturations correlate with adverse neurological outcomes. In a study of 26 infants and children undergoing surgery using DHCA, three patients had acute neurological changes:[46] one patient had seizures, and two patients had prolonged coma. All these patients had low rSO_2. In these three patients, the increase in rSO_2 was much less after the onset of CPB, and the duration of cooling before DHCA was shorter. In a retrospective study of multimodality neurological monitoring in 250 infants and children undergoing cardiac surgery with bypass, relative cerebral oxygen desaturation of more than 20 percent below prebypass baseline was associated with abnormal events in 58 percent of the patients.[21] If left untreated, 26 percent of these patients had adverse postoperative neurological events versus 6% of those who received treatment.

In a study of 16 patients undergoing neonatal cardiac surgery, with NIRS monitoring and pre- and postoperative brain MRI, 6 of 16 patients developed a new postoperative brain injury; these patients had a lower rSO_2 during aortic cross-clamp period versus those without new brain injury (48% vs 57%, $p = 0.008$).[47] In a recent study of 44 neonates undergoing the Norwood operation, who were tested at age 4 to 5 using a visual–motor integration test (VMI), the first 34 patients did not have NIRS monitoring, and the last 10 did have NIRS monitoring with a strict treatment protocol for low rSO_2 values, $< 50\%$.[48] No patients with NIRS monitoring had a VMI score < 85 (normal is 100), versus 6 percent without NIRS monitoring. Mean rSO_2 in the perioperative period was associated with VMI score, with no patient with mean $rSO_2 \geq 55\%$ having a VMI less than 96.

Toet and associates studied 20 neonates undergoing the arterial switch operation and monitored rSO_2 for 4 to 12 hours preoperatively, intraoperatively, and for 36 hours postoperatively.[49] Seven patients had a mean preoperative $rSO_2 \leq 35\%$,

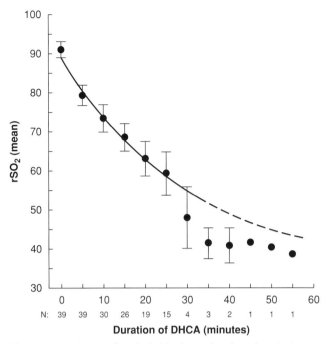

Figure 21.10. Pattern of cerebral rSO$_2$ during deep hypothermic circulatory arrest (DHCA) in 39 infants with D-transposition of the great arteries who underwent ≥ 5 minutes of DHCA. Data are presented as mean ± 1.96 SEM. The number of subjects (N) available for analysis at 5-minute intervals of DHCA is shown. The fitted nonlinear exponential decay curve (solid line) is base on data from 0 to 30 minutes with higher weight given to mean rSO$_2$ values calculated with more subjects. The fit is extrapolated beyond 30 minutes (dashed line). Reproduced with permission from ref. (50).

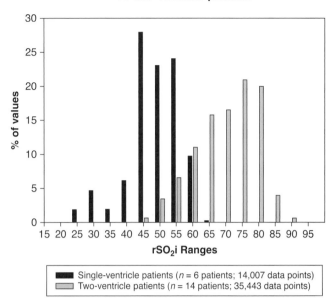

Figure 21.11. Frequency of rSO$_2$ values recorded at 1-minute intervals in the first 48 hours postoperatively in neonates undergoing repair of hypoplastic left heart syndrome (single-ventricle patients) or D-transposition of the great arteries (two-ventricle patients). Reproduced with permission from ref. (51).

and two of these patients had significantly abnormal Bayley Scales of Infant Development scores at 30 to 36 months: one to two standard deviations below the normal population mean.

Kussman and colleagues[50] studied 104 infants aged nine months or less undergoing complete two ventricle repair of transposition of the great arteries, tetralogy of Fallot, or ventricular septal defect to evaluate changes in rSO$_2$ and to determine association between low rSO$_2$ and early postoperative outcomes, including death, stroke, seizures, or choreoathetosis. pH stat blood gas management and hematocrit of 25 percent to 35 percent, along with brief DHCA and some low-flow bypass, were used. Bilateral NIRS was monitored during the intraoperative period and for 18 hours postoperatively; no interventions were made on the basis of rSO$_2$ values. An rSO$_2$ threshold of 45% was chosen as the cutoff for analysis. Eighty-one of 104 patients had no desaturation below 45%, 12 had brief desaturation below 45% for 1 to 39 minutes, and 11 had more prolonged desaturation of 60 to 383 minutes. Because no patient in the study died or suffered any neurologic complication, the relationship between low rSO$_2$ and early neurologic outcome could not be determined. There was also no relationship between low rSO$_2$ and postoperative cardiac index, lactate, severity of illness, or days ventilated, in the ICU or hospital. Thirty-nine of these patients had a period of DHCA, and important data about the rate of decline of rSO$_2$ under optimal CPB conditions were reported (Figure 21.10). The important finding is that brief periods of DHCA < 30 minutes did not result in nadir values of rSO$_2$, suggesting that this technique does not deplete the brain of oxygen stores and lending more credence to the idea that this practice is safe. The lack of an association between rSO$_2$ and early gross neurological outcomes is not unexpected, given that these were all two-ventricle patients, completely repaired, with normal arterial oxygen saturations postoperatively. The low incidence and severity of cerebral desaturation in this population has been previously described (Figure 21.11).[51]

Another potential benefit of routine NIRS monitoring is to avert the rare but very real and devastating potential neurological disaster from cannulation problems, in which rSO$_2$ declines dramatically from cannula malposition and cerebral arterial or venous obstruction, yet all other bypass parameters are normal.[52,53] In neonates and infants, it is clear that mixed venous saturation in the bypass circuit bears very poor association with cerebral saturation, emphasizing the point that intracerebral desaturation may go unnoticed.[54]

In a systematic review of 56 publications describing 1300 patients using NIRS monitoring for congenital heart disease in the operating room, intensive care unit, and cardiac catheterization laboratory, Hirsch and coworkers[55] concluded that the technology did serve as a reliable, continuous, noninvasive monitor of cerebral oxygenation; however, to date there have not been any published prospective, randomized, controlled studies of NIRS monitoring versus no NIRS monitoring, with short- or long-term follow-up, in pediatric patients.

Thus far most studies on cerebral oximetry are observational and descriptive, and the value of NIRS is difficult to establish definitively when evaluating the brain of neonates and children. Prospective randomized trials in infants and children are confounded by the duration of follow-up that is required and the multifactorial etiologies contributing to adverse neurologic outcomes. The single well-designed, prospective, adequately powered adult study gives strong evidence that NIRS monitoring is effective. In both adults and children, more prospective studies are needed to demonstrate the value of NIRS; however, it may be difficult for these studies to be performed owing to lack of equipoise for many centers that already use NIRS, and the complexity and cost of conducting trials requiring large sample sizes to achieve adequate statistical power to detect a difference in the incidence of relatively rare events.[13] Even though very large studies of changes in outcome through the use of pulse oximetry have never clearly demonstrated benefit, we would not practice without it.[56]

Complications and pitfalls of near-infrared oximetry

The noninvasive nature of NIRS monitoring obviates many of the problems seen with more invasive methods of measuring cerebral or somatic oxygenation, such as jugular venous bulb monitoring, pulmonary artery catheter placement, gastric tonometry, and lithium dilution cardiac output. It is possible to have skin irritation or pressure sores from the probes if the head is wrapped with a flexible bandage to apply the probe. If the probe is not securely applied, contamination of the NIRS signal with ambient light could alter the readings; however, the commercially available monitors all give an indication of signal strength and will not display a reading if this is the case. The reliability of NIRS monitors to display a valid reading during clinical use has not been specifically reported; in practice, however, the technology is extremely reliable and requires virtually no adjustment during use under a variety of conditions in operative and intensive care settings.

rSO_2 is a regional saturation; only a small portion of the frontal cerebral cortex is monitored, especially in adult patients, so it is entirely possible to have a hypoxic/ischemic condition in the contralateral hemisphere, or in parietal or occipital areas remote from the probe. In neonates, the light penetration is relatively deeper, given the smaller head circumference, and so this monitor assesses a larger cerebral volume for desaturation (Figure 21.12).

In the absence of absolute rSO_2 values (which is a limitation of two wavelength NIRS – see previous discussion), the Somanetics device especially must be regarded as a trend monitor, with each patient serving as his or her own control, and interventions made on the basis of a baseline value obtained under stable hemodynamic and respiratory conditions. In addition, differences in extracranial factors, such as skull and scalp thickness and edema, and venous stasis causing scalp venous desaturation, can affect the rSO_2 reading because the extracranial contribution may not be completely eliminated.[57] As with any other physiologic monitor, the data displayed must take into account

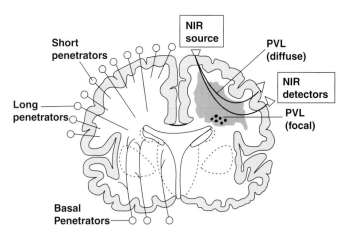

Figure 21.12. Areas of potential hypoxic–ischemic injury in the neonatal brain include moderate and deep cortical structures. The light path of an NIRS device applied to the forehead will traverse areas at risk between the short and long penetrating arteries in the frontoparietal lobes. More of these regions will be in the monitored field in neonates with small head dimensions, compared with the adult. PVL, periventricular leukomalacia. Reproduced with permission from ref. (60).

all the other variables contributing to the patient's physiologic status at the moment.

Specific situations that have been demonstrated to affect rSO_2 readings include icterus. Madsen and colleagues[58] studied 48 patients undergoing liver transplantation with varying degrees and durations of hyperbilirubinemia. rSO_2 was inversely proportional to serum bilirubin, with patients in the higher ranges of 300 to 600 mmol/L exhibiting very low rSO_2 of 15% to 40% despite adequate hemodynamics and mental status. This inverse correlation corrected only partially with lower serum bilirubin after transplant, suggesting that both bilirubin and its breakdown product, biliverdin, absorb near-infrared light in the path of the NIRS probe, affecting the rSO_2 readings. McDonaugh and associates describe five adult patients whose rSO_2 declined to a nadir of 6 percent to 12 percent below baseline and did not normalize for 20 to 40 minutes, after a standard injection of 5 mL (40 mg) IV indigo carmine.[59] Indigo carmine absorbs light at 700 nm, suggesting that this is the mechanism for the interference with the rSO_2 readings.

Training and credentialing for near-infrared spectroscopy

There is no credentialing process for NIRS monitoring. Following the manufacturer's instructions is a simple process, and because anesthesiologists are continually monitoring and responding to changes in physiological parameters such as SpO_2, the transition to rSO_2 monitoring is a natural one.

Practice parameters and guideline for near-infrared spectroscopy

There are currently no practice parameters or guidelines for NIRS monitoring; as of this writing, it cannot be considered an absolute standard of care in any setting. Any guidelines or parameters should be proposed only after more prospective outcome data are obtained, after a thorough review of available evidence and expert opinion.

References

1. Jobsis FF. Noninvasive, infrared monitoring of cerebral and myocardial oxygen sufficiency and circulatory parameters. *Science* 1977;**198**:1264–67.

2. Kurth CD, Steven JM, Nicolson SC, et al. Kinetics of cerebral deoxygenation during deep hypothermic circulatory arrest in neonates. *Anesthesiology* 1992;**77**:656–61.

3. Yoshitani K, Kawaguchi M, Tatsumi K, et al. A comparison of the INVOS 4100 and the NIRO 300 near infrared spectrophotometers. *Anesth Analg* 2002;**94**:586–590.

4. Kurth CD, Steven JL, Montenegro LM. Cerebral oxygen saturation before congenital heart surgery. *Ann Thorac Surg* 2001;**72**:187–92.

5. Watzman HM, Kurth CD, Montenegro LM, et al. Arterial and venous contributions to near-infrared cerebral oximetry. *Anesthesiology* 2000;**93**:947–53.

6. Dullenkopf A, Frey B, Baenziger O, et al. Measurement of cerebral oxygenation state in anaesthetized children using the INVOS 5100 cerebral oximeter. *Paediatr Anaesth* 2003;**13**:384–91.

7. Rais-Bahrami K, Rivera O, Short BL. Validation of a noninvasive neonatal optical cerebral oximeter in veno-venous ECMO patients with a cephalad catheter. *J Perinatol* 2006;**26**:628–35.

8. Daubeney PE, Pilkington SN, Janke E, et al. Cerebral oxygenation measured by near-infrared spectroscopy: comparison with jugular bulb oximetry. *Ann Thorac Surg* 1996;**61**:930–4.

9. Abdul-Khaliq H, Troitzsch D, Berger F, Lange PE. Regional transcranial oximetry with near infrared spectroscopy (NIRS) in comparison with measuring oxygen saturation in the jugular bulb in infants and children for monitoring cerebral oxygenation. *Biomed Tech (Berl)* 2000;**45**:328–32.

10. Cohn SM. Near infrared spectroscopy: potential clinical benefits in surgery. *J Am Coll Surg* 2007;**205**:322–32.

11. Hoffman GM, Stuth EA, Jacquiss RD, et al. Changes in cerebral and somatic oxygenation during stage I palliation of hypoplastic left heart syndrome using continuous regional cerebral perfusion. *J Thorac Cardiovasc Surg* 2004;**127**:223–33.

12. Meier SD, Eble BK, Stapleton GE, et al. Mesenteric oxyhemoglobin saturation improves with patent ductus arteriosus ligation. *J Perinatol* 2006;**26**:562–64.

13. Edmonds HL, Ganzel BL, Austin EH. Cerebral oximetry for cardiac and vascular surgery. *Semin Cardiothorac Vasc Anesth* 2004;**8**:147–66.

14. Roberts KW, Crnkowic AP, Linneman LJ. Near infrared spectroscopy detects critical cerebral hypoxia during carotid endarterectomy in awake patients. *Anesthesiology* 1998;**89**:A934.

15. Samra SK, Dy EA, Welch K, et al. Evaluation of a cerebral oximeter as a monitor of cerebral ischemia during carotid endarterectomy. *Anesthesiology* 2000;**93**:964–70.

16. Ramamoorthy C, Tabbutt S, Kurth CD. Effects of inspired hypoxic and hypercapnic gas mixtures on cerebral oxygen saturation in neonates with univentricular heart defects. *Anesthesiology* 2002;**96**:283–8.

17. Kurth CD, Levy WJ, McCann J. Near-infrared spectroscopy cerebral oxygen saturation thresholds for hypoxia-ischemia in piglets. *J Cereb Blood Flow Metab* 2002;**22**:335–41.

18. Hou X, Ding H, Teng Y, et al. Research on the relationship between brain anoxia at different regional oxygen saturations and brain damage using near-infrared spectroscopy. *Physiol Meas* 2007**6**;**28**:1251–65.

19. Kurth CD, McCann JC, Wu J, et al. Cerebral oxygen saturation-time threshold for hypoxic-ischemic injury in piglets. *Anesth Analg* 2009;**108**:1268–77.

20. Dent CL, Spaeth JP, Jones BV, et al. Brain magnetic resonance imaging abnormalities after the Norwood procedure using regional cerebral perfusion. *J Thorac Cardiovasc Surg* 2006;**131**:190–7.

21. Austin EH, III, Edmonds HL, Jr., Auden SM. Benefit of neurophysiologic monitoring for pediatric cardiac surgery. *J Thorac Cardiovasc Surg* 1997;**114**:707–15, 717.

22. Janelle GM, Mnookin S, Gravenstein N, et al. Unilateral cerebral oxygen desaturation during emergent repair of a DeBakey type 1 aortic dissection: potential aversion of a major catastrophe. *Anesthesiology.* 2002;**96**:1263–5.

23. Orihashi K, Sueda T, Okada K, Imai K. Near-infrared spectroscopy for monitoring cerebral ischemia during selective cerebral perfusion. *Eur J Cardiothorac Surg* 2004;**26**:907–11.

24. Orihashi K, Sueda T, Okada K, Imai K. Malposition of a selective cerebral perfusion catheter is not a rare event. *Eur J Cardiothorac Surg* 2007;**27**:644–48.

25. Santo KC, Barrios A, Dandekar U, et al. Near-infrared spectroscopy: an important monitoring tool during hybrid aortic arch replacement. *Anesth Analg* 2008;**107**:793–96.

26. Kurth CD, Steven JM, Nicolson SC. Cerebral oxygenation during pediatric cardiac surgery using deep hypothermic circulatory arrest. *Anesthesiology* 1995;**82**:74–82.

27. Greeley WJ, Kern FH, Ungerleider RM. The effect of hypothermic cardiopulmonary bypass and total circulatory arrest on cerebral metabolism in neonates, infants, and children. *J Thorac Cardiovasc Surg* 1991;**101**:783–794.

28. Wypij D, Newburger JW, Rappaport LA, et al. The effect of duration of deep hypothermic circulatory arrest in infant heart surgery on late neurodevelopment: the Boston Circulatory Arrest Trial. *J Thorac Cardiovasc Surg* 2003;**126**:1397–403.

29. Daubeney PE, Smith DC, Pilkington SN. Cerebral oxygenation during paediatric cardiac surgery: identification of vulnerable periods using near infrared spectroscopy. *Eur J Cardiothorac Surg* 1998;**13**:370–7.

30. Andropoulos DB, Diaz LK, Stayer SA, et al. Is bilateral monitoring of cerebral oxygen saturation necessary during neonatal aortic arch reconstruction? *Anesth Analg* 2004;**98**:1267–72.

31. Kussman BD, Wypij D, DiNardo JA, et al. An evaluation of bilateral monitoring of cerebral oxygen saturation during pediatric cardiac surgery. *Anesth Analg* 2005;**101**:1294–1300.

32. Moritz S, Kasprzak P, Arlt M, et al. Accuracy of cerebral monitoring during carotid endarterectomy: a comparison of transcranial Doppler sonography, near-infrared spectroscopy, stump pressure, and somatosensory evoked potentials. *Anesthesiology* 2007;**107**:563–9.

33. Bhatia R, Hampton T, Malde S, et al. The application of near infrared oximetry to cerebral monitoring during aneurysm embolization: a comparison with intraprocedural angiography. *J Neurosurg Anesthesiol* 2007;**19**:97–104.

34. Giacomuzzi C, Heller E, Mejak B, et al. Assessing the brain using near infrared spectroscopy during postoperative ventricular circulatory support. *Cardiol Young* 2005;**15**:154–8.

35. Tortoriello TA, Stayer SA, Mott AR, et al. A non-invasive estimation of mixed venous oxygen saturation using near infrared spectroscopy by cerebral oximetry in pediatric cardiac surgery patients. *Pediatr Anesth* 2005;**15**:495–503.

36. Bhutta AT, Ford JW, Parker JG, et al. Noninvasive cerebral oximeter as a surrogate for mixed venous saturation in children. *Pediatr Cardiol* 2007;**28**:34–41.

37. Smith J, Bricker S, Putnam B. Tissue oxygen saturation predicts the need for early blood transfusion in trauma patients. *Am Surg* 2008;**74**:1006–11.

38. Cohn SM, Nathens AB, Moore FA, et al. Tissue oxygen saturation predicts the development of organ dysfunction during traumatic shock resuscitation. *J Trauma* 2007;**62**:44–55.

39. Ives CL, Harrison DK, Stansby GS. Prediction of surgical site infections after major surgery using visible and near-infrared spectroscopy. *Adv Exp Med Biol* 2007;**599**:37–44.

40. Hoffman GM, Ghanayem NS, Mussatto KM, et al. Postoperative two-site NIRS predicts complications and mortality after stage 1 palliation of hypoplastic left heart syndrome. *Anesthesiology* 2007;**107**:A234.

41. Kaufman J, Almodovar MC, Zuk J, Freisen RH. Correlation of abdominal site near infrared spectroscopy with gastric tonometry in infants following surgery for congenital heart disease. *Pediatr Crit Care Med* 2008;**9**:62–8.

42. Nollert G, Möhnle P, Tassani-Prell P, et al. Postoperative neuropsychological dysfunction and cerebral oxygenation during cardiac surgery. *Thorac Cardiovasc Surg* 1995;**43**:260–4.

43. Yao FF, Tseng CA, Ho CA, et al. Cerebral oxygen desaturation is associated with early postoperative neuropsychological dysfunction in patients undergoing cardiac surgery. *J Cardiothorac Vasc Anesth* 2004;**18**:552–8.

44. Goldman S, Sutter F, Ferdinand F, Trace C. Optimizing intraoperative cerebral oxygen delivery using noninvasive cerebral oximetry decreases the incidence of stroke for cardiac surgical patients. *Heart Surg Forum.* 2004;**7**:E376–81.

45. Murkin JM, Adams SJ, Novick RJ, et al. Monitoring brain oxygen saturation during coronary bypass surgery: a randomized, prospective study. *Anesth Analg* 2007;**104**:51–8.

46. Kurth CD, Steven JM, Nicolson SC. Cerebral oxygenation during pediatric cardiac surgery using deep hypothermic circulatory arrest. *Anesthesiology* 1995;**82**:74–82.

47. McQuillen PS, Barkovich AJ, Hamrick SE, et al. Temporal and anatomic risk profile of brain injury with neonatal repair of congenital heart defects. *Stroke* 2007;**38** [part 2]:736–41.

48. Hoffman GM, Mussatto KM, Brosig CL, et al. Cerebral oxygenation and neurodevelopmental outcome in hypoplastic left heart syndrome. *Anesthesiology* 2008;**109**:A7 (Abstract).

49. Toet MC, Flinterman A, van de Laar I, et al. Cerebral oxygen saturation and electrical brain activity before, during, and up to 36 hours after arterial switch procedure in neonates without pre-existing brain damage: its relationship to neurodevelopmental outcome. *Exp Brain Res* 2005;**165**:343–50.

50. Kussman BD, Wypij D, DiNardo JA, et al. Cerebral oximetry during infant cardiac surgery: evaluation and relationship to early postoperative outcome. *Anesth Analg* 2009;**108**:1122–31.

51. Andropoulos DB, East DL, Stapleton GE, et al. Postoperative cerebral oxyhemoglobin saturation in neonates undergoing cardiac surgery with cardiopulmonary bypass. *Anesthesiology* 2005;**103**:A1340.

52. Gottlieb EA, Fraser CD, Andropoulos DB, Diaz LK. Bilateral monitoring of cerebral oxygen saturation results in recognition of aortic cannula malposition during pediatric congenital heart surgery. *Paediatr Anaesth* 2006;**16**:787–9.

53. Ing RJ, Lawson DS, Jaggers J, et al. Detection of unintended partial superior vena cava occlusion during a bidirectional cavopulmonary anastomosis. *J Cardiothorac Vasc Anesth* 2004;**18**:472–74.

54. Redlin M, Koster A, Huenbler M, et al. Regional differences in tissue oxygenation during cardiopulmonary bypass for correction of congenital heart disease in neonates and small infants: relevance of near infrared spectroscopy. *J Thorac Cardiovasc Surg* 2008;**136**:962–7.

55. Hirsch JC, Charpie JR, Ohye RG, Gurney JG. Near infrared spectroscopy: what we know and what we need to know – a systematic review of the congenital heart disease literature. *J Thorac Cardiovasc Surg* 2009;**137**:154–9.

56. Pedersen T, Pedersen BD, Moller AM. Pulse oximetry for perioperative monitoring. *Cochrane Database Syst Rev* 2003;**2**:CD002013.

57. Davies KJ, Janelle GM. Con: all cardiac surgical patients should not have intraoperative cerebral oxygenation monitoring. *J Cardiothorac Vasc Anesth* 2006;**20**:450–55.

58. Madsden PL, Skak C, Rasmussen A, Secher NH. Interference of cerebral near infrared oximetry in patients with icterus. *Anesth Analg* 2000;**90**:489–93.

59. McDonaugh DL, McDaniel MR, Monk TG. The effect of intravenous indigo carmine on near infrared cerebral oximetry. *Anesth Analg* 2007;**105**:704–6.

60. Hoffman GM. Neurological monitoring on cardiopulmonary bypass: What are we obligated to do? *Ann Thorac Surg* 2006;**81**:S273–80.

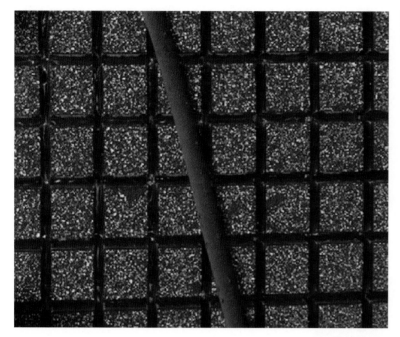

Plate I. Matrix array with 2500 independent elements representing the basis for real-time 3D scanning. Human hair is shown to better demonstrate dimensions. (See Figure 11.1.)

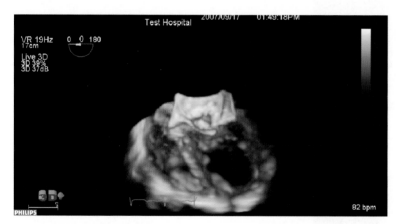

Plate II. Live 3D real-time scanning showing a 3D volume pyramid. (See Figure 11.2.)

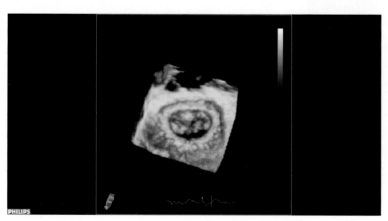

Plate III. 3D zoom mode. En face view of mitral valve after repair and annuloplasty. This view is real-time and devoid of ECG artifacts. (See Figure 11.3.)

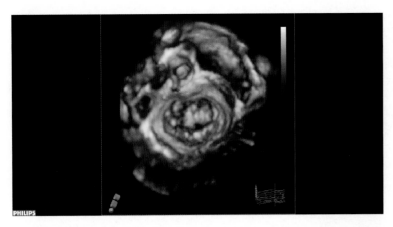

Plate IV. Full volume image. Four to eight ECG gated slabs are stitched together, enabling the acquisition of a larger volume without loss of frame rate or resolution. (See Figure 11.4.)

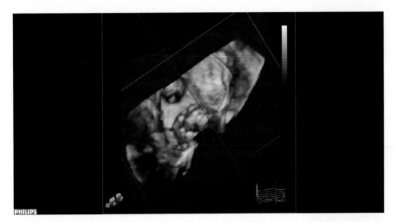

Plate V. Same image as shown in Figure 11.4. The operator has spatially reoriented the dataset and started to crop with the intent to better expose a region of interest. (See Figure 11.5.)

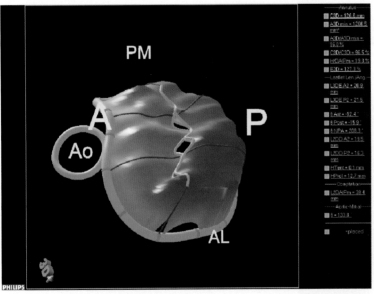

Plate VI. The 3D dataset can be quantified using semiautomatic software. The model created shows the relationship of the leaflet to the annular plane (red above, blue below). True volumes and unforeshortened distances can be measured. (See Figure 11.6.)

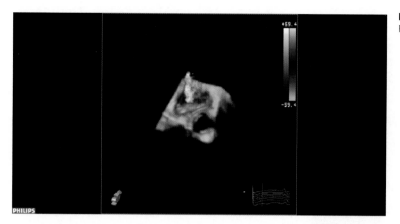

Plate VII. 3D color Doppler gated. Concentric jet originating from P2. Valve viewed from anterior to posterior. (See Figure 11.7.)

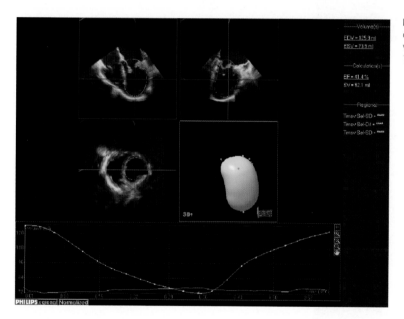

Plate VIII. Semiautomatic software with endocardial border detection capability enabling the measurement of true ventricular volumes and calculation of a true ejection fraction. (See Figure 11.25.)

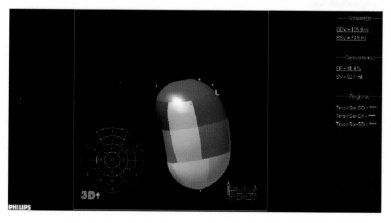

Plate IX. Myocardial segmental model of the left ventricle as reconstructed by software from a 3D dataset. (See Figure 11.27.)

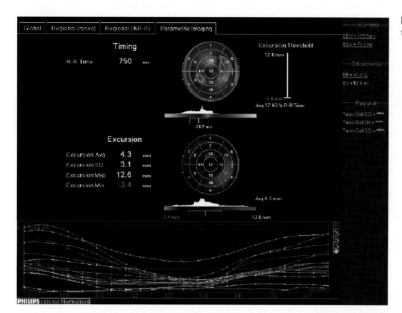

Plate X. Sixteen-segment model showing timing and excursion of the individual segments. (See Figure 11.28.)

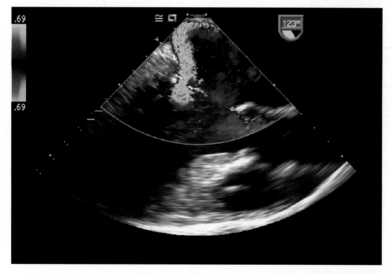

Plate XI. Eccentric mitral valve regurgitant jet. (See Figure 11.33.)

Perioperative monitoring of neuromuscular function

Aaron F. Kopman

Abbreviations

μQ	Microcoulombs
AMG	Acceleromyographic, acceleromyography
AP	Adductor pollicis
ASA	American Society of Anesthesiologists
CRE	Critical respiratory event
DBS	Double-burst stimulation
dTc	d-Tubocurarine
ECG	Electrocardiograph, electrocardiogram
EMG	Electromyographic, electromyogram
HL	Head lift (test)
Hz	Hertz (frequency); 1.0 Hz is one stimulus/sec. 0.10 Hz is one stimulus/10 sec.
ITS	Initial threshold for stimulation
KMG	Kinemyography
mA	Milliampere
MMG	Mechanomyographic, mechanomyogram
msec	Millisecond
NMBD	Neuromuscular blocking drug
PACU	Postanesthesia care unit
PMG	Acoustic or phonomyography
PNS	Peripheral nerve stimulator
PONB	Residual postoperative neuromuscular block
PTC	Posttetanic count
PTP	Posttetanic potentiation
SMS	Supramaximal stimulation
T1	Magnitude of an evoked single twitch response. The response to 0.10 Hz stimuli, or the first response of the train-of-four train.
TOF	Train-of-four
TOFC	TOF count

Introduction

In the years immediately following the introduction of d-tubocurarine (dTc) into the anesthesiologist's armamentarium in 1942,[1] considerable controversy arose concerning the indications for and the safety of this new class of drugs when used in day-to-day clinical practice. A tale (perhaps apocryphal) goes as follows: Emery Rovenstine, chairman of anesthesiology at Bellevue Hospital in New York, was given several vials of Intocostrin (curare, dTc), the commercial extract of *Chondrodendron tomentosum*, by the manufacturer (E. R. Squibb & Sons) to "try out." He ultimately returned several of the vials to the company unopened with the comment, "This drug has no future. It depresses ventilation."

Nevertheless, by the mid-1940s the use of dTc as adjunct to anesthesia was gaining considerable popularity and large case studies[2,3] began to appear. Review articles[4,5] followed soon afterward. However, little advice was offered to the clinician as to how to evaluate the depth of neuromuscular block or the adequacy of recovery. A 1953 paper by Morris and associates[6] probably accurately reflects the best clinical advice of the period: At the end of surgery, small doses of an anticholinesterase were administered until "ventilatory exchange seemed improved, and additional doses administered at 5 min intervals achieved no detectable change for the better." The ability of the patient to perform a "head lift" was considered evidence that he would continue to be able to take care of himself satisfactorily "without danger of hypoventilation and [airway] obstruction."

However, a 1954 paper by Beecher and Todd[7] again focused the attention of the specialty on the safety of all neuromuscular blocking drugs (NMBDs). In that now-notorious report, the authors suggested that these drugs had an inherent toxicity and were associated with a patient mortality rate six times that found in patients not receiving muscle relaxants. Although these conclusions were vigorously refuted,[8] they did serve a purpose. It became obvious that clinicians needed a better way of monitoring the perioperative effects of NMBDs. In 1958, Christie and Churchill-Davidson suggested that the indirectly evoked mechanical response to nerve stimulation might prove to be practical clinical tool in the diagnosis of prolonged apnea after the use of muscle relaxants and described a small battery-powered peripheral nerve stimulator (PNS) that they used for this purpose.[9] The following year, the same authors published what well may be the first objective study of the effects of various muscle relaxants and their acetylcholinesterase antagonists on neuromuscular transmission in anesthetized humans.[10]

However, it was not until the mid-1960s that the effort to move PNS devices into the operating room gained some critical mass. In 1965, two new commercially available PNS units were described,[11,12] and an editorial in *Anesthesiology*[13] opined, "The only satisfactory method of determining the degree of neuromuscular block is to stimulate a motor nerve with an electric current and observe the contraction of the muscles innervated by that nerve." Forty years later, another editorial in *Anesthesiology* presented this position more forcefully, that "it is time to introduce objective neuromuscular monitoring in all operating rooms. . . . [It] is an evidence-based practice and should consequently be used whenever a nondepolarizing neuromuscular blocking agent is administered. Such monitoring is noninvasive, has little risk, and there are strong reasons to believe that its use can improve patient outcome."[14]

Nevertheless, 50 years after PNSs were first suggested as aids in monitoring neuromuscular function, the utility of these instruments is still being argued.[15] In its published *Standards for Basic Anesthetic Monitoring* (last amended by the House of Delegates in October 2005), the American Society of Anesthesiologists (ASA) remained silent on the need for neuromuscular monitoring. The recent *Report of the ASA Task Force on Postanesthetic Care* stated, "Assessment of neuromuscular function primarily includes physical examination and on occasion *may* include neuromuscular monitoring."[16]

This chapter attempts to outline what we have learned in the last half-century about how to monitor neuromuscular function in the perioperative period and how we now define adequate recovery from nondepolarizing neuromuscular block. Finally, an attempt is made to address the apparent disconnect between "expert" editorial opinion and "official" practice guidelines.

The indirectly evoked response

Clinically used muscle relaxants have no effect on muscle contractility or on muscle membrane excitability. Hence, direct muscle stimulation will still result in a vigorous mechanical response, even when the level of drug-induced paralysis is profound. The depth of neuromuscular block must be measured by stimulating the motor nerve that innervates the muscle being studied and observing the indirectly evoked mechanical or electrical response.

The muscles of greatest interest to the anesthesiologist are the diaphragm, the masseter, the vocal cord abductors, and the accessory muscles of respiration. Unfortunately, all are technically difficult to study objectively and noninvasively. Because the ulnar nerve is quite superficial at the wrist and adduction of the thumb is easy to measure mechanically, the vast bulk of what we know about the clinical pharmacology of NMBDs comes from our study of this nerve–muscle group. As we will see later in this chapter, the evoked response of the adductor pollicis muscle (AP) has become a useful and reliable surrogate marker for other aspects of neuromuscular recovery such as respiratory mechanical reserve. For the remainder of this chapter, the reader should assume that the nerve–muscle group under discussion refers to the ulnar nerve and AP unless told otherwise.

Motor nerve stimulation

The electrical stimulus necessary to depolarize a single nerve fiber is a function of both the current applied to the cell

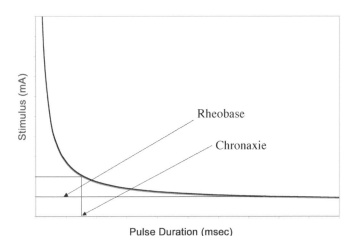

Figure 22.1. The electrical stimulus required for nerve depolarization is a product of the current delivered and the pulse duration. This is best expressed in microcoulombs, which is an expression of electrical charge. The shape of this stimulus–duration relationship approximates a rectangular parabola [$y = (k/x) + b$, where b is the rheobase and k is a constant]. The *rheobase* is that current below which depolarization will not occur regardless of the pulse duration. The *chronaxie* is the minimum time over which an electric current twice the strength of the rheobase needs to be applied to initiate depolarization.

membrane and the duration of that application (see Figure 22.1). Thus it is not the applied current that determines neural stimulation[17] but the electrical charge expressed in microcoulombs[1] (μQ) that is the determining factor.

Pulse durations greater than 0.30 msec should be avoided for several reasons. In large mammalian nerve fibers, the absolute refractory period is about 0.60 to 0.80 msec. Consequently, electrical pulses greater than 0.50 msec may result in repetitive firing.[18] In addition, excessively long pulses may result in direct muscle stimulation (see Figure 22.2).[19] Finally, because the chronaxie of unmyelinated C fibers approximates 0.40 msec,[20] pulse durations of this duration or greater are more likely to be painful in the conscious subject.

Very short pulse durations present a different problem. Chronaxie values in peripheral A-alpha fibers range from 0.05 to 0.10 msec[20] but may be as high as 0.17 msec in some motor nerves.[21] As a result, at pulse durations less than 0.10 msec, milliamperage (mA) requirements may rise exponentially. Thus, for entirely sound theoretical and practical reasons, most commercially available PNSs designed for use in the operating room employ a fixed 0.20-msec pulse duration. (In the following paragraphs, current will be given, rather than μQ, as a measure of the electrical stimulus because mA [at a pulse duration of 0.20 msec] is the value displayed by most PNS units.)

The typical motor nerve may contain thousands of individual nerve fibers. Although each axon is activated in an all-or-none fashion, the sensitivity or threshold required for depolarization varies from one to another in a normal distribution. Hence the number of axons firing (i.e. the force of contraction) has a Gaussian relationship to the stimulus delivered. This plots as a sigmoid curve (see Figure 22.3a). Figure 22.3b[22] is an actual

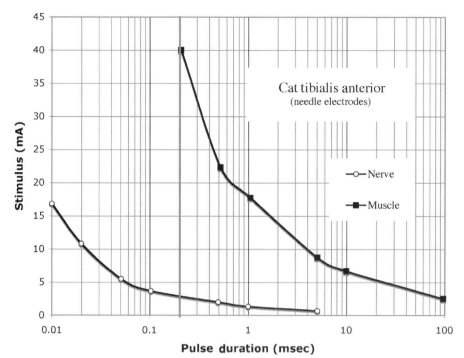

Figure 22.2. Stimulus–duration curve: direct vs. indirect muscle stimulation. As pulse duration increases above 0.20 msec (vertical gray line), direct muscle stimulation becomes more likely. Redrawn from ref. 19, with permission.

plot of the force generated at the thumb (AP muscle) when the ulnar nerve is stimulated by surface electrodes.

Several points are worth noting. Below a certain stimulus (in this case, 12 mA), no response is evoked. As delivered currents exceed this initial threshold for stimulation (ITS), small increases in current produce large increments in evoked force. Finally, a point is reached at which presumably the stimulus is of sufficient intensity to achieve activation of all fibers in the nerve bundle. An attempt is usually made to deliver an electric charge at least 20 percent greater than this (supramaximal maximal stimulation [SMS]) so the clinician can be confident that small decreases in the delivered stimulus will not result in significant changes in the evoked response. Using conventional ECG pre-gelled surface electrodes, typical SMS requirements for the ulnar nerve approximate 30 to 40 mA for a 60-kg female patient, but may reach 80 mA or more for a very obese or large individual. A good rough rule of thumb is to administer not less than 25 mA above the ITS.[23] This assumes proper electrode placement and polarity (negative electrode distal).[24–26] (Later is this chapter we discuss the usefulness and validity of using submaximal stimuli in certain clinical situations.)

Conventional nerve stimulators

By the mid 1980s, at least a half-dozen PNSs were being marketed to anesthesiologists for use in monitoring neuromuscular function. Unfortunately, the vast majority of these units were poorly suited to the task. Many of the early units had pulse durations in excess of 0.50 msec. Almost all were "constant voltage" devices. The user adjusted a dial (usually calibrated from

1 to10) connected to a potentiometer, which increased delivered voltage from zero to the unit's maximum output. For any given voltage setting, the delivered current was a function of skin/electrode resistance/impedance (I = E/R). The majority of these early units had maximum current outputs of <30 mA into a 470-ohm load,[17] and even less at the impedances (1–2 K ohms) encountered using pre-gelled surface electrodes.[27] Thus, for any given dial setting, delivered current might vary over time if skin or electrode impedance changed or battery output decreased. Top-of-the-line constant-voltage devices did, however, often incorporate a miniammeter, which gave the user some idea of the delivered current. Unfortunately, it is still possible to purchase constant-voltage units, which clearly are only of historic interest. Caveat emptor.

A more up-to-date PNS is the constant-current device.[28,29] With these units, the user selects the stimulus (in mA) to be delivered. The device then increases or decreases the voltage generated to compensate for changes in skin or electrode impedance. If the desired current cannot be delivered (e.g. because of a weak battery), an alarm is displayed to so inform the clinician. Most present-day PNS units are now rated to deliver at least 60 mA, and often 80 mA, into a 1000-ohm (1K) load with a pulse duration of 0.20 msec (some offer 0.30 msec as an option).

Patterns of stimulation

One of the hallmarks of nondepolarizing neuromuscular block is fade or decrement in force following repetitive nerve stimulation. This characteristic can be used for exploring the depth of paralysis.

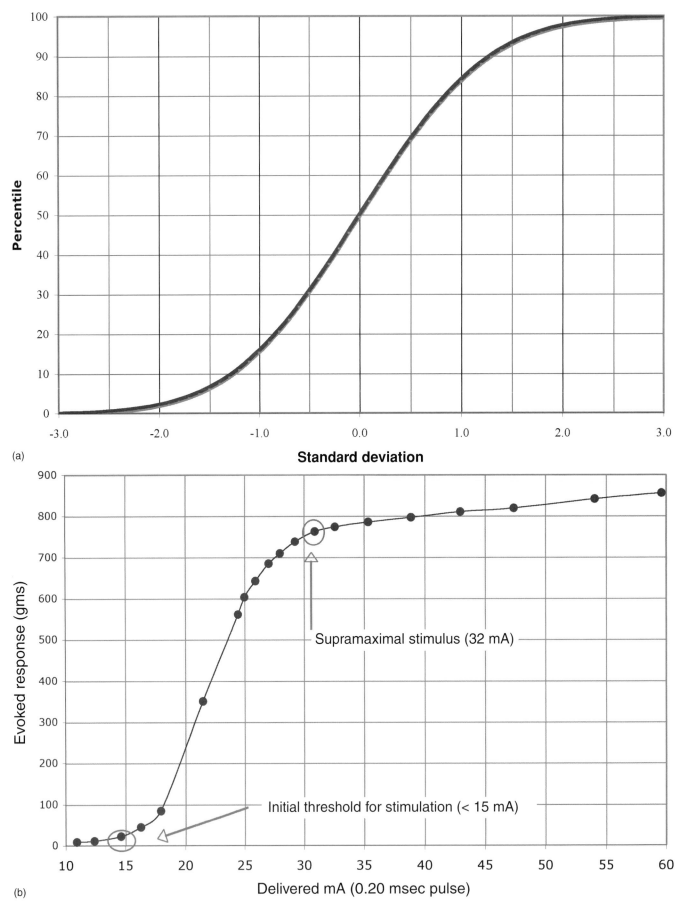

Figure 22.3. Although the normal distribution is usually plotted as a bell-shaped curve, it can also be expressed as percentile plot, which assumes a sigmoid shape (a). Note the similarity of (a) to (b), a sample plot that was obtained by stimulation of the ulnar nerve with surface electrodes and plotting the evoked response of the AP muscle (data from ref. 22). The rising plateau seen in (b) is probably the result of recruiting additional motor nerves at high delivered mA values.

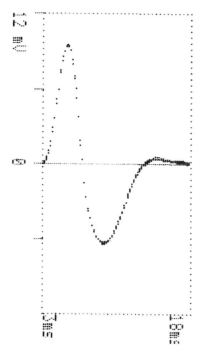

Figure 22.4. Printout from a Datex NMT 221 EMG Monitor. The trace starts at 3 msec after the stimulus and ends 15 msec later. The wave form has a duration of approximately 10.5 msec and total amplitude peak to peak of 16.3 mV. This control trace actually contains the data from four superimposed responses taken at 0.5 Hz. The fact that only one trace is visible demonstrates that the TOF ratio approximated 1.0.

Single twitch

Single stimuli at rates of 0.10 Hz (1 twitch every 10 sec) or slower show minimal or no fade upon repetition, even in the partially paralyzed subject. Thus, the single twitch (T1) response has been used as the standard when determining the potency of neuromuscular blocking drugs. If a 0.10 mg/kg dose of drug X reduces T1 to 5 percent of control in an average subject at a stimulation rate of 0.10 Hz, we say that this dose is the ED_{95} (effective dose to produce 95 percent twitch depression in an average

patient). However, 0.10 Hz stimulation is not very useful to the clinician unless the control response is first measured with an objective monitor, such as a force transducer or an electromyographic analyzer – instrumentation not available in most operating rooms. Subjective evaluation of the strength of the evoked response, as we will see later, is extremely unreliable.

Repetitive single stimuli

EMG recordings

The electromyographic (EMG) response lasts less than 20 msec (see Figure 22.4). Thus, at stimulation rates as high as 50 Hz, the evoked response to each stimulus is discrete and separate. In the unparalyzed subject, even at 50 Hz stimulation, the twitch response is well maintained. In the patient partially paralyzed with a nondepolarizing blocker, the magnitude of the evoked response decreases as the frequency increases (see Figure 22.5).[30] Frequencies greater than 5 Hz produce no further decrement.

Mechanical recordings

The mechanical response to repetitive stimulation is more complicated. In the absence of NMBDs, indirect muscle stimulation normally results in evoked responses that do not show any change in magnitude as the frequency of repetition is increased up to about 4 Hz. However, the mechanical response of the AP to a single SMS takes between 250 and 300 msec from the start of contraction to full relaxation of the muscle and return to baseline (see Figure 22.6). Thus, at frequencies ≥4 Hz, complete muscle relaxation cannot occur before the next stimulus is applied. The result is failure of the muscle to return to baseline between stimuli. At stimulus rates of 30 Hz to 50 Hz, the result is a sustained (tetanic) contraction.

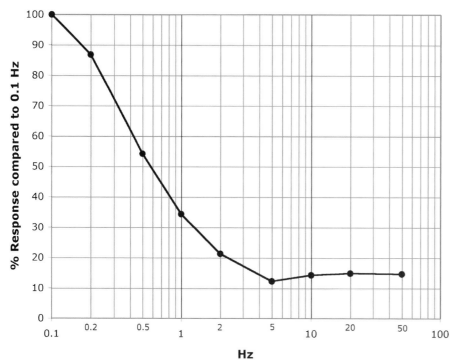

Figure 22.5. The effect of increasing twitch frequency on the evoked electromyographic response in man. In this study, T1 was decreased by 50% from control at 0.10 Hz by dTc. The y-axis represents the percent decrement from this value as the rate of stimulation increases. Maximum decrease is seen at 5 Hz. Note the lack of EMG tetanic response. Redrawn from ref. 30.

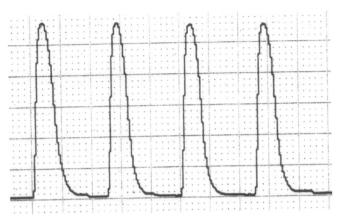

Figure 22.6. A control TOF. Four stimuli at 2 Hz (1 stimulus every 0.50 sec). The fourth response is 98% of the first, a TOF ratio of 0.98. Duration of each twitch response = approx. 300 μsec. This is a trace from a mechanomyographic recording.

Tetanic stimuli

In the unparalyzed individual, the mechanical response to 30- to 50-Hz stimulation of 5 sec duration is well sustained, the force of which is usually five to eight times greater than that generated by a single supramaximal stimulus. As stimulation rates increase above 50 Hz (up 250 Hz), the peak tetanic response remains unaltered, although tetanic fade now begins to appear. The higher the frequency, the greater the fade and the sooner it appears. At 200 Hz, even a 2-sec tetanus cannot be sustained.[31] A tetanic stimulus also has an effect on subsequent single-twitch responses; this effect depends on the tetanic frequency and the recording mode employed. When the force of contraction is measured (mechanomyography [MMG]) following a 30-Hz tetanus, there is usually some transient increase (20%–25%) in the height of the subsequently evoked twitch response. This posttetanic potentiation (PTP) or facilitation is not seen when the response is measured electromyographically, and represents a change in muscle contractility.[32] Following a 50-Hz tetanus, PTP is no longer seen with MMG recordings, and at even higher frequencies posttetanic twitch depression is the rule.[31]

In contrast with the control conditions just described, tetanic fade and PTP are prominent features of nondepolarizing block, even when measured electromyographically, and the tetanic frequency is as low as 30 Hz.[32] When T1 is reduced to 35 percent of control by dTc, a 30-Hz tetanus may fade by as much as 80 percent over five seconds, and PTP may transiently increase the reduced twitch height by more than 250 percent.[33]

Because stimuli greater than 50 Hz may demonstrate fade even in the absence of blocking agents, many experts feel that these stimuli are unphysiologic and should not be used to monitor perioperative neuromuscular function.[34] Kopman and colleages[35] found that when the train-of-four (TOF) fade ratio (discussed later in this chapter) indicated that recovery from nondepolarizing block was almost complete (a ratio of 0.80), a 2-sec 100-Hz tetanus still resulted in more than a 70 percent decrement in tetanic force. They concluded that 100 Hz was too

sensitive a test for routine clinical use. Using this parameter as a guide, a clinician might be led to administer reversal agents that are simply not required. This opinion is not universally shared; there are proponents of the utility of 100-Hz stimulation exactly because it is such a sensitive indicator of residual block.[36]

The posttetanic count

Measurement of twitch height has its limitations. As the level of neuromuscular block is intensified, the response to 0.10 Hz stimulation eventually disappears. How, then, is the clinician to tell if the patient is just 100 percent blocked or if, in fact, the level of paralysis is considerably more intense? A clever answer to this problem was devised by Viby-Mogensen and fellow researchers,[37] who noted that the phenomenon of PTP may be a useful tool when evaluating profound nondepolarizing block. They observed that, following a tetanus, it was often possible to briefly detect a response to single stimuli when no twitch was evident prior to the tetanus. They then suggested a stimulus sequence consisting of a 5-sec 50-Hz tetanus, a 3-sec pause, followed by 20 stimuli at one second intervals. As patients recover from deep neuromuscular block, initially only one posttetanic twitch can be detected (a posttetanic count of 1; PTC = 1). As recovery progresses, the PTC increases. They were able to show that the PTC gave a rough guide as to the time it would take for an evoked response to a single stimulus to recover in the absence of PTP. In general this occurs when the PTC has recovered to a value approximating 10 responses.[38]

Train-of-four stimulation

The literature on monitoring of neuromuscular function in the perioperative period can be divided into modern and premodern periods. The date for that division is 1970. It was in that year that Ali, Utting, and Gray suggested that four stimuli delivered at half-second intervals might prove useful to the clinician in diagnosing the extent of nondepolarizing block.[39] They recognized that "as the frequency of stimulation was increased there was a reduction in the amplitude of the recorded twitch response in curarized subjects, and that this reduction appeared to depend on the degree of curarization." Perhaps their most important insight was that this sequence did not require the clinician to first establish a control baseline to evaluate the evoked response.

In their initial paper, the authors raised several important issues. They noted that "the importance of particular levels of block as measured in this manner remain to be assessed," and "it is important … to establish the degree of reversal of neuromuscular block, which is compatible with safe return to the ward, and it seems probable that this can be achieved using the train-of-four stimuli."

The authors proceeded to provide initial answers to these questions with two now-classic studies the following year. In the first they defended the use of only four stimuli, noting that additional stimuli produced little or no additional fade.[40] Of greater importance, it was in this paper that they suggested

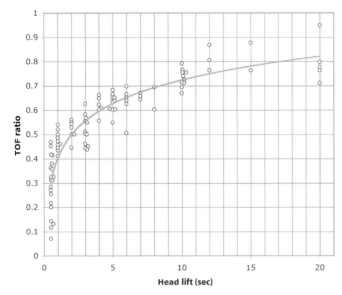

Figure 22.7. The relationship between the TOF ratio and the ability to perform a voluntary head lift after reversal of nondepolarizing block with neostigmine. Best-fit trendline added by the present author. Redrawn from ref. 41.

Table 22.1. The TOF ratio as a measure of mechanical respiratory reserve[†]

TOF ratio	Vital capacity*	Neg. insp. force*	Peak exp. flow rate*
0.60	91.2%	70.3%	95%
0.70	96.5	81.6	92.2
0.80	99.9	87.9	94.1
0.90	99.5	90.9	94.5
1.00	99.7	96.6	99.2

* Values expressed as % of control.
[†] From ref. 42.

that the important parameter to be measured was the height of the fourth response divided by the height of the first response (T4/T1), or the TOF ratio. In a companion paper,[41] they correlated this ratio with the ability of patients to perform a head lift maneuver. They concluded that obvious muscle weakness was associated with TOF values less than 0.60. However, it was not until the TOF ratio was 0.70 (see Figure 22.7) that patients could sustain a 10-sec head lift.

Ali and coworkers refined the clinical respiratory correlates of the TOF ratio four years later, in a paper that remains a classic in the neuromuscular literature.[42] In that study of eight volunteers, control vital capacity, peak expiratory flow rate, and the maximum negative inspiratory force that could be measured with an aneroid manometer were first recorded. These tests were employed as measures of mechanical respiratory reserve. Each subject was then administered small doses of dTc until the TOF ratio, measured mechanomyographically, was 0.60 or less. The tests of respiratory function were then repeated at this level of block and at frequent intervals as spontaneous recovery progressed. At a TOF ratio of 0.60, vital capacity and peak expiratory flow rate were still at 90 percent or greater of control values (see Table 22.1). Based on these data, the authors suggested that a TOF ratio ≥0.60 "would indicate that respiratory muscle function should be more than adequate for providing sustained spontaneous ventilation and pulmonary toilet." However, Ali later revised this value upward to 0.70, because he determined that a TOF ratio ≥0.70 "reliably indicates the recovery of single twitch to control height and a sustained response to tetanic stimulation at 50 Hz for 5 sec."[34] In addition, he and colleagues concluded that a TOF ratio of 0.70 correlates well with clinical signs of recovery in healthy[43] as well as ASA class III and IV patients.[44] As a result of these seminal studies, for the next two

decades a TOF ratio of 0.70 was accepted as defining adequate recovery from nondepolarizing neuromuscular block.

Although there is no reason to doubt the validity of Ali's volunteer data (Table 22.1), this study can be viewed more critically from today's perspective. First, the maximum negative inspiratory force did not return to 90 percent of control until the TOF ratio was 0.90. Of greater interest is anecdotal information that was never published. One of the volunteers studied by Ali related the following in a personal communication with this author: At a time when the subject's measured TOF ratio was 0.70, he felt distinctly unsteady on his feet and had difficulty flexing his knees. Even at a TOF ratio of 0.90, he did not feel "right." In fact, it took an additional three hours before he felt totally "normal." This conversation suggested that even though a TOF of 0.70 might represent adequate return of respiratory mechanics, it does not necessarily mean that it is synonymous with a patient being ready for discharge to home. This probably did not have much practical import in 1975 when ambulatory surgery was in its infancy. In the mid-1970s, an admission for repair of an inguinal hernia often meant the better part of a week in the hospital. Twenty years later, the issue of "street readiness" and the criteria for "satisfactory" recovery from nondepolarizing block became a subject of renewed interest.

By the early 1990s, evidence began to accumulate that adverse physiologic events might be associated with TOF ratios previously thought to represent adequate recovery. In an elegant study of awake volunteers partially paralyzed with vecuronium, Eriksson and colleagues[45] were able to establish that even modest levels of block might have unexpected consequences. They demonstrated conclusively that at a TOF ratio of 0.70, the ventilatory response to hypoxia was muted, presumably by an effect at the carotid body.

A subsequent paper from this group was even more disquieting.[46] In this study of 14 healthy awake volunteers, a catheter with embedded pressure transducers was placed via the nose with the tip in the cervical esophagus. Control pressure measurements during swallowing were obtained at the upper esophageal sphincter, the base of the tongue, and at two levels from the pharyngeal sphincter muscle. Then, during partial paralysis with vecuronium (TOF values 0.60 to 0.90), these pressures were again measured while simultaneous videoradiographic images were recorded as the subjects swallowed a radiopaque dye. Volunteers showed misdirected swallowing with episodes of aspiration at TOF ratios of 0.60 ($n = 4$), 0.70 ($n = 3$), and 0.80 ($n = 1$). All episodes showed penetration of the bolus contrast immediately above or to the level of the vocal cords (i.e. laryngeal penetration). The authors were also able to demonstrate changes in upper esophageal sphincter resting muscle tone, decreases in bolus transit time, and impaired coordination between esophageal sphincter relaxation and pharyngeal constrictor contraction at TOF levels of 0.60 to 0.80. They concluded that partial paralysis causes pharyngeal dysfunction and increased risk for aspiration at mechanical AP TOF ratios <0.90. In humans allowed to recover spontaneously, pharyngeal function is not normalized until an AP TOF ratio >0.90 is reached.

At about this time, the present author became interested in the question of "street-readiness." He and his coworkers recruited 10 healthy young volunteers for the following protocol.[47] Control measurements of grip strength in kilograms were obtained with a dynamometer. Arterial oxygen saturation was estimated by pulse oximetry. In addition, a standard wooden tongue depressor was placed between each subject's upper and lower incisor teeth, and the subject was told not to let the investigator remove it. All subjects were easily able to retain the device despite vigorous attempts to dislodge it. Control TOF values were obtained electromyographically; these values were continually recorded at 20-sec intervals for the remainder of the study. An infusion of mivacurium was then begun and was continued until the TOF ratio decreased to <0.70. It was then adjusted to keep it in the range of 0.65 to 0.75.

When infusion rates and the TOF ratio were stable for at least 10 minutes, grip strength and the tongue depressor test were repeated. In addition, the subjects were asked to perform a 5- and 10-sec head lift, to sip water from a straw, to attempt to visually track a moving object, and to report any symptoms that they felt were noteworthy. When these observations were complete, the infusion rate was decreased, the TOF ratio was then allowed to recover to a value of 0.85 to 0.90, and all the tests were repeated. The infusion was then stopped. TOF measurements were continued until a ratio of 1.0 was attained, when a final set of observations was recorded. No volunteer required intervention to maintain a patent airway, and arterial oxygen saturations while breathing room air were ≥96% at all times. However, a TOF ratio of 0.70 was accompanied by significant signs and symptoms of weakness. None of the subjects considered themselves even remotely "street ready" at this time. Grip strength was decreased to 57 ± 11 percent of control, and only one subject could retain the tongue depressor between his teeth when the investigator attempted to remove it (using only two fingers on the blade). Several subjects could not sip water through a straw because they could not make a tight seal around it with their lips. Most subjects had some difficulty in swallowing, and all experienced diplopia and difficulty in following a moving object at this level of block. However, all subjects could sustain a 5-sec head lift once the TOF ratio was 0.75. The tongue depressor test was not passed until the TOF ratio had returned

to a value, on average, of 0.85. As the level of block receded, so did symptoms, but even at a TOF ratio of 0.90 grip strength was depressed by an average of 16 percent and all subjects still reported visual disturbances.

As a result of these studies,[45–47] there has emerged a consensus[48] that a TOF ratio of 0.70 at the AP is no longer an acceptable standard of neuromuscular recovery. A value of 0.90 is now viewed as the minimum value synonymous with satisfactory return of neuromuscular function.

Subjective measurement of the TOF ratio, double burst stimulation, and tetanic fade

The preceding recommendations notwithstanding, the vast majority of anesthesia providers do not currently have access to the instrumentation necessary to measure the TOF ratio in real time (see the section on objective monitoring later in this chapter), and, unfortunately, evaluation of the TOF ratio, by either palpation of the thumb or by visual observation, is notoriously inaccurate. Subjective evaluation requires the observer to remember the magnitude of the first response in the train, ignore the next two responses, and then compare the fourth to the first evoked response. This is not easy to do. Once the TOF ratio exceeds 0.40, most clinicians cannot detect the presence of any fade at all.[49] Thus it is basically impossible to be sure, by subjective methods, whether the TOF ratio is 0.50 or 0.95. Subjective estimation of fade using 50-Hz stimulation is equally insensitive. Tetanic fade at this frequency is not reliably detected unless the TOF ratio is 0.30 or less.[50,51] Stimulation at 100 Hz is more sensitive, but the range of responses is so variable that it must be considered an unreliable parameter.[51]

In an attempt to help solve this dilemma, alternate stimulus patterns have been suggested. The sequence most widely investigated is double burst stimulation (DBS).[52] This consists of a brief 50-Hz tetanus (of three stimuli), a 0.75-sec pause, and another short 50-Hz sequence (see Figure 22.8). This pattern has two theoretical advantages over the TOF. First, because each stimulus represents a mini-tetanus, the evoked response is higher in amplitude than a single twitch would be and thus is easier to detect. Second, the observer has only to compare two "twitches," with no intervening responses to confuse the issue. Indeed, fade on DBS is easier to detect than fade on TOF stimulation. Unfortunately, once the TOF ratio exceeds 0.60 to 0.70, fade on DBS is also missed by most clinicians.[53] Thus, this sequence does not solve the problem of detecting TOF ratios <0.90. Some investigators have advocated a modified double burst sequence in which the second 50-Hz burst contains only two stimuli (DBS$_{3,2}$) as being even more sensitive than DBS$_{3,3}$.[54] However, this pattern has not been widely adopted by clinicians.

The train-of-four count

Despite the previously noted limitations in the subjective evaluation of the TOF ratio, intraoperative use of PNS devices still has

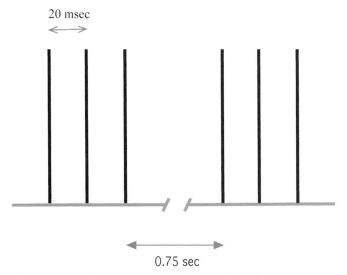

Figure 22.8. Double burst stimulation (DBS). The double burst sequence consists of three stimuli at 20-msec intervals (50 Hz), a 0.75-second pause, and a second brief 50-Hz tetanus.

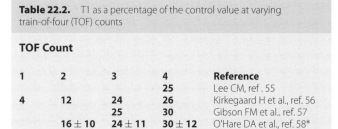

Table 22.2. T1 as a percentage of the control value at varying train-of-four (TOF) counts

TOF Count				
1	2	3	4	Reference
			25	Lee CM, ref . 55
4	12	24	26	Kirkegaard H et al., ref. 56
		25	30	Gibson FM et al.. ref. 57
	16 ± 10	24 ± 11	30 ± 12	O'Hare DA et al., ref. 58*
	19 ± 8	32 ± 9	41 ± 11	O'Hare DA et al., ref. 58**
5 ± 2	16 ± 5	27 ± 5	37 ± 8	Kopman AF, ref. 59
8 ± 4	20 ± 6	33 ± 9	44 ± 10	Kopman AF et al., ref . 60

* N_2O = enflurane anesthesia.
** N_2O = barbiturate anesthesia.

great clinical value. During modest nondepolarizing block, all four responses to TOF stimuli may be present (with fade). However, as the level of block deepens, eventually the fourth, third, second, and, finally, the initial response will disappear, and this progression reverses itself on recovery (see Figure 22.9). The number of evoked responses that can be detected (the TOF count) can be useful information. As a rough rule of thumb, TOF counts (TOFCs) of 1, 2, 3, and 4 correspond approximately to 5, 15, 25, and 35 percent of control twitch height (see Table 22.2).[55-60] Thus, the TOFC is an excellent guide for the clinician attempting to gauge both the depth of neuromuscular block during the intraoperative period and the necessity for administering additional blocking agents. For example, if

respiratory efforts resume despite a TOFC of 1, it is a pretty safe bet that what the patient requires is not additional muscle relaxant, but an additional dose of opioid.

The TOFC also provides key data in determining whether or not antagonism of the residual block will be successful. Anticholinesterases have a ceiling to the extent of the block that can be completely antagonized. When reversal of neuromuscular block greater than this level (twitch height <30% of control) is attempted, the peak effect of the antagonist is followed by a slow plateau phase, which represents the balance between diminishing anticholinesterase activity and spontaneous recovery of neuromuscular block.[61] Thus, in practical terms, the maximum depth of block that can be antagonized promptly by neostigmine corresponds approximately to the reappearance of the fourth response to TOF stimulation.[62] This situation will change to some degree with the introduction of sugammadex as a reversal agent, but even here, the TOFC will be a useful guide to sugammadex dosage.[63]

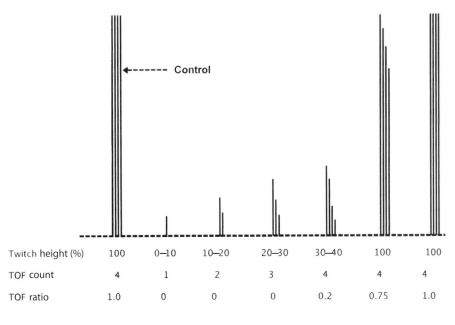

Figure 22.9. Twitch height (T1) as a function of the TOF ratio during recovery from nondepolarizing neuromuscular block. Redrawn from Beemer GH. Monitoring neuromuscular blockade. In *Clinical Anaesthesiology*, Vol. 8, No. 2 (Muscle Relaxants). Goldhill DR, Flynn PJ (eds.). Philadelphia: Bailliere Tindall, 1994.

Twitch height (%)	100	0–10	10–20	20–30	30–40	100	100
TOF count	4	1	2	3	4	4	4
TOF ratio	1.0	0	0	0	0.2	0.75	1.0

TOF stimuli at submaximal currents

Earlier in this chapter, it was suggested that when one is stimulating a peripheral nerve, supramaximal stimuli should be employed. When estimating single twitch depression, this is a sound principle, as it is necessary to have a stable control value to which to refer. However, one of the advantages of the TOF sequence is that no control value need be obtained. Because supramaximal stimuli may be unpleasant in the awake patient, it would be nice if TOF stimuli given at submaximal currents still produced accurate results. This issue was studied by Brull and associates in 12 unmedicated volunteers, 64 postanesthesia care unit (PACU) patients, and 28 anesthetized individuals.[64] As expected, the first twitch height (T1) increased significantly as delivered currents increased from 20 mA to 50 mA. However, as long as all four evoked responses were present, there was no statistical difference in the TOF ratios at 20, 30, or 50 mA. In the awake volunteers, median visual analog scale (VAS) pain scores were 2, 3, and 6 (on a scale of 1 to 10) at these delivered currents. The authors concluded that TOF testing can be done reliably in awake patients suspected of having residual weakness using currents that produce minimal discomfort. In fact, there is some evidence that visual assessment of fade may be improved by testing at low currents.[65] However, not all investigators are comfortable with these findings. Helbo-Hansen and colleagues,[23] although agreeing that some degree of submaximal stimulation is permissible, suggest that TOF monitoring in awake patients should be performed with currents 25 mA greater than that which produces the first detectable evoked response. This would usually dictate the use of currents of 40 mA or greater.

Objective measurement of indirectly evoked muscle responses

Subjective evaluation of the evoked response to indirect muscle stimulation has obvious clinical (as discussed earlier) as well as scientific limitations. Over the past half-century, although multiple techniques for accurately measuring and recording these responses in humans have evolved, few have shown themselves to have practical applicability in day-to-day use. Thus, although the investigator has a wide variety of tools from which to choose, the clinician is not so fortunate. The latter needs a device that is easy to set up, is rugged, gives real-time information, and – equally important – is affordable. Although the majority of the approaches to be discussed in this section are unlikely to have commercial potential, it is important to understand their principles if the neuromuscular literature is to be read with comprehension.

The mechanomyogram

Because of the technical difficulties involved in studying the EMG (discussed later), the vast majority of the early investigative work on the clinical pharmacology of neuromuscular blocking agents and their antagonists was done using a simpler and more accessible method: the measurement of the evoked muscle tension or isometric force generated by an indirect stimulus. (As noted earlier, the nerve–muscle preparation studied almost exclusively was the AP muscle response to ulnar nerve stimulation.)

The basic components needed for recording this mechanical response (mechanomyography [MMG]) are straightforward: a PNS; a force displacement transducer, such as the FT-03 or FT-10 (Grass Technologies; West Warwick, RI); a polygraph or strip recorder of modest bandwidth; and an arm board, which serves to immobilize the hand and to which the force transducer can be mounted. In addition, the transducer mount must be adjustable so that a preload (100–300 g) can be applied to the thumb, and the transducer oriented so the direction of thumb movement corresponds to the direction of displacement of the transducer cantilever.[66] This system has several virtues. Most of the parts are inexpensive. In the 1970s, a Grass transducer could be purchased for $300 ($945 in 2008), and a wide variety of recording devices were available to capture the generated analog signal. Thus, a very workable setup can be constructed by the interested clinician without a great deal of preexisting technical expertise.

A typical system had drawbacks as well. None of the first transducers employed was intended for clinical work. Thus, each investigator had to design and build his or her own unique armboard. These custom built devices were often time-consuming to set up. Satisfactory arm immobilization and transducer alignment might easily take 10 minutes. Thus, a two-person team was required to obtain data: one person to administer the patient's anesthetic and the other to concentrate on the monitoring setup. A commercial arm board, which was easier to use, was introduced in 1983,[67] but it cost $2000 and still did not solve the other major problem inherent in the MMG. Although mechanomyography could produce excellent waveform traces in real time (see Figure 22.10), they did not display either the twitch height as a percent of control (T_1/T_c) or the TOF ratio numerically. By the early to mid-1970s, attempts to accomplish this were described,[43,68] but none of these prototype neuromuscular analyzers was ever developed commercially. The first such device to achieve a modest distribution was the Myograph 2000 (Biometer; Odense, Denmark).[69] Despite its sophistication, the unit was bulky, expensive, and not suited for use in day-to-day clinical practice. The unit, first described in 1982, is no longer being manufactured, but it is still in use by many investigators. A more recent (1993) attempt to develop a compact neuromuscular analyzer was the Relaxometer,[70] a product of the University of Groningen in Holland. The university would build a unit for anyone on demand, and eventually software was developed that allowed the device to interface with a laptop computer. Nevertheless, the total number of Relaxometers actually delivered worldwide was less than a dozen (Ashraf Dahaba, personal communication). Thus, it does not appear likely that the MMG will ever achieve widespread use in the real world of actual clinical care. Nevertheless, the MMG is still considered by many authorities to be the gold standard by which other monitors of neuromuscular function must be compared.

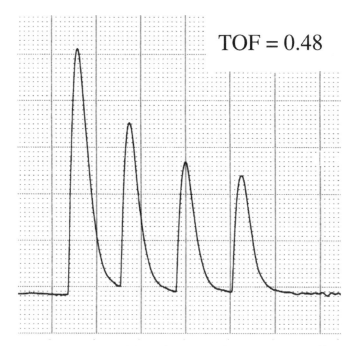

TOF = 0.48

Figure 22.10. TOF with fade. Mechanomyographic trace. T1 = 53 mm; T4 = 25.3 mm. TOF ratio = 25.3/53 = 0.48.

Electromyography

In theory, measuring the electrical response of muscle, rather than the mechanical response, as a barometer of neuromuscular transmission has much to recommend it. The electromyogram (EMG) is not affected by changes in muscle contractility, and tetanic responses are avoided at stimulation rates $\leq$50 Hz. In addition, it offers certain practical advantages. Immobilization of the muscle to be studied is not essential, and sites other than those of the hand are more easily studied. Nevertheless, technical complexity kept this method a strictly research tool until the early 1980s. The short duration of the EMG signal (<20 msec) presents several difficulties. A recording system must have a frequency bandpass of at least 10 to 1,000 Hz to capture this event. This precludes the use of mechanical recoding devices. Thus, early investigators were forced to employ a photographic recording system of some sort, either an oscilloscope camera or an oscillographic mirror galvanometer. Continuous recordings were also extremely wasteful of recording media and were difficult to handle. If stimuli at 0.10 Hz were being administered, 99.8 percent of the recording trace would consist of electrical silence. The latter issue was addressed in some degree by Epstein and coworkers.[71] They recorded the EMG on frequency-modulated magnetic tape running at 30 inches per second and later, using a 16-to-1 speed reduction, played back the signal on a direct-writing polygraph. A major problem with this approach (aside from complexity) was that the TOF signal still could not be analyzed in real time.

In 1977, Lee and colleagues[72] employed then-emerging computer technology to begin to solve the previously noted problems. Briefly, they digitized the evoked EMG signal, stored the waveform in memory, and then, with time expansion, printed out an analog reconstruction of the signal in real time. This device represented a major breakthrough. Although it was never produced commercially, it was undoubtedly the model for other units that followed soon thereafter.

A prototype for what would eventually become a commercial product was first described in 1981.[73] By 1984, at least one such series of units (the Datex Relaxograph or NMT monitor) became clinically available and achieved modest commercial success.[74] Unfortunately, these units are no longer being manufactured, and to the best of this author's knowledge, no easy-to-use, freestanding EMG units aimed at the anesthesiologist are currently on the market. Datex-Ohmeda Inc. (Madison, WI) manufactures an EMG NeuroMuscular Transmission Module (the E-NMT); however, it is expensive and works only when interfaced with the company's S/5 or S/3 monitoring systems. Thus, at present, it does not seem likely that EMG will achieve widespread clinical utilization. However, many Datex units are still serviceable, and studies employing this technology will certainly continue to appear from time to time. For this reason, and because a great number of important contributions to our understanding of neuromuscular pharmacology are based on this monitoring method, an acquaintance with the basics of EMG is still important if the neuromuscular literature is to be read with comprehension. The agreement between EMG recordings and other methods of monitoring neuromuscular function has been studied extensively.[75-79] Although evoked EMG and MMG responses show minor dissimilarities, for practical clinical purposes the two can be used interchangeably. An excellent review of this subject may be found in a dissertation by Jens Engbæk.[80]

A technical note: Early EMG studies used the peak-to-peak amplitude of the evoked response to measure twitch height. Most computer-based systems, such as the Relaxograph, instead use the integrated the area under the waveform curve (positive and negative) to represent twitch height. These two methods give interchangeable results.[81]

Acceleromyography

Because of the technical (and commercial) difficulties encountered in introducing mechanomyography and electromyography as neuromuscular monitors into the operating room, other approaches have been sought. An elegant and very promising solution was first described by Viby-Mogensen and colleagues in 1988.[82,83] Their rationale was based on Newton's second law of motion which states that force = mass × acceleration. Presumably the mass of the thumb remains constant, so acceleration is directly proportional to force. For measurement of acceleration, a piezoelectric ceramic wafer is fixed to the thumb. When an evoked mechanical response of the thumb is elicited, an electrical signal proportional to the acceleration is generated. This signal can then be digitized, processed, and displayed electronically in real time. Although early models of the accelograph were bulky, a hand-held battery-operated version using the same principle (the TOF-Guard)[84,85] was soon

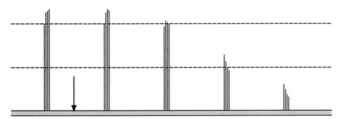

Figure 22.11. Computer screen shot from TOF-Watch Monitor software. The control acceleromyographic TOF response is at the extreme left. The initial TOF ratio is 1.16 (T1 = 100%, T2 = 112%, T4 = 116%). The T4/T2 ratio at this time is 1.04. Onset of neuromuscular block becomes evident at arrow.

introduced. The latter unit was replaced in 1997 by the TOF-Watch monitor (Organon Teknika B.V.; Boxtel, the Netherlands). As of 2008, this unit was available in several models and has achieved considerable commercial success and scientific acceptance. The advantages of acceleromyography are many. It provides an objective measurement of neuromuscular function in real time, setup time is rapid, it has a simple user interface, no preload or arm immobilization is required, the acquisition cost is low, and it is highly portable. In addition, the TOF-Watch SX allows computer capture of evoked responses via a fiberoptic link to an excellent data management program.

Early reports suggested that acceleromyographically (AMG) measured evoked responses were basically interchangeable with EMG or MMG values.[76,77] More recent information indicates that subtle, but important, differences exist between these modalities. With MMG and EMG recordings, a TOF ratio of 0.75 indicates at least 95 percent recovery of T1 twitch height.[66] However, with AMG recordings at a TOF ratio of 0.70, T1 averages only about 70 percent of control, and a TOF ratio of 0.90 is required to ensure 90 percent recovery of T1.[86] Similarly, at an AMG TOF ratio of 0.70, the simultaneous recorded EMG values is only 0.60. If an EMG TOF value of 0.90 is sought, then AMG TOF ratios of 0.95 to 1.0 must be obtained.[87] Thus, the AMG tends to overestimate recovery, compared with the MMG or EMG. In part, these discrepancies may result from an idiosyncrasy of the AMG, which is poorly understood. In contrast to the MMG and EMG, in which the control TOF ratio in the unparalyzed subject approximates a value of 1.00 (T4 is 100% of T1), the control AMG is more likely to be 110 percent, and values as high as 120 percent are not uncommon (see Figure 22.11).[87] Because of this phenomenon, it has been suggested that AMG TOF ratios should be normalized.[88] For example, if the control TOF ratio is 110 percent, a displayed value of 0.90 should be read as 82 percent (90/110 = 0.82). The problem with this approach is that the control TOF ratio may not be known.

The manufacturer of the TOF-Watch has taken an alternate approach to solving this problem. The TOF-Watch and TOF-Watch-S models, which are intended for routine clinical use, employ an algorithm that corrects for this effect. If T2 is greater than T1, the unit displays the T4/T2 ratio rather than the T4/T1 ratio. In addition, TOF ratios greater than 100 percent are never displayed. In practice, the error created by this modification has few clinical implications and does make the user interface less

confusing.[89] The TOF-Watch-SX, which is aimed at investigators, continues to display the actually measured TOF ratio. For a more complete discussion of acceleromyography as a research and clinical tool, the reader is referred to a recent critical review by Claudius and Viby-Mogensen.[90]

Kinemyography

A different approach to the use of a piezoelectric motion sensor was suggested by Kern and colleagues.[91] To cite the authors, "Deformation of a piezoelectric substance causes a redistribution of charge in the material which leads directly to electron flow to balance the charge. The electron flow produces a voltage which is measured by electrodes placed across the piezo material. The charge is rapidly dissipated owing to internal resistance; thus only dynamic changes can be measured when using these devices."[92] In contrast to an accelerometer, which uses a piezoelectric ceramic wafer to measure acceleration of a fixed mass in the transducer, the authors employed a flexible piezoelectric film that has no fixed mass acting against it. Sensor output occurs when the film spans a movable joint; muscle movement from evoked stimulation bends the piezoelectric film, which generates a voltage proportional to the amount of bending. To distinguish this technology from acceleromyography, several authors refer to this mode of monitoring as kinemyography (KMG).

The first commercial unit to employ this strategy was the ParaGraph (Vital Signs; Totowa, NJ). The unit had several virtues. It was small, easy to set up, and had a a simple interface. However, the limits of agreement to MMG-evoked TOF ratios were quite wide. Of interest, in a study of 10 individuals, control KMG TOF ratios exceed 1.00, whereas MMG values did not.[93] This "reverse fade" was similar in nature to that described earlier with AMG. In a study comparing the ParaGraph to a MMG transducer, using simultaneously recorded values from opposite arms, Dahaba and colleagues observed very little overall bias as to twitch height depression or TOF fade. However, the limits of agreement for individual subjects was quite wide. The authors concluded that the two monitors could not be used interchangeably. The ParaGraph did not see great commercial success, perhaps in part because it employed a proprietary disposable sensor. Thus, if the supply of sensors became depleted, the device was inoperable.

More recently, kinemyography has been adopted by another manufacturer using a slightly different (and reusable) sensor/transducer. The Datex-Ohmeda MechanoSensor (M-NMT) plugs into the same module as the E-NMT described earlier (see electromyography). The M-NMT is a boomerang-shaped device that contains a piezoelectric foil membrane. The unit is placed between the thumb and the forefinger. Thumb movement bends the sensor and, as described earlier, generates an electrical signal, which is then processed. This unit has several practical limitations. It must be used as part of the Datex-Ohmeda AS/5 aesthesia monitoring system; a freestanding version is not available. Of greater concern is that the direction in which the boomerang transducer bends does not match the natural vector of thumb movement as driven by the AP muscle. Consequently, the device is a poor fit for many individuals, especially those with small hands. An analysis of the correlation between the M-NMT monitor and the MMG concluded that because of the wide limits of agreement between the two monitors, they cannot be used interchangeably.[94]

In summary, although KMG gives measurements that are repeatable and gives good enough correspondence with a force transducer that they can be used clinically to assess recovery of neuromuscular blockade, the wide limits of agreement with MMG and EMG rule out research applications.[95]

Other methods of measurement

Another interesting line of attack is acoustic or phonomyography (PMG).[96] This method is based on the fact that muscle contraction evokes low-frequency sounds that can be recorded using special microphones. Initially, this method was called *acoustic myography* and used an air-chamber interface between the skin and the microphone. It shows good agreement for several muscles with the gold standard of monitoring (MMG).[97,98] In addition, it can be employed at muscle sites at which other technologies may not be applicable.[99] However, again, these units are not commercially available.

Because each of the previously described approaches to the objective monitoring of neuromuscular function when moved into the operating room for routine clinical use has some practical or theoretical drawbacks, it is not surprising that new ideas keep emerging.[100] A comprehensive catalog of all of these approaches is beyond the scope of this chapter.

All muscles are not the same

As noted earlier, the strength of the AP per se has little clinical importance. This muscle is used as a surrogate for others that have more immediate clinical relevance, such as the diaphragm, the masseter, and the adductors of the vocal cords. Unfortunately, the sensitivities to blocking drugs of these latter muscles are often quite different from those of the hand. In addition, the times to onset of effect and rates of recovery often vary significantly from muscle to muscle. Although the vast literature on this subject is beyond the scope of this chapter, certain significant differences between various muscle groups must be noted.

Diaphragm

The diaphragm is considerably more resistant to the effects of muscle relaxants than is the AP muscle. The dose of nondepolarizing blocker required to produced comparable degrees of block is 1.5 to 2.0 times greater at the diaphragm.[101–103] It is not uncommon to see spontaneous respiration resume at a time when twitch depression at the hand is still quite profound. Thus, the resumption of respiratory effort by itself should not by itself be considered as a signal that muscle relaxation is inadequate and that additional blocking agents should be administered.

More often than not, what the patient is requesting is augmented ventilation or supplementary doses of opioid and/or hypnotic – perhaps all three.

Despite the diaphragm's greater resistance to relaxants, onset of paralysis is usually faster at the diaphragm than at the muscles of the hand.[104,105] This apparent contradiction results from the greater circulatory perfusion that the diaphragm receives. Following a rapid intravenous bolus, the diaphragm is exposed initially to a much higher blood concentration of blocker than is the AP. However, as expected, recovery of neuromuscular function at the diaphragm precedes that at the hand.

Larynx

The sensitivity to blocking drugs, as well as the onset/offset profile, of the adductor muscles of the larynx more closely matches those of the diaphragm than those of the AP. The dose required for comparable levels of paralysis is 1.75 times higher at the larynx than at the AP.[106,107] As with the diaphragm, the times to onset of effect are shorter and recovery rates faster than observed at the AP. For example, after rocuronium 0.5 mg/kg, the onset time was also more rapid at the vocal cords (1.4 ± 0.1 min) than at the AP (2.4 ± 0.2 min). Maximum blockade was 77 ± 5 percent and 98 ± 1 percent, respectively, and time to 90 percent T1 recovery was 22 ± 3 min and 37 ± 4 min, respectively.[107]

Failure to achieve adequate neuromuscular block at the laryngeal adductors clearly has implications as to the clinical success of tracheal intubation. Unfortunately, the response of the thumb to ulnar nerve stimulation is a poor prognosticator of conditions for intubation. Excellent conditions may be present at a time when evoked responses at the thumb are still present. Some authors have suggested that a better surrogate for the state of block at the larynx is the corrugator supercilii muscle (see section on facial muscles).[108] Hemmerling and Donati have published a comprehensive review of this subject.[113]

The previous discussion notwithstanding, in the real world of daily clinical practice it is doubtful whether many clinicians routinely monitor the evoked response of the facial muscles as a guide to readiness for tracheal intubation. This author has found that the clock on the wall is equally useful and much more convenient.

Alternate monitoring sites

Observing the indirectly evoked response of the muscles of the hand to ulnar nerve stimulation is the traditional site for monitoring neuromuscular function in the perioperative period. However, the arm is not always accessible during surgery, and other sites for monitoring neuromuscular function have been sought by clinicians.

Facial muscles

A common and convenient choice is stimulation the facial nerve at the angle of the jaw or just anterior to the earlobe and observing the response of the periorbital muscles.

More than 20 years ago, Caffrey and coworkers[109] convincingly demonstrated that the facial muscles were a poor surrogate for the muscles of the hand. Following a dose of atracurium that completely abolished twitch response at both the AP and (what may have been erroneously reported as) the orbicularis oculi, they allowed spontaneous recovery to take place. At a time when the facial muscles had returned to a TOFC of four with fade, the AP still showed no response to TOF stimulation. Early recovery of the orbicularis oculi compared with the muscles of the hand has subsequently been observed by multiple investigators.[110–112]

However, the periorbital muscular response to facial nerve stimulation reflects the contraction of corrugator supercilii muscle as well as the orbicularis oculi. The orbicularis oculi are the muscles of the eyelids, the corrugator supercilii is the muscle of the superciliary arch (the eyebrow). Differences between these two muscles in their responses to blocking agents have frequently not been appreciated, and this has resulted in some confusion in the literature. Although early investigators invariably described responses of the muscles surrounding the eye as effects on the orbicularis oculi, it is possible that often they were, in fact, measuring the corrugator supercilii muscle.[113] More recent data suggest that the orbicularis oculi's rate of return from nondepolarizing block is not appreciably shorter than that of the AP, and that the corrugator supercilii recovers first.[114,108]

From a practical point of view, these fine distinctions are perhaps less than helpful in daily practice. Visually differentiating between the response of the orbicularis oculi and the corrugator supercilii is probably asking too much of the clinician. From this author's perspective, it seems safer to assume that the evoked response to facial nerve stimulation overestimates neuromuscular recovery as measured at the AP muscle.

Flexor hallucis brevis

When the hand is not available to the clinician, Sopher and associates[115] suggest that the response of the flexor hallucis brevis (plantar flexion of the foot) to posterior tibial nerve stimulation at the ankle provides responses that are not statistically different from those measured simultaneously at the AP. This report has not yet been validated by other investigators.

Bedside or clinical tests of neuromuscular recovery

The preceding discussion of methods for measuring and evaluating the evoked responses to indirect muscle stimulation is perhaps misleading. The fact is that even conventional peripheral nerve stimulators are far from universally used by clinicians. A recent survey[116] from the United Kingdom is rather depressing. The authors reported that 60 percent of anesthetists surveyed never use a PNS of any kind, and fewer than 10 percent have access to an "objective" monitor of neuromuscular function. The situation is little different in Denmark[117] or Germany.[118] Thus, a large percentage of clinicians apparently

still rely primarily on such clinical signs as tidal volume, grip strength, tongue protrusion, and negative inspiratory force as measures of the adequacy of neuromuscular recovery. This approach presents several problems. First, bedside tests require an awake and cooperative patient. The decision to antagonize residual neuromuscular block should not have to wait until the patient emerges from anesthesia. More importantly, most bedside tests are simply unreliable indicators of neuromuscular recovery.[119]

Probably the most widely cited clinical test is the ability to elevate the head off the bed or pillow for at least five seconds (a 5-sec head-lift [HL]). El Mikatti and colleagues,[120] in a study of seven awake volunteers given small increments of pipecuronium, reported that at an EMG TOF ratio of 0.50, six of seven individuals could still sustain a 5-sec HL, and that this test was accomplished by all seven at a TOF ratio of 0.60. Engbæk and coworkers[121] found the HL somewhat more sensitive in a clinical setting but still found that 8 of 16 patients could perform a 5-sec HL at a TOF value of 0.60. Therefore considerable residual weakness may exist despite the ability of a patient to execute the most widely employed bedside test of clinical recovery.

Does neuromuscular monitoring reduce residual postoperative neuromuscular block?

Ultimately, the goal of perioperative neuromuscular monitoring is to decrease the incidence of residual postoperative neuromuscular block (PONB). There is abundant evidence that undetected PONB is still a frequent occurrence. Recent studies (from 2000 or later) report that the incidence of PONB ranges from a low of 16 percent of individuals arriving in the PACU following a single dose of relaxant[122] to as many as 70 percent of patients who still have TOF values <0.70 at the time of extubation.[123] Other reports are equally alarming.[124–126] These observations raise an obvious question: Does neuromuscular monitoring actually decrease the incidence of PONB? Common sense suggests that even conventional PNS units, which require subjective evaluation of the evoked response, should prove superior to bedside tests (especially when the patient is not able to cooperate with the clinician).

A recent study by Naguib and colleagues that examined this hypothesis, however, found that the peer-reviewed literature does not necessarily support this premise.[127] Their analysis was not able to demonstrate that the use of conventional PNSs decreased the incidence of PONB. Unfortunately, in this meta-analysis, most of the studies cited that failed to demonstrate that monitoring had a favorable effect in reducing PONB were poorly designed to do so. To give just two examples: In a study by Pedersen and coworkers,[128] patients received either vecuronium or pancuronium. In half the patients, the degree of intraoperative blockade was assessed by tactile evaluation of the TOF response at the thumb. In the other half, the degree of block was evaluated solely by clinical criteria. The use of a PNS had no effect on the dose of relaxant given or on the incidence of PONB evaluated clinically. In the clinical criteria groups, reversal of residual paralysis was not attempted until spontaneous respiration or other indication of muscle activity was observed. However, the authors' protocol almost guaranteed that results in the monitored group would be less than optimal. Anesthetists were instructed to maintain the TOF count at one or two detectable responses and antagonism of residual block with neostigmine was initiated at this level of block. There is ample evidence that prompt and satisfactory anticholinesterase-induced antagonism at this level of block is simply not a realistic goal. Intraoperative neuromuscular monitoring should be used to help the clinician titrate doses of relaxant to avoid this level of block at the end of surgery, not the converse.

Hayes and associates[125] focused on the frequency of PONB on arrival in the PACU in patients who received blockers of intermediate duration. Residual block was considered present in patients with a TOF ratio <0.80. The overall incidence of PONB was 52 percent. Intraoperative neuromuscular monitoring was used in only 41 percent of patients, and reversal of residual block was omitted in one-third of the patients. The authors were not able to demonstrate that the incidence of PONB was significantly less in patients in whom a PNS was used. Nevertheless, because several of their patients (no PNS device used) arrived in the PACU with TOF counts of less than four detectable responses, it is difficult to accept the premise that even rudimentary monitoring would not have been helpful.

Papers such as those cited previously expose a basic lack of knowledge on the part of clinicians more than they indicate a lack of utility of conventional PNS devices. Although it is true that subjective evaluation of the TOF ratio is subject to considerable error, the tactile TOF count is still a very useful parameter. If the TOF count at the time reversal is initiated is known, the clinician at least has a rough ballpark estimate of when satisfactory return of neuromuscular may be expected. If the TOF count has recovered to one detectable response following the administration of cisatracurium or rocuronium, then neostigmine 0.05 mg/kg will take approximately 20 minutes to restore the TOF ratio to a value of about approximately 0.80 (with considerable individual variation).[129] In practical terms, the maximum depth of block that can be promptly ($\leq$10 min) reversed by anticholinesterase antagonists corresponds approximately to the reappearance of the fourth response to TOF stimulation.[62]

In knowledgeable hands, the use of conventional PNS units will usually provide adequate information for the safe and rational administration of neuromuscular blockers and their antagonists. However, there are circumstances under which objective devices (monitors that display the TOF ratio in real time) are clearly preferable to conventional PNS units.

The case for objective neuromuscular monitors

Reversal agents are not without their own potential side effects. Even though early concerns about lethal catastrophes following anticholinesterase administration were clearly alarmist,[130,131]

it is also true that atropine, glycopyrrolate, neostigmine, and edrophonium all have potentially unwanted cardiovascular and other side effects. Neostigmine may actually enhance TOF fade if given to the patient who has fully recovered spontaneously.[133,132] Thus, if satisfactory spontaneous recovery of neuromuscular function has occurred, there are cogent reasons to avoid administering unnecessary antagonists. Unfortunately, subjective evaluation of the TOF ratio is unreliable,[46] and the passage of time is not an adequate guarantee that sufficient neuromuscular recovery has occurred.[133,122] Thus, it is hard to argue with the dictum that residual neuromuscular block should always be reversed unless there is objective evidence that the TOF ratio has recovered to acceptable levels.[134]

Objective monitoring is also strongly indicated when reversing profound neuromuscular block. If the TOF count is less than 2, prompt recovery of neuromuscular function cannot be ensured by anticholinesterase administration. Nevertheless, neostigmine antagonism of deep block may result in the rapid return of all four evoked responses to TOF stimulation with minimal or no subjectively detectable fade (a TOF ratio >0.40). Thus, a prolonged period may exist during which the TOF ratio is above 0.40 but below satisfactory recovery levels.[129] In the absence of an objectively measured TOF ratio, tracheal extubation may be undertaken when it is clearly inappropriate.[135]

There is now increasing evidence that objective monitoring does decrease the incidence of residual weakness in the PACU. When compared with patients monitored using only clinical criteria of neuromuscular recovery, all available studies indicate that the intraoperative use of objective neuromuscular monitors reduces the incidence of PONB.[136,137] In the only paper comparing outcomes in patients monitored intraoperatively with conventional PNS units versus objective monitors,[138] PONB was credibly reduced in the latter group.

Perhaps the most convincing evidence that the use of objective neuromuscular monitors (combined with a strong educational effort at the departmental level) can decrease the incidence of PONB comes from two studies by Baillard and colleagues. The first[139] was a prospective study of the incidence of PONB following the administration of vecuronium in 568 consecutive patients over a three-month period in 1995. As was customary in the authors' department, no anticholinesterase antagonists were given, and PNS devices were rarely used intraoperatively. PONB (indicated by an acceleromyographic TOF ratio of <0.70) in the PACU was found in 42 percent of patients. Of 435 patients who had been extubated in the operating room, the incidence of PONB was 33 percent. As a result of these rather alarming findings, Baillard's department placed acceleromyographic monitors in all operating rooms shortly after the completion of the 1995 study. In addition, the department instituted an educational program about the use of neuromuscular monitoring and the indications for neostigmine administration. The results of their findings regarding the incidence of PONB were distributed to their staff. They then conducted repeat three-month surveys of clinical practice in the years 2000 ($n = 130$), 2002 ($n = 101$), and 2004 ($n = 218$) to determine the success of their educational efforts.[140] In the nine-year interval between the first and last of these studies, the use of intraoperative monitoring of neuromuscular function rose from 2 percent to 60 percent, and reversal of residual antagonism increased from 6 percent to 42 percent of cases. As a result of these changes in clinical practice, the incidence of PONB (acceleromyographic TOF ratio of <0.90) in this department decreased from 62 percent to less than 4 percent. These results clearly show that the incidence of PONB can be reduced to very low levels when nondepolarizing neuromuscular blocking drugs are administered by knowledgeable clinicians who employ objective neuromuscular monitors as adjuncts to their care and administer anticholinesterase antagonists on indication.

Does residual neuromuscular block have clinical consequences?

In a 1989 editorial, Miller[141] noted that there were no outcome data available assessing what role residual paralysis might play in adverse respiratory events in the PACU or on postoperative morbidity. Two decades later, there is still only limited outcome information to suggest that PONB represents a frequent cause of major morbidity. As pointed out by Shorten,[142] several factors work against obtaining reliable information. First, it is unlikely that most postoperative complications can be attributed to a single cause. Second, an ethical dilemma exists. If postoperative neuromuscular function is judged to be inadequate, the investigator is obliged to intervene, and in doing so, has altered the course that otherwise would have transpired. Finally, the incidence of serious adverse events associated with the administration of muscle relaxants is unknown, but probably small. When designing an outcome study, this presents a serious problem related to statistical power. For example, if the incidence of serious pulmonary sequelae in the absence of residual block is 1 percent and rises to 2 percent in the presence residual motor weakness, a sample size approaching 1600 subjects would be needed for achieve statistical significance at the $P < 0.05$ level (beta = 50%). Few well-designed investigations of this magnitude have been attempted.

A recent study by Murphy and coworkers[143] adds credence to the hypothesis that residual neuromuscular block may have clinical consequences. The authors collected data over a one-year period of all cases of critical respiratory events (CREs) that occurred within the first 15 minutes following admission to their PACU. TOF ratios were immediately measured in these patients using AMG. A total of 7459 patients received a general anesthetic during the study period; of these, 61 developed a CRE. The most common events were severe hypoxemia (22 of 42 patients) and upper-airway obstruction (15 of 42 patients). There were no significant differences between the CRE cases and a match control group in any measured preoperative or intraoperative variables. Mean ($\pm$SD) TOF ratios were 0.62 ($\pm$0.20) in the CRE cases, with 73.8 percent of the cases having TOF ratios <0.70. In contrast, TOF values in the controls were 0.98 ($\pm$0.07; $P < 0.0001$), and no control patients were observed to have TOF values <0.70. These findings strongly suggest that incomplete neuromuscular recovery can be an important contributing factor in the development of adverse respiratory events in the PACU.

However, these observations may also explain why so many clinicians appear to view the risk of PONB as minimal (failure to use even conventional peripheral nerve stimulators and/or failure to administer reversal agents at the end of anesthesia). There is ample evidence that PONB on arrival in the PACU is not a rare occurrence.[116–120] If we define PONB conservatively as a TOF ratio less than an AMG value of 0.90, then the actual incidence of PONB on arrival to today's recovery rooms is probably not less than 20 percent and is most likely more. Thus, in Murphy's study, perhaps 1500 subjects had some degree of PONB but did not suffer a noticeable adverse respiratory event. Put differently, Murphy's data suggest that PONB may be associated with a frequency of short-term critical respiratory events of only 4 percent to 5 percent, and the incidence of actual long-term morbidity is likely to be significantly lower than that. Hence, most patients appear to tolerate residual block of modest extent without untoward results. This is not to diminish the importance of Murphy's work. There is no reason to accept even infrequent adverse events if they can be prevented.

Does neuromuscular monitoring have a future?

As this chapter is written (the summer of 2008), acetylcholinesterase inhibitors are the only antagonists of nondepolarizing neuromuscular block available to clinicians. Because these agents have limited efficacy, it is important to know the depth of preexisting block when reversal is contemplated. Prompt and satisfactory antagonism of residual paresis is unreliable at best when the TOFC is 3 or less.[56,123,144]

However, the introduction of sugammadex into our armamentarium has the potential to change the way we think about and administer neuromuscular blocking agents.[145] It appears that we may have, for the first time, the ability to rapidly and completely reverse deep nondepolarizing neuromuscular block. If sugammadex is given in the proper dosage, the TOF ratio can be returned to values approximating 0.90 within three minutes even if rocuronium 1.2 mg/kg was administered only five minutes earlier.[146] At this moment, it is unclear what the drug's acquisition cost will be. It is not likely to be cheap. Thus, economic considerations will undoubtedly play a role in how physicians will ultimately use this drug. If the lowest effective (and least expensive) dose is to be selected, it will still be important to know the extent of neuromuscular block prior to its administration. However, knowledge of the TOFC or the PTC may be sufficient information on which to base sugammadex dosage. Thus, the arguments for objective monitoring of neuromuscular function may be less compelling if and when sugammadex becomes available. Objective measurement of the TOF ratio may be most helpful when determining whether antagonism of residual block is actually required.

Endnotes

1   1 ampere × 1 second = 1 coulomb (Q). Thus, 50 mA × 0.20 msec = 10 μQ.

2   As of September 2008, sugammadex had been approved for use by the European Union. However, in the United States the FDA was withholding approval, and its future status in this country is uncertain.

References

1. Griffith HR, Johnson GE. The use of curare in general anesthesia. *Anesthesiology* 1942;**3**:412–20.

2. Cole F. The use of curare in anesthesia; a review of 100 cases. *Anesthesiology* 1945;**6**:48–56.

3. Prescott F, Organe G, Rowbotham S. Tubocurarine chloride as an adjunct to anesthesia. *Lancet* 1946;**2**:80–4.

4. Cullen SC. Curare: its past and present. *Anesthesiology* 1947;**8**:479–88.

5. Robbins BH, Lundy JS. Curare and curare-like compounds: a review. *Anesthesiology* 1947;**8**:252–65 (part 1) and *Anesthesiology* 1947;8:348–58 (part 2).

6. Morris LE, Schilling EA, Frederickson EL. The use of Tensilon with curare and nitrous oxide anesthesia. *Anesthesiology* 1953;**14**:117–25.

7. Beecher HK, Todd DP. A study of the deaths associated with anesthesia and surgery. *Ann Surg* 1954;**140**:2–35.

8. Abajian J Jr, Arrowood JG, Barrett RH, et al. Critique of "A study of deaths associated with anesthesia and surgery." *Ann Surg* 1955;**142**:138–41.

9. Christie TH, Churchill-Davidson HC. The St. Thomas's hospital nerve stimulator in the diagnosis of prolonged apnea. *Lancet* 1958;**1**:776.

10. Churchill-Davidson HC, Christie TH. The diagnosis of neuromuscular block in man. *Br J Anaesth* 1959;**31**:290–301.

11. Churchill-Davidson HC. A portable peripheral nerve stimulator. *Anesthesiology* 1965;**26**:224–6.

12. Katz RL. A nerve stimulator for the continuous monitoring of muscle relaxant action. *Anesthesiology* 1965;**26**:832–33.

13. Churchill-Davidson HC. The d-tubocurarine dilemma. *Anesthesiology* 1965;**26**:132–3.

14. Eriksson LI. Evidence-based practice and neuromuscular monitoring: It's time for routine quantitative assessment. *Anesthesiology* 2003;**98**:1037–9.

15. Naguib M, Kopman AF, Ensor JE. Neuromuscular monitoring and postoperative residual curarisation: a meta-analysis. *Br J Anaesth* 2007;**98**:302–16.

16. American Society of Anesthesiologists Task for on Postanesthesia Care. Practice Guidelines for Postanesthetic Care. *Anesthesiology* 2002;**96**:742–52.

17. Mylrea KC, Hameroff SR, Calkins JM, Blitt CD, Humphrey LL. Evaluation of peripheral nerve stimulators and relationship to possible errors in assessing neuromuscular blockade. *Anesthesiology* 1984;**60**:464–6.

18. Horcholle-Bossavit G, Jami L, Petit J, Scott JJ. Activation of cat motor units by paired stimuli at short intervals. *J Physiol* 1987;**387**:385–99.

19. Mortimer JT. Motor prosthesis. In *American Handbook of Physiology*, vol. II, section I. Brooks VB, ed. 1981, Bethesda, American Physiological Society, pp. 155–87.

20. Pither CE, Raj PP, Ford DJ. The use of peripheral nerve stimulators for regional anesthesia. *Reg. Anesth* 1985;**10**:49–58.

21. Voorhees CR, Voorhees WD 3rd, Geddes LA, Bourland JD, Hinds M. The chronaxie for myocardium and motor nerve in the dog with chest-surface electrodes. *IEEE Trans Biomed Eng* 1992;**39**:624–8.

22. Kopman AF, Lawson D. Milliamperage requirement for supramaximal stimulation of the ulnar nerve with surface electrodes. *Anesthesiology* 1984;**61**:83–5.

23. Helbo-Hansen HS, Bang U, Nielsen HK, Skovgaard LT. The accuracy of train-of-four monitoring at varying stimulating currents. *Anesthesiology* 1992;**76**:199–203.

24. Berger JJ, Gravenstein JS, Munson ES. Electrode polarity and peripheral nerve stimulation. *Anesthesiology* 1982;**56**:402–4.

25. Rosenberg H, Greenhow DE. Peripheral nerve stimulator performance: The influence of output polarity and electrode placement. *Can Anaesth Soc J* 1978;**25**:424–6.

26. Brull SJ, Silverman DG. Pulse width, stimulus intensity, electrode placement, and polarity during assessment of neuromuscular block. *Anesthesiology* 1995;**83**:702–9.

27. Pierce PA, Mylrea KC, Watt RC, Hameroff SR, Cork RV, Calkins JM. Effects of pulse duration on neuromuscular blockade monitoring: implications for supramaximal stimulation. *J Clin Monit* 1986;**2**:169–73.

28. Pollmaecher T, Steiert H, Buzello W. A constant current nerve stimulator (Neurostim T4). Description, and evaluation in volunteers. *Br J Anaesth* 1986;**58**:1443–6.

29. Viby-Mogensen J, Hansen PH, Jørgensen BC, Ording H, Kann T, Fries B. A new nerve stimulator (myotest). *Br J Anaesth* 1980;**52**:547–50.

30. Lee CM, Katz RL. Fade of neurally evoked compound EMG during neuromuscular block by d-tubocurarine. *Anesth Analg* 1977;**56**:271–5.

31. Stanec A, Heyduk J, Stanec G, Orkin LR. Tetanic fade and post tetanic potentiation in the absence of neuromuscular blocking agents in anesthetized man. *Anesth Analg* 1978;**57**:102–7.

32. Epstein RM, Epstein RA. The electromyogram and the mechanical response of indirectly stimulated skeletal muscle in anesthetized man following curarization. *Anesthesiology* 1973;**38**:212–23.

33. Gissen AJ, Katz RL. Twitch, tetanus, and post-tetanic potentiation as indices of neuromuscular block in man. *Anesthesiology* 1969;**30**:481–7.

34. Ali HH, Savarese JJ, Lebowitz PW, Ramsey FM. Twitch, tetanus, and train-of-four as indices of recovery from nondepolarizing neuromuscular blockade. *Anesthesiology* 1981;**54**:294–7.

35. Kopman AF, Epstein RH, Flashburg MH. Use of 100 hertz tetanus as an index of recovery from pancuronium-induced nondepolarizing neuromuscular blockade. *Anesth Analg* 1982;**61**:439–41.

36. Baurain MJ, Hennart DA, Godschalx A, et al. Visual evaluation of residual curarization in anesthetized patients using one hundred-hertz, five-second tetanic stimulation at the adductor pollicis muscle. *Anesth Analg* 1998;**87**:185–9.

37. Viby-Mogensen J, Howardy-Hansen P, Chræmmer-Jorgensen B, Ørding H, Engbæk J, Nielsen A. Posttetanic count (PTC): a new method of evaluating an intense nondepolarizing block. *Anesthesiology* 1981;**55**:458–61.

38. El-Orbany MI, Joseph NJ, Salem MR. The relationship of posttetanic count and train-of-four responses during recovery from intense cisatracurium-induced neuromuscular blockade. *Anesth Analg* 2003;**97**:80–84.

39. Ali HH, Utting JE, Gray TC. Stimulus frequency in the detection of neuromuscular block in man. *Br J Anaesth* 1970;**42**:967–78.

40. Ali HH, Utting JE, Gray TC. Quantitative assessment of residual antidepolarizing Block (Part I). *Br J Anaesth* 1971;**43**:473–7.

41. Ali HH, Utting JE, Gray TC. Quantitative assessment of residual antidepolarizing Block (Part II). *Br J Anaesth* 1971;**43**:478–85.

42. Ali HH, Wilson RS, Savarese JJ, Kitz RJ. The effect of d-tubocurarine on indirectly elicited train-of-four muscle response and respiratory measurements in humans. *Br J Anaesth* 1975;**47**:570–4.

43. Ali HH, Kitz RJ. Evaluation of recovery from non-depolarizing neuromuscular blockade using a digital neuromuscular analyzer: Preliminary report. *Anesth Analg* 1973;**52**:740–4.

44. Brand JB, Cullen DJ, Wilson NE, Ali HH. Spontaneous recovery from nondepolarizing neuromuscular blockade: correlation between clinical and evoked responses. *Anesth Analg* 1977;**56**:55–58.

45. Eriksson LI, Sato M, Severinghaus JW. Effect of a vecuronium-induced partial neuromuscular block on hypoxic ventilatory response. *Anesthesiology* 1993;**78**:693–9.

46. Eriksson LI, Sundman E, Olsson R, et al. Functional assessment of the pharynx at rest and during swallowing in partially paralyzed humans. Simultaneous videomanometry and mechanomyography of awake human volunteers. *Anesthesiology* 1997;**87**:1035–43.

47. Kopman AF, Yee PS, Neuman GG. Correlation of the train-of-four fade ratio with clinical signs and symptoms of residual curarization in awake volunteers. *Anesthesiology* 1997;**86**:765–71.

48. Capron F, Alla F, Hottier C, Meistelman C, Fuchs-Buder T. Can acceleromyography detect low levels of residual paralysis?: A probability approach to detect a mechanomyographic train-of-four ratio of 0.9. *Anesthesiology* 2004;**100**:1119–24.

49. Viby-Mogensen J, Jensen NH, Engbæk J, Ording H, Skovgaard LT, Chraemmer-Jorgensen B. Tactile and visual evaluation of the response to train-of-four nerve stimulation. *Anesthesiology* 1985;**63**:440–3.

50. Dupuis JY, Martin R, Tessonnier JM, Tétrault JP. Clinical assessment of the muscular response to tetanic nerve stimulation. *Can J Anaesth* 1990;**37**:397–400.

51. Capron F, Fortier L, Racine S, Donati F. Tactile fade detection with hand or wrist stimulation using train-of-four, double-burst stimulation, 50-hertz tetanus, 100-hertz tetanus, and acceleromyography. *Anesth Analg* 2006;**102**:1578–84.

52. Engbæk J, Østergaard D, Viby-Mogensen J. Double burst stimulation (DBS): a new pattern of nerve stimulation to identify residual neuromuscular block. *Br J Anaesth* 1989;**62**:274–8.

53. Drenck NE, Ueda N, Olsen NV, et al. Manual evaluation of residual curarization using double burst stimulation: A comparison with train-of-four. *Anesthesiology* 1989;**70**:578–81.

54. Ueda N, Muteki T, Tsuda H, Inoue S, Nishina H. Is the diagnosis of significant residual neuromuscular blockade improved by using double burst nerve stimulation? *Eur J Anaesthesiol* 1991;**8**:213–8.

55. Lee CM. Train-of-four quantitation of competitive neuromuscular block. *Anesth Analg* 1975;**54**:649–53.

56. Kirkegaard H, Heier T, Caldwell JE. Efficacy of tactile-guided reversal from cisatracurium-induced neuromuscular block. *Anesthesiology* 2002;**96**:45–50.

57. Gibson FM, Mirakhur RK, Clarke RS, Brady MM. Quantification of train-of-four responses during recovery of block from non-depolarizing muscle relaxants. *Acta Anaesthesiol Scand* 1987;**3**:655–7.

58. O'Hara DA, Fragen RJ, Shanks CA. Comparison of visual and measured train-of-four recovery after vecuronium-induced neuromuscular blockade using two anesthetic techniques. *Br J Anaesth* 1986;**58**:1300–1302.

59. Kopman AF. Tactile evaluation of train-of-four count as an indicator of reliability of antagonism from vecuronium or atracurium-induced neuromuscular blockade. *Anesthesiology* 1991;**75**:588–93.

60. Kopman AF, Mallhi MU, Justo MD, Rodricks P, Neuman GG. Antagonism of mivacurium-induced neuromuscular blockade in humans. Edrophonium dose requirements at threshold train-of-four count of 4. *Anesthesiology* 1994;**81**:1394–1400.

61. Beemer GH, Bjorksten AR, Dawson PJ, Dawson RJ, Heenan PJ, Robertson BA. Determinants of the reversal time of competitive neuromuscular block by anticholinesterases. *Br J Anaesth* 1991;**66**:469–75.

62. Beemer GH, Goonetilleke PH, Bjorksten AR. The maximum depth of an atracurium neuromuscular block antagonized by edrophonium to effect adequate recovery. *Anesthesiology* 1995;**82**:852–8.

63. Suy K, Morias K, Cammu G, et al. Effective reversal of moderate rocuronium- or vecuronium-induced neuromuscular block with sugammadex, a selective relaxant binding agent. *Anesthesiology* 2007;**106**:283–8.

64. Brull SJ, Ehrenwerth J, Dewan DM. Stimulation with submaximal current for train-of-four stimulation. *Anesthesiology* 1990;**72**:629–32.

65. Brull SJ, Silverman DG. Visual assessment of train-of-four and double burst-induced fade at submaximal stimulating currents. *Anesth Analg* 1991;**73**:627–32.

66. Ali HH, Savarese JJ. Monitoring of neuromuscular function. *Anesthesiology* 1976;**45**:216–49.

67. Stanec A, Stanec G. The adductor pollicis monitor apparatus and method for the quantitative measurement of the isometric contraction of the adductor pollicis muscle. *Anesth Analg* 1983;**62**:602–5.

68. Perry IR, Worsley R, Sugai N, Payne JP. The use of a digital computer for the on-line real-time assessment of neuromuscular blockade in anaesthetized man. *Br J Anaesth* 1975;**47**:1097–1100.

69. Viby-Mogensen J. Clinical assessment of neuromuscular transmission. *Br J Anaesth* 1982;**54**:209–23.

70. Rowaan CJ, Vandenbrom RHG, Wierda JMKH. The Relaxometer: a complete and comprehensive computer controlled neuromuscular transmission measurement system. *J Clin Monit* 1993;**9**:38–44.

71. Epstein RM, Epstein RA, Lee ASJ. A recording system for continuous evoked EMG. *Anesthesiology* 1976;**38**:287–9.

72. Lee CM, Katz RL, Lee ASJ, Glaser B. A new instrument for continuous recording of the evoked compound electromyogram in the clinical setting. *Anesth Analg* 1977;**56**:260–70.

73. Lam HS, Cass NM, Ng KC. Electromyographic monitoring of neuromuscular block. *Br J Anaesth* 1981;**53**:1351–7.

74. Carter JA, Arnold R, Yate PM, Flynn PJ. Assessment of the Datex Relaxograph during anesthesia and atracurium-induced neuromuscular blockade. *Br J Anaesth* 1986;**58**:1447–52.

75. Katz RL. Comparison of electrical and mechanical recording of spontaneous and evoked muscle activity. *Anesthesiology* 1965;**26**:204–11.

76. Weber S, Muravchick S. Electrical and mechanical train-of-four responses during depolarizing and nondepolarizing neuromuscular blockade. *Anesth Analg* 1986;**65**:771–6.

77. Weber S. Integrated electromyography: is it the new standard for clinical monitoring of neuromuscular blockade? *Int J Clin Monit Comp* 1987;**4**:53–57.

78. Kopman AF. The dose-effect relationship of metocurine: the integrated electromyogram of the first dorsal interosseous muscle and the mechanomyogram of the adductor pollicis compared. *Anesthesiology* 1988;**68**:604–7.

79. Donati F, Bevan DR. Muscle electromechanical correlations during succinylcholine infusion. *Anesth Analg* 1984;**63**:891–4.

80. Engbæk J. Monitoring of neuromuscular transmission by electromyography during anaesthesia. A comparison with mechanomyography in cat and man. *Dan Med Bull* 1996;**43**:301–16.

81. Pugh ND, Kay B, Healy TEJ. Electromyography in anaesthesia. *Anaesthesia* 1984;**39**:574–7.

82. Viby-Mogensen J, Jensen E, Werner M, Kirkegaard Neilsen H. Measurement of acceleration: a new method of monitoring neuromuscular function. *Acta Anaesthesiol Scand* 1988;**32**:45–48.

83. Jensen E, Viby-Mogensen J, Bang U. The accelograph: a new neuromuscular transmission monitor. *Acta Anaesth Scand* 1988;**32**:49–52.

84. Loan PB, Paxton LD, Mirakhur RK, Connolly FM, McCoy EP. The TOF-Guard neuromuscular monitor. A comparison with the Myograph 2000. *Anaesthesia* 1995;**50**:699–702.

85. Dahaba AA, Rehak PH, List WF. Assessment of acceleromyography with the TOF-GUARD: a comparison with electromyography. *Eur J Anaesthesiol* 1997;**14**:623–9.

86. Kopman AF, Klewicka MM, Neuman GG: The relationship between acceleromyographic train-of-four fade and single twitch depression. *Anesthesiology* 2002;**96**:583–7.

87. Kopman AF. Chin WA. A dose-response study of rocuronium. Do acceleromyographic and electromyographic monitors produce the same results? *Acta Anaesthesiologica Scandinavica.* 2005;**49**:323–7.

88. Kopman AF. Normalization of the acceleromyographic train-of-four fade ratio. *Acta Anaesthesiol Scand* 2005;**49**:1575–6.

89. Kopman AF, Kopman DJ. The TOF-watch algorithm for modifying the displayed train-of-four fade ratio: an analysis. *Acta Anaesthesiol Scand* 2006;**50**:1313–4.

90. Claudius C, Viby-Mogensen J. Acceleromyography for use in scientific and clinical practice: a systematic review of the evidence. *Anesthesiology* 2008;**108**:1117–40.

91. Kern SE, Johnson JO, Westenskow DR, Orr JA. An effectiveness study of a new piezoelectric sensor for train-of-four measurement. *Anesth Analg* 1994;**78**:978–82.

92. Johnson JO, Kern SE. A piezoelectric neuromuscular monitor. *Anesth Analg* 1994;**79**:1210–11.

93. Dahaba AA, Von Klobucar F, Rehak PH, List WF. Comparison of a new piezoelectric train-of-four neuromuscular monitor, the ParaGraph, and the Relaxometer mechanomyograph. *Br J Anaesth* 1999;**82**:780–2.

94. Dahaba AA, von Klobucar F, Rehak PH, List WF. The neuromuscular transmission module versus the Relaxometer mechanomyograph for neuromuscular block monitoring. *Anesth Analg* 2002;**94**:591–6.

95. Motamed C, Kirov K, Combes X, Duvaldestin P. Comparison between the Datex-Ohmeda M-NMT module and a force-displacement transducer for monitoring neuromuscular blockade. *Eur J Anaesthesiol.* 2003;**20**:467–9.

96. Dascalu A, Geller E, Moalem Y, Manoah M, Enav S, Rudick Z. Acoustic monitoring of intraoperative neuromuscular block. *Br J Anaesth* 1999;**83**:405–9.

97. Hemmerling TM, Michaud G, Tragger G, Deschamps S, Babin D, Donati F. Phonomyography and mechanomyography can be used interchangeably to measure neuromuscular block at the adductor pollicis muscle. *Anesth Analg* 2004;**98**:377–81.

98. Hemmerling TM, Michaud G, Trager G, Deschamps S. Phonomyographic measurements of neuromuscular blockade are similar to mechanomyography for hand muscles. *Can J Anaesth* 2004;**51**:795–800.

99. Hemmerling TM, Michaud G, Trager G, Donati F. Simultaneous determination of neuromuscular blockade at the adducting and abducting laryngeal muscles using phonomyography. *Anesth Analg* 2004;**98**:1729–33.

100. Dahaba AA, Bornemann H, Holst B, Wilfinger G, Metzler H. Comparison of a new neuromuscular transmission monitor compressomyograph with mechanomyograph. *Br J Anaesth* 2008;**100**:344–50.

101. Donati F, Antzaka C, Bevan DR. Potency of pancuronium at the diaphragm and the adductor pollicis muscle in humans. *Anesthesiology* 1986;**65**:1–5.

102. Cantineau JP, Porte F, d'Honneur G, Duvaldestin P. Neuromuscular effects of rocuronium on the diaphragm and adductor pollicis in anesthetized patients. *Anesthesiology* 1994;**81**:585–90.

103. Laycock JRD, Donati F, Smith CE, Donati DR. Potency of atracurium and vecuronium at the diaphragm and the adductor pollicis muscle. *Br J Anaesth* 1988;**61**:286–91.

104. Derrington MC, Hindocha N. Comparison of neuromuscular blockade in the diaphram and the hand. *Br J Anaesth* 1988;**61**:279–85.

105. Chauvin M, Lebrault C, Duvaldestin P. The neuromuscular blocking effect of vecuronium on the human diaphragm. *Anesth Analg* 1987;**66**:117–22.

106. Donati F, Meistelman C, Plaud B. Vecuronium neuromuscular blockade at the adductor muscles of the larynx and the adductor pollicis. *Anesthesiology* 1991;**74**:833–7.

107. Meistelman C, Plaud B, Donati F. Rocuronium (ORG 9426) neuromuscular blockade at the adductor muscles of the larynx and adductor pollicis in humans. *Can J Anaesth* 1992;**39**:665–9.

108. Plaud B, Debaene B, Donati F. The corrugator supercilii, not the orbicularis oculi, reflects rocuronium neuromuscular blockade at the laryngeal adductor muscles. *Anesthesiology* 2001;**95**:96–101.

109. Caffrey RR, Warren ML, Becker KE. Neuromuscular blockade monitoring comparing the orbicularis oculi and adductor pollicis muscles. *Anesthesiology* 1986;**65**:95–97.

110. Donati F, Meistelman C, Plaud B. Vecuronium neuromuscular blockade at the diaphragm, the orbicularis oculi, and the adductor pollicis muscle. *Anesthesiology* 1990;**73**:870–5.

111. Sharpe MD, Moote CA, Lam AM, Manninen PH. Comparison of integrated evoked EMG between the hypothenar and facial muscle groups following atracurium and vecuronium administration. *Can J Anaesth* 1991;**38**:318–23.

112. Paloheimo MPJ, Wilson RC, Edmonds HL, Lucas LF, Triantafillou AN. Comparison of neuromuscular blockade in upper facial and hypothenar muscles. *J Clin Monit* 1988;**4**:256–9.

113. Hemmerling TM, Donati F. Neuromuscular blockade at the larynx, the diaphragm and the corrugator supercilii muscle: a review. *Can J Anaesth* 2003;**50**:779–94.

114. Hemmerling TM, Schmidt J, Hanusa C, Wolf T, Schmitt H. Simultaneous determination of neuromuscular block at the larynx, diaphragm, adductor pollicis, orbicularis oculi and corrugator supercilii muscles. *Br J Anaesth* 2000;**85**:856–60.

115. Sopher MJ, Sears DH, Walts LF. Neuromuscular function monitoring comparing the flexor hallucis brevis and adductor pollicis muscles. *Anesthesiology* 1988;**69**:129–31.

116. Grayling M, Sweeney BP. Recovery from neuromuscular blockade: a survey of practice. *Anaesthesia* 2007;**62**: 806–9.

117. Sorgenfrei IF, Viby-Mogensen J, Swiatek FA. Does evidence lead to a change in clinical practice? Danish anaesthetists' and nurse anesthetists' clinical practice and knowledge of postoperative residual curarization. *Ugeskr Laeger* 2005;**167**:3878–82.

118. Fuchs-Buder T, Hofmockel R, Geldner G, Diefenbach C, Ulm K, Blobner M. The use of neuromuscular monitoring in Germany. *Anaesthesist* 2003;**52**:522–6.

119. Beemer GH, Rozental P. Postoperative neuromuscular function. *Anaesth Intensive Care* 1986;**14**:41–45.

120. El Mikatti N, Wilson A, Pollard BJ, Healy TEJ. Pulmonary function and head lift during spontaneous recovery from pipecuronium neuromuscular block. *Br J Anaesth* 1995;**74**:16–19.

121. Engbæk J, Østergaard D, Viby-Mogensen J, Skovgaard LT. Clinical recovery and train-of-four measured mechanically and electromyographically following atracurium. *Anesthesiology* 1989;**71**:391–5.

122. Debaene B, Plaud B, Dilly MP, Donati F. Residual paralysis in the PACU after a single intubating dose of nondepolarizing muscle relaxant with an intermediate duration of action. *Anesthesiology* 2003;**98**:1042–8.

123. McCaul C, Tobin E, Boylan JF, McShane AJ. Atracurium is associated with postoperative residual curarization. *Br J Anaesth* 2002;**89**:766–9.

124. Baillard C, Gehan G, Reboul-Marty J, Larmignat P, Samama CM, Cupa M. Residual curarization in the recovery room after vecuronium. *Br J Anaesth* 2000;**84**:394–5.

125. Hayes AH, Mirakhur RK, Breslin DS, Reid JE, McCourt KC. Postoperative residual block after intermediate-acting neuromuscular blocking drugs. *Anaesthesia* 2001;**56**: 312–8.

126. Kim KS, Lew SH, Cho HY, Cheong MA. Residual paralysis induced by either vecuronium or rocuronium after reversal with pyridostigmine. *Anesth Analg* 2002;**95**:1656–60.

127. Naguib M, Kopman AF, Ensor JE. Neuromuscular monitoring and postoperative residual curarisation: a meta-analysis. *Br J Anaesth* 2007;**98**:302–16.

128. Pedersen T, Viby-Mogensen J, Bang U, Olsen NV, Jensen E, Engbæk J. Does perioperative tactile evaluation of the train-of-four response influence the frequency of postoperative residual neuromuscular blockade? *Anesthesiology* 1990;**73**:835–9.

129. Kopman AF, Kopman DJ, Ng J, Zank LM. Antagonism of profound cisatracurium and rocuronium block: the role of

130. Mackintosh RR. Death following injection of neostigmine. *Br Med J* 1949;**1**:852.

131. Pooler HE. Atropine, neostigmine, and sudden deaths. *Anaesthesia* 1957;**12**:198–202.

132. Payne JP, Hughes R, Al Azawi S. Neuromuscular blockade by neostigmine in anesthetized man. *Br J Anaesth* 1981;**52**:69–76.

133. Caldwell JE. Reversal of residual neuromuscular block with neostigmine at one to four hours after a single intubating dose of vecuronium. *Anesth Analg* 1995;**80**:1168–74.

134. Viby-Mogensen J. Postoperative residual curarization and evidence-based anaesthesia. *Br J Anaesth* 2000;**84**:301–3.

135. Kopman AF, Sinha N. Acceleromyography as a guide to anesthetic management. A case report. *J Clin Anesth* 2003;**15**:145–8.

136. Gatke MR, Viby-Mogensen J, Rosenstock C, Jensen FS, Skovgaard LT. Postoperative muscle paralysis after rocuronium: less residual block when acceleromyography is used. *Acta Anaesthesiol Scand* 2002;**46**:207–13.

137. Mortensen CR, Berg H, El-Mahdy A, Viby-Mogensen J. Perioperative monitoring of neuromuscular transmission using acceleromyography prevents residual neuromuscular block following pancuronium. *Acta Anaesthiol Scand* 1995;**39**:797–801.

138. Murphy GS, Szokol JW, Marymount JH, et al. Intraoperative acceleromyography monitoring reduces the risk of residual neuromuscular blockade and adverse respiratory events in the postanesthesia care unit. *Anesthesiology* 2008;**109**:389–98.

139. Baillard C, Gehan G, Reboul-Marty J, Larmignat P, Samama CM, Cupa M. Residual curarization in the recovery room after vecuronium. *Br J Anaesth* 2000;**84**:394–5.

140. Baillard C, Clec'h C, Catineau J, et al. Postoperative residual neuromuscular block: a survey of management. *Br J Anaesth* 2005;**95**:622–6.

141. Miller RD. How should residual neuromuscular blockade be detected? *Anesthesiology* 1989;**70**:379–80.

142. Shorten GD. Postoperative residual curarisation: incidence, aetiology and associated morbidity. *Anaesth Intensive Care* 1993;**21**:782–9.

143. Murphy GS, Szokol JW, Marymount JH, Greenberg SB, Avram MJ, Vender JS. Residual neuromuscular blockade and critical respiratory events in the postanesthesia care unit. *Anesth Analg* 2008;**107**:130–7.

144. Kopman AF, Zank LM, Ng J, Neuman GG. Antagonism of cisatracurium and rocuronium block at a tactile train-of-four count of 2: Should quantitative assessment of neuromuscular function be mandatory? *Anesth Analg* 2004;**98**:102–6.

145. Kopman AF. Sugammadex: a revolutionary approach to neuromuscular antagonism. *Anesthesiology* 2006;**104**:631–3.

146. de Boer H, Driessen JJ, Marcus MAE, Kerkkamp H, Heeringa M, Klimek M. Reversal of rocuronium-induced (1.2 mg/kg) profound neuromuscular block by sugammadex: a multicenter, dose-finding and safety study. *Anesthesiology* 2007;**107**:239–44.

Critical care testing in the operating room
Electrolytes, glucose, acid–base, blood gases

Lakshmi V. Ramanathan, Judit Tolnai, and Michael S. Lewis

Overview

Homeostasis requires maintenance of the normal physiologic balance of bodily fluids and their composition; major disturbances in fluid and electrolyte balance can rapidly alter cardiovascular, neurologic, endocrine, and neuromuscular function. In some cases, a disturbance of the normal composition of bodily fluids provides vital information regarding the function (or dysfunction) of major organ systems. Thus, measurements of electrolytes, blood gases, acid–base status, glucose, hemoglobin, hematocrit, parameters of coagulation, and indices of renal, cardiac, and hepatic function must be rapidly available to perioperative practitioners because the patient's condition may change rapidly and dramatically during the course of the procedure and the immediate postoperative period. Such measurements can be provided by a central laboratory, a dedicated stat lab, or point-of-care instruments.

The focus of this chapter is electrolytes, fluid balance, acid–base status, and blood gases. A review of bodily fluids and electrolyte composition is followed by a discussion of preanalytical factors that influence test results and regulatory issues. Reference ranges and critical values for routinely monitored parameters are provided. The chapter concludes with a presentation of several commonly used point-of-care testing platforms and technologies that are available in the operating room.

Body fluid and electrolyte composition

Total body water in an adult male represents approximately 60 percent of the body weight; the remainder is composed of 7 percent minerals, 18 percent protein, and 15 percent fat.[1] For females, there is a slightly increased body fat content and decreased water content to 50 percent. The distribution of water is either extracellular or intracellular, with the two compartments separated by semipermeable membranes. Extracellular fluid (ECF) comprises about one-third of the total body water and body weight. ECF is further divided between blood volume (8% of body weight), plasma (5% body weight), and interstitial fluid (15% body weight). The other two-thirds represent intracellular fluid (ICF), which is approximately 40 percent of body weight. Table 23.1 illustrates the distribution of the electrolytes in different bodily fluids.[1]

Sodium and chloride dominate the extracellular fluid, whereas potassium and phosphorus are predominant in the intracellular fluid. The type of surgery being performed (e.g. minimal vs large blood losses, minimal vs large evaporative losses from open bodily cavities) and the anesthetic chosen (e.g. vasodilatory central neuraxial blockade vs general anesthesia) have varying effects on patient hemodynamics and often play a large role in determining the amount of fluid replacement that is needed. The type of fluid provided is generally determined by the illness present and the needs of the individual patients, based on their specific fluid losses. The physiology of the perioperative period also mandates certain fluid choices (e.g. isotonic replacement fluids in the operating room vs physiologic maintenance fluids in the perioperative period). Local custom may also influence the choice of intravenous fluids used.

Sodium

Sodium is the major cation of extracellular fluid. As it represents the bulk of inorganic cations in plasma, it plays a central role in maintaining the normal distribution of water and the osmotic pressure in the ECF compartment.[1] The normal reference range for serum sodium ranges from 135 to 145 mEq/L.

Hyponatremia

Hyponatremia occurs when sodium is less than 135 mEq/L. Clinically, the symptoms tend to occur at levels less than 130 mEq/L. These include headache, confusion, and lethargy. More severe symptoms, including stupor, seizures, and coma, occur when the sodium is less than 120 mEq/L.

Causes of hyponatremia can be described by the osmolarity of the ECF. The differential diagnosis includes hypoosmolar hyponatremia, normoosmolar hyponatremia, and hyperosmolar hyponatremia.

Hypoosmolar hyponatremia is the most common and is caused by either sodium loss or water gain. Normoosmolar hyponatremia is usually the result of hyperlipidemia and hyperproteinemia. The plasma component of blood is composed of water and nonaqueous protein and lipid. If proteins or lipids are elevated, the sodium concentration measured is less than its true concentration. Hyperosmolar hyponatremia is usually the result of increases in nonsodium solutes that remain mostly in

Table 23.1. Electrolyte content and daily volumes of body fluids and secretions

Fluid	Na$^+$ (mEq/L)	K$^+$ (mEq/L)	H$^+$ (mEq/L)	Cl$^-$ (mEq/L)	HCO$_3^-$ (mEq/L)	Adult volume (mL/day)
Saliva	60	20	0	15	50	1500
Gastric	20–120	15	60	130	0	2500
Pancreatic	140	5	0	70	70	1000
Biliary	140	5	0	140	44	600
Ileostomy	120	20	0	100	40	3000
Diarrhea	100	20	0	100	40	Variable

the ECF. Hyperglycemia and mannitol are common causes of this condition. Other solutes, including ethanol, methanol, and ethylene glycol, can cause hyperosmolar hyponatremia. Sodium decreases by 1.5 to 2.0 mEq/L for every 100 mg/dL increase in blood glucose.[1]

Free water restriction is the first-line therapy in hypervolemic hyponatremia. Hypertonic saline (1.8% or 3%) is indicated for the treatment of severe hyponatremia. When such treatment is employed, the sodium values should be closely followed, and the increase in measured sodium should not exceed 1 to 2 mEq/L/hour.

Hypernatremia

Hypernatremia occurs when sodium is greater than 145 mEq/L. Symptoms are typically seen with levels >150 mEq/L. These patients have neuromuscular irritability, lethargy, and ataxia that can progress to confusion, coma, and seizures as the sodium approaches 180 mEq/L. Hypernatremia is caused by water loss or a primary sodium gain. Water loss can be the result of either diabetes insipidus or osmotic diuresis. Nonrenal losses are from the GI tract and from insensible losses (the use of a warming device or warming blanket during long operating room cases can contribute to significant insensible losses). Hypernatremia may also occur from administration of hypertonic saline and sodium bicarbonate.

The treatment relies on the calculation of the free water deficit,[2] which can be calculated as indicated below:

Free water deficit (liters)

= (total body water)

×[(plasma sodium concentration − 140)/140],

where total body water = 0.6 × body weight in kilograms.

Half the deficit is replaced over the first 24 hours, and the remainder over the next 24 to 48 hours. Overcorrection of sodium can result in coma, seizures, and intracerebral edema. The sodium values, therefore, should be closely followed, and the decline of measured sodium should not exceed 1 to 2 mEq/L/hr.

Potassium

Potassium plays an important role in cell membrane physiology by maintaining cell membrane potential. Potassium is actively transported into cells by Na/K ATPase, which maintains an intracellular K$^+$. Normal serum or plasma potassium concentrations range from 3.5 to 5.5 mEq/L. Body potassium stores are primarily intracellular; about 2 percent of the total potassium is found in ECF.[2] Although both hyper- and hypokalemia can be detrimental, it is often the rate of change of serum potassium (as opposed to the absolute level) that causes problems (e.g. dysrhythmias).

Hyperkalemia

Hyperkalemia can result from renal failure, hypoadrenal-cortisolism (Addison syndrome), rhabdomyolysis, potassium supplements, and medications such as penicillin-K, heparin, aldosterone antagonists, ACE inhibitors, and succinylcholine. Pseudohyperkalemia as a laboratory error can occur as a result of hemolysis in the sample, an elevated platelet count (>600,000/mm^3), or leukocytosis. Clinically, hyperkalemia causes ECG changes that may include tall peaked T waves, a widened QRS, and a widened PR interval.

Management of hyperkalemia can be challenging. When severe hyperkalemia is present, K$^+$ can be driven into the ICF compartment by giving insulin, 0.1 unit regular insulin/kg (usually with dextrose, 0.5–1.0 g/kg to prevent hypoglycemia). Temporary, mild hyperventilation can be helpful as well in emergent situations as respiratory alkalosis will drive potassium intracellularly. Additionally, the adverse manifestations of hyperkalemia can be immediately counteracted electrically by the administration of a judicious amount of calcium chloride (5 mg/kg). Sodium polystyrene sulfonate in 20 percent sorbitol by mouth or per rectum can additionally remove 1 mEq/g of K$^+$; however, it adds approximately 1.7 mEq of Na$^+$/g. Diuretics (e.g., furosemide 20 mg, IV) can be employed where acceptable to assist with the removal of potassium from the body. Hemodialysis is a definitive management of severe hyperkalemia where necessary.

Hypokalemia

Hypokalemia is defined as a serum potassium concentration of less than 3.5 mEq/L. It can occur by one of three mechanisms: intracellular shift, reduced intake, and increased loss owing to several conditions, including primary and secondary aldosteronism.[2] As the intracellular K$^+$ concentration is much greater than the extracellular concentration, the potassium shift into the cells can cause severe hypokalemia, with little change in the extracellular concentration.[2] Clinical manifestations of hypokalemia include muscle weakness, cardiac arrhythmias, cardiac U waves, inverted and flattened T waves, prolonged QT interval, paresthesias, and ileus. Hypokalemia can precipitate rhabdomyolysis, increase renal ammonia production, and worsen hepatic encephalopathy. K^+ supplementation can be provided by the oral or parenteral routes.

Chloride

Chloride is the major anion in extracellular fluid. Together with sodium, it is involved in the maintenance of water distribution, osmotic pressure, and the anion–cation balance in the extracellular fluid compartment. The chloride concentration in ICF is 45 to 54 mEq/L; in serum, the normal concentration is 95 to 105 mEq/L.

Chloride is a strong ion that is completely or nearly completely dissociated, as is sodium. An increase in sodium relative to chloride increases the dissociation and, hence, the pH. The opposite effect, a decrease in the pH, occurs when the sodium and chloride concentrations move closer together. Chloride becomes the body's strongest tool for adjusting the plasma pH. A common form of metabolic alkalosis is the loss of chloride from gastric fluid. When a strong anion, such as chloride, is lost in gastric secretions, there is an increase in the ionic difference between anions and cations, resulting in a decrease in the amount of free water dissociation into H^+ and OH^-. This results in a decrease in the H^+ concentration.

Hypochloremia

Hypochloremia, or decreased serum chloride less than 95 mEq/L, is observed in salt-losing nephritis associated with chronic pyelonephritis, as well as in metabolic acidosis caused by increased production, as in diabetic ketoacidosis, or decreased excretion, as in renal failure. Other conditions include aldsteronism, bromide intoxication, cerebral salt wasting after head injury, syndrome of inappropriate antidiuretic hormone (SIADH), and conditions associated with expansion of extracellular fluid volume.[2]

The treatement of hypochloremic metabolic alkalosis is to replenish chloride. Two treatments are usually given: saline and potassium chloride. Saline gives back equal parts of sodium and chloride. The chloride concentration is always much lower that serum sodium; thus, chloride will increase more rapidly when large amounts of saline are administered. Potassium chloride is generally more effective, as much of the potassium moves intracellularly, leaving much of the chloride in the plasma.

Hyperchloremia

Hyperchloremia (chloride greater than 105 mEq/L) is seen in dehydration, renal tubular acidosis, and acute renal failure. It is also observed in metabolic acidosis associated with prolonged diarrhea, loss of sodium bicarbonate in diabetes insipidus, adrenocortical hyperfunction, and salicylate intoxication.

Calcium

Plasma calcium is present in three forms: protein-bound (50%), ionized (45%), and a nonionized and diffusible fraction (5%). The nonionized form is complexed with phosphate, bicarbonate, and citrate. The normal range for serum calcium is 8.8 to 10.4 mg/dL; this represents the protein-bound component. Normal ionized calcium is 4.8 to 7.2 mg/dL or 1.1 to 1.3 mmol/L. About 90 percent of the protein that binds calcium is albumin. An increase or decrease in albumin of 1g/dL is associated with a decline or rise of the serum calcium by 0.8 mg/dL.[2] Ionized calcium is critical for

1. Proper function of the heart, brain, and other organs;
2. Myocardial contraction and conduction;
3. Smooth vascular muscle tone and the normal function of metabolic systems; and
4. Intracellular messenger and biochemical modulator for various organ systems.

Hypocalcemia

Several factors can contribute to ionized hypocalcemia, including hypomagnesemia, elevated circulating cytokines, resistance to PTH or vitamin D calcium binding and chelation, or cellular distribution and sequestration.[2]

Hypocalcemia is manifested with skeletal muscle spasm, tetany, paresthesias, cramps, hyperreflexia, confusion, seizures, and coma. Cardiovascular signs include peripheral vasodilation, hypotension, ventricular tachycardia, and prolonged QT interval. The skeletal muscle spasm and tetany are a result of decreased threshold for neuronal excitability. Latent tetany can be demonstrated in a patient by eliciting the Chvostek or Trousseau sign.

Postoperative hypocalcemia may occur following thyroidectomy or parathyroidectomy, usually within 24 to 36 hours after surgery, and in patients with pancreatic insufficiency and/or malnutrition. Many blood products (particularly packed red blood cells) contain citrate as an additive, which will bind ionized calcium in the patient. The effect of blood transfusion is most pronounced in patients with hepatic and renal failure where citrate clearance is reduced. Hypocalcemia is worsened by alkalosis that could be seen in a patient who is hyperventilating because of pain. Alkalosis results in increased calcium binding to albumin, causing a precipitous fall in plasma calcium. Treatment should be reserved for symptomatic patients and for those with ionized calcium levels below 0.8 mmol/L.

Hypercalcemia

Hypercalcemia is a relatively common metabolic abnormality. The most common reason for hypercalcemia is primary hyperparathyroidism caused by a parathyroid adenoma. The clinical manifestations of hypercalcemia are often described by the following collection of symptoms: "bones, stone, abdominal groans, and psychiatric overtones." The individual symptoms include hypotonia, weakness, hyporeflexia, seizures, confusion, psychosis, coma, anorexia, vomiting, constipation, polyuria, and nephrocalcinosis; fractures, osteopenia, hypovolemia, and hypotension; and QT shortening, cardiac arrhythmias, and heart block. Hypercalcemia is defined as ionized serum calcium concentration greater than 1.3 mmol/L or serum calcium levels greater than 10.5 mg/dL. Patients are asymptomatic with mild symptoms until serum calcium levels are above 11.5 mg/dL. Immediate management is to use normal saline at 250 to 500 mL/hr to correct volume depletion and to dilute the ionized calcium. Calcium and inhibit calcium reabsorption increases sodium excretion via the kidneys.

Magnesium

The active form of magnesium is ionized, and normal levels are 1.6 to 2.6 mEq/L. Approximately 1 percent of total magnesium stores are in the ECF, with the majority being in the bone, muscle, and cells. Serum magnesium levels are therefore not reflective of total body stores. Magnesium is important in cardiac conduction, neuromuscular function, and metabolic pathways, and as a cofactor in enzyme metabolism.

Hypomagnesemia

Hypomagnesemia occurs when serum concentration is less than 1.2 mEq/L; it presents clinically with neurologic manifestations. These include paresthesias, fasciculations, tetany, hyperreflexia, seizures, and numerous cardiac manifestations. The cardiac symptoms include premature ventricular contractions, atrial fibrillation, ventricular arrythmias including torsades de pointes, prolonged PR and QT intervals, premature atrial contractions, and superventricular tachycardias. Neurologically, the patients have ataxia, confusion, and coma. Hypomagnesemia can potentiate digoxin toxicity and congestive heart failure. It is caused most commonly by inadequate gastrointestinal absorption, magnesium loss, or failure of renal magnesium conservation. Hypomagnesemia has been associated with prolonged nasogastric suctioning, gastrointestinal or biliary fistulas, and drains.

Hypermagnesemia

Hypermagnesemia occurs when serum concentration is greater than 2.5 mg/dL; most cases result from iatrogenic administration of antacids, enemas, and total parenteral nutrition. Often this is found in patients with impaired renal function. Hypermagnesemia impairs the release of acetylcholine at the neuromuscular junction; the result is decreased skeletal muscle function and neuromuscular blockade. Clinically, patients exhibit lethargy, drowsiness, nausea and vomiting, flushing, and diminished deep tendon reflexes when the magnesium level is 5.0 to 7.9 mg/dL. When the magnesium levels are above 7.0 mg/dL, the patient experiences somnolence, hypotension, and ECG changes, which progress to heart block, apnea, and paralysis when the magnesium levels are greater than 12.0 mg/dL. Immediate treatment is through the use of IV calcium (5 to 10 mEq) to delay toxicity while definitive therapy is instituted. This includes stopping the source of the magnesium and expanding the extracellular volume with saline and then inducing diuresis with furosemide.

Glucose

Glucose can be derived from either endogenous or exogenous sources. The exogenous sources of glucose include enteral or parenteral nutrition and intravenous fluids. Plasma glucose normally ranges from 60 to 100 mg/dL before meals and up to 150 mg/dL after meals.

Hypoglycemia

Hypoglycemia is usually defined as a glucose level less than 50 mg/dL; however, a significant portion of normal individuals, particularly healthy young women, may have glucose levels that fall to <50 mg/dL. Initial symptoms include nervousness, blurred vision, diaphoresis, nausea, and tachycardia. Additionally, hypoglycemia can present acutely as a result of seizures or cardiac arrest. It is a contributing factor of agitation, somnolence, and mental status changes. Severe hypoglycemia can precipitate a myocardial infarction or encephalopathy. Patients at risk include those with depleted glycogen stores or impaired glycogenolysis, as well as those with malnutrition, cirrhosis, renal failure, and alcoholic ketoacidosis. Commonly used drugs that lead to hypoglycemia include pentamidine, moxifloxacin, salicylates, haloperidol, and trimethoprim-sulfamethoxazole.[2]

Hyperglycemia

Hyperglycemia can be divided into three clinically relevant categories: mild hyperglycemia (glucose range of 110–180 mg/dL), moderate hyperglycemia (180–400 mg/dL), and severe or diabetic ketoacidosis (>400 mg/dL).

Hyperglycemia is clinically associated with diabetes mellitus, insulin resistance, diabetic ketoacidosis, or nonketotic hyperosmolar states. In the hospitalized patient, stress and medications may lead to elevated glucose levels. Pseudohyperglycemia may also occur in the setting of a blood sample drawn from a peripheral IV line where the patient is receiving D_5W or parenterally administered nutritional supplementation (e.g. total parenteral nutrition). Relative insulin resistance can occur after administration of catecholamines or glucocorticoids. Hyperglycemia also produces dehydration and electrolyte imbalances as a result of a relative hyperosmolar state and the subsequent osmotic diuresis. Hyperglycemia is undesirable after cardiac arrest as a consequence of increasing the level of intraneural lactic acidosis.

Hyperglycemia in hospitalized patients has been associated with increased rates of infection; tight glucose control has been shown to reduce mortality when the glucose was kept between 80 and 110 mg/dL.

Hemoglobin/hematocrit

Red cell analysis is part of a complete blood count (CBC). Normal red blood cell (RBC) count for males is 4.6 to $6.0 \times 10^6/\mu L$ and females is 4.1 to $5.4 \times 10^6/\mu L$. Red blood cells and white blood cells are analyzed together. This does not pose a problem until the white blood cell count is greater than 50,000/μL. Additionally, patients with large platelets may have falsely elevated hematocrits.

Normal values for hemoglobin concentration is 14 to 18 g/dL for males and 12 to 16 g/dL for females. However, the normal hemoglobin value for patients with chronic disease (sickle cell, myelodysplasias) is often significantly lower, 6 to 7 g/dL.[3] Although most analyzers are able to measure hemoglobin optically between 478 and 672 nm, it is also calculated from the measured hematocrit. Increased sample turbidity from paraproteins, lipids, TPN, hemoglobinopathies, and nucleated cells (including nucleated red cells and leukemias) can lead to falsely elevated hemoglobins.

The normal reference range for mean corpuscular volume (MCV) is 80 to 100 fL, which is the average measurement of red cell volume or size. Proteins or antibodies can coat red cells, causing them to agglutinate and falsely elevate the MCV. The MCV is the average value of all cells counted.

The normal reference range for hematocrit is 42 percent to 53 percent in males and 34 percent to 48 percent in females. This represents a percentage of blood volume occupied by red blood cells.[3] Overdilution of the sample by an IV with saline or lactated Ringer solution will result in a hemodilution. A similar laboratory error can occur if there is too much anticoagulant in the collection tube relative to the amount of sample drawn into it. A pseudohemoconcentration can occur by collection of blood from a prolonged tourniquet application.

Lactic acid

Lactic acid is converted to pyruvic acid in the presence of lactate dehydrogenase. Molecular oxygen is required for the conversion of pyruvate to acetyl-Coenzyme A, which is subsequently metabolized in the tricarboxylic acid cycle to produce 36 mmol of adenosine triphosphate (ATP). When oxygen is lacking, pyruvate concentration rises and it is converted to lactate. During hypoxia, glucose metabolism yields only 2 mmol of ATP. The relationship among oxygen delivery, oxygen consumption, and blood lactate levels is well demonstrated, as blood lactate levels rise with a decrease in oxygen consumption. Persistent tissue hypoxia is associated with organ failure and ultimately death in surgical and medical emergency patients.[4]

Lactate is available on most blood gas analyzers, as well as in a point-of-care test. Arterial specimens are usually used, with the measurements being performed immediately. If there is difficulty obtaining an arterial sample, blood specimens should be collected in a gray-top tube that uses sodium fluoride as an additive that prevents glycolysis.

Blood gases and acid–base equilibrium

Internal respiration of tissue cells consumes oxygen and produces carbon dioxide and organic acid metabolites of biochemical substrates. The major buffer system of the extracellular

Table 23.2. Reference ranges

	Arterial	Venous
pH	7.35–7.43	7.33–7.43
pCO_2	35–45 mmHg	40–50 mmHg
pO_2	80–105 mmHg	20–50 mmHg
Base excess	–2.3 to 2.3 mmol/L	–3 to 3 mmol/L
HCO_3	20–29 mEq/L	20–27 mEq/L
TCO_2	24–32 mEq/L	24–32 mEq/L
O_2 saturation	90–100%	0–75%
Hematocrit		42–55% male, 34–48% female
Glucose	60–120 mg/dL	60–120 mg/dL
Sodium	135–145 mEq/L	135–145 mEq/L
Potassium	3.5–5.0 mEq/L	3.5–5.0 mEq/L
Calcium, ionized	1.14–1.29 mmol/L	1.14–1.29 mmol/L
Lactate	0.5–2.2 mmol/L	0.5–2.2 mmol/L

fluid is the bicarbonate system, which interacts with CO_2 and physically dissolved CO_2 in the blood. The definitive acid–base equation is the Henderson–Hasselbalch[5] equation:

$$pH = 6.1 + \log(HCO_3^-)/(0.03 \times PaCo_2),$$

where 6.1 = the pKa of carbonic acid and 0.03 is the solubility coefficient in blood of carbon dioxide.

A clear understanding of a patient's acid–base status involves the integration of information obtained from measurements of arterial blood gases, electrolytes, and often, the history of the present illness. The first step is to determine whether a patient is acidemic (pH < 7.35) or alkalemic (pH > 7.45). One then needs to determine whether the arterial blood gas results are consistent with a simple or complex, acute or chronic, respiratory or metabolic alkalosis or acidosis. Often, a mixed picture is present in complex surgical patients that requires a teasing apart of acute from chronic disturbances, taking physiologic compensation and the effects of acute patient management into account (e.g. mechanical ventilation or diuresis). In general, mild acidosis is better tolerated than alkalosis, because of the improved oxygen kinetics in acidosis. With the notable exception of the pulmonary vasculature, all vascular beds vasodilate in response to acidosis. Normal reference ranges used at the Mount Sinai Hospital (New York, NY) for blood gases and electrolytes are displayed in Table 23.2.

As discussed in a subsequent section, proper specimen collection is essential for correct interpretation of the acid–base status of the patient. It is important to note that if the specimen is not placed on ice, arterial pCO_2 rises 3 to 10 mmHg/hr, with a fall in the pH. If a sample is left at room temperature, pseudohypoxemia and pseudoacidosis occur because of active metabolism in the sample. Pseudohypocarbia and falsely elevated arterial pO_2 can occur with trapped air bubbles.

Diagnostic indicators for vital functions

For the critical care patient, the parameters we have discussed play a major role in vital body functions that are summarized in Table 23.3, Blood gases, glucose, and electrolytes are involved in acid–base balance; energy and physiologic processes such as conduction, contraction, and perfusion; and maintenance of

Table 23.3. Critical care test profiles

Vital function	Diagnostic indications	Mount Sinai alert/critical values
Acid–base	pH	<7.20 or >7.60
	pCO_2	<20 mmg or ≫70 mmHg
	CO_2 content	<10 mEq/L or >40 mEq/L
	Bicarbonate	<10 mEq/L or >40 mEq/L
Energy	Glucose	Adults <40 mg/dL; newborns >400 mg/dL
	Hemoglobin	Adults <6 g/dL; newborns <6.6 g/dL
	pO_2	<40 mmHg (arterial only)
	Oxygen saturation	
Conduction	Potassium	Adults <2.5 mEq/L or >6.5 mEq/L
		Newborns <2.5 mEq/L or >8.0 mEq/L
	Sodium	<120 mEq/L or >160 mEq/L
	Ionized calcium	<0.8 or >1.54 mmol/L
	Ionized magnesium	<0.40 mmol/L
Contraction	Ionized calcium	<0.8 or >1.54 mmol/L
	Ionized magnesium	<0.40 mmol/L
Perfusion	Lactate	<5.0 mmol/L
Osmolality	Measured osmolality	<250 or >335 mOsm/kg
	Calculated osmolality	<250 or >335 mOsm/kg
Hemostasis	Hematocrit	Adult <15%; newborn <20%
	Prothrombin time (PT; international normalized ratio, INR)	PT >43 sec; INR >5.0
	Activated partial thromboplastin time (APTT)	>100 sec
	Activated clotting time (ACT)	N/A
	Platelet count and function	
	D-Dimer	N/A
Homeostasis	Creatinine urea nitrogen	Creat >9.9 mg/dL; BUN >40 mg/dL
	White blood cell count	<2500 or >40,000
	Glycosolated hemoglobin, fructosamine	N/A

osmolality, hemostasis, and homeostasis.[5] Many of these tests are available at the bedside using different point-of-care testing platforms. Included in Table 23.3 is a list of the critical values used at the Mount Sinai Hospital.

Preanalytical factors in critical care testing

Proper specimen collection is essential for the interpretation of blood gas and electrolyte analyses. These tests, especially pO_2, are very sensitive to preanalytic effects that include collection techniques, volume of (liquid) anticoagulant used, exposure to air and air bubbles, time of sample handling, and temperature and agitation of the sample. Blood gas measurements are done exclusively on heparinized whole blood samples, usually of arterial origin. Anaerobic collection technique is essential to successful blood gas measurements. As air has a much lower pCO_2 and higher pO_2 than blood, exposure at any time affects these results. Air bubbles are easily entrapped when blood is collected in a syringe. If the air bubble is disturbed when the sample is agitated or transported in a pneumatic tube, the pO_2 value can be significantly affected.[3] A 0.2-mL air bubble, for example, can increase the pO_2 by 100 mmHg.[5] Additionally, if a blood gas specimen remains at room temperature for more than 15 minutes, the pO_2 decreases.[5]

It is preferable that blood samples be collected using lyophilized heparin rather than liquid heparin.[6] Liquid heparin in sufficient volume can alter the PCO_2 result when either the syringes are not completely filled or there is too much heparin.

If the correct amount of heparin is not used, samples usually clot, making them unsuitable for analysis.

Apart from heparinized syringes, if specimens must be sent to the laboratory, the order of drawing blood tubes for various tests to obtain accurate results[7] is as follows:

1. Blood culture (yellow) SPS sterile top tube.
2. Light blue (buffered sodium citrate) tube for prothrombin time/international normalized ratio/activated clotting time.
3. Plain gold or speckled top with or without separator for chemistry tests.
4. Green or light green sodium or lithium heparin with or without separator for potassium.
5. Lavender top (EDTA) for complete blood count.
6. Pink, white, or royal blue top (EDTA).
7. Gray, sodium fluoride/potassium oxalate for glucose and lactate.
8. Dark blue top for fibrin degradation products.

Role of the laboratory

Laboratory support in a critical care setting, specifically the operating room, is vital to outcomes and patient care. Several institutions have rapid-response, stat, or acute laboratories in the immediate vicinity of the operating room. These laboratories are usually operated by licensed medical technologists. The testing menu is usually limited to blood gases, electrolytes, hematocrit, hemoglobin, prothrombin times, and other tests, depending on the needs of the institution. The turnaround time depends on the test and the vicinity of the laboratory to the operating room. For the Stat Lab at Mount Sinai Medical Center, which is connected to the operating room by a pneumatic tube, the turnaround time for a blood gas, once received, is 10 minutes.

On the other hand, tests performed at the patient location are known as point-of-care (POC) testing. The evolution of technologies in this area has enabled operating room personnel to operate relatively simple devices at the bedside with oversight from the laboratory. We present here an overview of the POC testing program with special reference to regulatory, technical, and competency aspects.

Regulatory requirements and credentialing

Although tests are often conducted outside a traditional laboratory setting, testing procedures and documentation requirements are governed by regulatory agency guidelines, hospital policy, and procedure manuals for each instrument. Licensing for POC tests is under the central or core laboratory, with the medical director of the labs being responsible for all procedures followed.

Regulations governing the procedures for POC testing are established by the following agencies:[8]

1. Health Care Financing Organization (HCFA)
2. Clinical Laboratory Improvement Amendments of 1988 (CLIA'88)
3. College of American Pathologists (CAP)
4. Joint Commission, formerly the Joint Commission on Accreditation of Health Care Organizations (JCAHO)
5. Individual state departments of health that require separate licenses (e.g. New York and California)

In Mount Sinai's operating room, POC tests conducted are considered by CLIA'88 regulations as moderately complex. This requires that operators have a minimum of a bachelor of science degree, and procedures for testing must follow guidelines as outlined by CLIA'88, CAP, and JCAHO regulations. These include proficiency testing for accuracy, reference range validation, calibration verification, linearity, and annual competency of testing personnel. Proficiency testing involves analysis of unknown samples provided by CAP or other commercial sources. It is conducted by nonlaboratory personnel to ensure performance of the device as well as the technique of the operator. The results are submitted to CAP, which compares the values to a nationwide pool of the same device and methodology. If a problem is noted, corrective action is taken; in some cases, this may mean that the operator is retrained.

Point-of-care devices

Recent advances in POC testing have resulted in smaller and more accurate devices, with a wide menu of tests.[9] The most widely used POC tests are bedside glucose testing, critical care

Table 23.4. Partial list of critical care instruments

Vendor	Instrument
Abbott (i-STAT)	i-STAT
Bayer	200,300 800 series, Rapidpoint
Diametrics	IRMA
Instrumentation Lab	1600, 1700 series, GEM series
NOVA	Stat profile series, CCX
Radiometer	ABL series
Roche (AVL)	900 series, Omni and Opti series
ITC	Hemochron, Response
Medtronic	Hepcon Series
Accumetrics	Verify Now series
Haemoscope	Thromboelastograph

analysis, urinalysis, coagulation, occult blood, and urine pregnancy testing. Other selected tests include cardiac markers, drugs of abuse, influenza A and B, Rapid Strep A, urine microalbumin, and creatinine. Table 23.4 gives a partial list of critical care instruments that can be used either in the laboratory or the point-of-care setting such as the operating room.

Methodologies/instrumentation used in critical care testing

Blood gas electrodes are electrochemical devices used to measure pH and blood gases directly. pH is measured using a hydrogen ion (H^+)-selective glass electrode. The sample diffuses into the H^+-selective glass membrane, creating a change in potential between the buffer and the sample. The change in electrical potential is measured with respect to a reference electrode of constant potential. Blood pCO_2 is determined using the same principles, in which CO_2 in dissolved blood diffuses across a semipermeable membrane covering the glass electrode. The change in pH of the buffer under the membrane is measured. pO_2 is determined using the Clark electrode, at which changes in electrical current are measured across a semipermeable membrane. This amperometric method is also used in the measurement of urea, nitrogen, fructose, lactate, creatinine, ketones, and other substances.[10]

i-STAT analyzer

Single-use sensors have been constructed using thin-film technology, the most commercial example being the i-STAT analyzer (Abbott Point of Care; Princeton, NJ; Figure 23.1). This is a hand-held blood gas device that measures electrolytes, glucose, creatinine, and certain coagulation parameters. The electrodes are wafer structures constructed with thin metal oxide films using microfabrication techniques directly comparable with those used in the computer industry. The results are small, single-use cartridges containing an array of electrochemical sensors that operate in conjunction with a hand-held analyzer to be used at the bedside. As the sensor layer is thin, blood can permeate quickly and the sensor cartridge can be used immediately after it is unwrapped from its packaging. This is

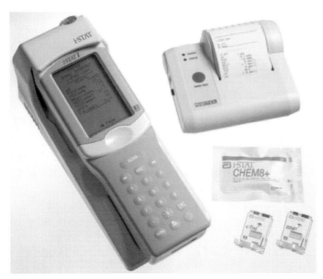

Figure 23.1. The i-STAT point of care analyzer (Abbott, Princeton, NJ).

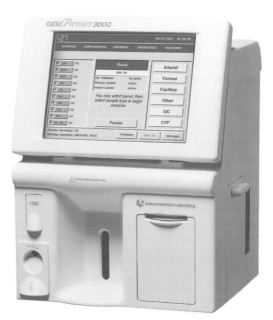

Figure 23.2. GEM 3000 (Instrumentation Laboratories, Bedford, MA).

an advantage over devices using thick-film sensors that require an equilibration time period before they can be used on patient samples.

The i-STAT consists of a hand-held analyzer and a data transmitter (including a battery charger) commonly called a downloader. The instrument uses a single cartridge for each sample. The cartridges are manufactured in several configurations, and each cartridge can test for multiple analytes. Blood gases, electrolytes, lactate, and ionized calcium can be measured by using specific cartridges.[11]

The analyzer is a microprocessor-controlled electromechanical device that moves the sample through the cartridge, in which it reacts with the reagent(s) and produces electrical signals to be analyzed by the microprocessor. The cartridge also contains quality control solutions. Automatic internal checks are performed with each cartridge.[11]

The sequence of actions that take place in the analyzer is as follows:

1. Makes electrical contact with the cartridge.
2. Identifies the cartridge type.
3. Injects calibration fluid over reference sensors.
4. Mixes the reagents and the samples.
5. Heats the sensors to 37°C.
6. Measures the electrical signals generated by the sensors and calibration fluid.
7. Measures the electrical signals generated by the sensors and the sample.
8. Calculates, displays, and stores the results.

The relative ease of transport of the i-STAT to the bedside makes it extremely attractive to the operating room staff. The disadvantage is the waste caused by managing the different cartridges that are available during the procedure.

GEM 3000

Devices such as the GEM 3000 (Instrumentation Laboratories; Bedford, MA; Figure 23.2) used in critical care testing include thick-film sensors or electrodes in strips to measure glucose, lactate, and blood gases. These are reusable. The sensors contain reagents and calibrators packed into a small cartridge that is placed in the body of the GEM 3000. The reagent pack can measure a specific number of samples. It has an expiration date. The GEM 3000 analyzer provides measurements of pH, pCO_2, pO_2, Na, K, ICa, glucose, and lactate on whole blood samples using a disposable cartridge.[12] Several other parameters are calculated from the measured analytes. Cartridges can test multiple samples and are manufactured with capacities ranging for 75 to 600 samples.[12]

The GEM Premier 3000 Pak Disposable Cartridge contains the system's reagents, sensors pump tubing, and waste container. The central component of the cartridge is the sample chamber, which is in a thermal block that maintains all components, including the sample being tested, at 37°C. Within the blocks is a sensor card that contains the reference sensors and analyte-specific membranes. The basic principle is that an electrical potential/current can be established across a membrane that is selectively permeable to a specific ion.

Other key features include development of liquid calibration systems that use a combination of aqueous base solution and conductance measurements, to calibrate the pH and pCO_2 electrodes. Oxygen is calibrated with oxygen-free solution and room air. In addition, all sensors, electronics, and fluidics are continuously monitored to ensure that specifications are met at all times. If any of the analytes does not meet specification, the analyzer will disable the test, ensuring that no samples can be analyzed. This safety feature of the GEM 3000 ensures accurate test reporting.

Interfering substances on the GEM 3000

Samples with abnormally elevated osmolalities, high protein concentrations, or high lipid values should not be used. Benzalkonium chloride and benzalkonium heparin may elevate Na and ICa readings. Thiopental sodium may interfere with Na, K, pCO_2, and ICa readings. Halothane may produce unreliable pO_2 readings. Flaxedil at ≥ 2 mg/dL and ethanol at ≥ 350 mg/dL may lower glucose and lactate readings. Acetaminophen at ≥ 15 mg/dL, isoniazide at ≥ 2 mg/dL, thiocyanate at ≥ 10 mg/dL, and hydroxyurea at ≥ 15 mg/dL can elevate glucose and lactate readings. Sodium fluoride at ≥ 1 g/dL and potassium oxalate at ≥ 1 g/dL can cause lower glucose and lactate readings.[12]

Minimally invasive devices

There is a smaller group of devices that are minimally invasive. This requires continuous monitoring devices, for which sensors are inserted into the bloodstream. These are confined to blood gases using optical technology, but electrochemical applications have been developed for both blood gases and glucose.[13]

To overcome the disadvantages of intermittent arterial blood sampling, blood gas monitors were developed to measure pH, pCO_2, and pO_2 without permanently removing blood samples. Optical sensors are used to monitor blood gas levels. The signal from the sensing element is used to calculate blood gas values.

Extraarterial and intraarterial blood gas monitors have been developed for blood gas analysis at the bedside. Extraarterial blood gas monitors are on-demand catheters that allow direct blood gas analysis at the bedside, and are not continuous measurements. Blood is drawn up the arterial line tubing, when needed, into a cassette containing optodes, to measure pH, pCO_2, and pO_2.

Intraarterial blood gas monitors, on the other hand, offer continuous measurement of arterial blood gases. Although the tests are based on the same optode technology, the sensor is inserted directly into the arterial bloodstream in this case. The continuous monitoring systems consist of a sterile disposable fiberoptic sensor introduced through a 20-gauge arterial catheter, a microprocessor-controlled monitor with a self-contained calibration unit and a detectable display and control panel. The consistency and reliability of this platform are questionable, however, as significant malfunctions and inconsistencies are attributed to the intraarterial environment.

CDI 500 Blood Parameter Monitoring System

The CDI 500 Blood Parameter Monitoring System (Terumo Cardiovascular Systems; Ann Arbor, MI) is designed to continuously monitor pH, pCO_2, pO_2, potassium, oxygen saturation, hematocrit, hemoglobin, and temperature during cardiopulmonary bypass (CPB).[13] The system uses optical flurometric and reflectance technologies, as well as disposable sensors placed in the extracorporeal circuit. It agrees with traditional laboratory analyzers[14] using electrochemical technology to measure these parameters at certain intervals on demand.

The blood parameter module measures pH, pO_2, pCO_2, and potassium, and the H/S probe measures hematocrit, hemoglobin, and oxygen saturation. The pH, pCO_2, and pO_2 are measured every second, whereas the potassium is measured every six seconds. Sensors for pH, pCO_2, and pO_2 are calibrated with a two-point tonometered calibration system similar to the electrodes in traditional blood gas analyzers.

Regulatory agencies, such as CAP, have developed guidelines for laboratory oversight of alternative test systems to include transcutaneous and in vitro monitoring devices. Guidelines state that systems must be in place to ensure accurate results, as traditional approaches to management, quality control, and so forth may not be applicable.[15]

Limitations and complications

Reliable intravascular blood gas analyses depend on many mechanical, electrical, and physicochemical properties of the probes used, as well as the conditions of the vessel into which the probe is inserted.[9] Mechanical factors relating to the intraarterial probe and the artery itself, interferences from electrocautery, and ambient changes in endoscopic light may lead to false measurements.[9] Although continuous intravascular blood gas monitoring has potential advantages, additional cost/benefit studies need to be evaluated.

References

1. Tietz NW, Pruden EL, Siggard-Andersen O. Electrolytes. In Burtis CA, Ashwood EL, eds. *Tiets Textbook of Clinical Chemistry*. Philadelphia: W. B. Saunders, 1994, pp. 1354–1374.
2. Papadakos PJ, Szalados JE. Fluid, electrolyte, blood, and blood product management. In *Critical Care, the Requisites in Anesthesiology*. Philadelphia: Elsevier Mosby, 2005, pp. 59–72.
3. Perkins SL, Hussong JW. Hematology. In Jones SL, ed. *Clinical Laboratory Pearls*. Philadelphia: Lippincott Williams & Williams, 2001, pp. 61–161.
4. Elshanydoh A, Cork RC. Blood gas measurments. In Webster SG, ed. *Encyclopedia of Medical Devices and Instrumentation*. Hoboken, NJ: John Wiley & Sons, 2006, pp. 18–28.
5. Pruden EL, Siggard-Andersen O., Tietz NA. Blood gases and pH. In Burtis CA, Ashwood EL, eds. *Tietz Textbook of Clinical Chemistry*. Philadelphia: W. B. Saunders, 1994, pp. 1375–1410.
6. Hutchison AS, Ralston SH, Drybungh FJ, et al. Too much heparin: possible sources of error in blood gas analysis. *Br Med J* 1983;**287**:1131–2.
7. Miller H, Lifshitz MS. Pre-analysis. In McPherson RA, Pincus MR, eds. *Henry's Clinical Diagnosis and Management by Laboratory Methods*. Philadelphia: W. B. Saunders, 2007, pp. 175–207.
8. Ehrmeyer S, Laessig RH. Regulation, accreditation and education for point of care testing. In Kost G, ed. *Principles and Practice of*

Point-of-Care Testing. Philadelphia: Lippincott Williams & Wilkins, 2002, pp. 434–443.

9. Ramanathan L, Sarkozi L. Analytical methods, automated. In Webster SG, ed. *Enclopedia of Medical Devices and Instrumentation.* Hoboken, NJ: John Wiley & Sons, 2006, p. 9.

10. Tang Z, Louie RF, Kost GJ. Principles and performance of point-of-care testing instruments. In Webster JG, ed. *Encyclopedia of Medical Devices and Instrumentation.* Hoboken, NJ: John Wiley & Sons, 2006, pp. 67–99.

11. iStat, Abbott Point of Care Operator's Manual, 2008.

12. Gem Premier 3000 Operator's Manual, 2007.

13. CD1 500 Blood Parameter Monitoring System. Terumo Cardiovascular Systems Operator's Manual, 2004.

14. Trowbridge C, Stammers A, et al. The effects of continuous blood gas monitoring during cardiopulmonary bypass: A prospective randomized study: Parts 1 and 11. *J. Extra-Corp Tech,* 2000;**32**:120–37.

15. College of American Pathologists. Point of care checklist. 2007.

Chapter 24

Laboratory-based tests of blood clotting

Nathaen Weitzel, Tamas Seres, and Glenn P. Gravlee

Introduction

Laboratory tests of blood clotting range from simple and routine to complex and rare. The simpler tests are more commonly used and generally provide the most useful information to the anesthesiologist, surgeon, and intensive care physician. Whole blood bedside point-of-care (POC) versions exist for several of the tests, as discussed in the second part of this chapter.

This part of the chapter will present laboratory-based tests in the context of their use in monitoring coagulation function in the operating rooms or in patients who are acutely bleeding. An exception is that the whole blood viscoelastic tests Sonoclot and thromboelastograph are sometimes located in the central laboratory and at other times near the bedside, but when used as POC tests they are most often performed by an experienced laboratory technician in a satellite laboratory; thus, the term *laboratory tests* remains appropriate. Tests that have the greatest utility in diagnosis of common blood clotting disturbances are presented. This includes activated partial thromboplastin time, prothrombin time, thrombin time, fibrinogen,

platelet count, fibrin degradation products, D-dimers, thromboelastogram (TEG), and Sonoclot. A variety of other tests are less useful because of nonspecificity, imprecision, or lack of prompt availability. These include template bleeding time and any of several platelet function tests. POC platelet function tests other than TEG and Sonoclot are discussed in the second part of this chapter.

Overview of blood clotting

In the past, blood clotting was viewed as a series of "silos" containing independent components such as plasma-based coagulation, platelet adhesion and aggregation, and fibrinolysis. More recently, the interdependence of these processes has been recognized, as depicted in Figure 24.1.[1] Aside from being a more accurate depiction of the biologic clotting process, the newer model underscores synergistic "explosive" interactions among plasma coagulation factors and platelets and shows that the majority of the plasma coagulation activity occurs on the surface of platelets.[1] The term *cell-based clotting* is often used to

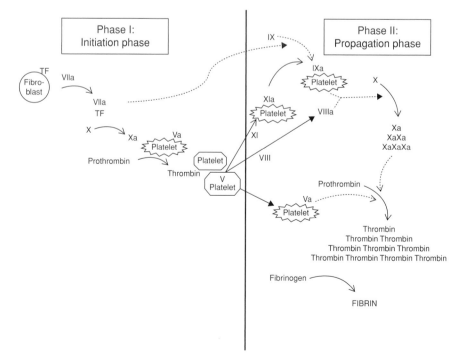

Figure 24.1. The two-phase model of coagulation. In the initiation phase of coagulation, tissue factor (TF), exposed on a subendothelial fibroblast after vessel injury, complexes with small amounts of factor VIIa present in the circulation. This complex then activates a small amount of factor X to Xa in the presence of an activated platelet. The platelet-bound Xa converts a tiny amount of prothrombin to thrombin. This small amount of thrombin then sparks the propagation phase of coagulation. Thrombin activates factors XI, VIII, and V at or near the activated platelet. Factor IX is activated by either factor XIa or the TF-VIIa complex. Factor IXa complexes with the factor VIIIa activated by thrombin, and on the platelet surface generates factor Xa with remarkable kinetic efficiency. The platelet-bound factor Xa complexes with factor Va, which converts prothrombin to explosive amounts of thrombin. This thrombin in turn converts fibrinogen to fibrin, thereby sealing the vessel injury beneath. From ref. 1, with permission.

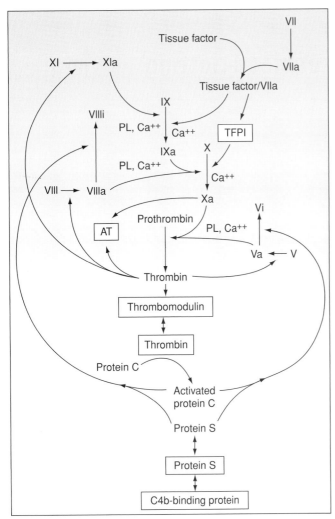

Figure 24.2. The diagram depicts the natural plasma intrinsic (partially) and extrinsic coagulation pathways to the level of thrombin production along with natural inhibitors of the coagulation pathways. The natural inhibitors are depicted as boxes at the site of their inhibition in the pathway, and include antithrombin (AT), tissue factor pathway inhibitor (TFPI), and the various components of the thrombomodulin/protein C and protein S pathway. Abbreviations not described above: Roman numerals represent coagulation factors in their inactivated (e.g. IX) or activated states (e.g. IXa), PL = phospholipid, C4b = complement 4b, Ca^{++} = ionized calcium. From ref. 2, with permission.

describe this model. In the context of this paradigm, whole-blood–based global tests of clotting function, such as the thromboelastogram and Sonoclot, offer appeal. Nevertheless, silo tests such as the activated partial thromboplastin time (PTT), prothrombin time (PT), and platelet count at times can offer greater specificity in diagnosing and treating blood clotting deficiencies.

Several endogenous mechanisms provide built-in protection against runaway blood clotting, as depicted in Figure 24.2.[2] For example, tissue factor (TF) is one of the most potent stimuli to blood clotting, so it is fortunate that TF resides principally in the extravascular space. Should TF overflow into the vascular space, its action can be potently inhibited by tissue factor pathway inhibitor (TFPI).[2] Other commonly recognized

endogenous anticoagulants include antithrombin III and proteins C and S, significant deficiencies of which predispose to intravascular thrombosis. The silo tests lack sensitivity to the hypercoagulable states associated with these deficiencies. Once an intravascular clot has been formed, the fibrinolytic system breaks it down; this system also has appropriate checks and balances, because overactive fibrinolysis may inappropriately lyse clots necessary to hemostasis in the face of injury or surgery.

The need for monitoring blood clotting

Blood clotting monitoring falls principally into two categories: monitoring the effects of an administered anticoagulant drug, such as heparin or warfarin, and checking for the presence of a clinically significant clotting disturbance in a patient who is bleeding. In the operating room milieu, POC tests are most often used to assess heparin-induced anticoagulation, but these tests often fall short of optimal precision in the diagnosis of clinical coagulopathy. In patients undergoing surgery, changes in the composition of the circulating blood can occur rapidly as the patient bleeds and blood volume is sustained with crystalloids, colloids, and blood products. Red blood cell salvage devices centrifuge and wash the collected spilled blood to provide a product that is nearly devoid of plasma and platelets. Surgeons and anesthesiologists often have difficulty assessing whether bleeding is caused by insufficient surgical hemostasis or by pathologic microvascular bleeding, which will be called *coagulopathy* in this chapter.

During surgery, the diagnosis of coagulopathy principally involves observation of surgical wounds and suture lines, invoking clinical judgment about which similarly astute observers can reasonably disagree. Monitoring laboratory tests of blood clotting augments bedside observation by providing objective gauges to support or refute bedside observations about surgical hemostasis versus coagulopathy.

As compared with POC blood clotting tests, central laboratory tests generally offer greater accuracy and precision at the expense of a slower response time. Although it is possible to provide centralized laboratory results for such tests as PT, activated PTT, and platelet count within 10 to 15 minutes, such factors as transport of blood samples to the laboratory and prioritization of testing in the laboratory most often result in turnaround times (interval from drawing the blood sample to having access to the test result) of 30 to 90 minutes. Hence, despite good intentions, central laboratory response times often are too slow to affect patient care, because the patient's coagulopathy or volume of bleeding dictates a need for blood component or pharmacologic therapy before results are obtained.

Unfortunately, this clinical reality can discourage the appropriate use of laboratory tests, and it sets the stage for disagreements between the operating room team and the blood bank about sufficiency of documentation to justify the administration of blood components such as fresh frozen plasma and platelet concentrates. The TEG and Sonoclot tests may take as much as 30 to 60 minutes to complete, but useful information

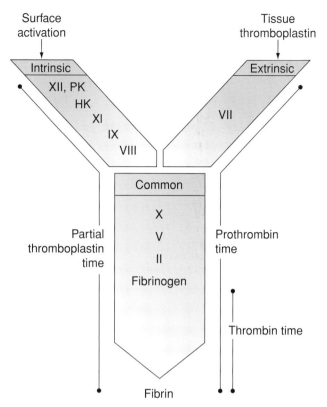

Figure 24.3. Schematic depiction of the coagulation system showing extrinsic, intrinsic, and common pathways. The pathways tested by partial thromboplastin time, prothrombin time, and thrombin time are also depicted. Roman numerals represent coagulation factors. Other abbreviations: PK = prekallikrein, HK = high molecular weight fibrinogen. From ref. 2, with permission.

about plasma coagulation and platelet function is usually available within 15 to 30 minutes.

Plasma or serum-based laboratory coagulation tests

Prothrombin time

PT is probably the most commonly used laboratory test for assessing the function of plasma coagulation factors. Plasma coagulation tests depend on the preservation of intact plasma from the time of whole blood collection until it is centrifuged to separate plasma from the buffy coat and red blood cells. This is almost universally achieved by placing the blood sample immediately into a test tube that contains citrate, which binds calcium to prevent plasma coagulation. After isolation of plasma, excess calcium is added to reverse the effects of the citrate, thereby restoring the plasma sample to its presumed natural state.[3] Because the plasma clotting process lacks a physiologic stimulant at that point, additives are used to isolate the desired pathways depicted in Figure 24.3.[2] In the case of the prothrombin time, the activant is animal-derived or recombinant tissue thromboplastin, which is analogous to endogenous tissue factor.[2] The added thromboplastin initiates the coagulation

pathways, and the laboratory machine then automatically detects the formation of a gel (i.e. clear plasma clot). The time taken for this to occur is detected automatically and constitutes the PT.

PT assesses the extrinsic and common pathways, representing a physiologic mechanism that comes into play principally when a blood vessel is disrupted, which exposes extravascular blood to TF. This is a rapid response pathway both physiologically and in the laboratory, which explains why the reference range (normal values) for PT in most laboratories is 11 to 15 seconds.[4] As depicted in Figure 24.2, the physiologic extrinsic pathway actually provides two routes into the common pathway, and it is likely that the inhibitory effect of TFPI favors the route through factor IX.[2]

The laboratory PT test overwhelms TFPI with an excess of TF, thereby bypassing factor IX, so one could argue that the laboratory test fails to accurately reproduce the physiologic extrinsic pathway except when an abundance of TF is present. In a patient who is undergoing surgery or who is experiencing blunt or penetrating trauma, this is most often the case. Assuming that coagulopathy during surgery derives principally from failure to form clots around injured blood vessels, then PT theoretically should be the best silo test to assess plasma coagulation competency. PT is also used to monitor warfarin therapy, because the vitamin K-dependent factors inhibited by that drug reside principally in the extrinsic and common pathways, and because depletion of factor VII is critical to warfarin-induced inhibition of clotting. Even though the activated PTT also measures the common pathway, PT is more sensitive to warfarin than PTT is.

Different tissue thromboplastin reagents are used in different laboratories as activants for PT.[2,3] Not surprisingly, different activants produce different reference ranges for PT. In response to this problem, the laboratory medicine community has embraced a parameter known as the *International Normalized Ratio* (INR), which exists for the sole purpose of correcting for variations in the administration of the PT test to provide a standardized number that is interchangeable across laboratories.[5] To calculate INR, one must know the International Sensitivity Index (ISI) for the thromboplastin reagent used for a PT test. ISI calibrates the degree of responsiveness of each reagent to the vitamin-K–dependent coagulation factors; this value enters into an equation that yields INR as a corrected ratio of the patient's PT value to the normal PT value for that laboratory. The reference range for INR is 0.9 to 1.1 at the University of Colorado Hospital. INR was created principally for and achieves its greates utility in monitoring warfarin-induced anticoagulation.[2,4]

Activated partial thromboplastin time

As shown in Figure 24.3,[2] the activated PTT measures the speed of clotting via the intrinsic and common pathways. Blood sample collection and processing are identical to that for PT up to the point of adding the activant. In the case of PTT, the intrinsic pathway is activated by exposure of plasma to foreign surfaces, such as glass or plastic, so this pathway will proceed even in the absence of an additional activant such as phospholipid. The activant speeds the process without sacrificing diagnostic information, so the activated version of the test is the clinical standard.[2,3] (Commonly, the activated version of the test is abbreviated as APTT or aPTT, but because the activated test is the only one used clinically, the abbreviation PTT is used exclusively in this chapter to represent the activated version of the test.) Because the extrinsic pathway is activated in the presence of a foreign surface, theoretically this pathway would seldom be invoked in vivo, although nonendothelialized intravascular foreign surfaces, such as intravascular stents, calcium deposits, or arteriosclerotic plaques, may initiate it. As noted earlier, the integrated clotting model involving platelets and plasma coagulation factors most often applies to these situations, which explains why pharmacotherapy with platelet inhibitors alone effectively deters clotting in the presence of intravascular stents.

The fact that the extrinsic pathway is slower than the intrinsic pathway (PTT reference range 25–35 seconds)[4] may teleologically reflect a more urgent survival advantage to forming a clot around a disrupted, leaking blood vessel than to forming one around a foreign body introduced into a previously intact vascular tree iatrogenically, accidentally, or as a result of a disease process. Accordingly, the extrinsic pathway is less critical than the intrinsic pathway to physiologic hemostasis. If the extrinsic pathway lacked any importance, however, hemophiliacs would not develop hemarthroses and other manifestations of insufficient blood clotting.

As a preoperative screening tool, PTT is limited by the fact that, in the absence of a symptomatic bleeding disturbance, isolated PTT prolongation is most often caused by conditions such as the presence of lupus anticoagulant or isolated factor XII deficiency, neither of which induces coagulopathy. In the case of lupus anticoagulant, the prolonged PTT represents an inhibitor, and the patient is paradoxically at increased risk for thrombosis rather than bleeding. In the case of factor XII deficiency, the abnormality is clinically insignificant aside from its adverse impact on monitoring of heparin anticoagulation.[2]

In hospitalized patients who are not undergoing surgery, PTT is used principally to monitor the effect of intravenous unfractionated heparin. Although heparin's anticoagulant effect resides principally in the common pathway, it also inhibits Factors IX and XI, which probably explains why PTT is more sensitive to heparin than PT is. In theory, one could use PTT to monitor heparin-induced anticoagulation intraoperatively, but doing so incurs two significant disadvantages. First, it takes more time and costs more to send a sample to a central laboratory. Second, most PTT tests are calibrated to detect lower levels of anticoagulation than those achieved when heparin is administered intraoperatively for vascular or cardiac surgical procedures. After a patient undergoing vascular or cardiac surgery receives 100 to 400 USP units/kg of heparin, the PTT would most often become unclottable – that is, infinitely prolonged.

This limitation holds for most POC whole blood versions of the PTT as well.

The activated clotting time, a less sophisticated and precise test than the PTT, offers the convenience of POC testing and preservation of a reasonably linear dose–response relationship at the higher heparin concentrations used for surgical procedures (see the second part of this chapter). In the absence of heparin, PT alone most often offers as much diagnostic information as the combination of PT and PTT, yet most clinicians order both tests when assessing intraoperative or postoperative coagulopathy.

Thrombin time

Thrombin time (TT) assesses the final step in the common pathway (Figure 24.3). Blood samples are handled in the same fashion as PT until the activant is added, which in the TT is thrombin itself. Therefore, the test measures the capacity to convert fibrinogen to fibrin. The reference range is typically 11 to 18 seconds,[4] but it is best to check the reference range for one's local laboratory. TT is prolonged in the absence of sufficient normal fibrinogen, in the presence of dysfunctional fibrinogen, or in the presence of a potent thrombin inhibitor such as heparin.[3] The presence of large quantities of fibrin degradation products (FDPs) reduces sensitivity to the added thrombin, so TT becomes prolonged.[3] A TT variant known as the reptilase time is not prolonged by heparin or FDPs,[3] so an elevated reptilase time diagnoses quantitative or qualitative fibrinogen deficiency.

There are few intraoperative situations in which TT provides useful diagnostic information that is not also provided by either the PT or PTT. PTT is exquisitely sensitive to heparin, and both PT and PTT are almost as sensitive to deficient or dysfunctional fibrinogen as TT is. Most central laboratories can measure and report plasma fibrinogen concentration as quickly as TT, so it is usually preferable to monitor fibrinogen concentration without TT. A whole blood version of the TT can be useful as a heparin monitor, as discussed later in this chapter.

Fibrinogen concentration

Plasma fibrinogen concentration is typically determined by using a variation of the thrombin time using serial dilutions, because fibrinogen becomes the limiting factor in clot formation under those conditions.[3] Plasma fibrinogen concentrations of 200 to 400 mg/dL are considered normal in most laboratories.[4] A critical plasma fibrinogen concentration that would unequivocally call for fibrinogen administration in the form of fresh frozen plasma, cryoprecipitate, or an isolated fibrinogen concentrate (not available in the United States) has not been established. There is general agreement that concentrations exceeding 100 mg/dL are sufficient for normal coagulation, and that those below 75 mg/dL merit intervention. At plasma fibrinogen concentrations between 75 and 100 mg/dL, clinical circumstances should guide therapy.

In surgical patients, decreased plasma fibrinogen concentrations are seldom observed in isolation, so this test may serve best as a marker for either the degree of global plasma protein dilution or as a marker for the degree of clotting factor consumption in the presence of disseminated intravascular coagulation. In either case, one can argue that fresh frozen plasma is as appropriate as cryoprecipitate, because there is a global clotting factor deficiency. In the face of coagulopathy accompanied by plasma fibrinogen concentrations below 75 mg/dL, however, the administration of cryoprecipitate (or other fibrinogen concentrate) in addition to fresh frozen plasma is reasonable. At fibrinogen concentrations below 50 mg/dL, the need for cryoprecipitate becomes compelling.

Fibrin degradation products and D-dimers

These tests are used to diagnose fibrinolysis, and they are performed on serum rather than plasma because they require the formation of a clot before analysis. FDPs serve as generic markers for plasmin hyperactivity, which can occur in situations of primary or secondary fibrinolysis.[2,3] In primary fibrinolysis, both soluble (i.e. normal circulating) fibrinogen and insoluble fibrin (i.e. clot) are broken down by plasmin, so a marked elevation in FDP with normal or modest elevation in D-dimers suggests primary fibrinolysis,[3] which may merit treatment with an antifibrinolytic agent such as aminocaproic acid or tranexamic acid. D-dimers are formed by lysis of fibrin, whereas FDPs can be formed by lysis of either fibrinogen or fibrin. The reference range for FDP is <10 μg/mL[4] and for D-dimers is <500 fibrinogen equivalency units (University of Colorado Hospital Clinical Laboratory).

Secondary fibrinolysis derives from formation of extravascular clots that are dissolving or from pathologic disseminated intravascular coagulation (DIC), either of which elevates serum concentrations of both FDPs and D-dimers. Especially in the case of DIC, treatment with antifibrinolytic agents is likely to induce harm by inhibiting plasmin-mediated clot dissolution. With the possible exceptions of liver transplantation and the milieu following circulatory arrest or prolonged hypothermic cardiopulmonary bypass, little evidence supports routine intraoperative monitoring of FDP or D-dimers. Primary fibrinolysis, which is relatively rare, seldom presents de novo intraoperatively, and the need to specifically diagnose DIC intraoperatively is debatable. The most common causes of intraoperative DIC are shock and acidosis, and the use of FDP or D-dimers to diagnose the presence or severity of the shock state or to guide therapy lacks evidence-based support. Thromboelastography and Sonoclot can also be used to diagnose fibrinolysis (as discussed later).

Whole blood traditional laboratory test
Platelet count

Platelet count is usually performed in conjunction with a complete blood count, but it can be performed separately.[3] Normal values are between 150,000 and 450,000 platelets per microliter, which is equivalent to 150 to 450 × 10^9 platelets per liter.[4] As noted previously, central laboratory tests of platelet function are seldom available with sufficient rapidity to guide perioperative diagnosis or treatment of coagulopathy.

Intervention thresholds for traditional laboratory tests
PT and PTT intervention thresholds

Massive transfusion studies from the 1970s and 1980s support a correlation between clinical bleeding and PT or PTT levels at or above 1.5 times the control level.[6,7] The control level may be best defined as the patient's baseline value, but because this value is often lacking, it may also be defined as the midpoint of an individual laboratory's normal range – that is, approximately 14 seconds for PT and 30 seconds for PTT. As with any laboratory test, sensitivity increases and specificity decreases as the PT or PTT threshold for diagnosing abnormality decreases. Hence, in the presence of coagulopathy, abnormalities in the range of 1.3 times the midpoint of the normal range probably justify transfusion with fresh frozen plasma. Conversely, values as high as 2.0 times the control level may not merit intervention in the face of adequate clinical hemostasis, which, although unlikely, can be present even at values that high. Consequently, one should treat the patient rather than the numbers, but the bedside definition of clinical coagulopathy can understandably be biased by the receipt of abnormal clotting test results. Operations inside closed spaces such as the cranial vault or the orbit merit lower intervention thresholds than those in less confined spaces, because small hematomas in those spaces are more likely to induce clinically significant functional deficits.

Platelet count intervention thresholds

As with PT and PTT, the threshold for intervention is subject to flexible interpretation. In surgical patients who have normal platelet function, the most widely recommended intervention threshold is 50,000/μL.[7,8] However, if clinical coagulopathy exists in the presence of a normal PT and PTT, transfusing platelet concentrates may be appropriate with a platelet count even higher than 100,000/μL, because the coagulopathy serves as presumptive evidence that a platelet functional deficit is present. After cardiac surgery using cardiopulmonary bypass (CPB), a platelet count intervention threshold of 100,000/μL is commonly used, because there is considerable evidence that platelet function is compromised by CPB.[9,10] Platelet counts can also be used as a crude diagnostic marker for DIC, as Reed and colleagues showed in 1986.[11] In patients undergoing massive transfusion who started with a mean platelet count of 160,000/μL, average platelet counts were 110,000/μL after 10 units of blood, 85,000/μL after 20 units, and 55,000/μL after 30 units. These platelet counts far exceeded the expected decay curve, because the bone marrow and spleen possess the capacities to acutely mobilize platelets. By deductive reasoning, a platelet count below 80,000/μL after 10 units of RBCs suggests DIC.

Viscoelastic whole blood clotting tests
Sonoclot coagulation and platelet function analyzer

The Sonoclot Analyzer (Sienco Inc.; Arvada, CO) is a POC or laboratory-based coagulation testing system similar to the TEG in that it measures whole blood coagulation by viscoelastic measurements to provide the user with real-time coagulation analysis. Sonoclot applications include the clinical and research laboratory, along with POC uses such as in the operating room, intensive care unit, interventional radiology and cardiology, and possibly even in outpatient clinics.

Historical perspective

The concept of using blood viscosity to measure clotting ability dates back to 1889, when Georges Hayem, a French physician and early founder of hematology, suggested that viscosity might form the basis of a test for coagulation.[12,13] This concept lay dormant for more than 20 years until Koffman developed the coaguloviscometer, which provided the ability to measure viscosity changes in blood.[13,14] Further scientific advancements over the ensuing 40 years led to the early form of the thromboelastograph in 1948 by Hartert.[15,16] In 1975, von Kaulla and Ostendorf published the initial description of the Sonoclot device,[17] which initially was called the impedance machine. Sonoclot measures changing impedance during fibrin clot formation on a vibrating probe.

Principles of analysis

The Sonoclot Analyzer (Figure 24.4) responds to mechanical changes in the blood sample and converts this into an analog signal that is converted to a graphic tracing. A tubular probe that oscillates vertically is placed in a disposable

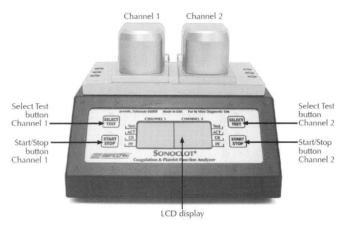

Figure 24.4. Sonoclot Analyzer 2 channel machine. Photograph provided courtesy of Sienco Inc, Arvada, CO.

cuvette containing the blood sample and an activator (Figure 24.5).[18] The probe oscillates a distance of 1 μm at a frequency of 200 Hz in a 360-μL sample.[13] As fibrin formation occurs, the sample exerts viscous drag on the probe tip, which mechanically impedes the vibration. The electronic circuit attached to the probe converts this resistance into an output signal on paper, which represents the developing clot.[13,19] This output signal, also called the Sonoclot signature, is broken into three distinct phases: onset or activated clotting time (ACT), clot rate (CR), and time to peak (TP, also called platelet function; Figure 24.6).[18] The Sonoclot signature provides these three quantitative values along with the qualitative graphic printout. Multiple types of assays are available from the manufacturer, depending on the clinical application (Table 24.1).

The phases of the Sonoclot signature represent distinct processes of coagulation. The ACT is the time in seconds until the generation of fibrin, which corresponds to the ACT measured

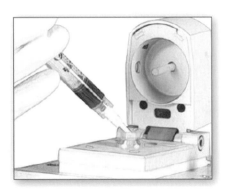

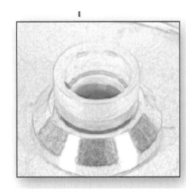

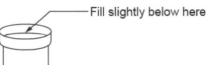

Fill slightly below here

Figure 24.5. Sonoclot Analyzer demonstrating disposable cup used for sample analysis. Notice the vertical probe tip, which will oscillate vertically in the sample to measure whole blood viscosity changes. Photographs provided courtesy of Sienco Inc, Arvada CO.

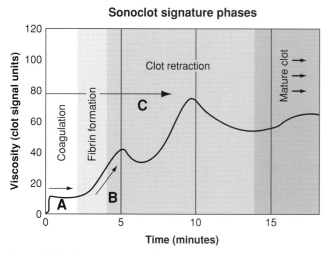

Figure 24.6. Sonoclot signature phases. A: Onset time or activated clotting time (ACT). B: Clot rate. C: Time to peak, also known as platelet function time. With permission from Sienco Inc, Arvada, CO.

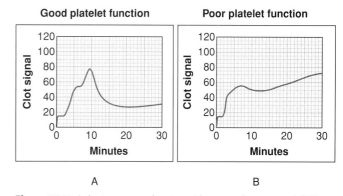

Figure 24.7. A depicts a normal tracing with a normal time to peak (TP) shown at approximately 10 minutes. B depicts a greatly delayed TP, representing poor platelet function. With permission from Sienco Inc, Arvada, CO.

via the Hemochron (International Technidyne; Edison, NJ) method.[20] These values for ACT are shorter than the R values obtained via the TEG, as the TEG R parameter measures a more developed and later stage of fibrin clot development.[21,22] The CR phase encompasses a single or double peak on the tracing that represents the maximal slope based on the rate of fibrin formation. Finally, the TP develops once the fibrin clot matures, at which time the clot retracts from the probe. TP represents overall platelet function and it is prolonged or absent in the presence of severe platelet dysfunction, severe thrombocytopenia, or combinations of platelet dysfunction or thrombocytopenia (Figure 24.7, Table 24.2).[13,21,23] Typically, the Sonoclot analysis is stopped prior to normal fibrinolysis; however, in fibrinolytic states, the Sonoclot signature curve will decay faster than predicted.

Sonoclot versus conventional coagulation testing

Conventional central laboratory coagulation testing is carried out on plasma samples rather than the whole blood sample used for the Sonoclot. Most conventional laboratory tests of coagulation conclude with the development of fibrin strands, whereas this point represents the ACT time from the Sonoclot Analyzer; thus, much more information may be gained with the full Sonoclot analysis. Conventional central laboratory studies lack evaluation of platelet function, which may explain limited correlations between conventional laboratory abnormalities and perioperative blood loss.[13] Platelet counts lack an assessment of platelet function, and most platelet function tests are too slow, expensive, and complex for practical perioperative use. Sonoclot, much like TEG, provides a functional assay of platelet function that correlates well with perioperative bleeding in both cardiac and liver transplant surgery.[24,25] The sensitivity of Sonoclot in predicting postoperative bleeding following cardiopulmonary bypass was reported as 74 percent.[25] The TP parameter correlates well with platelet function as measured by platelet aggregation studies; however, prolonged TP may reflect not only poor platelet function, but also inadequate clotting factors or fibrinogen.[23]

Sonoclot correlates well with current ACT testing modalities (see the second half of this chapter for ACT information) along with assessment of platelet function in the presence of GP IIb/IIIa inhibitors.[20–22,26–28] Sonoclot can be used to monitor standard heparin therapy and to evaluate heparin neutralization following CPB.[20,26,29]

Table 24.1. Types of assays available

Assay type	Activator	Indication
kACT	Kaolin	High-dose heparin monitoring; not intended for platelet function testing
gbACT	Glass bead	General coagulation testing including platelet function, in setting of low levels of heparin
Nonactivated	No activator	Custom design coagulation testing, allowing for research on specific activators
SonoACT	Celite	General coagulation testing including platelet function in moderate to high levels of heparin
aiACT	Celite blend (clay)	ACT monitoring of high-dose heparin levels in presence of aprotinin

Table adapted from Sienco Inc. (Arvada, CO) product summary, with permission.

Table 24.2. Normal values: SonoACT test

Result:	Normal Range
ACT/onset	85–145 seconds
Clot rate (CR)	15–45 clot signal units/minute
Time to peak (TP)	<30 minutes

Information provided courtesy of Sienco Inc. (Arvada, CO).

Fibrinolysis, commonly detected by measuring FDP, can contribute importantly to perioperative bleeding. Sonoclot assessment of fibrinolysis is comparable in accuracy to FDP for detecting fibrinolysis; however, it may generate faster results.[13] Sonoclot CR correlates well with measured fibrinogen concentrations based on two studies; therefore, a reduced CR represents inadequate quantitative fibrinogen or dysfunctional fibrinogen.[23,30]

Sonoclot clinical applications

Viscoelastic measures have been investigated most extensively in liver transplantation and CPB, and there are more studies looking at the use of TEG (discussed in the following section), than Sonoclot. However, several studies show that Sonoclot predicts excessive bleeding after CPB,[21,24,25,31,32] although one study found standard coagulation testing to be superior to both TEG and Sonoclot in predicting post-CPB bleeding.[33] Initial studies criticized Sonoclot for variability attributable to age, gender, and platelet count, along with suboptimal reproducibility.[34-36] Subsequent studies have refuted this to some degree, especially when using fresh whole blood rather than citrated blood samples for later analysis.[23,32] Although there are transfusion algorithms using TEG analysis (see the following section), there are no published algorithms using Sonoclot.

During liver transplantation, TEG has been widely accepted and used as a guide to transfusion and coagulation analysis.[37] Sonoclot correlates well with TEG as well as with standard coagulation studies in liver transplantation.[24] Chapin and colleagues concluded that both TEG and Sonoclot effectively analyze platelet dysfunction, clotting factor deficiency, and defective fibrinolysis, and can be used to guide intraoperative blood product therapy.[24]

Additional applications and future considerations

As more clinicians become aware of the utility of viscoelastic coagulation testing, Sonoclot analysis may well find applications outside the arena of liver transplantation and cardiac surgery. Much like TEG, Sonoclot has the potential to detect hypercoagulable states; however, no studies to date have investigated this possibility. An important emerging area of interest is monitoring antiplatelet therapy. Sonoclot reliably detects GPIIb/IIIa inhibition[19] and could be applied to monitor aspirin or clopidogrel therapy, although currently this is not available. One additional area of interest is the use of Sonoclot to help guide factor VIIa (rVIIa) treatment. Initial research indicates that the Sonoclot may be useful in this application.[38]

Thromboelastography

Background

Perioperative coagulation monitoring can predict the risk of bleeding, diagnose potential causes of hemorrhage, and guide hemostatic therapies during surgical procedures. The value of commonly used central laboratory-based tests has been questioned in the acute perioperative setting because of delays, the use of plasma rather than whole blood, the absence of information about platelet function, and the use of a standard temperature of 37°C rather than the patient's own temperature.[21] Based on the the Society of Thoracic Surgeons and Society of Cardiovascular Anesthesiologists Clinical Practice Guideline, it is reasonable to transfuse non–red-cell hemostatic blood products based on clinical evidence of bleeding and POC tests that assess hemostatic function in a timely and accurate manner.[39]

TEG, rotation thromboelastometry (ROTEM, a modified TEG), and Sonoclot analysis can be used as POC coagulation tests to assess the viscoelastic properties of whole blood and overcome several limitations of routine coagulation tests. POC testing allows faster turnaround times, and the coagulation status is assessed in whole blood, allowing interactions of the coagulation factors with platelets to provide information on platelet function. Furthermore, clot development can be visually displayed in real time and the coagulation analysis can be performed at the patient's temperature.[21] For these tests to provide sufficient precision, they should performed by individuals who have received detailed training in their operation and who perform the tests frequently, so their application at the POC should be considered in that context.

The balance among clot formation, retraction, and lysis in a viscoelastic clotting test may reflect the ability of the hemostatic plug to perform its in vivo hemostatic function. Thus, by measuring various properties of the clot formation in vitro, one can potentially detect a number of acquired and congenital platelet and coagulation factor abnormalities. However, despite the advantages of viscoelastic clotting tests, a significant difference between in vitro and in vivo blood clotting must be considered: viscoelastic coagulation tests measure the clotting status under low shear conditions without the the complex dynamic effects of tissue injury present on the operating field. Therefore, results obtained from these tests must be carefully interpreted after considering the clinical conditions and possible risk factors for bleeding.[21]

TEG was developed by Hartert as a research tool in 1948.[16] Its entry into clinical practice was pioneered by Kang and coworkers in the setting of liver transplantation in 1985, and it was introduced by Spiess and associates for use in cardiac surgery two years later.[37,40] Both surgeries are commonly associated with coagulopathy and massive blood loss. TEG measures the viscoelastic and mechanical properties of a developing clot. With the exception of fibrinolytic activity, TEG typically takes 15 to 30 minutes to assess all phases of the hemostatic activity from a single sample of whole blood. The computerized TEG analyzer automatically measures the shear elasticity and mechanical properties of a developing clot and its subsequent lysis.

Principles and technical aspects of TEG

The TEG tracing graphically represents clot formation and lysis. Clot formation is the net result of interaction between the platelets and coagulation proteins. The test is performed using a small quantity (0.36 mL) of whole blood placed into a heated

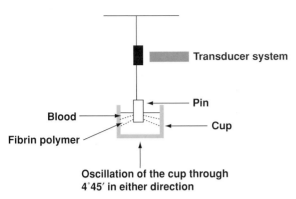

Figure 24.8. The working parts of the thrombelastography device. The TEG device monitors clot formation and lysis. To measure the elastic shear modulus of the sample, the cup oscillates through an angle of 4°45′. The rotation cycle lasts 10 seconds. The torque of the oscillating cup is transmitted to the pin through clot formation in the cup. The transducer system of the device transforms the torsion of the wire to an electrical signal, which is processed and displayed by a computer.

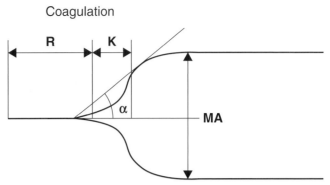

Figure 24.9. Standard parameters of TEG during clot formation. Blood clotting is characterized by R time, K parameter, alpha angle (α), and maximum amplitude (MA). R time (measured in millimeters, or minutes, which equal 1/2 × mm) is the period of time from blood placement in the TEG until initial clot formation (divergence of the lines to 2 mm). K parameter (also called K time) is measured from R until the level of clot firmness reaches 20 mm (divergence of the lines from 2 mm to 20 mm). The alpha angle is the slope of the tangent of the TEG tracing. As does K, α denotes the speed at which a solid clot forms. MA (maximum divergence of the lines) is the measurement of maximum strength of the developed clot.

cup. The cup oscillates through an angle of 4°45′. Each rotation cycle lasts 10 seconds. A pin that is suspended freely in the blood by a torsion wire is monitored for motion. The torque of the rotation cup is transmitted to the immersed pin only after fibrin–platelet bonding has linked the cup and pin together (Figure 24.8). The rotation movement of the pin is converted by a mechanical–electrical transducer to an electrical signal, finally being displayed as the typical TEG tracing. The clot's physical properties may suggest whether the patient has normal hemostasis or a tendency to bleed or to develop thrombosis. Initially, when no clot exists, the oscillation of the cup does not affect the pin and a straight-line trace is recorded. The strength and rate of formation of fibrin–platelet bonds affect the magnitude of the pin motion. As the clot lyses, these bonds are broken and the transfer of cup motion is again diminished.

Blood sampling and activants for TEG

TEG analysis in whole blood provides useful results if it is processed within six minutes of sampling.[41] If transport and handling time of the blood exceeds six minutes, however, sodium citrate should be used for anticoagulation and recalcification should be achieved before performing TEG.[42] In healthy controls, citrated whole blood may be used in the TEG when stored at room temperature for 30 minutes or at 4°C up to 150 minutes, giving results that do not differ significantly from those obtained with fresh whole blood.[43]

Although whole blood provides the most physiologic sample for evaluation of clot formation, this is not practical because of the long coagulation time. The addition of activators such as celite, kaolin, or tissue factor has been implemented to reduce the time to tracing generation. Diatomaceous earth acts as a contact surface activator in the celite-activated TEG. Celite increases the rapidity with which results become available and improves test reproducibility by activating factor XII and platelets to induce the intrinsic pathway of coagulation.[44]

Hydrated aluminum silicate, called *kaolin*, activates the intrinsic pathway of coagulation in a way similar to celite. Coagulation activated by kaolin is less sensitive to the inhibitory effect of aprotinin on the intrinsic pathway of coagulation most likely because of binding of aprotinin to kaolin.[45,46] Recombinant tissue factor has been suggested as an activator for TEG. This may provide a more accurate model for blood clotting because it activates the extrinsic coagulation pathway, which probably provides the major impetus for clot formation during surgery.[46–48] In tissue factor-activated TEG, tissue factor together with factor VIIa activates factors IX and X to initiate the extrinsic coagulation pathway.

Heparinase I, derived from *Flavobacterium heparinum*, is an enzyme that rapidly and specifically neutralizes the anticoagulant effect of heparin. Addition of heparinase to the blood sample during TEG analysis allows diagnosis of developing coagulopathies during CPB that would otherwise be masked by heparin.[49] Heparinase can also help to distinguish between residual heparin effect and other causes of coagulopathies after heparin neutralization with protamine.[50,51]

Measured TEG parameters

Four principal clot formation parameters are measured by TEG: reaction time (R), kinetics of clot formation (K parameter, or K), α angle, and maximum amplitude (MA) (Figure 24.9). Clot lysis is characterized by the clot lysis index (CLI) at 30 and 60 min, the estimated percent lysis (EPL) and the percent lysis at 30 and 60 min (LY_{30} and LY_{60}; Figure 24.10).

Reaction Time (R)

Reaction time, or latency time, is defined as the time from placing blood in the cup until the clot begins to form and reaches a tracing amplitude of 2 mm. This denotes the time taken for initial fibrin formation. Normal values are 10 to 14 mm or

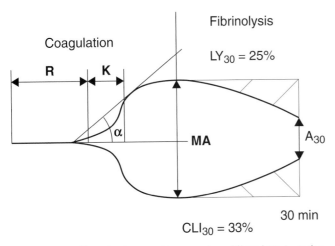

Figure 24.10. Thromboelastographic parameters of fibrinolysis. A_{30} is the amplitude of the TEG tracing 30 min after MA measurement. The figure shows the calculated clot lysis index, CLI_{30} (A_{30}/MA × 100%) is about 33%. LY_{30} measures the percent lysis based on the reduction of the area under the TEG tracing from the time of MA measurement until 30 min. In the figure, the decrease of the area at 30 min, LY_{30}, is about 25%.

5 to 7 min in celite- or kaolin-activated TEG, and 4 to 6 mm or 2 to 3 min in tissue factor-activated TEG (2 mm = 1 minute) (Haemoscope Corp., Niles, IL). Prolonged R may represent the effect of an anticoagulant (heparin or warfarin) or deficiencies of factors involved in the coagulation pathway (Figure 24.11). R also prolongs in the case of severe platelet dysfunction. In clinical practice, protamine, vitamin K, or fresh frozen plasma serve as potential interventions for prolonged R time. After intervention, a repeat TEG analysis assesses efficacy and helps

Heart transplantation
TEG before CPB
Kaolin-activated TEG without heparinase

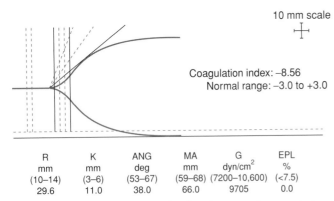

10 mm scale

Coagulation index: −8.56
Normal range: −3.0 to +3.0

R mm (10–14)	K mm (3–6)	ANG deg (53–67)	MA mm (59–68)	G dyn/cm² (7200–10,600)	EPL % (<7.5)
29.6	11.0	38.0	66.0	9705	0.0

Figure 24.11. A kaolin-activated TEG without heparinase from a patient who received warfarin before heart transplantation. The R time (R) and K parameter (K) are prolonged, the α (angle) is small, but the maximum amplitude (MA) and G parameter (G) are normal. Coagulation index is low, and estimated percent lysis (EPL) is listed as 0.0% because clot lysis had not commenced at the time of analysis. This pattern represents coagulation factor deficiency with normal platelet function and, most likely, a normal plasma fibrinogen concentration. Fresh frozen plasma would be an appropriate intervention if microvascular bleeding were present.

LVAD
After CPB
Celite-activated TEG without heparinase

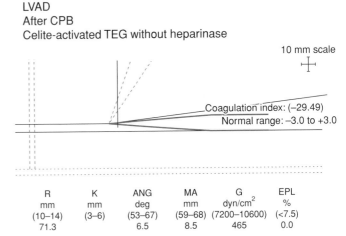

10 mm scale

Coagulation index: (−29.49)
Normal range: −3.0 to +3.0

R mm (10–14)	K mm (3–6)	ANG deg (53–67)	MA mm (59–68)	G dyn/cm² (7200–10600)	EPL % (<7.5)
71.3		6.5	8.5	465	0.0

Figure 24.12. Celite-activated TEG without heparinase from a patient undergoing left ventricular assist device (LVAD) placement after cardiopulmonary bypass (CPB) and protamine administration. R time (R) was prolonged; K parameter (K) could not be measured because the MA never reached 20 mm. α (angle), maximum amplitude (MA), G parameter (G), and coagulation index were very low. Estimated percent lysis (EPL) could not be determined. Assuming adequate heparin neutralization, this pattern exemplifies severe clotting factor deficiency and platelet dysfunction.

plan further intervention. R time is shortened in hypercoagulable states.

K parameter (K)

K parameter is defined as the time between the TEG trace reaching 2 mm and the tracing reaching 20 mm. K characterizes the rate of fibrin polymerization based on the interaction between clotting factors and platelets. Normal values are 3 to 6 mm or 1.5 to 3 min in celite- or kaolin-activated TEG, and 2 to 4 mm or 1 to 2 min in tissue factor-activated TEG (Haemoscope Corp., Niles, IL). Prolonged K represents low fibrinogen concentration, the presence of anticoagulants, factor deficiency (accompanied by prolonged R), or possibly low platelet count or reduced platelet function. Consequently, administration of fresh frozen plasma, cryoprecipitate, or platelet concentrates may improve a prolonged K, depending on the clinical situation. K is shortened in hypercoagulable conditions.

Alpha angle

Alpha (α) is defined as the angle between the line representing the center of the TEG tracing and the line tangential to the developing TEG tracing. Alpha is closely related to K time and represents the kinetics of fibrin crosslinking and the rate of clot strengthening. The α angle is more comprehensive than K time because there are hypocoagulable conditions in which the final level of clot firmness does not reach the amplitude of 20 mm (in which case K is not defined; Figure 24.12). Normal α values are 53 to 67 degrees in celite- or kaolin-activated TEG, and 62 to 73 degrees in tissue factor-activated TEG (Haemoscope Corp., Niles, IL). As with the K parameter, α can be small in the presence of a variety of conditions, including low plasma concentrations of fibrinogen, anticoagulants, clotting factor deficiencies, low platelet count, and reduced platelet function. Fresh frozen plasma, platelet concentrates, or cryoprecipitate may improve the altered angle, depending on the clinical situation. The α angle is wide in hypercoagulable conditions.

Maximum amplitude (MA)

MA is the greatest amplitude of the TEG trace, which represents the maximum strength of the developed clot. Gottumukkala and colleagues found that the contribution of fibrinogen and platelets to the MA were 45 percent and 55 percent, respectively.[52] Normal MA values are 59 to 68 mm in celite- or kaolin-activated TEG, and 61 to 69 mm in tissue factor-activated TEG (Haemoscope Corp, Niles, IL). A small MA represents thrombocytopenia, or reduced platelet function. In the presence of aspirin MA is normal, but inhibitors of GPIIb/IIIa receptors decrease MA. MA can be low in severe factor or fibrinogen deficiencies as well. Administration of platelet concentrates is the first choice to improve MA, but fresh frozen plasma or cryoprecipitate can be effective when fibrinogen concentration is low. MA is high in hypercoagulable conditions, especially when platelets are activated.

Clot lysis parameters

The process of fibrinolysis dissolves clots, thereby decreasing clot strength. This is represented by decrease in TEG tracing amplitude after MA is reached. CLI at 30 or 60 min (CLI_{30} and CLI_{60}) represent fibrinolytic status 30 and 60 minutes after MA is reached. These parameters are derived from the amplitudes (mm) of the TEG tracing at 30 minutes (A_{30}) or 60 minutes (A_{60}) after MA measurement. The CLI represents A_{30} or A_{60} as percentage of MA and is calculated as follows:

$$CLI_{30} = 100 \times (A_{30}/MA) \text{ (Figure 24.10)}$$
$$CLI_{60} = 100 \times (A_{60}/MA)$$

Normal values for CLI_{30} are 92 percent to 100 percent and those for CLI_{60} are 85 percent to 100 percent (Haemoscope Corp., Niles, IL).

Decrease in area

LY_{30} or LY_{60} measure the percent lysis based on the reduction of the area under the TEG tracing from the time of MA measurement until 30 (LY_{30}; Figure 24.10) or 60 minutes (LY_{60}). LY_{30} and LY_{60} represent the fibrinolytic process during the entire 30 and 60 minutes after MA is reached, whereas the CLI represents the degree of clot lysis attained at single time points 30 and 60 minutes after reaching MA. The normal range for LY_{30} is < 7.5 percent and for LY_{60} is < 15% (Haemoscope Corp., Niles IL).

Estimated percent lysis (EPL) is automatically computed beginning 30 sec after MA and is continually updated until 30 minutes, when the EPL becomes equal to LY_{30}. This parameter gives a value of the percent lysis prior to 30 minutes after MA. EPL is computed by finding the slope connecting MA to any point between MA and 30 minutes after MA, then extrapolating LY_{30}. In clinical conditions in which EPL is greater than

7.5 percent and the patient is bleeding, further administration of antifibrinolytics should be considered.

Other TEG parameters

The TEG parameters mentioned here are the ones most commonly used to measure clot formation, but some other parameters are occasionally used by clinicians.

A is the amplitude of the TEG tracing at any time point. The amplitude (A) can be transformed into a physical measurement of clot firmness (shear elastic modulus strength, or SEMS) called the *G parameter* (G), which is measured in dynes per square centimeter (dynes/cm²). G can be calculated from A as follows:

$$G = 5000 \times A/(100 - A)$$

where A = amplitude.

Normal values are calculated at MA and are: 7200 to 10,600 dynes/cm² in celite- or kaolin-activated TEG, and 7800 to 11,100 dynes/cm² in tissue factor-activated TEG (Haemoscope Corp., Niles, IL). Changes in G follow changes in MA.

Coagulation index (CI) describes the patient's overall coagulation status. It is derived from the R, K, MA, and α angle of native or celite-activated whole blood tracings and has no units.

In celite-activated whole blood, CI is calculated as follows:

$$CI = (-0.3258 \times R) - (0.1886 \times K) + (0.1224 \times MA) + (0.0759 \times \alpha) - 7.7922.$$

Normal values are -3 to $+3$ (Haemoscope Corp., Niles, IL).

In hypercoagulable conditions CI is higher than 3, whereas in hypocoagulable conditions it is less than -3.

TEG in cardiac surgery

After CPB, coagulation abnormalities, platelet dysfunction, and fibrinolysis can occur, creating a situation in which the integrity of hemostasis must often be accurately assessed and restored. The complex processes of anticoagulation with heparin, heparin neutralization by protamine, and post-CPB hemostasis therapy are best guided by tests that assess hemostatic function in a timely and accurate manner.[39] In routine cardiac surgery, impaired hemostasis identified by TEG does not inevitably lead to postoperative hemorrhage. However, patients with normal test results are unlikely to demonstrate coagulopathic bleeding; thus, bleeding in such patients is probably caused by inadequate surgical hemostasis. TEG's high negative predictive value therefore facilitates targeted treatment of post-CPB bleeding by distinguishing surgical bleeding from clinically significant coagulopathy.[53] The use of TEG for component therapy algorithms in cardiac surgery is described later.

TEG in liver transplantation

Patients undergoing orthotopic liver transplantation (OLT) often have significant deterioration in their coagulation. Defective liver function leads to impaired hemostasis and hyperfibrinolysis. Disseminated intravascular coagulation may further complicate a preexisting coagulopathy as a result of inadequate hepatic synthetic function.[54] Marked changes in hemostasis occur during the anhepatic phase of OLT and immediately after organ reperfusion. These changes may result from hyperfibrinolysis from the accumulation of tissue plasminogen activator in the absence of normal hepatic clearance and from the release of exogenous heparin and endogenous heparinlike substances. In this clinical scenario, TEG or other rapidly available coagulation tests play an important role in monitoring the dynamic changes of hemostasis.[21,55,56] As noted earlier, hemostatic management of OLT was one of the first clinical applications of TEG. A transfusion algorithm was introduced based on TEG results.[37] For R time >15 minutes, two units of FFP were administered, whereas for MA <40 mm, 10 units of platelet concentrates were given.

Aside from optimizing blood product administration, TEG can monitor the effects of therapeutic interventions, such as recombinant activated factor VII or aminocaproic acid, on the clotting process.[57] Although the use and value of TEG in management of patients undergoing OLT was established in the 1980s, a 2002 survey of United States liver transplantation centers showed that only one-third of OLT programs in the United States routinely used viscoelastic coagulation devices.[58–61] In addition to the hemorrhagic risk associated with OLT, hypercoagulability and thrombotic complications have been described in the postoperative period, and the propensity for these conditions can also be assessed with TEG. Even when traditional laboratory tests suggest hypocoagulability, TEG monitoring showed unexpected hypercoagulability in the majority of the subjects after hepatectomy for living-donor liver transplantation.[62] TEG monitoring could also be useful in the perioperative management of living donors and recipients to guide antithrombotic treatment and increase the safety of the procedure.[63]

Other applications for TEG

TEG may have role in evaluating patients for orthopedic or trauma surgery, as well as in high-risk pregnancy patients.

Femoral neck fracture is associated with a hypercoagulable state that can be detected by TEG. A significant correlation between hypercoagulability and the development of deep venous thrombosis has been demonstrated.[64] Hyperactivation of clotting, as monitored by TEG, predominates in bilateral total knee arthroplasty after releasing the tourniquet of the second leg and returns to baseline 24 h postoperatively.[65] Disturbance of fibrinogen/fibrin polymerization, as diagnosed by TEG, is the primary problem triggering dilutional coagulopathy during major orthopedic surgery.[66] The magnitude of clot firmness reduction is determined by the type of fluid used, with hydroxyethyl starch showing the most pronounced effects and Ringer lactate solution the least. These undesirable effects can be reversed by administering fibrinogen concentrate even during continuing blood loss and intravascular volume replacement.[66]

Trauma-associated coagulation abnormalities can lead to either hypercoagulability or hypocoagulability. In this perspective, TEG plays an important role together with traditional laboratory tests to evaluate and treat the coagulation process in a timely manner.[67] Hypothermia (temperature <34°C) associated with trauma disrupts fibrin polymerization and platelet–fibrin interaction, but patients with core temperature ≥34°C demonstrated hypercoagulability.[68]

Normal pregnancy is a hypercoagulable state, as has been confirmed in TEG studies showing significant decreases in R and K and increases in MA and α.[69] TEG has shown that women with mild forms of preeclampsia may be more hypercoagulable than pregnant women who are not preeclamptic.[70] As preeclampsia becomes more severe, clot formation becomes impaired.[71] Fluid preloading with 500 mL of 6% hetastarch in healthy parturients prior to spinal anesthesia for cesarean delivery induced mild coagulation defects, as measured with TEG (longer R and K).[40] No TEG changes were observed following preloading with 1500 mL of lactated Ringer solution.[71]

Usual TEG applications and activants are unable to detect impairment in platelet function induced by aspirin or by ADP receptor antagonists, because coagulation activants such as kaolin and celite override inhibition of platelet ADP and arachidonic acid pathways. A sophisticated TEG test called Platelet Mapping has recently been developed to specifically determine platelet function in the presence of antiplatelet agents. This novel modification of the TEG assay appears to be a useful POC whole-blood assay for monitoring the effects of ADP and thromboxane A_2-receptor–inhibiting drugs on platelets.[72]

Platelet mapping measures reduction in platelet function resulting from the use of antiplatelet drugs by using the individual's maximum platelet function as a control. Maximum platelet function is determined by measuring MA using kaolin-activated whole blood (MA_{kaolin}). Additional TEG assays are performed in the presence of heparin to eliminate the effect of thrombin to unmask the effect of arachidonic acid (AA) inhibition in patients treated with aspirin. A heparinized blood sample is treated with a direct fibrinogen activator with or without AA, and the resulting MA values generated from AA (MA_{AA}) and from the fibrinogen activator alone (MA_F) are recorded. The aspirin effect on platelet function is calculated as follows:

$$[(MA_{AA} - MA_F)/(MA_{kaolin} - MA_F)] \times 100(\%).$$

The aspirin effect is recorded as a percent reduction of maximum platelet function.

In 75 patients undergoing CPB, Carroll and colleagues found that both glass bead platelet adhesion and TEG platelet mapping showed significant dysfunction 15 minutes after protamine neutralization of heparin, yet neither of these abnormalities correlated significantly with postoperative chest tube drainage.[73] Low body mass, lowest core body temperature during CPB, and longer duration of aortic crossclamping correlated strongly with postoperative chest tube drainage.[73] The patients of Carroll and coworkers were not at high risk for excessive postoperative bleeding and were not taking aspirin or clopidogrel, so it would be interesting to assess the diagnostic capabilities of platelet mapping in cardiac surgical patients whose platelets remain under the influence of aspirin or clopidogrel at the time of surgery. As compared with traditional platelet function tests, such as optical platelet aggregation, platelet mapping can be used to rapidly assess the effects of antiplatelet agents on ex vivo blood clotting, thus giving a measurement that is both timely and relevant to in vivo responses. Platelet mapping needs more rigorous evaluation, but it represents a potentially powerful tool to assess response of individual patients to antiplatelet therapy.[74,75]

Blood component transfusion algorithms

Blood component transfusion algorithms using clotting tests have been compared prospectively with other transfusion therapy methods in cardiac surgery patients in six studies since 1994.[33,49,76,78–80] This population is known for its propensity for postoperative coagulopathy. It is surprising that transfusion algorithms have not been prospectively compared with laboratory-based testing or empiric therapy in liver transplantation or massive bleeding from trauma or elective noncardiac surgery, although a TEG-based algorithm has been evaluated and recommended in liver transplantation.[37]

The transfusion algorithm studies performed in post-CPB cardiac surgical patients have typically included 50 to 100 patients randomly assigned to a transfusion algorithm using a battery of traditional clotting tests (e.g. PT, PTT, platelet count, fibrinogen concentration, FDP),[76,80] thromboelastogram,[78,81] or both.[33,79] Avidan and colleagues also assessed an automated platelet function analyzer.[79] With the exception of the study of Capraro and associates,[80] each algorithm used an objective method for assessing and neutralizing any residual heparin effect. Avidan and coworkers compared a historical control group using central laboratory-based tests to two prospective POC algorithm groups, one assessing thromboelastography and the other POC INR, PTT, and platelet count.[79] A lower percentage of patients in both POC groups received RBCs fresh-frozen plasma, and platelet concentrates, but there was no difference in postoperative chest tube drainage among the three groups. Despotis and coworkers prospectively compared POC whole blood PT, PTT, and platelet counts to laboratory-based PT, PTT, fibrinogen, FDPs, thrombin time, and platelet counts, and found that the POC group experienced less blood loss and received fewer units of red blood cells, fresh frozen plasma, and platelet concentrates.[76]

Figure 24.13 demonstrates the algorithm of the Despotis group as subsequently modified to emphasize heparin neutralization assessment and add fibrinolysis and platelet function.[76,77] The original algorithm commenced with the box labeled "platelet count." The modified version replaces PLAT count with PLAT function and is important to rule out unneutralized heparin before initiating post CPB blood component therapy along with assessment of platelet function. Capraro and colleagues compared POC PT, PTT, laboratory-based platelet counts, and bedside template bleeding times with empiric therapy, and found a reduction in the number of patients receiving platelet concentrates without any difference in blood loss, total donor exposure, or red blood cells or fresh frozen plasma transfused.[80] Their study is the only one of the six in which algorithm implementation awaited patient arrival in the ICU, which probably is too late and may explain findings less favorable to algorithm utilization.

Nuttall and colleagues compared empiric treatment of coagulopathy with the use of POC PT, PTT, platelet count, and TEG, using abnormalities in any of these tests as triggers for component therapy.[33] The algorithm patients experienced less bleeding and fewer surgical reexplorations, and received fewer intraoperative transfusions with fresh frozen plasma or platelet concentrates.

Shore-Lesserson and associates prospectively compared TEG-based and traditional laboratory-based tests for the treatment of coagulopathy after cardiopulmonary bypass (Figure 24.14).[78] The TEG algorithm patients needed to fulfill both TEG and platelet count criteria before receiving platelet concentrates. The TEG algorithm patients received fewer units of red blood cells, fresh frozen plasma, and platelet concentrates despite the absence of a difference in chest tube drainage. The differences in fresh frozen plasma and platelet transfusion occurred postoperatively, at which time the algorithm was no longer used. These fresh frozen plasma and platelet transfusion differences may therefore have been attributable to less perceived coagulopathy or to the effect that faster availability of TEG results had on targeted ordering and transfusion of fresh frozen plasma and platelets.

Royston and associates prospectively compared heparinase TEG-guided transfusion to empiric blood component therapy in patients who were at increased risk for postoperative coagulopathy.[49] The TEG-guided group received fewer units of fresh frozen plasma and platelets as well as fewer total blood components. The studies varied in their use of prophylactic antifibrinolytic agents, which was not standardized except in the Royston (no antifibrinolytic agents) and Shore-Lesserson (aminocaproic acid) studies.[49,78]

Taken together, algorithm studies in cardiac surgery strongly suggest merit to the use of algorithm-driven blood component therapy for patients experiencing post-CPB coagulopathy. The most effective algorithms initiate laboratory assessment intraoperatively before or soon after heparin neutralization using either POC whole blood versions of traditional clotting tests (PT, PTT, platelet count) or TEG criteria. These tests appear most helpful if applied selectively intraoperatively to patients with persistent coagulopathy (i.e. microvascular bleeding) after confirmation of complete heparin neutralization. Typical POC criteria for fresh frozen plasma transfusion were PT, INR, or PTT equal to or greater than 1.5 times the mean laboratory control value. Typical POC criteria for platelet transfusion were a platelet count below 100,000/μL, although two studies supported the use of desmopressin prior to platelet concentrates for platelet counts between 50,000/μL and

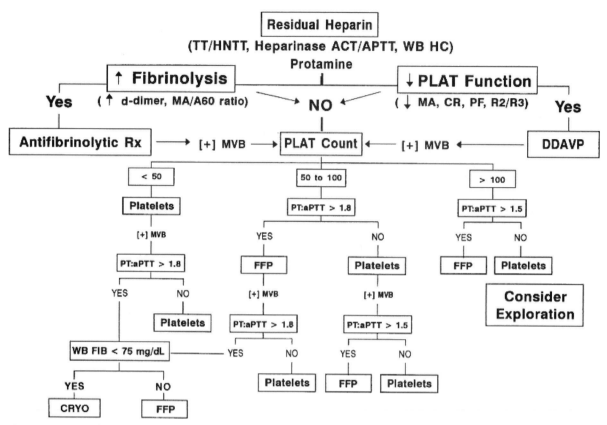

Figure 24.13. Modified Despotis algorithm for patients with microvascular bleeding after cardiopulmonary bypass. The modification introduced a quantitative assessment of the presence or absence of unneutralized heparin, the presence or absence of fibrinolysis, and a quantitative assessment of platelet function, as well as treatment options for those abnormalities if presence. The original algorithm began at platelet count, and was the only portion that was prospectively compared with traditional empiric therapy. The PT/aPTT intervention threshold for fresh frozen plasma was higher if platelet count was below 100,000/μL. Abbreviations listed from top to bottom: TT/HNTT = whole blood unmodified thrombin time combined with whole blood heparin-neutralized thrombin time, Heparinase ACT/APTT = activated clotting time or activated partial thromboplastin time with and without heparinase, WB HC = whole blood heparin concentration, MA/A60 Ratio = thromboelastographic ratio of maximum amplitude (MA) to amplitude 60 minutes after MA, MA = thromboelastographic maximum amplitude, CR = clot ratio (HemoSTATUS, Hepcon, Medtronic Co.), PF = platelet force measurement (Hemodyne Instrument), R2/R3 = R2 and R3 slope ratios (Sonoclot, Sienco, Inc.), MVB = microvascular bleeding, PLAT = platelet, DDAVP = desmopressin, PT = prothrombin time, aPTT = activated partial thromboplastin time, FFP = fresh frozen plasma, Platelets = platelet concentrates, WB FIB = whole blood fibrinogen test (Hemochron), CRYO = cryoprecipitate. From ref. 77, with permission; copyright Elsevier, 2000.

100,000/μL.[33,76] Typical TEG criteria for fresh frozen plasma varied from an R time greater than 10 minutes to one greater than 20 minutes.[78,79] The TEG threshold for desmopressin or platelet concentrate administration was an MA value less than either 48 mm or 45 mm.[49,78] TEG presence of a $LY_{30} > 7.5\%$

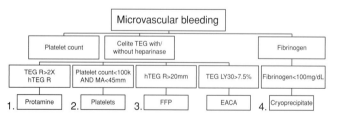

Figure 24.14. Shore-Lesserson thromboelastography-based algorithm for microvascular bleeding after cardiopulmonary bypass. Abbreviations, from top to bottom: TEG = thromboelastogram, TEG R = Reaction (R) time from TEG, h TEG R = Reaction time from TEG with added heparinase, MA = maximum amplitude from TEG, TEG LY30 = thromboelastogram percent lysis 30 minutes after MA, FFP = fresh frozen plasma, EACA = epsilon aminocaproic acid. From ref. 78, with permission.

was used as an indication for an antifibrinolytic agent whether or not one was already in use.[49,78,79]

Laboratory-based clotting tests were effective when compared with empiric therapy,[79] but the time delays incurred placed them at a disadvantage when compared with similar POC tests.[76] A recent review of transfusion algorithms in cardiac surgery notes that considerable variation in transfusion practice in cardiac surgery continues to exist and supports the use of algorithms to reduce unnecessary transfusions.[81] It seems plausible that the algorithms established in cardiac surgery would also apply to liver transplantation and to massive bleeding in elective noncardiac surgical patients.

Conclusions

When used selectively, laboratory-based traditional clotting tests and viscoelastic tests play an important role in monitoring blood clotting in surgical patients. Although intervention thresholds can be debated, reasonable component-specific guidelines have been established for PT, PTT, platelet count, and for the TEG parameters R time and MA. Sonoclot may be as useful as TEG, but its clinical applications have not been tested as well as those for TEG.

Transfusion algorithms in cardiac surgical patients who have coagulopathy after CPB reduce bleeding and transfusion, and it appears likely that, with slight modification, such algorithms would apply also to liver transplantation and to other operations in which major bleeding is occurring. These algorithms show the greatest promise when the test results can be rapidly obtained and when they are applied to patients soon after coagulopathy commences.

References

1. Rinder CS. Hematologic effects and coagulopathy. In Gravlee GP, Davis RF, Stammers AH, Ungerleider RM, eds. *Cardiopulmonary Bypass: Principles and Practice*, 3rd ed. Philadelphia: Lippincott Williams & Wilkins, 2008, pp. 439–58.

2. Schmaier AH, Thornburg CD, Pipe SW. Coagulation and fibrinolysis. In Miller JL, ed. *McPherson & Pincus: Henry's Clinical Diagnosis and Management by Laboratory Methods*, 21st ed. Philadelphia: W. B. Saunders Elsevier, 2006, accessed via www.mdconsult.com, 2009, Elsevier Inc.

3. Horrow JC, Mueksch JN. Coagulation testing. In Gravlee GP, Davis RF, Stammers AH, Ungerleider RM, eds. *Cardiopulmonary Bypass: Principles and Practice*, 3rd ed. Philadelphia: Lippincott Williams & Wilkins, 2008, pp. 459–71.

4. Appendix: Reference intervals and laboratory values. In Goldman L, Ausiello D, eds. *Cecil Medicine*, 23rd ed. Philadelphia: Saunders Elsevier, 2008, accessed via www.mdconsult.com, 2009, Elsevier Inc.

5. Fink LM, Marlar RA, Miller JL. Antithrombotic therapy. In Miller JL, ed. *McPherson & Pincus: Henry's Clinical Diagnosis and Management by Laboratory Methods*, 21st ed. Philadelphia: W. B. Saunders Elsevier, 2006, accessed via www.mdconsult.com, 2009, Elsevier Inc.

6. Counts RB, Haish C, Simon TL, et al. Hemostasis in massively transfused trauma patients. *Ann Surg* 1979;**190**:91–99.

7. Mannucci PM, Federici AB, Sirchia G. Hemostasis during massive blood replacement: a study of 172 cases. *Vox Sang* 1982;**42**:113–23.

8. Miller RD, Robbins TO, Tong MJ, Barton SL. Coagulation defects associated with massive blood transfusions. *Ann Surg* 1971;**174**:795–801.

9. Harker LA, Malpass TW, Branson HE, Hessel EA 2nd. Mechanism of abnormal bleeding in patients undergoing cardiopulmonary bypass: acquired transient platelet dysfunction associated with selective α-granule release. *Blood* 1980;**56**:824–34.

10. Slaughter TF, Sreeram G, Sharma AD, El-Moalem H, et al. Reversible shear –medicated platelet dysfunction during cardiac surgery as assessed by the PFA-100 platelet function analyzer. *Blood Coagul Fibrinolysis* 2001;**12**:85–93.

11. Reed RL III, Heimbach DM, Counts RB, Baron L, et al. Prophylactic platelet administration during massive transfusion: a prospective, randomized, double-blind clinical study. *Ann Surg* 1986;**203**:40–48.

12. Hayem G. *Du sang et de ses altérations anatomiques*. G. Masson, 1889.

13. Hett DA, Walker D, Pilkington SN, Smith DC. Sonoclot analysis. *Br J Anaesth* 1995;**75**:771–6.

14. Koffmann K. Der Koaguloviskosimeter mit spezieller Beruecksichtigung seiner klinischen verwendbarkeit fuer gerinnungsestimmungen des Blutes. *Zeitschrift Klinische Medizin* 1910;**59**:415–21.

15. Hartert H. Thrombelastography, a method for physical analysis of blood coagulation. *Z Gesamte Exp Med* 1951;**117**:189–203.

16. Hartert H. Blutgerinnungsstudien mit der thromboeslastographic, einen neven untersuchungsver fahren. *Klin Wochenschr* 1948;**26**:577–83.

17. von Kaulla KN, Ostendorf P, von Kaulla E. The impedance machine: a new bedside coagulation recording device. *J Med* 1975;**6**:73–88.

18. Sienco Inc. The Sonoclot Coagulation and Platelet Function Analyzer Owners Manual. 1996–2006.

19. Ganter MT, Hofer CK. Intensive care medicine; point-of-care coagulation monitoring: current status of viscoelastic techniques. In Vincent J-L, ed. *Intensive Care Medicine Annual Update 2007*, Springer Berlin/Heidelberg, 2007, pp. 834–46.

20. Ganter MT, Monn A, Tavakoli R, et al. Monitoring activated clotting time for combined heparin and aprotinin application: in vivo evaluation of a new aprotinin-insensitive test using Sonoclot. *Eur J Cardiothorac Surg* 2006;**30**:278–84.

21. Ganter MT, Hofer CK. Coagulation monitoring: current techniques and clinical use of viscoelastic point-of-care coagulation devices. *Anesth Analg* 2008;**106**:1366–75.

22. Tanaka KA, Szlam F, Sun HY, Taketomi T, Levy JH. Thrombin generation assay and viscoelastic coagulation monitors demonstrate differences in the mode of thrombin inhibition between unfractionated heparin and bivalirudin. *Anesth Analg* 2007;**105**:933–9.

23. Miyashita T, Kuro M. Evaluation of platelet function by Sonoclot analysis compared with other hemostatic variables in cardiac surgery. *Anesth Analg* 1998;**87**:1228–33.

24. Chapin JW, Becker GL, Hulbert BJ, et al. Comparison of thromboelastograph and Sonoclot coagulation analyzer for assessing coagulation status during orthotopic liver transplantation. *Transplant Proc* 1989;**21**:3539.

25. Tuman KJ, Spiess BD, McCarthy RJ, Ivankovich AD. Comparison of viscoelastic measures of coagulation after cardiopulmonary bypass. *Anesth Analg* 1989;**69**:69–75.

26. Ganter MT, Dalbert S, Graves K, Klaghofer R, Zollinger A, Hofer CK. Monitoring activated clotting time for combined heparin and aprotinin application: an in vitro evaluation of a new aprotinin-insensitive test using Sonoclot. *Anesth Analg* 2005;**101**:308–14.

27. Tucci MA, Ganter MT, Hamiel CR, Klaghofer R, Zollinger A, Hofer CK. Platelet function monitoring with the Sonoclot analyzer after in vitro tirofiban and heparin administration. *J Thorac Cardiovasc Surg* 2006;**131**:1314–22.

28. Ganter MT, Monn A, Tavakoli R, Klaghofer R, Zollinger A, Hofer CK. Kaolin-based activated coagulation time measured by Sonoclot in patients undergoing cardiopulmonary bypass. *J Cardiothorac Vasc Anesth* 2007;**21**:524–8.

29. Dalbert S, Ganter MT, Furrer L, Klaghofer R, Zollinger A, Hofer CK. Effects of heparin, haemodilution and aprotinin on kaolin-based activated clotting time: in vitro comparison of two different point of care devices. *Acta Anaesthesiol Scand* 2006;**50**:461–8.

30. Sugiura K, Ikeda Y, Ono F, Watanabe K, Ando Y. Detection of hypercoagulability by the measurement of the dynamic loss modulus of clotting blood. *Thromb Res* 1982;**27**:161–6.

31. Stern MP, DeVos-Doyle K, Viguera MG, Lajos TZ. Evaluation of post-cardiopulmonary bypass Sonoclot signatures in patients

taking nonsteroidal anti-inflammatory drugs. *J Cardiothorac Anesth* 1989;**3**:730–3.

32. Saleem A, Blifeld C, Saleh SA, et al. Viscoelastic measurement of clot formation: a new test of platelet function. *Ann Clin Lab Sci* 1983;**13**:115–24.

33. Nuttall GA, Oliver WC, Ereth MH, Santrach PJ. Coagulation tests predict bleeding after cardiopulmonary bypass. *J Cardiothorac Vasc Anesth* 1997;**11**:815–23.

34. McKenzie ME, Gurbel PA, Levine DJ, Serebruany VL. Clinical utility of available methods for determining platelet function. *Cardiology* 1999;**92**:240–7.

35. Horlocker TT, Schroeder DR. Effect of age, gender, and platelet count on Sonoclot coagulation analysis in patients undergoing orthopedic operations. *Mayo Clin Proc* 1997;**72**:214–9.

36. Ekback G, Carlsson O, Schott U. Sonoclot coagulation analysis: a study of test variability. *J Cardiothorac Vasc Anesth* 1999;**13**:393–7.

37. Kang YG, Martin DJ, Marquez J, et al. Intraoperative changes in blood coagulation and thrombelastographic monitoring in liver transplantation. *Anesth Analg* 1985;**64**:888–96.

38. Ganter MT, Schmuck S, Hamiel CR, et al. Monitoring recombinant factor VIIa treatment: efficacy depends on high levels of fibrinogen in a model of severe dilutional coagulopathy. *J Cardiothorac Vasc Anesth* 2008;**22**:675–80.

39. Ferraris VA, Ferraris SP, Saha SP, et al. Perioperative blood transfusion and blood conservation in cardiac surgery: the Society of Thoracic Surgeons and The Society of Cardiovascular Anesthesiologists clinical practice guideline. *Ann Thorac Surg* 2007;**83**(5 Suppl):S27–S86.

40. Spiess BD, Tuman KJ, McCarthy RJ, et al. Thromboelastography as an indicator of post-cardiopulmonary bypass coagulopathies. *J Clin Monit* 1987;**3**:25–30.

41. Camenzind V, Bombeli T, Seifert B, et al. Citrate storage affects thrombelastograph analysis. *Anesthesiology* 2000;**92**:1242–9.

42. Chandler WL. The thromboelastography and the thromboelastograph technique. *Semin Thromb Hemost* 1995;**21**:1–6.

43. Bowbrick VA, Mikhailidis DP, Stansby G. The use of citrated whole blood in thromboelastography. *Anesth Analg* 2000;**90**:1086–8.

44. Yamakage M, Tsujiguchi N, Kohro S et al. The usefulness of celite-activated thromboelastography for evaluation of fibrinolysis. *Can J Anaesth* 1998;**45**:993–6.

45. Dietrich W, Jochum M. Effect of celite and kaolin on activated clotting time in the presence of aprotinin: activated clotting time is reduced by binding of aprotinin to kaolin. *J Thorac Cardiovasc Surg* 1995;**109**:177–8.

46. Johansson PI, Bochsen L, Andersen S, Viuff D. Investigation of the effect of kaolin and tissue-factor-activated citrated whole blood, on clot-forming variables, as evaluated by thromboelastography. *Transfusion* 2008;**48**:2377–83.

47. Khurana S, Mattson JC, Westley S, et al. Monitoring platelet glycoprotein IIb/IIIa-fibrin interaction with tissue factor-activated thromboelastography. *J Lab Clin Med* 1997;**130**:401–11.

48. Boisclair MD, Lane DA, Philippou H, et al. Mechanisms of thrombin generation during surgery and cardiopulmonary bypass. *Blood* 1993;**82**:3350–7.

49. Royston D, von Kier S. Reduced haemostatic factor transfusion using heparinase-modified thrombelastography during cardiopulmonary bypass. *Br J Anaesth* 2001;**86**:575–8.

50. Tuman KJ, McCarthy RJ, Djuric M, et al. Evaluation of coagulation during cardiopulmonary bypass with a heparinase-modified thromboelastographic assay. *J Cardiothorac Vasc Anesth* 1994;**8**:144–9.

51. Despotis GJ, Summerfield AL, Joist JH, et al. In vitro reversal of heparin effect with heparinase: evaluation with whole blood prothrombin time and activated partial thromboplastin time in cardiac surgical patients. *Anesth Analg* 1994;**79**:670–4.

52. Gottumukkala VN, Sharma SK, Philip J. Assessing platelet and fibrinogen contribution to clot strength using modified thromboelastography in pregnant women. *Anesth Analg* 1999;**89**:1453–5.

53. Cammerer U, Dietrich W, Rampf T, et al. The predictive value of modified computerized thromboelastography and platelet function analysis for postoperative blood loss in routine cardiac surgery. *Anesth Analg* 2003;**96**:51–57.

54. Papatheodoridis GV, Patch D, Webster GJ, et al. Infection and hemostasis in decompensated cirrhosis: a prospective study using thrombelastography. *Hepatology* 1999;**29**:1085–90.

55. Senzolo M, Cholongitas E, Thalheimer U, et al. Heparin-like effect in liver disease and liver transplantation. *Clin Liver Dis* 2009;**13**:43–53.

56. Agarwal S, Senzolo M, Melikian C, et al. The prevalence of a heparin-like effect shown on the thromboelastograph in patients undergoing liver transplantation. *Liver Transpl* 2008;**14**:855–66.

57. Hendriks HG, Meijer K, de Wolf JT, et al. Effects of recombinant activated factor VII on coagulation measured by thromboelastography in liver transplantation. *Blood Coagul Fibrinolysis* 2002;**13**:309–13.

58. Coakley M, Reddy K, Mackie I, Mallett S. Transfusion triggers in orthotopic liver transplantation: a comparison of the thromboelastometry analyzer, the thromboelastogram, and conventional coagulation tests. *J Cardiothorac Vasc Anesth* 2006;**20**:548–53.

59. Gillies BS. Thromboelastography and liver transplantation. *Semin Thromb Hemost* 1995;**21Suppl** 4:45–49.

60. Schumann R. Intraoperative resource utilization in anesthesia for liver transplantation in the United States: a survey. *Anesth Analg* 2003;**97**:21–28.

61. Fuchs RJ, Levin J, Tadel M, Merritt W. Perioperative coagulation management in a patient with afibrinogenemia undergoing liver transplantation. *Liver Transpl* 2007;**13**:752–6.

62. Stahl RL, Duncan A, Hooks MA, et al. A hypercoagulable state follows orthotopic liver transplantation. *Hepatology* 1990;**12**:553–8.

63. Cerutti E, Stratta C, Romagnoli R, et al. Thromboelastogram monitoring in the perioperative period of hepatectomy for adult living liver donation. *Liver Transpl* 2004;**10**:289–94.

64. Wilson D, Cooke EA, McNally MA, et al. Changes in coagulability as measured by thrombelastography following surgery for proximal femoral fracture. *Injury* 2001;**32**:765–70.

65. Hsu HW, Huang CH, Chang Y et al. Perioperative alterations of the thromboelastography in patients receiving one-stage bilateral total knee arthroplasty. *Acta Anaesthesiol Sin* 1996;**34**:129–34.

66. Mittermayr M, Streif W, Haas T et al. Hemostatic changes after crystalloid or colloid fluid administration during major orthopedic surgery: the role of fibrinogen administration. *Anesth Analg* 2007;**105**:905–17.

67. Kaufmann CR, Dwyer KM, Crews JD, et al. Usefulness of thrombelastography in assessment of trauma patient coagulation. *J Trauma* 1997;**42**:716–22.

68. Watts DD, Trask A, Soeken K, et al. Hypothermic coagulopathy in trauma: effect of varying levels of hypothermia on enzyme speed, platelet function, and fibrinolytic activity. *J Trauma* 1998;**44**:846–54.

69. Sharma SK, Philip J, Wiley J. Thromboelastographic changes in healthy parturients and postpartum women. *Anesth Analg* 1997;**85**:94–98.

70. Sharma SK, Philip J, Whitten CW, et al. Assessment of changes in coagulation in parturients with preeclampsia using thromboelastography. *Anesthesiology* 1999;**90**:385–90.

71. Butwick A, Carvalho B. The effect of colloid and crystalloid preloading on thromboelastography prior to Cesarean delivery. *Can J Anaesth* 2007;**54**:190–5.

72. Craft RM, Chavez JJ, Bresee SJ, et al. A novel modification of the thrombelastograph assay, isolating platelet function, correlates with optical platelet aggregation. *J Lab Clin Med* 2004;**143**:301–9.

73. Carroll RC, Chavez JJ, Snider CC, et al. Correlation of perioperative platelet function and coagulation tests with bleeding after cardiopulmonary bypass surgery. *J Lab Clin Med* 2006;**147**:197–204.

74. Hobson AR, Agarwala RA, Swallow RA, et al. Thrombelastography: current clinical applications and its potential role in interventional cardiology. *Platelets* 2006;**17**:509–18.

75. Lev EI, Ramchandani M, Garg R, et al. Response to aspirin and clopidogrel in patients scheduled to undergo cardiovascular surgery. *J Thromb Thrombolysis* 2007;**24**:15–21.

76. Despotis GJ, Santoro SA, Spitznagel E, Kater KM, et al. Prospective evaluation and clinical utility of on-site monitoring of coagulation in patients undergoing cardiac operation. *J Thorac Cardiovasc Surg* 1994;**107**:271–9.

77. Despotis GJ, Goodnough LT. Management approaches to platelet-related microvascular bleeding in cardiothoracic surgery. *Ann Thorac Surg* 2000;**70**:S20–S32.

78. Shore-Lesserson L, Manspeizer H, DePerlo M, et al. Thromboelastography-guided transfusion algorithm reduces transfusions in complex cardiac surgery. *Anesth Analg* 1999;**88**:312–9.

79. Avidan MS, Alcock EL, Da Fonseca J, Ponte J, et al. Comparison of structured use of routine laboratory tests or near-patient assessment with clinical judgement in the management of bleeding after cardiac surgery. *Br J Anaesth* 2004;**92**:178–86.

80. Capraro L, Kuitunen A, Salmenpera M, Kekomaki R. On-site coagulation monitoring does not affect hemostatic outcome after cardiac surgery. *Acta Anaethesiol Scand* 2001;**45**:200–6.

81. Steiner ME, Despotis GJ. Transfusion algorithms and how they apply to blood conservation: the high-risk cardiac surgical patient. *Hematol Oncol Clin North Am* 2007;**21**:177–84.

Chapter 25

Coagulation and hematologic point-of-care testing

Liza J. Enriquez and Linda Shore-Lesserson

Introduction

For many years, the majority of laboratory testing was performed in a central facility. With advanced technology, testing has emerged from the laboratory to the patient's bedside. Point-of-care (POC) testing provides the caregiver with immediate access to laboratory results that can be used for the optimal management of the patient. This rapid turnaround time is particularly useful in the operating room as well as in other sites, including the emergency room, critical care units, and interventional cardiology and radiology suites, for monitoring therapy and hemostasis. POC assessment guides the practitioner to provide appropriate pharmacologic and transfusion interventions.[1] Outcome studies have proven that POC testing has resulted in a reduction in blood loss and transfusion requirements, cost, and complication rates.[2-4] In addition, it has shown improved timely patient care and clinical outcomes, as well as a reduction in length of stay. The majority of the POC devices used today can perform multiple coagulation tests depending on which cartridge or test tube is selected.

This chapter will cover the various modalities for POC coagulation and platelet function testing.

Monitoring anticoagulation

Heparin monitoring

Heparin is the most widely used anticoagulant drug for the treatment and prevention of thromboembolic disorders.[5] In addition, it is used for the diagnosis and treatment of acute and chronic consumption coagulopathies – disseminated intravascular coagulation (DIC). In the operating room and interventional suites, heparin is used for prevention of clotting in cardiac and arterial surgery. The activated clotting time (ACT) is the most commonly used functional point-of-care test to measure heparin anticoagulation especially when high blood concentrations (>1 IU/mL) cannot be accurately measured by aPTT.[6-8] An automated variation of the Lee–White clotting time, it uses an activator such as celite or kaolin to activate clotting, then measures clotting time in a test tube.[9] Hattersley first described the ACT in 1966 using whole blood placed in a warmed test tube with diatomaceous earth as an activator.[10] The tubes were tilted back and forth manually until evidence of a clot appeared.

Currently, the two most commonly used ACT devices are the Hemochron (International Technidyne Inc.; Edison, NJ) and the HemoTec (Medtronic HemoTec; Parker, CO). The Hemochron system consists of a precision aligned magnet within a test tube and a magnet detector located within the well. Whole blood is added into a test tube containing an activator (celite, kaolin, glass beads, or a combination of these) and placed in the well. As a clot begins to form, the magnet is lifted within the tube, displacing the magnet from the magnet detector. The clotting time is the time the clot takes to displace the magnet in a given distance. The HemoTec device uses a two-chamber cartridge containing kaolin as an activator. Blood (0.4 mL) is placed into each chamber and a daisy-shaped plunger rises and falls into the chamber. The formation of a clot will slow the rate of descent of the plunger, and the decrease in velocity of the plunger is detected by a photooptical system that signals the end of the ACT test. Each ACT analyzer is consistent in its ability to reproducibly measure the clotting time using its specific methodology.[11] There are intrinsic biases built into some of the measurement devices, but repeatability within a given device is high.

ACT monitoring of heparinization has been criticized because it is highly susceptible to variation.[9,12] The main limiting factor is that it correlates poorly with anti-Xa measures of heparin activity,[13] or with heparin concentration during cardiopulmonary bypass (CPB) as a result of hypothermia and hemodilution.[13,14] This is especially true for pediatric patients,[15,16] whose consumption of heparin is increased. Other factors altering ACT include thrombocytopenia, presence of platelet inhibitors, platelet membrane receptor antagonists, and the use of the antifibrinolytic aprotinin (celite only).[17-19]

Heparin concentration

Quantitative heparin testing uses the Hepcon HMS system (Medtronic HemoTec; Parker, CO). The Hepcon HMS system measures whole blood heparin using an automated protamine titration technique based on the fact that protamine neutralizes heparin in 1 mg:100 U ratio. Because CPB increases the sensitivity of ACT, the quantitative measure of whole blood heparin concentration can supplement the functional measure of heparin anticoagulation (ACT) and provide a means of stable anticoagulation. Because ACT increases when CPB is initiated, and heparin concentrations remain stable (or decrease), maintenance of stable heparin *concentrations* during CPB require additional doses of heparin. This is considered beneficial, as it implies a more profound degree of anticoagulation.[20] Heparin concentration monitoring is also advantageous because heparin concentrations during CPB have been shown to more closely correlate with anti-Xa measurements than does the ACT.[14]

It has been demonstrated that when heparin concentration monitoring is used in conjunction with transfusion algorithms, there is less postoperative bleeding and fewer transfusions of allogeneic blood products.[21,22] This reduction in bleeding using heparin concentration monitoring has not been replicated in other studies, mostly as a result of untreated heparin rebound.[23]

High dose thrombin time, or HiTT (International Technidyne Inc.; Edison, NJ), is a functional test of heparin anticoagulation that overcomes some of the limitations of the standard ACT. HiTT is not altered by hemodilution or hypothermia, and has been shown to correlate better with heparin concentration than the ACT during CPB.[24] The HiTT exhibits less artifactual modulation, because it measures the effects of heparin at the level of thrombin.[25] With HiTT, a large dose of thrombin is added into the test tube and binds a significant proportion of the heparin–antithrombin 3 (AT3) complexes present during heparinization. The remaining AT3-unbound heparin prolongs the time required for fibrin to form, and is measured as HiTT. The Hemochron testing platform allows the performance of HiTT. In contrast to the ACT during CPB, HiTT decreases with heparin concentration and is not affected by aprotinin. It also is affected less than ACT by the heparin resistance seen in patients placed on preoperative heparin infusions. Its use has not become the standard of care in cardiac surgery because more research is necessary to confirm its reliability and precision for every day use. In addition, the reagents in the tube were lyophilized and required prehydration prior to use.

Cascade POC system

A completely different technology for measuring the effect of heparin is used by the Cascade POC analyzer (Helena, Beaumont, TX; formerly Rapid Point coagulation analyzer, Bayer Diagnostics, Tarrytown, NY). This test system contains disposable cards with celite activator for the measure of heparin activity. This variation of the ACT is called the heparin management test (HMT). The card contains paramagnetic iron oxide particles that move in response to an oscillating magnetic field within the device. When clot formation is detected, movement of the iron oxide particles is decreased, and the end of the test is signaled. This system is capable of measuring prothrombin time (PT) and activated partial thromboplastin time (aPTT), which will be discussed later. The suitability of this platform for the monitoring of ACT during cardiac surgery has been demonstrated in a variety of clinical studies.[26,27] Suitability for monitoring heparinization in the interventional cardiology laboratory has also been reported.[28] HMT correlates well with anti-Xa heparin activity in CPB patients and is less variable than

standard ACT measures.[29] In a comparison with ACT, the coefficients of variation were similar between the tests at baseline but were three times higher for the ACT during heparinization. This degree of agreement with plasma anti-Xa measurements has not been demonstrated universally when studying blood from patients undergoing CPB.[30]

Individualized heparin dosing

In vitro techniques have been introduced that measure the patient dose–response to heparin.[31] These assays measure a patient's heparin sensitivity to a known quantity of heparin and generate a dose–response curve that will enable calculation of the heparin dose required to attain the target goal. Blood loss and transfusion requirements in cardiac surgical patients may be reduced with more accurate control of heparin anticoagulation and its reversal. These assays measure a patient's heparin sensitivity to a known quantity of heparin and generate a dose–response curve that will enable calculation of the heparin dose required to attain the target goal. Similarly, a protamine dose–response curve is generated using an in vitro sample with a known quantity of protamine, thus enabling protamine dosing to be based only on the level of *circulating* heparin. The Hemochron RxDx (International Technidyne Corp.; Edison, NJ) system is an ACT-based heparin dose–response assay. The patient heparin requirement is measured by the heparin response test (HRT), and the required protamine dose is measured by the protamine response test (PRT); a zero value indicates that heparin is adequately neutralized. A separate test, the protamine dose assay (PDA-O), can be used to measure the residual heparin in the blood. Using this system, other investigators have been able to significantly lower protamine doses only,[32] and some have reported significantly reduced transfusions and chest tube drainage in the group that received individualized dosing with RxDx.[33]

Another in vitro individualized heparin dose–response assay is the Hepcon (Medtronic) Heparin Dose Response (HDR), which constructs a three-point heparin dose–response curve using the baseline, 1.5 IU/mL, and 2.5 IU/mL of heparin. From this curve, extrapolation to the desired ACT or heparin concentration will yield the indicated dose of heparin to be given. These dose–response assays are used less frequently than weight-based heparin dosing because the latter technique is faster, less expensive, and extremely safe, if monitored. It is not clear from the literature that individualized heparin dosing alone, in the absence of individualized protamine dosing, has any effect on perioperative blood loss and transfusions in cardiac surgery.[34]

See Table 25.1 for a list of heparin monitoring devices and their attributes.

Point-of-care monitoring of coagulation status (PT, INR, aPTT)

Several POC coagulation analyzers are currently available for use. The former Thrombolytic Assessment System (TAS)

Table 25.1. Tests for monitoring large-dose heparin

Device (manufacturer)	Assay	Activators available	Dose–response
Hemotec (Medtronic Hemotec; Parker, CO)	ACT	Kaolin, celite, glass beads	No
Hemochron (International Technidyne Inc.; Edison, NJ)	ACT	Kaolin, celite	Yes – Hemochron RxDx
Hepcon HMS system (Medtronic Hemotec; Parker, CO)	Heparin concentration	Kaolin	Yes – HDR (heparin dose response test)
HiTT (International Technidyne Inc.; Edison, NJ)	Thrombin time	Human thrombin	No
Cascade POC analyzer (Helena; Beaumont, TX)	Heparin management test (HMT)	Celite	Yes – HRT (heparin response test)

(Pharmanetics Inc.; Raleigh, NC), also known as the Rapid-Point (Bayer Diagnostics; Tarrytown, NY), has been acquired by Helena (Beaumont, TX) as the Cascade POC (discussed under heparin management systems). This device, in addition to measuring the HMT, also measures PT and aPTT using citrated whole blood or plasma. The sample is added to a cartridge containing paramagnetic iron oxide particles, which oscillate in a magnetic field as described. Specific reagents are used for each analyte. The analytes used include rabbit brain thromboplastin for PT, aluminum magnesium silicate for aPTT, and celite for HMT. The blood moves by capillary action and mixes with the paramagnetic iron oxide particles and reagent within the testing chamber. The decreased movement of the particles is detected optically as the sample clots and the resultant time is displayed in seconds, and as International Normalized Ratios (INRs) for PT.

The CoaguChek Pro DM monitor (Roche Diagnostics, Mannheim, Germany), formerly CoaguChek-plus, and formerly Ciba Corning Biotrack 512 monitor, uses a whole blood sample added to a test cartridge that contains a soybean activator and phospholipids. As the sample clots, the decrease in blood flow is optically monitored by a laser, and the resultant clotting time is displayed in seconds for PT and aPTT, and as a ratio for INR. The accuracy of this aPTT as compared with plasma aPTT was deemed unacceptable in a series of surgical intensive care unit patients.[35] However, this device has been studied in cardiac surgical patients and the PT result compared favorably with laboratory plasma based assays at most perioperative time points.[36] The aPTT result also correlated with plasma-based samples but was slightly less accurate and had a significant bias.[36]

The same authors used the former Biotrack 512 POC coagulation monitor to define normal versus abnormal aPTT and PT values after CPB. Using these data, they predicted which patients were more likely to have bleeding based on sensitivity, specificity, and receiver operating characteristic curves.[37] In addition, this POC device has been used in various transfusion algorithms to direct transfusion of fresh frozen plasma after cardiac surgery.[22,38]

The Hemochron (International Technidyne Corp.; Edison, NJ) coagulation tests are performed on small POC devices that use cuvette technology. These are whole blood coagulation analyzers that monitor PT, aPTT, and ACT via optical detection of clot formation. They have not been as extensively studied as the former Biotrack 512 PT and aPTT for use in transfusion algorithms in cardiac surgery.

Thrombin time and heparin neutralized thrombin time

Thrombin time/heparin neutralized thrombin time (TT/HNTT) tests can also be run after protamine administration to identify the presence of heparin rebound or abnormal fibrinogen function. The Hemochron (International Technidyne Corp.; Edison, NJ) device offers these tests. The TT is a very sensitive measure of low-level residual heparin activity or abnormal fibrinogen activity. The HNTT is a TT test tube with protamine included so that the effects of heparin will be neutralized. If the HNTT is significantly shorter than the TT, one can assume that residual heparin activity exists. This method of detection of residual heparinization has been used successfully in a number of studies.[33,39]

Monitoring platelet function

The past decade has seen the introduction into clinical practice of many new anticoagulants, antiplatelet agents, and procoagulants in the treatment of cardiovascular disease. Patients taking these medications who present to the operating room render the safe practice of anesthesia and surgery very challenging. Monitoring hemostasis is crucial to ensure an appropriate balance between the risk of thrombosis and the risk of hemorrhage. Perioperative use of platelet function analyzers is helpful in the prediction of blood loss, especially in cardiac surgery.[40] Algorithms for perioperative coagulation management based on POC testing permit a fast diagnostic and goal-directed therapy of coagulation and functional platelet disorders. This helps reduce the empiric usage of blood components, reducing the mortality of patients and subsequently the overall cost for their hospital stay. Some of these algorithms and their use in reducing bleeding and transfusions are covered in the laboratory testing portion of this chapter.

POC tests of fibrinogen level

A number of assays of plasma fibrinogen have been described in the laboratory. Most laboratories use the Clauss method of detection, which is a functional assay based on the time for fibrin clot formation. An excess amount of thrombin is added to a plasma sample, and the time to fibrin clot formation is measured. This excess of thrombin substrate ensures that fibrinogen will have enough substrate on which to act and that small concentrations of heparin will not interfere with the assay.

Whole blood assays are also available that measure fibrinogen level. The Hemochron system uses a test tube that contains human thrombin, snake venom, calcium, and protamine (to neutralize any heparin). Diluted whole blood is added to the test tube and the time for clot formation, as detected by the Hemochron platform, is measured. This test has been validated in adult fibrinogen assays but has been shown to correlate poorly with plasma-based measurements in the pediatric population.[41] The thromboelastograph (TEG) modification measurement technique for fibrinogen level will be described in the TEG section of this chapter.

Traditional tests of platelet function

Bleeding time

The bleeding time is a bedside test to measure both platelet number and function. The test is performed by creating a skin incision and measuring the time to clot formation by way of the platelet plug. The use of bleeding time has fallen out of favor because the test is neither sensitive nor specific and is subject to patient and operator variability. In addition, this test is not a useful predictor of the risk of hemorrhage associated with surgical procedures.

Platelet aggregometry

Platelet aggregometry remains the gold standard when evaluating platelet function. A photooptical instrument is used to measure light transmittance through a sample of platelet-rich plasma. When exposed to a platelet agonist, the light transmittance will be increased as a result of integrin $\alpha IIb\beta 3$ (GP IIb/IIIa)–dependent platelet-to-platelet aggregation. Light transmittance aggregometry is almost always considered a laboratory test rather than a POC test, as it is time-consuming and requires centrifugation, pipetting, and large photooptical systems.

Platelet aggregation can also be measured in whole blood at the POC by using an electrical impedance technique.[40,42–44] The whole blood aggregometer uses an electrode pair immersed in a sample of blood.[45] As the platelets aggregate, the voltage change or impedance is measured; this correlates with platelet function. Impedance aggregometry has been modified to include activators such as arachidonic acid (AA) and ADP and can be used to measure platelet inhibition in response to the drugs aspirin (AA) and clopidogrel (ADP), respectively.[46–49] The whole blood impedance platform described for drug-induced platelet function testing is called the Multiplate Analyzer (Dynabyte; Munich, Germany). It is currently approved for use in many European countries but is not yet approved by the US Food and Drug Administration.

POC platelet function tests

Platelet Function Analyzer (PFA-100)

The Platelet Function Analyzer (PFA-100) monitor (Siemens; Deerfield, IL) conducts a modified in vitro bleeding time under high-shear conditions. Whole blood is placed on a test cartridge and, by vacuum, blood is perfused across a collagen-coated aperture in the presence of an agonist, either epinephrine (EPI) or adenosine diphosphate (ADP). This coating activates the platelets in the moving sample and promotes platelet adherence and aggregation. The time it takes for a clot to form inside the glass tube and prevent further blood flow is measured as the closure time. This device is able to identify drug-induced abnormalities, von Willebrand disease, and other acquired and congenital platelet defects.[44,50,51] It has been used in clinical studies of aspirin resistance and to monitor GP IIB/IIIa antagonists.[52–55] However, the PFA-100 is not recommended for monitoring clopidogrel therapy.[56] In cardiac surgical patients, the PFA-100 closure time has only a high negative predictive value and thus may help in identifying patients who are unlikely to need platelet transfusions to reduce bleeding.[40,57] Its positive predictive value is low and thus it is not very useful in transfusion algorithms to direct transfusion therapy. (Table 25.2.).

VerifyNow

The VerifyNow system (formerly marketed as Ultegra; Accumetrics, San Diego, CA) mixing chamber contains a platelet agonist (thrombin receptor-activating peptide, arachidonic acid, or ADP) and fibrinogen-coated beads. After anticoagulated whole blood is added to the mixing chamber, the platelets become activated.[58] The activated glycoprotein (GP) IIb/IIIa receptors on the platelets bind via the fibrinogen on the beads and cause agglutination of the platelets and the beads. Light transmittance through the chamber is measured and increases as the agglutinated platelets and beads fall out of the solution. Drug effects cause a diminished agglutination (measured by light transmittance) and thus the degree of platelet inhibition can be quantified. Direct pharmacologic blockade of GP IIb/IIIa receptors with a GP IIb/IIIa antagonist is detected with a very high accuracy using this device.[59–61]

The indirect prevention of GPIIb/IIIa expression is accomplished by aspirin[62,63] through inhibition of AA and by clopidogrel through ADP P2Y12 receptor inhibition.[56,64–67] Each of these drug effects can be measured using the appropriate cartridge of the VerifyNow device. Aspirin resistance, which can be present in 5 percent to 50 percent of the population, can be detected by the VerifyNow and identified even more resistant patients than light-transmittance aggergometry.[68] This has been critically important in the interventional cardiology laboratory, where 30-day adverse outcomes were shown to correlate with the degree of preprocedure platelet reactivity measured by the VerifyNow.[69]

Table 25.2. Tests for evaluation of platelet function

Device	Agonists available	Clinical use
Bleeding time	No (collagen)	Screening
Platelet aggregometry PRP	Yes – all	Screening and diagnostic
Whole blood aggregation	Yes – all	Efficacy of antiplatelet therapy
Platelet function Analyzer-100 (Siemens; Deerfield, IL)	Yes – Epi, ADP	Screening, vWD, aspirin therapy
Verify Now (formerly marketed as Ultegra; Accumetrics; San Diego, CA)	Yes – ADP, AA	Efficacy of antiplatelet therapy (aspirin, clopidogrel)
Plateletworks (Helena Labs; Beaumont, TX)	Yes – ADP, Collagen, Epinephrine	Efficacy of antiplatelet therapy (aspirin, clopidogrel)
Hemostatus (Medtronic; Parker, CO)	Yes – PAF	Not currently
Sonoclot (Sienco Inc.; Wheat Ridge, CO)	No	Cardiac surgery
		Liver transplant surgery
		Vascular surgery
		Orthopedic surgery
		Obstetrics/neonate care
		Cardiology trauma and hemostasis research
Thromboelastograph assay (TEG) (Haemonetics; Braintree, MA)	Yes – ADP, AA	Cardiac surgery
		Liver transplant surgery
		Vascular surgery
		Orthopedic surgery
		Obstetrics/neonate care
		Cardiology trauma and hemostasis research
		DIC
ROTEM ((Pentapharm; Munich, Germany	Yes – ADP, AA	Cardiac surgery
		Liver transplant surgery
Clot Signature Analyzer	Yes	None
Impact Cone and Plate(let)	No	Screening
Analyzer (DiaMed Cressier, Switzerland)		Efficacy of antiplatelet therapy

Platelet Works

Platelet Works (Helena Laboratories; Beaumont, TX) is a whole blood assay that uses the principle of the platelet count ratio to assess platelet reactivity. The instrument is a Coulter counter that compares platelet counts in a standard ethylenediaminetetraacetic acid (EDTA)-tube with platelet counts in a citrate tube after aggregation with either ADP or collagen. When blood is added to these agonist tubes, it causes the platelets to activate, adhere to the tube, and be effectively eliminated from the platelet count. The ratio of the activated platelet count to the nonactivated platelet count is a function of the reactivity of the platelets (Figure 25.1). Early investigation indicates that this assay is useful for providing a platelet count and is capable of measuring the platelet dysfunction induced by the GPIIb/IIIa receptor inhibitors and by clopidogrel.[70,71] Further investigation is warranted to determine whether PlateletWorks can be used as a monitor during coronary interventions or afterward as a monitor of inhibition by antithrombotic drugs.[72]

HemoSTATUS

The HemoSTATUS (Medtronic Inc., Parker, CO) is a device that measures the platelet-activated clotting time. It measures the ACT without platelet activator and compares this value to the ACT obtained when increasing concentrations of a platelet-activating factor (PAF) are added. The percentage of reduction of the ACT caused by the addition of PAF is related to the ability of the platelets to be activated and to shorten the clotting time. This assay was performed using a specific Medtronic cartridge for the HMS machine. It was approved by the US Food and Drug Administration for monitoring platelet function during cardiac surgery, and was used in transfusion algorithms. The ability of HemoSTATUS to correlate with bleeding after cardiac surgery was demonstrated by some,[73] but not universally in all studies.[74-77] This POC platelet function assay is no longer supported commercially.

Sonoclot

The Sonoclot Analyzer (Sienco Inc.; Arvada, CO) is a test of the viscoelastic properties of blood that provides accurate information on the entire hemostasis process, including coagulation, fibrin gel formation, clot retraction (platelet function), and fibrinolysis.[44,78] This device consists of a tubular probe that oscillates up and down within a blood sample. The detection mechanism responds to mechanical changes that occur within the blood sample. The electronic drive and detection circuitry sense the resistance to motion that the probe encounters from the blood sample as it clots. This generates an analog electronic signal that is processed by a microcomputer within the analyzer and is reported as the clot signal. The Sonoclot Analyzer measures these properties by graphically recording the dynamics of clot formation as a Sonoclot signature, and yields quantitative results. The Sonoclot signature is the plotted values of the clot signal value versus time. The quantitative results of the Sonoclot signature include a lag period (SonACT) that corresponds to ACT (seconds), and a wave that occurs as a result of crosslinkage of fibrin (clot rate). Other parameters in the tracing indicate platelet–fibrin binding, fibrin formation, and clot retraction (time to peak TP; Figure 25.2) Hemostasis abnormalities

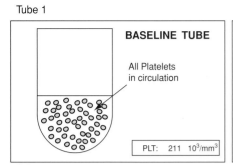

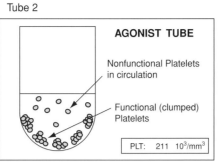

Figure 25.1. The PlateletWorks assay is a Coulter counter platelet count ratio that compares the baseline platelet count with an activated platelet count. Note the baseline platelet count tube on the left, compared with the activated (reduced) platelet count on the right. See text for full details. Courtesy of Helena Laboratories, Beaumont, TX.

Baseline Platelet Count − Agonist Platelet Count x 100 = % aggregation
Baseline Platelet Count

$$\frac{211 - 8 \times (100)}{211} = 96.2\%$$

Users may refer to the % Aggregation Chart in each box of PlateletWorks tubes.

including platelet dysfunction, factor deficiencies, anticoagulant effects, hyperfibrinolysis, and hypercoagulable states can be detected using the Sonoclot.

The Sonoclot has been used in cardiac surgery applications to measure a modified activated clotting time.[79,80]

Thromboelastograph

The thromboelastograph (Haemoscope, Niles, IL; now Haemonetics, Braintree, MA) was invented in 1947 and is another test of the viscoelastic properties of blood that examines the time of initiation through acceleration, control, and eventual lysis. A small amount of blood (0.36 mL) is placed in an oscillating cuvette and a piston is lowered into the blood sample. The cuvette oscillates at an arc angle of $4°45'$. As the blood begins to clot, the elastic force exerted on the piston is translated to a signature tracing (thromboelastogram) that reveals information

about fibrin formation, platelet–fibrin interactions, platelet clot strength, and fibrinolysis. With the current disposables, an activator is needed because the onset to coagulation varies, and the time to clot formation can conveniently be accelerated so the test is useful in POC settings. Celite, kaolin, or tissue factor have all been used to activate the TEG.

There are five parameters to the TEG tracing that measure different stages of clot development: R, K, alpha angle, MA, and MA_{60} (Figure 25.3) In addition, clot lysis indices are measured at 30 and 60 minutes after MA (LY_{30} and LY_{60}). Normal values vary depending on the type of activator used.

The R value is a measure of clotting time, which is the period of time from the start of the bioassay test to the initial fibrin formation. R time can be prolonged by factor deficiency,

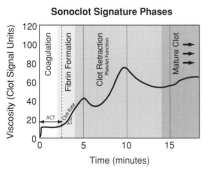

Figure 25.2. The Sonoclot Signature tracing is demonstrated. Note the different waves and plateaus that correspond to the coagulation factor function, platelet activity, platelet–fibrin binding, and clot retraction. Courtesy of Sienco Inc., Arvada, CO.

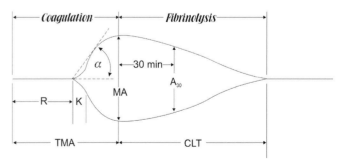

Figure 25.3. The typical TEG tracing is shown. Note the tracing components that correspond to coagulation factor function (R time), fibrin–platelet interaction (alpha angle), platelet function (maximal amplitude, MA), and fibrinolysis (A_{30}). Courtesy of Haemoscope, Niles, IL, now Haemonetics, Braintree, MA.

anticoagulation, severe thrombocytopenia, and hypofibrinogenemia. Low levels of heparin can prolong the R time, and higher levels of heparin can prolong the test indefinitely such that no measurements can be made. To eliminate any effect that heparin might have on the coagulating sample, a heparinase cup can be used to measure the TEG.[81] R time can be shortened by hypercoagulability states.

The K value represents clot kinetics, measuring the speed to reach a specific level of clot strength. It is the time from beginning of clot formation (the end of R time) until the amplitude reaches 20 mm. K time can be increased by factor deficiency, hypofibrinogenemia, thrombocytopenia, and thrombocytopathy. It is decreased in hypercoagulable states.

The alpha angle is an angle between the horizontal line in the middle of the TEG tracing and the line tangential to the developing body of the TEG tracing at 2 mm amplitude. The alpha angle represents the acceleration (kinetics) of fibrin buildup and crosslinking (clot strengthening). It is increased in hypercoagulable states and is decreased in thrombocytopenia and hypofibrinogenemia.

The maximum amplitude (MA) reflects the ultimate strength of the clot, which depends on number and function of platelets and the interaction with fibrin. It is increased in hypercoagulable states and decreased in thrombocytopenia, thrombocytopathy, and hypofibrinogenemia. The MA is the parameter most frequently measured, because it correlates with platelet dysfunction in cardiac surgery.[77] The MA is used as a marker for platelet function and has thus been incorporated into transfusion algorithms used to reduced platelet and other transfusions given to patients after CPB.[82-85] These transfusion algorithms are discussed in a separate part of this chapter.

LY_{30}, or the lysis index at 30 minutes after MA, is increased in conjunction with fibrinolysis.

A limitation of the TEG is that it is unable to detect impairment in platelet function induced by antiplatelet agents unless specific modifications are made (see the section on platelet mapping assay).

TEG modifications

Fibrinogen assay

Initial modifications of the TEG assay included the addition of a potent platelet antagonist (abciximab [Reopro], Lilly) to eliminate all platelet contribution to the maximum amplitude. The remaining amplitude was contributed almost solely by the functional fibrinogen in the blood sample. This early test correlated well with laboratory-based measures of fibrinogen.[86] More recently, another modification of the TEG MA has been studied as a measure of fibrinogen level. This assay creates a fibrinogen clot using reptilase and factor XIII in the absence of thrombin, much like the one the platelet mapping assay uses (see next section). In healthy volunteers, the clot strength of this fibrinogen clot correlated well with fibrinogen levels.[87]

Platelet mapping assay

The development of the platelet mapping assay overcomes some of the shortcomings of the TEG in that it allows for the thromboelastographic measurement of platelet function in patients on antiplatelet medication. Platelet mapping uses three cuvettes. One incorporates thrombin to activate platelets and overrides the inhibition of other activation pathways, such as arachidonic acid, ADP, and GP IIb/IIIa. A second cuvette contains reptilase plus factor XIII to create a fibrinogen clot, or a thrombin-less clot. This clot strength will be smaller and will not have the contribution of thrombin-activated platelets. The third cuvette incorporates the fibrinogen clot and adds back ADP or AA to stimulate the platelets. The ability of the MA to increase in response to ADP (clopidogrel) or AA (aspirin) is a measure of drug-induced platelet function. This POC test correlates well with the gold standard optical aggregometry.[88]

ROTEM

ROTEM (rotational thromboelastometry, Pentapharm, Munich, Germany) gives a viscoelastic measurement of clot strength in whole blood. A small amount of blood and coagulation activators is added to a disposable cuvette that is then placed in a heated cuvette holder. A disposable pin (sensor) that is fixed on the tip of a rotating shaft is lowered in the whole blood sample. The loss of elasticity upon clotting of the sample leads to changes in the rotation of the shaft that is detected by the reflection of light on a small mirror attached to the shaft. A detector records the axis rotation over time; this rotation is translated into a graph or thromboelastogram.

The main descriptive parameters associated with ROTEM are the following:

- Clotting time (CT), corresponding to the time in seconds from the beginning of the reaction to an increase in amplitude of thromboelastogram of 2 mm. It represents the initiation of clotting, thrombin formation, and start of clot polymerization.
- Clotting formation time (CFT), the time in seconds between an increase in amplitude of thromboelastogram from 2 to 20 mm. This identifies the fibrin polymerization and stabilization of the clot with platelets and factor XIII.
- Maximum clot firmness (MCF), the maximum amplitude in millimeters reached in thrombelastogram, which correlates with platelet count, platelet function, and the concentration of fibrinogen.
- Alpha (α) angle, the tangent to the clotting curve through the 2-mm point.
- Maximum lysis (ML), the percentage of MCF. This represents a reduction of clot firmness after MCF in relation to MCF.
- Maximum velocity (maxVel), the maximum of the first derivative of the clot curve.
- Time to maximum velocity (t-maxVel), the time from the start of the reaction until maximum velocity is reached.

– Area under curve (AUC), defined as the area under the velocity curve – that is, the area under the first derivative curve ending at a time point that corresponds to MCF.

ROTEM is also being evaluated for its ability to measure drug-induced platelet dysfunction in a way similar to the platelet mapping assay.[89]

Clot Signature Analyzer

Hemostatometry is a methodology that allows ex vivo assessment of multiple aspects of hemostasis in whole blood. The technique uses shear stress and collagen to initiate hemostasis in blood that is perfused through a small tube. Hemostatic plug formation within the tube causes a characteristic pattern of pressure changes that can be detected and quantified by the hemostatometer. The Clot Signature Analyzer (CSA; Xylum Corp., Scarsdale, NY) is a hemostatometer modified for POC use. The device measures ex vivo hemostasis using three separate assays: (a) the time to collagen-induced thrombus formation (CITF); (b) the platelet-mediated hemostasis time (PHT); and (c) the clotting time (CT). The CITF and PHT may be measures of platelet function because they detect defects caused by platelet inhibitors such as aspirin, prostacyclin, and antibodies to platelet glycoproteins IIb-IIIa (fibrinogen receptor) and Ib-IX (von Willebrand receptor). The CT appears to assess fibrin stability because inhibitors of fibrin formation and fibrinolytics (e.g. heparin, warfarin, and streptokinase) prolong this measurement. The CSA has been studied by Faraday and colleagues in the setting of postcardiac surgery bleeding. The CITF had a very high predictive value for identifying bleeding patients and those who would require transfusion of FFP and platelets.[90] This test remains a research tool and has not been advanced into clinical use.

Impact Cone and Plate(let) Analyzer

In the Impact Cone And Plate(let) Analyzer (DiaMed Cressier, Switzerland), whole blood is exposed to uniform shear by the spinning of a cone in a standardized cup. This allows for platelet function testing under conditions that mimic physiological blood flow, thus achieving the most accurate and authentic pattern of platelet function. After automated staining, platelet adhesion to the cup is evaluated by image analysis software.[91,92] Studies have demonstrated the success of the Impact in screening for congenital primary hemostasis abnormalities and testing platelet response to GPIIb-IIIa antagonists, aspirin, and clopidogrel.[93,94]

Conclusions

POC hemostasis monitoring has evolved to the point that measures of coagulation factor function and platelet activity can be obtained on whole blood in a matter of minutes. This development of rapid-turnaround, user-friendly laboratory testing has

enabled the early detection of hemostasis problems and appropriate treatment. Use of POC testing in transfusion algorithms in cardiac surgery has helped to decrease transfusion requirements, blood loss, length of stay, and overall costs of medical care in this high-risk population of patients.

References

1. Despotis GJ, Joist JH, Goodnough LT. Monitoring of hemostasis in cardiac surgical patients: impact of point-of-care testing on blood loss and transfusion outcomes. *Clin Chem* 1997;**43**:1684–96.

2. Harle CC. Point-of-care platelet function testing. *Semin Cardiothorac Vasc Anesth* 2007;**11**:247–51.

3. Kozek-Langenecker S. Management of massive operative blood loss. *Minerva Anestesiol* 2007;**73**:401–15.

4. von Kier S, Smith A. Hemostatic product transfusions and adverse outcomes: focus on point-of-care testing to reduce transfusion need. *J Cardiothorac Vasc Anesth* 2000;**14**:15–21; discussion 37–38.

5. Bull BS, Huse WM, Brauer FS, Korpman RA. Heparin therapy during extracorporeal circulation. II. The use of a dose-response curve to individualize heparin and protamine dosage. *J Thorac Cardiovasc Surg* 1975;**69**:685–9.

6. Dougherty KG, Gaos CM, Bush HS et al. Activated clotting times and activated partial thromboplastin times in patients undergoing coronary angioplasty who receive bolus doses of heparin. *Cathet Cardiovasc Diagn* 1992;**26**:260–3.

7. Hattersley PG. Heparin and the activated partial thromboplastin time. *Am J Clin Pathol* 1979;**71**:480–1.

8. Hattersley PG, Hayse D. The effect of increased contact activation time on the activated partial thromboplastin time. *Am J Clin Pathol* 1976;**66**:479–82.

9. Bull MH, Huse WM, Bull BS. Evaluation of tests used to monitor heparin therapy during extracorporeal circulation. *Anesthesiology* 1975;**43**:346–53.

10. Hattersley PG. Activated coagulation time of whole blood. *JAMA* 1966;**196**:436–40.

11. Bosch YP, Ganushchak YM, de Jong DS. Comparison of ACT point-of-care measurements: repeatability and agreement. *Perfusion* 2006;**21**:27–31.

12. Zucker ML, Jobes C, Siegel M, et al. Activated clotting time (ACT) testing: analysis of reproducibility. *J Extra Corpor Technol* 1999;**31**:130–4.

13. Despotis GJ, Summerfield AL, Joist JH, et al. Comparison of activated coagulation time and whole blood heparin measurements with laboratory plasma anti-Xa heparin concentration in patients having cardiac operations. *J Thorac Cardiovasc Surg* 1994;**108**:1076–82.

14. Despotis GJ, Joist JH, Goodnough LT, et al. Whole blood heparin concentration measurements by automated protamine titration agree with plasma anti-Xa measurements. *J Thorac Cardiovasc Surg* 1997;**113**:611–3.

15. Horkay F, Martin P, Rajah SM, Walker DR. Response to heparinization in adults and children undergoing cardiac operations. *Ann Thorac Surg* 1992;**53**:822–6.

16. Codispoti M, Ludlam CA, Simpson D, Mankad PS. Individualized heparin and protamine management in infants and children undergoing cardiac operations. *Ann Thorac Surg* 2001;**71**:922–7; discussion 927-8.

17. Despotis GJ, Joist JH, Joiner-Maier D, et al. Effect of aprotinin on activated clotting time, whole blood and plasma heparin measurements. *Ann Thorac Surg* 1995;**59**:106–11.

18. Despotis GJ, Levine V, Joist JH, et al. Antithrombin III during cardiac surgery: effect on response of activated clotting time to heparin and relationship to markers of hemostatic activation. *Anesth Analg* 1997;**85**:498–506.

19. Gravlee GP, Whitaker CL, Mark LJ, et al. Baseline activated coagulation time should be measured after surgical incision. *Anesth Analg* 1990;**71**:549–53.

20. Despotis GJ, Joist JH, Hogue CW Jr, et al. More effective suppression of hemostatic system activation in patients undergoing cardiac surgery by heparin dosing based on heparin blood concentrations rather than ACT. *Thromb Haemost* 1996;**76**:902–8.

21. Despotis GJ, Filos KS, Zoys TN, et al. Factors associated with excessive postoperative blood loss and hemostatic transfusion requirements: a multivariate analysis in cardiac surgical patients. *Anesth Analg* 1996;**82**:13–21.

22. Despotis GJ, Joist JH, Hogue CW Jr, et al. The impact of heparin concentration and activated clotting time monitoring on blood conservation. A prospective, randomized evaluation in patients undergoing cardiac operation. *J Thorac Cardiovasc Surg* 1995;**110**:46–54.

23. Gravlee GP, Rogers AT, Dudas LM, et al. Heparin management protocol for cardiopulmonary bypass influences postoperative heparin rebound but not bleeding. *Anesthesiology* 1992;**76**:393–401.

24. Shore-Lesserson L, Manspeizer HE, Bolastig M, et al. Anticoagulation for cardiac surgery in patients receiving preoperative heparin: use of the high-dose thrombin time. *Anesth Analg* 2000;**90**:813–8.

25. Wang JS, Lin CY, Karp RB. Comparison of high-dose thrombin time with activated clotting time for monitoring of anticoagulant effects of heparin in cardiac surgical patients. *Anesth Analg* 1994;**79**:9–13.

26. Wallock M, Jeske WP, Bakhos M, Walenga JM. Evaluation of a new point of care heparin test for cardiopulmonary bypass: the TAS heparin management test. *Perfusion* 2001;**16**:147–53.

27. Kim YS, Murkin JM, Adams SJ. In vivo and in vitro evaluation of the heparin management test versus the activated coagulation time for monitoring anticoagulation level in aprotinin-treated patients during cardiac surgery. *Heart Surg Forum* 2004;**7**:E599–604.

28. Tsimikas S, Beyer R, Hassankhani A. Relationship between the heparin management test and the HemoTec activated clotting time in patients undergoing percutaneous coronary intervention. *J Thromb Thrombolysis* 2001;**11**:217–21.

29. Fitch JC, Geary KL, Mirto GP, et al. Heparin management test versus activated coagulation time during cardiovascular surgery: correlation with anti-Xa activity. *J Cardiothorac Vasc Anesth* 1999;**13**:53–7.

30. Flom-Halvorsen HI, Ovrum E, Abdelnoor M, et al. Assessment of heparin anticoagulation: comparison of two commercially available methods. *Ann Thorac Surg* 1999;**67**:1012–6; discussion 1016–7.

31. Doty DB, Knott HW, Hoyt JL, Koepke JA. Heparin dose for accurate anticoagulation in cardiac surgery. *J Cardiovasc Surg (Torino)* 1979;**20**:597–604.

32. Shore-Lesserson L, Reich DL, DePerio M. Heparin and protamine titration do not improve haemostasis in cardiac surgical patients. *Can J Anaesth* 1998;**45**:10–18.

33. Jobes DR, Aitken GL, Shaffer GW. Increased accuracy and precision of heparin and protamine dosing reduces blood loss and transfusion in patients undergoing primary cardiac operations. *J Thorac Cardiovasc Surg* 1995;**110**:36–45.

34. Slight RD, Buell R, Nzewi OC, et al. A comparison of activated coagulation time-based techniques for anticoagulation during cardiac surgery with cardiopulmonary bypass. *J Cardiothorac Vasc Anesth* 2008;**22**:47–52.

35. Ferring M, Reber G, de Moerloose P, et al. Point of care and central laboratory determinations of the aPTT are not interchangeable in surgical intensive care patients. *Can J Anaesth* 2001;**48**:1155–60.

36. Nuttall GA, Oliver WC Jr, Beynen FM, et al. Intraoperative measurement of activated partial thromboplastin time and prothrombin time by a portable laser photometer in patients following cardiopulmonary bypass. *J Cardiothorac Vasc Anesth* 1993;**7**:402–9.

37. Nuttall GA, Oliver WC, Beynen FM, et al. Determination of normal versus abnormal activated partial thromboplastin time and prothrombin time after cardiopulmonary bypass. *J Cardiothorac Vasc Anesth* 1995;**9**:355–61.

38. Despotis GJ, Santoro SA, Spitznagel E, et al. Prospective evaluation and clinical utility of on-site monitoring of coagulation in patients undergoing cardiac operation. *J Thorac Cardiovasc Surg* 1994;**107**:271–9.

39. Reich DL, Yanakakis MJ, Vela-Cantos FP, et al. Comparison of bedside coagulation monitoring tests with standard laboratory tests in patients after cardiac surgery. *Anesth Analg* 1993;**77**:673–9.

40. Hertfelder HJ, Bos M, Weber D, et al. Perioperative monitoring of primary and secondary hemostasis in coronary artery bypass grafting. *Semin Thromb Hemost* 2005;**31**:426–40.

41. Matthews DR, Ecklund JM, Hennein H. Clinical comparison of patient-side fibrinogen assay and common laboratory analyzer in pediatric cardiopulmonary bypass. *J Extra Corpor Technol* 1995;**27**:126–31.

42. Elwood PC, Beswick AD, Sharp DS, et al. Whole blood impedance platelet aggregometry and ischemic heart disease. The Caerphilly Collaborative Heart Disease Study. *Arteriosclerosis* 1990;**10**:1032–6.

43. Zeidan AM, Kouides PA, Tara MA, Fricke WA. Platelet function testing: state of the art. *Expert Rev Cardiovasc Ther* 2007;**5**:955–67.

44. McKenzie ME, Gurbel PA, Levine DJ, Serebruany VL. Clinical utility of available methods for determining platelet function. *Cardiology* 1999;**92**:240–7.

45. Velik-Salchner C, Maier S, Innerhofer P, et al. Point-of-care whole blood impedance aggregometry versus classical light transmission aggregometry for detecting aspirin and clopidogrel: the results of a pilot study. *Anesth Analg* 2008;**107**:1798–806.

46. Breugelmans J, Vertessen F, Mertens G, et al. Multiplate whole blood impedance aggregometry: a recent experience. *Thromb Haemost* 2008;**100**:725–6.

47. Mueller T, Dieplinger B, Poelz W, Haltmayer M. Utility of the PFA-100 instrument and the novel multiplate analyzer for the assessment of aspirin and clopidogrel effects on platelet function in patients with cardiovascular disease. *Clin Appl Thromb Hemost* 2009;**15**:652–9.

48. Sibbing D, Braun S, Jawansky S, et al. Assessment of ADP-induced platelet aggregation with light transmission aggregometry and multiple electrode platelet aggregometry before and after clopidogrel treatment. *Thromb Haemost* 2008;**99**:121–6.

49. Mueller T, Dieplinger B, Poelz W, et al. Utility of whole blood impedance aggregometry for the assessment of clopidogrel action using the novel Multiplate analyzer–comparison with two flow cytometric methods. *Thromb Res* 2007;**121**:249–58.

50. Van Der Planken MG, Claeys MJ, Vertessen FJ, et al. Comparison of turbidimetric aggregation and in vitro bleeding time (PFA-100) for monitoring the platelet inhibitory profile of antiplatelet agents in patients undergoing stent implantation. *Thromb Res* 2003;**111**:159–64.

51. Ziegler S, Maca T, Alt E, et al. Monitoring of antiplatelet therapy with the PFA-100 in peripheral angioplasty patients. *Platelets* 2002;**13**:493–7.

52. Kotzailias N, Elwischger K, Sycha T, et al. Clopidogrel-induced platelet inhibition cannot be detected by the platelet function analyzer-100 system in stroke patients. *J Stroke Cerebrovasc Dis* 2007;**16**:199–202.

53. Mani H, Linnemann B, Luxembourg B, et al. Response to aspirin and clopidogrel monitored with different platelet function methods. *Platelets* 2006;**17**:303–10.

54. Pidcock M, Harrison P. Can the PFA-100 be modified to detect P2Y12 inhibition? *J Thromb Haemost* 2006;**4**:1424–6.

55. Mueller T, Haltmayer M, Poelz W, Haidinger D. Monitoring aspirin 100 mg and clopidogrel 75 mg therapy with the PFA-100 device in patients with peripheral arterial disease. *Vasc Endovascular Surg* 2003;**37**:117–23.

56. Paniccia R, Antonucci E, Gori AM, et al. Different methodologies for evaluating the effect of clopidogrel on platelet function in high-risk coronary artery disease patients. *J Thromb Haemost* 2007;**5**:1839–47.

57. Slaughter TF, Sreeram G, Sharma AD, et al. Reversible shear-mediated platelet dysfunction during cardiac surgery as assessed by the PFA-100 platelet function analyzer. *Blood Coagul Fibrinolysis* 2001;**12**:85–93.

58. van Werkum JW, Harmsze AM, Elsenberg EH, et al. The use of the VerifyNow system to monitor antiplatelet therapy: a review of the current evidence. *Platelets* 2008;**19**:479–88.

59. Selvaraj CL, Van De Graaff EJ, Campbell CL, et al. Point-of-care determination of baseline platelet function as a predictor of clinical outcomes in patients who present to the emergency department with chest pain. *J Thromb Thrombolysis* 2004;**18**:109–15.

60. Wheeler GL, Braden GA, Steinhubl SR, et al. The Ultegra rapid platelet-function assay: comparison to standard platelet function assays in patients undergoing percutaneous coronary intervention with abciximab therapy. *Am Heart J* 2002;**143**:602–11.

61. Steinhubl SR, Talley JD, Braden GA, et al. Point-of-care measured platelet inhibition correlates with a reduced risk of an adverse cardiac event after percutaneous coronary intervention: results of the GOLD (AU-Assessing Ultegra) multicenter study. *Circulation* 2001;**103**:2572–8.

62. Dichiara J, Bliden KP, Tantry US, et al. Platelet function measured by VerifyNow identifies generalized high platelet reactivity in aspirin-treated patients. *Platelets* 2007;**18**:414–23.

63. Gurbel PA, Bliden KP, DiChiara J, et al. Evaluation of dose-related effects of aspirin on platelet function: results from the Aspirin-Induced Platelet Effect (ASPECT) study. *Circulation* 2007;**115**:3156–64.

64. Lordkipanidze M, Pharand C, Nguyen TA, et al. Assessment of VerifyNow P2Y12 assay accuracy in evaluating clopidogrel-induced platelet inhibition. *Ther Drug Monit* 2008;**30**:372–8.

65. Jakubowski JA, Payne CD, Li YG, et al. The use of the VerifyNow P2Y12 point-of-care device to monitor platelet function across a range of P2Y12 inhibition levels following prasugrel and clopidogrel administration. *Thromb Haemost* 2008;**99**:409–15.

66. Malinin A, Pokov A, Swaim L, et al. Validation of a VerifyNow-P2Y12 cartridge for monitoring platelet inhibition with clopidogrel. *Methods Find Exp Clin Pharmacol* 2006;**28**:315–22.

67. Collet JP, Silvain J, Landivier A, et al. Dose effect of clopidogrel reloading in patients already on 75-mg maintenance dose: the Reload with Clopidogrel Before Coronary Angioplasty in Subjects Treated Long Term with Dual Antiplatelet Therapy (RELOAD) study. *Circulation* 2008;**118**:1225–33.

68. Kim KE, Woo KS, Goh RY, et al. Comparison of laboratory detection methods of aspirin resistance in coronary artery disease patients. *Int J Lab Hematol* 2010;**140**:123–6.

69. Patti G, Nusca A, Mangiacapra F, et al. Point-of-care measurement of clopidogrel responsiveness predicts clinical outcome in patients undergoing percutaneous coronary intervention results of the ARMYDA-PRO (Antiplatelet therapy for Reduction of MYocardial Damage during Angioplasty-Platelet Reactivity Predicts Outcome) study. *J Am Coll Cardiol* 2008;**52**:1128–33.

70. Craft RM, Chavez JJ, Snider CC, et al. Comparison of modified Thrombelastograph and Plateletworks whole blood assays to optical platelet aggregation for monitoring reversal of clopidogrel inhibition in elective surgery patients. *J Lab Clin Med* 2005;**145**:309–15.

71. van Werkum JW, Kleibeuker M, Postma S, et al. A comparison between the Plateletwork-assay and light transmittance aggregometry for monitoring the inhibitory effects of clopidogrel. *Int J Cardiol* 2010;**140**:123–6.

72. Mobley JE, Bresee SJ, Wortham DC, et al. Frequency of nonresponse antiplatelet activity of clopidogrel during pretreatment for cardiac catheterization. *Am J Cardiol* 2004;**93**:456–8.

73. Despotis GJ, Levine V, Filos KS, et al. Evaluation of a new point-of-care test that measures PAF-mediated acceleration of coagulation in cardiac surgical patients. *Anesthesiology* 1996;**85**:1311–23.

74. Shore-Lesserson L, Ammar T, DePerio M, et al. Platelet-activated clotting time does not measure platelet reactivity during cardiac surgery. *Anesthesiology* 1999;**91**:362–8.

75. Isgro F, Rehn E, Kiessling AH, et al. Platelet function test HemoSTATUS 2: tool or toy for an optimized management of hemostasis? *Perfusion* 2002;**17**:27–31.

76. Ereth MH, Nuttall GA, Santrach PJ, et al. The relation between the platelet-activated clotting test (HemoSTATUS) and blood loss after cardiopulmonary bypass. *Anesthesiology* 1998;**88**:962–9.

77. Ereth MH, Nuttall GA, Klindworth JT, et al. Does the platelet-activated clotting test (HemoSTATUS) predict blood loss and platelet dysfunction associated with cardiopulmonary bypass? *Anesth Analg* 1997;**85**:259–64.

78. Ganter MT, Hofer CK. Coagulation monitoring: current techniques and clinical use of viscoelastic point-of-care coagulation devices. *Anesth Analg* 2008;**106**:1366–75.

79. Ganter MT, Monn A, Tavakoli R, et al. Monitoring activated clotting time for combined heparin and aprotinin application: in vivo evaluation of a new aprotinin-insensitive test using Sonoclot. *Eur J Cardiothorac Surg* 2006;**30**:278–84.

80. Ganter MT, Dalbert S, Graves K, et al. Monitoring activated clotting time for combined heparin and aprotinin application: an in vitro evaluation of a new aprotinin-insensitive test using SONOCLOT. *Anesth Analg* 2005;**101**:308–14.

81. Tuman KJ, McCarthy RJ, Djuric M, et al. Evaluation of coagulation during cardiopulmonary bypass with a heparinase-modified thromboelastographic assay. *J Cardiothorac Vasc Anesth* 1994;**8**:144–9.

82. Taneja R, Fernandes P, Marwaha G, et al. Perioperative coagulation management and blood conservation in cardiac surgery: a Canadian survey. *J Cardiothorac Vasc Anesth* 2008;**22**:662–9.

83. Ronald A, Dunning J. Can the use of thromboelastography predict and decrease bleeding and blood and blood product requirements in adult patients undergoing cardiac surgery? *Interact Cardiovasc Thorac Surg* 2005;**4**:456–63.

84. Avidan MS, Alcock EL, Da Fonseca J, et al. Comparison of structured use of routine laboratory tests or near-patient assessment with clinical judgement in the management of bleeding after cardiac surgery. *Br J Anaesth* 2004;**92**: 178–86.

85. Royston D, von Kier S. Reduced haemostatic factor transfusion using heparinase-modified thrombelastography during cardiopulmonary bypass. *Br J Anaesth* 2001;**86**:575–8.

86. Kettner SC, Panzer OP, Kozek SA, et al. Use of abciximab-modified thrombelastography in patients undergoing cardiac surgery. *Anesth Analg* 1999;**89**:580–4.

87. Carroll RC, Craft RM, Chavez JJ, et al. Measurement of functional fibrinogen levels using the Thrombelastograph. *J Clin Anesth* 2008;**20**:186–90.

88. Tantry US, Bliden KP, Gurbel PA. Overestimation of platelet aspirin resistance detection by thrombelastograph platelet mapping and validation by conventional aggregometry using arachidonic acid stimulation. *J Am Coll Cardiol* 2005;**46**:1705–9.

89. Scharbert G, Auer A, Kozek-Langenecker S. Evaluation of the platelet mapping assay on rotational thromboelastometry ROTEM. *Platelets* 2009;**20**:125–30.

90. Faraday N, Guallar E, Sera VA, et al. Utility of whole blood hemostatometry using the clot signature analyzer for assessment of hemostasis in cardiac surgery. *Anesthesiology* 2002;**96**: 1115–22.

91. Jilma-Stohlawetz P, Horvath M, Eichelberger B, et al. Platelet function under high-shear conditions from platelet concentrates. *Transfusion* 2008;**48**:129–35.

92. Savion N, Varon D. Impact – the cone and plate(let) analyzer: testing platelet function and anti-platelet drug response. *Pathophysiol Haemost Thromb* 2006;**35**:83–8.

93. Shenkman B, Einav Y, Salomon O, et al. Testing agonist-induced platelet aggregation by the Impact-R [Cone and plate(let) analyzer (CPA)]. *Platelets* 2008;**19**:440–6.

94. Shenkman B, Matetzky S, Fefer P, et al. Variable responsiveness to clopidogrel and aspirin among patients with acute coronary syndrome as assessed by platelet function tests. *Thromb Res* 2008;**122**:336–45.

Chapter 26

Cardiac biomarkers for perioperative management

Anoushka Afonso and Eric Adler

Introduction

Assessment and management of patients with cardiovascular disease in the perioperative period is one of the primary tasks of the cardiac anesthesiologist and has become progressively more challenging as patients getting surgery become increasingly older and more morbid. This problem is compounded by the limited amount of time providers have to assess patients, particularly prior to emergent surgeries. Biomarkers have emerged in the past 20 years to help screen, diagnose, prognosticate, and manage patients benefiting from intervention. With effective treatment at hand, rapid and accurate diagnosis is of major medical importance. As the number of cardiovascular biomarkers expands, it is critical to understand each one's specific strengths and limitations.[1] Furthermore, it is critical that all biomarkers are not used as stand-alone tests. They must be interpreted in their appropriate clinical context and do not replace other parts of the examination, such as physical examination or imaging modalities.

Scrutiny of new biomarkers must include validating analytical imprecision and detection limits, calibrator characterization, assay specificity and standardization, preanalytical issues, and appropriate reference interval studies.[2] An ideal biomarker should aid the clinician in diagnosis, prognosis, and treatment. It should be readily available and adequately tested; have established reference values, compared with a gold standard; have known sensitivity and specificity; have low turnaround time; and not be costly.[2,3]

The rates of liberation of specific biomarkers differ depending on their intracellular location and molecular weight, as well as local blood and lymphatic flow. The temporal pattern of protein release is of diagnostic importance. Therefore, patients' baseline clinical status can affect biomarker clearance and must be taken into account for appropriate interpretation.

In this chapter we review multiple biomarkers, including those used to acutely diagnose and prognosticate patients with suspected myocardial ischemia and infarction as well as decompensated heart failure. We also discuss novel biomarkers that are not currently in routine practice but are often used in research settings and likely to become the standard of care in the near future.

Commonly used biomarkers

Creatine phosphokinase (CK), CK-MP

Creatine phosphokinase (CK) is an enzyme present in muscle, brain, and other tissues that catalyzes the reversible conversion of adenosine diphosphate (ADP) and phosphocreatine into adenosine triphosphate (ATP) and creatine. Serving as an energy reservoir to many tissues, such as skeletal muscle, brain, and smooth muscle, CK regenerates ATP rapidly. Because it is ubiquitous, however, an important limitation is its lack of specificity. Total CK level is too insensitive and nonspecific of a test to be used to diagnose acute myocardial infarction (AMI), although data correlating irreversible ischemic injury and the release of creatine kinase are strong.[4]

Creatine kinase MB (CK-MB) isoenzyme is considered more specific over total CK, as it is present in higher concentrations in cardiac tissue. The CK-MB isoenzyme, which has a molecular mass of approximately 87 kDa, accounts for 5 percent to 50 percent of total CK activity in myocardium. In skeletal muscle, by contrast, it normally accounts for less than 1 percent, with CK-MM being the dominant form, although the percentage can be as high as 10 percent in conditions reflecting skeletal muscle injury and regeneration.[5]

Total CK is elevated in a variety of conditions, including myocardial infarction, renal failure, hypothyroidism, or any type of muscle damage, to name a few. CK-MB is used to determine infarction or reinfarction timing, as the isozyme normalizes by 24 to 36 hours, although it loses its specificity after skeletal muscle injury or cardiac surgery, when the CK-MB also can be elevated.[6] Overall, CK-MB is a less useful as a biomarker than cardiac troponin. It has fallen out of favor, although many still use it along with other biomarkers.

Higher periprocedural CK-MB levels during a percutaneous coronary intervention (PCI) had significantly higher rates of adverse clinical events at 12 months, including death and late thrombosis.[7] Studies have shown a link between an elevation of CK-MB after coronary intervention and increased mortality.[8]

CK-MB usually rises within four hours of injury and normalizes within 24 to 36 hours. However, one measurement of CK-MB cannot rule out, or even confirm, an AMI. The pattern of serial CK-MB measurements over a 24-hour period is more sensitive and specific than the initial CK-MB measurement alone.[9] Assays of CK-MB isoform have better diagnostic value at six or more hours after the onset of chest pain than at four hours.[10]

Troponin

Troponins are a complex of regulatory proteins that are involved in skeletal and cardiac muscle contraction. The three regulatory proteins involved are troponin I, C, and T, each having different functions in muscular contraction. Troponin I (TnI) and T (TnT) are very specific and sensitive indicators of myocardial damage, and thus have been supported for routine use by the ACC/AHA 2007 guidelines.[11] It is well established that TnI and TnT are superior compared with other biomarkers such as CK-MB, and are the preferred markers in diagnosing myocardial damage.[12]

Cardiac troponins are measured by immunoassays,[13] with TnI having multiple assays measuring different epitopes and fragments of this troponin subtype. This has caused a problem of heterogeneity and has made standardization difficult,[14–16] which is not the case in TnT, with only one assay. The recommendation for the preferred markers (cTnI and cTnT) and for CK-MB is that the upper limit be defined as the 99th percentile. This is approximately three standard deviations above the mean for the normal range. This information should be available from peer-reviewed information published for each of these assays, along with an acceptable level (<10%) of analytical variability in precision at this level of detection.[3]

Elimination of these cardiac troponin markers occurs in the kidney, liver, pancreas, and reticuloendothelial system; thus, any impaired clearance leads to prolonged increase of troponin level.[17] Data have shown that patients with end-stage renal disease (ESRD) have higher troponin levels, even in asypmtomatic cases without any evidence of coronary artery disease.[18] However, recent data demonstrate TnT predicting long-term cardiac pathology and death in patients undergoing hemodialysis.[19–23]

Troponin levels rise normally within 4 to 12 hours after initial myocardial damage, with a peak 12 to 48 hours from onset of initial symptoms. Troponin is highly sensitive and specific for diagnosis of AMI up to two weeks after onset of myocardial ischemia.[1,24–31] In fact, troponins have a prolonged window of time during which they are elevated, allowing clinicians to detect a larger patient population at future risk for subsequent adverse cardiovascular events.[25,28–31] Looking at troponin patterns is important in trying to decipher whether the myocardial damage is acute or chronic in ESRD patients.

As troponin levels have a high cardiac specificity, it is common to see elevations in any condition that affects the heart. Mechanical injury,[32] ablation,[33] direct trauma to the heart,[34] congestive heart failure, pulmonary embolism, and sepsis[35] are just a few of the conditions that can elevate troponin levels without any evidence of cardiac ischemia. It is important to recognize the limitations of any biomarker when using it to guide decision making.

Both TnT and TnI are superior to previous cardiac biomarkers not only in detection, but also in prognosis. Troponin (TnI or TnT) level has been shown to correlate with infarct size,[36] as well as predicting risk of morbidity and mortality.[37] Risk stratification using TnI predicted outcome in patents presenting with chest pain and coronary artery disease as well as guiding therapy. In fact, TnI- and TnT-positive patients treated with tirofiban, an antiplatelet drug, significantly lowered the risk of death and MI at 30 days.[38] Another study showed elevated TnI correlated with a higher risk of recurrent ischemia requiring revascularization by 48 hours and two weeks. There was a benefit of enoxaparin in unstable angina in patients with elevated TnI levels.[39] Early assessment of coronary reperfusion after thrombolytic therapy showed the utility of TnT levels.[40–42] Thus, troponin levels have been used to guide targeted therapy in high-risk patients.

It is not uncommon to see patients after cardiac surgery with troponin and CK-MB release. TnI levels (even minor elevations) in postoperative patients following vascular surgery, along with CK-MB, have been shown to be independent and complementary predictors of long-term mortality.[23] The higher the value, the worse the associated injury, and high values precede adverse cardiac events. Elevations have been related to the cross-clamp and bypass time,[43] the nature of cardioplegia, and procedure (valves and coronaries vs coronary artery bypass grafting alone) as well as surgical approach.[44] Lasocki and colleagues showed that TnI concentration measured 20 hours after the end of surgery is an independent predictor of in-hospital death after cardiac surgery. In addition, elevated concentrations of cTnI are associated with a cardiac cause of death and with major postoperative complications.[45]

Guidelines suggest that troponin be the first biomarker checked when there is clinical suspicion of myocardial injury and or infarction. Given their high sensitivity but lack of specificity, they need to be interpreted in the context of the patient's clinical status.

B type natriuretic peptide (BNP) and pro-BNP

The natriuretic peptides are a class of hormones released in response to an extracellular fluid load and cause vasodilation, natriuresis, and diuresis. They bind to the natriuretic peptide receptor, which can be found on multiple different cell types, in particular on endothelial and smooth muscle cells throughout the vasculature, as well on myocytes and renal tubules. Activation of these receptors results in opposition to the vasoconstriction, sodium retention, and antidiuretic effects of the activated renin-angiotensin-aldosterone system.

B type natriuretic peptide (BNP) was first isolated from porcine brain tissue in 1988.[46] Although it was initially referred to as brain natriuretic peptide, it was soon noted to be released by cardiac ventricular myocytes in response to stretch; hence, it is preferably referred to as B type. It is initially produced as a pre-pro-BNP, which is first cleaved to pro-BNP and ultimately into its biologically active form BNP and its terminal fragment N-terminal pro-BNP. Commercially available assays for the multiple forms of BNP exist, but levels cannot be used interchangeably, as they have notably different cutoff values. For the purposes of this section, we will refer to BNP levels, as they are more commonly used and studied.

Natriuretic peptide level measurement was initially studied as a tool for differentiating cardiac from noncardiac causes of dyspnea. In a landmark 2002 study, Maisel and associates demonstrated that the test had a sensitivity for detecting heart failure of more than 90 percent in patients with acute dyspnea presenting to the emergency room when compared to blinded physicians who assessed the probability that the patient had congestive heart failure as a cause of their symptoms.[47] The utility of BNP in an emergency room setting was confirmed in several subsequent studies as well.[48]

A recent consensus algorithm was created in which patients with BNP <100 were felt to have a very improbable (2%) chance of heart failure, whereas when BNP was >400, heart failure was felt to be very probable (>95%).[49] Some recent studies suggest that in an intensive care unit (ICU) setting, the cutoff level of BNP should be slightly higher, roughly 150 pg/mL. BNP levels may be elevated in septic shock; therefore, caution must be used in its interpretation in an ICU setting.

In clinical practice, we find low levels of BNP very helpful in ruling out the presence of significant heart failure. One confounding element is measurement in the very obese patient, who may have low levels even in heart failure.[50] High levels of BNP may represent acute heart failure, although BNP levels may also be elevated in the elderly and in patients with chronic heart failure, renal failure, sepsis, and pulmonary disease that results in right heart strain, such as pulmonary embolism. BNP is generally not helpful diagnostically when the level is between 100 and 400.

BNP has demonstrated utility as a prognostic marker. Inpatient mortality is related to admission levels in a linear manner.[51] It may be equally useful as a measurement prior to discharge, where high levels (BNP >350) are highly predictive of readmission.[52] In optimal situations, a patient should have a BNP level below 350 prior to discharge. In some patients with chronic stage C–D heart failure, this may be difficult to achieve. Ideally, providers will be aware of their patient's "dry" BNP level and try to achieve a level no more than 25 percent higher than this prior to discharge.

The utility of BNP in preoperative assessment has been validated in patients undergoing cardiovascular surgery. In a 2004 study, BNP was found to be a powerful predictor of postoperative complications in patients undergoing heart surgery.[53] More recently, patients undergoing emergent surgery for type A aortic dissection were found to have significantly higher mortality if they had elevated NT–pro-BNP levels.[54] It is not clear whether the elevated levels reflect the severity of the dissection or merely baseline cardiovascular function, yet they may help providers prognosticate patients prior to surgery nonetheless.

BNP also may have some utility in assisting with ventilator weaning in patients with heart failure. In a recent study, BNP levels were higher in patients who failed a weaning trial compared with those with successful weaning.[55]

BNP has been firmly established as a powerful diagnostic and prognostic tool. Though it has primarily been used diagnostically in patients with dyspnea of unclear etiology, it must be interpreted in the appropriate clinical context. Although there are far fewer data, the test may be useful in preoperative assessment and critical care management as well, and further study is warranted.

C-reactive protein, high-sensitivity C-reactive protein

Produced by the liver, C-reactive protein (CRP) is an acute-phase reactant. CRP is cleared and catabolized exclusively by hepatocytes, with a similar half-life regardless of the presence of disease or even circulating CRP concentrations. Thus, the synthesis rate of CRP is the only determinant of plasma concentrations.[56,57] Many cytokines – in particular, interleukin 6 (IL-6) – stimulate the production of acute-phase reactants in response to different stimuli.[58]

As with most inflammatory markers, CRP is not specific. Increased levels are seen in a variety of infectious, neoplastic, and other systemic inflammatory conditions, such as lupus.[58] Levels of CRP rise during inflammatory processes, such as atherosclerosis and its acute manifestations.[59] High-sensitivity CRP (hsCRP) assays are now available for commercial use and are inexpensive as well. The Reynolds risk score, a prediction model designed to calculate cardiovascular risk, added hsCRP and family history, thus making its accuracy of prediction higher and reclassifying 40 percent to 50 percent of women who were initially intermediate-risk into higher or lower categories.[60] In fact, many population-based prospective studies report an association between coronary heart disease and prolonged increases in baseline CRP,[61] although a recent report suggested that the modest CRP predictive value disappeared after adjusting for common clinical values.[62]

Most evidence regarding CRP and utility are in reference to their use in the treatment of patients with atherosclerosis. Statins have been shown to lower CRP levels, regardless of cardiovascular risk factors. In a primary prevention trial of 1702 patients, compared with placebo, pravastatin reduced median CRP levels by 16.9 percent ($P < 0.001$) at 24 weeks, whereas no change in CRP levels was observed in the placebo group.[63] Patients who have low CRP levels after statin therapy have better clinical outcomes than those with higher CRP levels, regardless of the resultant level of LDL cholesterol.[64] These data suggest statin level titration based on CRP levels, using CRP in therapeutic decision-making. The JUPITER trial looked at 17,802 healthy individuals and assessed whether treatment with rosuvastatin reduces cardiovascular risk among individuals with elevated hsCRP and no overt hyperlipidemia. Rosuvastatin reduced LDL cholesterol levels by 50 percent and hsCRP levels by 37 percent.[65]

There is much debate about the utility of CRP, as one can see race and gender differences in levels,[66] as well as high levels in critically sick patients. Levels above 10 mg/dL on ICU admission are correlated with an increased risk of organ failure and death, with persistently high CRP concentrations associated with a poorer outcome.[67] Again, the utility of CRP must be used in an additive strategy for risk stratification, and by itself, it does have limitations.

Novel biomarkers

Myeloperoxidase

Myeloperoxidase (MPO) is an enzyme expressed by activated leukocytes. MPO is responsible for catalyzing the conversion of chloride and hydrogen peroxide to hypochlorite. MPO, a hemoprotein, is stored in the granules of polymorphonuclear neutrophils and macrophages. It is secreted in large amounts in inflammatory states[68] and oxidizes LDL and HDL by binding to apolipoprotein A1 in atherosclerosis, causing plaque vulnerability.[69–71]

Unlike many of the other traditional biomarkers, MPO can be measured early after the occurrence of symptoms. It can be used early to measure plaque destabilization. Baldus and coworkers implied that MPO release actually precedes myocardial injury and that MPO elevation identifies patients with unstable atherosclerotic plaque formation even before complete microvascular obstruction occurs. MPO release is a prerequisite, rather than a consequence, of myocardial injury, as evidenced by ECG with myocardial ischemia not correlating with MPO levels.[72] Therefore, MPO predicts at-risk patients even before myocardial injury has taken place.

This enzyme has been shown to be predictive of risk in patients with acute coronary syndromes extending prognostic information by these biomarkers. Serum MPO levels were assessed in 1090 patients with ACS. Patients with elevated MPO levels (>350 μg/L; 31.3%) experienced a markedly increased cardiac risk (adjusted hazard ratio [HR] 2.25 [1.32–3.82]; P = 0.003). In particular, MPO serum levels identified patients at risk who had TnT levels below 0.01 μg/L.[72] MPO is a significant value-added factor for the diagnosis of acute coronary syndromes and for the identification of high-risk subgroups among patients treated for acute chest pain with non-ST elevation ECGs. It has proven to have significant predictive value for adverse cardiac events, with an elevated sensitivity. It presents an eightfold increase for a final diagnosis of AMI when the MPO level is greater than or equal to 100 pM.[73] In fact, admission MPO level concentration is an independent predictor of in-hospital mortality in patients with ST-segment myocardial infarctions (STEMIs) presenting with cardiogenic shock. This was independent of the extent of coronary artery disease.[74] Brennan and coworkers showed a direct relationship between MPO admission levels and degree of risk of adverse events within one and six months in a series of 604 patients, even among those with negative TnT values.[75] This is an important

finding in terms of risk stratification and has significant long-term prognostic value.

Not only is MPO giving more insight into the development of coronary artery disease, but it also has been implicated in the progression of congestive heart failure. Tang and colleagues showed the mean plasma MPO levels in the heart failure cohort were significantly elevated compared with those of control patients. In addition, mean plasma MPO levels increased in parallel with increasing NYHA class, showing a relationship between severity of heart failure and MPO. An MPO level of 230 pM identified heart failure with 72 percent sensitivity and 77 percent specificity (p < 0.0001) in patients. Furthermore, MPO levels were shown to be predictors of heart failure independent of BNP.[76]

As MPO is a leukocyte-derived enzyme, it is not uncommon to see this marker increased in other noncardiac conditions, such as in infection,[77] inflammation, and infiltrative conditions.[78] Although this marker is promising in the evaluation of patients with coronary syndromes, the lack of specificity of this marker is a limitation. Further investigation is under way to increase our knowledge base about the utility of this promising marker.

Ischemia-modified albumin

Approved by the FDA for measurement of cardiac ischemia, the novel marker ischemia-modified albumin (IMA) is measured by the albumin cobalt binding test. This test is based on the reduced in vitro binding of exogenous cobalt to the N-terminus of human serum albumin in the presence of myocardial ischemia. In fact, Bar-Or and associates showed that there are structural changes of the N-terminus portion of albumin.[79]

This assay is reported to be positive, even before levels of creatinine kinase isoenzyme (CK-MB) and troponin become positive, and remains positive within minutes of ischemia and for many hours later.[80]

In emergency room patients with myocardial infarction and early onset of unstable angina,[81] it was demonstrated that ischemia-modified albumin (IMA), based on this albumin cobalt binding assay, is positive if there was a reduced binding of albumin to cobalt.

An investigative study by Sinha and colleagues looked at patients who develop ST segment changes and chest pain during percutaneous coronary intervention and found IMA to be a more consistent marker of ischemia, as compared with 8-iso prostaglandin F2-A (a marker of oxidative stress).[82] Additionally, IMA is a sensitive tool to demonstrate PCI-induced ischemia. However, recent data have been conflicting, and more investigation needs to be done to look at this biomarker.

Several clinical studies show IMA as a poor predictor of serious cardiac outcomes in the short term,[83] with poor diagnostic accuracy and low specificity.[84] Additionally, IMA also seems to be influenced by serum levels of albumin.[85] Given conflicting clnical data, more study is required before it is used clinically.

Pregnancy-associated plasma protein A

Originally isolated from the serum of pregnant women, pregnancy-associated plasma protein A (PAPP-A) has been used in prenatal genetic screening, with low levels associated with problems such as trisomy 21, premature delivery, and stillbirth. This zinc-binding metalloproteinase cleaves insulin-factor–binding proteins and is also thought to be involved in proliferative processes.[86] In fact, PAPP-A has been recently thought of as a marker involved in plaque rupture.

This novel biomarker has been associated in the early phases of acute coronary syndrome. PAPP-A levels were found to be higher in unstable plaques, with elevated levels in acute coronary syndrome (ACS).[87] This study demonstrated high levels of expression of PAPP-A in patients with acute coronary syndrome. It showed histologic evidence from patients who died of sudden cardiac death who expressed PAPP-A in ruptured and eroded plaques, but minimally in stable plaques.

Lund and colleagues examined 200 ACS patients who were troponin-negative and followed PAPP-A levels on admission, after 6 to12 hours, and at 24 hours. This study showed PAPP-A as an independent predictor of adverse cardiac events in TnI-negative ACS patients. PAPP-A levels greater or equal to 2.9 mIU/L were associated with a 4.6-fold higher adjusted risk of adverse outcome, compared with patients whose circulating PAPP-A levels were less than 2.9 mIU/L. In particular, 20 of 26 (77%) of all cardiovascular deaths, MIs, and revascularizations during the six-month follow-up occurred in patients with PAPP-A greater than 2.9 mIU/L.[88]

There is a poor correlation between CK-MB levels and troponin levels to PAPP-A, demonstrating that PAPP-A levels increased even before cardiac damage occurred. Iversen and associates showed that PAPP-A levels are elevated in more than 90 percent of patients presenting with STEMIs if measured less than six hours after the onset of symptoms or less than two hours after primary percutaneous coronary intervention. PAPP-A seems to be a much more sensitive marker of myocardial infarction than CK-MB and TnT, more so in the early stages of a myocardial infarction.[89] Free PAPP-A does not increase with age and seems to be a more sensitive assay than assays that measure the sum of free and complexed PAPP-A.[90]

PAPP-A remains a promising marker in combination with other markers in multimarker strategy for early risk stratification. More studies are needed to further investigate the role of this novel cardiac biomarker.

Soluble CD40 ligand

Soluble CD 40 ligand is released by platelets after stimulation.[91,92] This platelet activation marker encourages coagulation by tissue factor expression on monocytes[93] and has a role in ACS. Not only is CD40 ligand a platelet agonist, but it has also been demonstrated to be an IIb3 (glycoprotein IIb/IIIa) ligand and is essential for arterial thrombus formation.[94]

Recent trials have demonstrated that patients with unstable angina had higher levels of soluble CD40 ligand than did the controls or patients with stable angina.[95] In a prospective study of healthy middle-aged women, those who had markedly elevated soluble CD40 ligand had a higher increased risk of cardiovascular events in a four-year follow-up.[96]

Heeschen and colleagues[97] showed soluble CD40 ligand to have an independent predictive value with regard to risk of ischemic events. This study also proved a benefit of antiplatelet (glycoprotein IIb/IIIa receptor antagonist) therapy with those patients with elevated soluble CD40 ligand levels. Thus, not only is soluble CD40 ligand seen as a prognostic marker, but it also gives insight into the effects of treatment.

A limitation of this marker is the lack of specificity, as it is seen in other inflammatory conditions and autoimmune conditions.[98] However, this novel marker has potential to be used in a multimarker strategy in the future.

Conclusions

Despite the large number of existing and novel biomarkers for cardiovascular disease, no one marker has enough sensitivity and specificity to be evaluated in isolation. Therefore a multi-biomarker strategy is likely to be the most useful for clinical decision making.[99] In fact, most patients with ACS have multiple processes occurring simultaneously; these biomarkers can help detect distinct points in the pathway of development of ACS.[100]

It is possible that the sheer number of biomarkers that are abnormal may have prognsotic significance that exceeds that of any one abnormal biomarker. Bodi and coworkers measured different biomarkers (troponin, CRP, and others) in 557 patients with non-ST elevation acute coronary syndromes to determine if risk for major events (death or nonfatal myocardial infarction) at first month and first year follow-up were significant. This study found that the number of biomarkers was an independent risk predictor of major events.[101]

In summary, biomarkers may be of assistance in the perioperative evaluation and management of patients with suspected or known cardiovascular disease. Each individual marker should be interpreted in the appropriate clinical context. A plethora of novel markers is currently being studied. Whether they become clinically useful remains to be determined.

References

1. Wu AH, Apple FS, Gibler WB, Jesse RL, Warshaw MM, Valdes R **Jr**. National Academy of Clinical Biochemistry Standards of Laboratory Practice: recommendations for the use of cardiac markers in coronary artery diseases. *Clin Chem* 1999;**45**(7):1104–21.
2. Apple FS, Wu AH, Mair J, et al. Future biomarkers for detection of ischemia and risk stratification in acute coronary syndrome. *Clin Chem* 2005;**51**(5):810–24.
3. Jaffe AS, Babuin L, Apple FS. Biomarkers in acute cardiac disease: The present and the future. *J Am Coll Cardiol* 2006;**48**(1):1–11.
4. Ishikawa Y, Saffitz JE, Mealman TL, Grace AM, Roberts R. Reversible myocardial ischemic injury is not associated with

increased creatine kinase activity in plasma. *Clin Chem* 1997;**43**(3):467–75.

5. Apple FS, Preese LM. Creatine kinase-MB: Detection of myocardial infarction and monitoring reperfusion. *J Clin Immunoassay* 1994;**17**:24–9.

6. Rajappa M, Sharma A. Biomarkers of cardiac injury: an update. *Angiology* 2005;**56**(6):677–91.

7. Ajani AE, Waksman R, Sharma AK, et al. Usefulness of periprocedural creatinine phosphokinase-MB release to predict adverse outcomes after intracoronary radiation therapy for in-stent restenosis. *Am J Cardiol* 2004;**93**(3):313–7.

8. Brener SJ, Lytle BW, Schneider JP, Ellis SG, Topol EJ. Association between CK-MB elevation after percutaneous or surgical revascularization and three-year mortality. *J Am Coll Cardiol* 2002;**40**(11):1961–7.

9. Gibler WB, Lewis LM, Erb RE, et al. Early detection of acute myocardial infarction in patients presenting with chest pain and nondiagnostic ECGs: serial CK-MB sampling in the emergency department. *Ann Emerg Med* 1990;**19**(12):1359–66.

10. Karras DJ, Kane DL. Serum markers in the emergency department diagnosis of acute myocardial infarction. *Emerg Med Clin North Am* 2001;**19**(2):321–37.

11. Cohen M, Diez JE, Levine GN, et al. Pharmacoinvasive management of acute coronary syndrome: Incorporating the 2007 ACC/AHA guidelines: The CATH (cardiac catheterization and antithrombotic therapy in the hospital) clinical consensus panel report–III. *J Invasive Cardiol* 2007;**19**(12):525,38; quiz 539–40.

12. Gerhardt W, Ljungdahl L. Rational diagnostic strategy in diagnosis of ischemic myocardial injury. S-troponin T and S-CK MB (mass) time series using individual baseline values. *Scand J Clin Lab Invest Suppl* 1993;**215**:47–59.

13. Melanson SE, Tanasijevic MJ, Jarolim P. Cardiac troponin assays: a view from the clinical chemistry laboratory. *Circulation* 2007;**116**(18):501–4.

14. Panteghini M, Pagani F, Yeo KT, et al. Evaluation of imprecision for cardiac troponin assays at low-range concentrations. *Clin Chem* 2004;**50**(2):327–32.

15. Apple FS. Clinical and analytical standardization issues confronting cardiac troponin I. *Clin Chem* 1999;**45**(1):18–20.

16. Panteghini M, Gerhardt W, Apple FS, Dati F, Ravkilde J, Wu AH. Quality specifications for cardiac troponin assays. *Clin Chem Lab Med* 2001;**39**(2):175–9.

17. Ellis K, Dreisbach AW, Lertora JL. Plasma elimination of cardiac troponin I in end-stage renal disease. *South Med J* 2001;**94**(10):993–6.

18. Han SH, Choi HY, Kim DK, et al. Elevated cardiac troponin T predicts cardiovascular events in asymptomatic continuous ambulatory peritoneal dialysis patients without a history of cardiovascular disease. *Am J Nephrol* 2009;**29**(2):129–35.

19. Needham DM, Shufelt KA, Tomlinson G, Scholey JW, Newton GE. Troponin I and T levels in renal failure patients without acute coronary syndrome: A systematic review of the literature. *Can J Cardiol* 2004;**20**(12):1212–8.

20. Havekes B, van Manen JG, Krediet RT, et al. Serum troponin T concentration as a predictor of mortality in hemodialysis and peritoneal dialysis patients. *Am J Kidney Dis* 2006;**47**(5):823–9.

21. Dierkes J, Domrose U, Westphal S, et al. Cardiac troponin T predicts mortality in patients with end-stage renal disease. *Circulation* 2000;**102**(16):1964–9.

22. de Filippi C, Wasserman S, Rosanio S, et al. Cardiac troponin T and C-reactive protein for predicting prognosis, coronary atherosclerosis, and cardiomyopathy in patients undergoing long-term hemodialysis. *JAMA* 2003;**290**(3):353–9.

23. Landesberg G, Shatz V, Akopnik I, et al. Association of cardiac troponin, CK-MB, and postoperative myocardial ischemia with long-term survival after major vascular surgery. *J Am Coll Cardiol* 2003;**42**(9):1547–54.

24. Adams JE 3rd, Bodor GS, Davila-Roman VG, et al. Cardiac troponin I. A marker with high specificity for cardiac injury. *Circulation* 1993;**88**(1):101–6.

25. Katus HA, Schoeppenthau M, Tanzeem A, et al. Non-invasive assessment of perioperative myocardial cell damage by circulating cardiac troponin T. *Br Heart J* 1991;**65**(5):259–64.

26. Apple FS, Falahati A, Paulsen PR, Miller EA, Sharkey SW. Improved detection of minor ischemic myocardial injury with measurement of serum cardiac troponin I. *Clin Chem* 1997;**43**(11):2047–51.

27. Jaffe AS, Landt Y, Parvin CA, Abendschein DR, Geltman EM, Ladenson JH. Comparative sensitivity of cardiac troponin I and lactate dehydrogenase isoenzymes for diagnosing acute myocardial infarction. *Clin Chem* 1996;**42**(11):1770–6.

28. Galvani M, Ottani F, Ferrini D, et al. Prognostic influence of elevated values of cardiac troponin I in patients with unstable angina. *Circulation* 1997;**95**(8):2053–9.

29. Hamm CW, Heeschen C, Goldmann B, et al. Benefit of abciximab in patients with refractory unstable angina in relation to serum troponin T levels. c7E3 fab antiplatelet therapy in unstable refractory angina (CAPTURE) study investigators. *N Engl J Med* 1999;**340**(21):1623–9.

30. Stubbs P, Collinson P, Moseley D, Greenwood T, Noble M. Prognostic significance of admission troponin T concentrations in patients with myocardial infarction. *Circulation* 1996;94(6):1291–7.

31. Hamm CW, Goldmann BU, Heeschen C, Kreymann G, Berger J, Meinertz T. Emergency room triage of patients with acute chest pain by means of rapid testing for cardiac troponin T or troponin I. *N Engl J Med* 1997;**337**(23):1648–53.

32. Dworschak M, Franz M, Khazen C, Czerny M, Haisjackl M, Hiesmayr M. Mechanical trauma as the major cause of troponin T release after transvenous implantation of cardioverter/defibrillators. *Cardiology* 2001;**95**(4):212–4.

33. Gupta A, Halankar S, Vora AM, Lokhandwala YY. Does radiofrequency ablation increase creatine kinase and troponin-T? *Indian Heart J* 1999;**51**(4):418–21.

34. Jackson L, Stewart A. Best evidence topic report. Use of troponin for the diagnosis of myocardial contusion after blunt chest trauma. *Emerg Med J* 2005;**22**(3):193–5.

35. Missov E, Calzolari C, Pau B. Circulating cardiac troponin I in severe congestive heart failure. *Circulation* 1997;**96**(9):2953–8.

36. Remppis A, Ehlermann P, Giannitsis E, et al. Cardiac troponin T levels at 96 hours reflect myocardial infarct size: a pathoanatomical study. *Cardiology* 2000;**93**(4):249–53.

37. Antman EM, Tanasijevic MJ, Thompson B, et al. Cardiac-specific troponin I levels to predict the risk of mortality in patients with acute coronary syndromes. *N Engl J Med* 1996;**335**(18):1342–9.

38. Heeschen C, Hamm CW, Goldmann B, Deu A, Langenbrink L, White HD. Troponin concentrations for stratification of patients with acute coronary syndromes in relation to therapeutic efficacy of tirofiban. PRISM study investigators: platelet receptor inhibition in ischemic syndrome management. *Lancet* 1999;**354**(9192):1757–62.

39. Morrow DA, Antman EM, Tanasijevic M, et al. Cardiac troponin I for stratification of early outcomes and the efficacy of enoxaparin in unstable angina: A TIMI-11B substudy. *J Am Coll Cardiol* 2000;**36**(6):1812–7.

40. Apple FS, Henry TD, Berger CR, Landt YA. Early monitoring of serum cardiac troponin I for assessment of coronary reperfusion following thrombolytic therapy. *Am J Clin Pathol* 1996;**105**(1):6–10.

41. Giraldi F, Grazi S, Guazzi MD. Early evaluation of results from systemic thrombolysis in acute myocardial infarct: The value of troponin I. *Cardiologia* 1998;**43**(5):485–91.

42. Tanaka H, Abe S, Yamashita T, et al. Serum levels of cardiac troponin I and troponin T in estimating myocardial infarct size soon after reperfusion. *Coron Artery Dis* 1997;**8**(7):433–9.

43. Vermes E, Mesguich M, Houel R, et al. Cardiac troponin I release after open heart surgery: A marker of myocardial protection? *Ann Thorac Surg* 2000;**70**(6):2087–90.

44. Jaffe AS, Ravkilde J, Roberts R, et al. It's time for a change to a troponin standard. *Circulation* 2000;**102**(11):1216–20.

45. Lasocki S, Provenchere S, Benessiano J, et al. Cardiac troponin I is an independent predictor of in-hospital death after adult cardiac surgery. *Anesthesiology* 2002;**97**(2):405–11.

46. Sudoh T, Minamino N, Kangawa K, Matsuo H. Brain natriuretic peptide-32: N-terminal six amino acid extended form of brain natriuretic peptide identified in porcine brain. *Biochem Biophys Res Commun* 1988;**155**(2):726–32.

47. Maisel AS, Krishnaswamy P, Nowak RM, et al. Rapid measurement of B-type natriuretic peptide in the emergency diagnosis of heart failure. *N Engl J Med* 2002;**347**(3):161–7.

48. Mueller C, Scholer A, Laule-Kilian K, et al. Use of B-type natriuretic peptide in the evaluation and management of acute dyspnea. *N Engl J Med* 2004;**350**(7):647–54.

49. Maisel A, Mueller C, Adams K Jr, et al. State of the art: using natriuretic peptide levels in clinical practice. *Eur J Heart Fail* 2008;**10**(9):824–39.

50. Horwich TB, Hamilton MA, Fonarow GC. B-type natriuretic peptide levels in obese patients with advanced heart failure. *J Am Coll Cardiol* 2006;**47**(1):85–90.

51. Fonarow GC, Heywood JT, Heidenreich PA, Lopatin M, Yancy CW, ADHERE Scientific Advisory Committee and Investigators. Temporal trends in clinical characteristics, treatments, and outcomes for heart failure hospitalizations, 2002 to 2004: Findings from Acute Decompensated Heart Failure National Registry (ADHERE). *Am Heart J* 2007;**153**(6):1021–8.

52. Dokainish H, Zoghbi WA, Lakkis NM, et al. Incremental predictive power of B-type natriuretic peptide and tissue Doppler echocardiography in the prognosis of patients with congestive heart failure. *J Am Coll Cardiol* 2005;**45**(8):1223–6.

53. Hutfless R, Kazanegra R, Madani M, et al. Utility of B-type natriuretic peptide in predicting postoperative complications and outcomes in patients undergoing heart surgery. *J Am Coll Cardiol* 2004;**43**(10):1873–9.

54. Sodeck G, Domanovits H, Schillinger M, et al. Pre-operative N-terminal pro-brain natriuretic peptide predicts outcome in type A aortic dissection. *J Am Coll Cardiol* 2008;**51**(11):1092–7.

55. Mekontso-Dessap A, de Prost N, Girou E, et al. B-type natriuretic peptide and weaning from mechanical ventilation. *Intensive Care Med* 2006;**32**(10):1529–36.

56. Vigushin DM, Pepys MB, Hawkins PN. Metabolic and scintigraphic studies of radioiodinated human C-reactive protein in health and disease. *J Clin Invest* 1993;**91**(4):1351–7.

57. Hutchinson WL, Noble GE, Hawkins PN, Pepys MB. The pentraxins, C-reactive protein and serum amyloid P component, are cleared and catabolized by hepatocytes in vivo. *J Clin Invest* 1994;**94**(4):1390–6.

58. Gabay C, Kushner I. Acute-phase proteins and other systemic responses to inflammation. *N Engl J Med* 1999;**340**(6):448–54.

59. Ross R. Atherosclerosis – an inflammatory disease. *N Engl J Med* 1999;**340**(2):115–26.

60. Ridker PM, Buring JE, Rifai N, Cook NR. Development and validation of improved algorithms for the assessment of global cardiovascular risk in women: the Reynolds risk score. *JAMA.* 2007 Feb 14;**297**(6):611–9.

61. Emerging Risk Factors Collaboration, Danesh J, Erqou S, Walker M, et al. The Emerging Risk Factors Collaboration: analysis of individual data on lipid, inflammatory and other markers in over 1.1 million participants in 104 prospective studies of cardiovascular diseases. *Eur J Epidemiol* 2007;**22**(12):839–69.

62. Bogaty P, Boyer L, Simard S, et al. Clinical utility of C-reactive protein measured at admission, hospital discharge, and 1 month later to predict outcome in patients with acute coronary disease. the RISCA (Recurrence and Inflammation in the Acute Coronary Syndromes) study. *J Am Coll Cardiol* 2008;**51**(24):2339–46.

63. Albert MA, Danielson E, Rifai N, Ridker PM, PRINCE Investigators. Effect of statin therapy on C-reactive protein levels: the Pravastatin Inflammation/CRP Evaluation (PRINCE): a randomized trial and cohort study. *JAMA* 2001;**286**(1):64–70.

64. Ridker PM, Cannon CP, Morrow D, Rifai N, Rose LM, McCabe CH, et al. C-reactive protein levels and outcomes after statin therapy. *N Engl J Med* 2005;**352**(1):20–8.

65. Ridker PM, Danielson E, Fonseca FA, et al. Rosuvastatin to prevent vascular events in men and women with elevated C-reactive protein. *N Engl J Med* 2008;**359**(21):2195–207.

66. Khera A, McGuire DK, Murphy SA, et al. Race and gender differences in C-reactive protein levels. *J Am Coll Cardiol* 2005;**46**(3):464–9.

67. Lobo SM, Lobo FR, Bota DP, et al. C-reactive protein levels correlate with mortality and organ failure in critically ill patients. *Chest* 2003;**123**(6):2043–9.

68. Loria V, Dato I, Graziani F, Biasucci LM. Myeloperoxidase: A new biomarker of inflammation in ischemic heart disease and acute coronary syndromes. *Mediators Inflamm* 2008;**2008**:135625.

69. Malle E, Marsche G, Arnhold J, Davies MJ. Modification of low-density lipoprotein by myeloperoxidase-derived oxidants and reagent hypochlorous acid. *Biochim Biophys Acta* 2006;**1761**(4):392–415.

70. Nambi V. The use of myeloperoxidase as a risk marker for atherosclerosis. *Curr Atheroscler Rep* 2005;**7**(2):127–31.

71. Young IS, McEneny J. Lipoprotein oxidation and atherosclerosis. *Biochem Soc Trans* 2001;**29**(Pt 2):358–62.

72. Baldus S, Heeschen C, Meinertz T, et al. Myeloperoxidase serum levels predict risk in patients with acute coronary syndromes. *Circulation* 2003;**108**(12):1440–5.

73. Esporcatte R, Rey HC, Rangel FO, et al. Predictive value of myeloperoxidase to identify high-risk patients admitted to the hospital with acute chest pain. *Arq Bras Cardiol* 2007;**89**(6):377–84.

74. Dominguez-Rodriguez A, Samimi-Fard S, Abreu-Gonzalez P, Garcia-Gonzalez MJ, Kaski JC. Prognostic value of admission myeloperoxidase levels in patients with ST-segment elevation myocardial infarction and cardiogenic shock. *Am J Cardiol* 2008;**101**(11):1537–40.

75. Brennan ML, Penn MS, Van Lente F, et al. Prognostic value of myeloperoxidase in patients with chest pain. *N Engl J Med* 2003;**349**(17):1595–604.

76. Tang WH, Brennan ML, Philip K, et al. Plasma myeloperoxidase levels in patients with chronic heart failure. *Am J Cardiol* 2006;**98**(6):796–9.

77. Bresser P, Out TA, van Alphen L, Jansen HM, Lutter R. Airway inflammation in nonobstructive and obstructive chronic bronchitis with chronic haemophilus influenzae airway infection. comparison with noninfected patients with chronic obstructive pulmonary disease. *Am J Respir Crit Care Med* 2000;**162**(3 Pt 1):947–52.

78. Roncucci L, Mora E, Mariani F, et al. Myeloperoxidase-positive cell infiltration in colorectal carcinogenesis as indicator of colorectal cancer risk. *Cancer Epidemiol Biomarkers Prev* 2008;**17**(9):2291–7.

79. Bar-Or D, Curtis G, Rao N, Bampos N, Lau E. Characterization of the Co(2+) and Ni(2+) binding amino-acid residues of the N-terminus of human albumin. An insight into the mechanism of a new assay for myocardial ischemia. *Eur J Biochem* 2001;**268**(1):42–7.

80. Bar-Or D, Winkler JV, Vanbenthuysen K, Harris L, Lau E, Hetzel FW. Reduced albumin-cobalt binding with transient myocardial ischemia after elective percutaneous transluminal coronary angioplasty: a preliminary comparison to creatine kinase-MB, myoglobin, and troponin I. *Am Heart J* 2001;**141**(6):985–91.

81. Bar-Or D, Lau E, Winkler JV. A novel assay for cobalt-albumin binding and its potential as a marker for myocardial ischemia-a preliminary report. *J Emerg Med* 2000;**19**(4):311–5.

82. Sinha MK, Gaze DC, Tippins JR, Collinson PO, Kaski JC. Ischemia modified albumin is a sensitive marker of myocardial ischemia after percutaneous coronary intervention. *Circulation* 2003;**107**(19):2403–5.

83. Worster A, Devereaux PJ, Heels-Ansdell D, et al. Capability of ischemia-modified albumin to predict serious cardiac outcomes in the short term among patients with potential acute coronary syndrome. *CMAJ* 2005;**172**(13):1685–90.

84. Keating L, Benger JR, Beetham R, et al. The PR.IMA study: Presentation ischaemia-modified albumin in the emergency department. *Emerg Med J* 2006;**23**(10):764–8.

85. Howie-Esquivel J, White M. Biomarkers in acute cardiovascular disease. *J Cardiovasc Nurs* 2008;**23**(2):124–31.

86. Lawrence JB, Oxvig C, Overgaard MT, et al. The insulin-like growth factor (IGF)-dependent IGF binding protein-4 protease secreted by human fibroblasts is pregnancy-associated plasma protein-A. *Proc Natl Acad Sci USA* 1999;**96**(6):3149–53.

87. Bayes-Genis A, Conover CA, Overgaard MT, et al. Pregnancy-associated plasma protein A as a marker of acute coronary syndromes. *N Engl J Med* 2001;**345**(14):1022–9.

88. Lund J, Qin QP, Ilva T, et al. Circulating pregnancy-associated plasma protein A predicts outcome in patients with acute coronary syndrome but no troponin I elevation. *Circulation* 2003;**108**(16):1924–6.

89. Iversen KK, Teisner AS, Teisner B, et al. Pregnancy associated plasma protein A, a novel, quick, and sensitive marker in ST-elevation myocardial infarction. *Am J Cardiol* 2008;**101**(10):1389–94.

90. Wittfooth S, Qin QP, Lund J, et al. Immunofluorometric point-of-care assays for the detection of acute coronary syndrome-related noncomplexed pregnancy-associated plasma protein A. *Clin Chem* 2006;**52**(9):1794–801.

91. Lee Y, Lee WH, Lee SC, et al. CD40L activation in circulating platelets in patients with acute coronary syndrome. *Cardiology* 1999;**92**(1):11–6.

92. Henn V, Steinbach S, Buchner K, Presek P, Kroczek RA. The inflammatory action of CD40 ligand (CD154) expressed on activated human platelets is temporally limited by coexpressed CD40. *Blood* 2001;**98**(4):1047–54.

93. Mach F, Schonbeck U, Bonnefoy JY, Pober JS, Libby P. Activation of monocyte/macrophage functions related to acute atheroma complication by ligation of CD40: Induction of collagenase, stromelysin, and tissue factor. *Circulation* 1997;**96**(2):396–9.

94. Andre P, Prasad KS, Denis CV, et al. CD40L stabilizes arterial thrombi by a beta3 integrin–dependent mechanism. *Nat Med* 2002;**8**(3):247–52.

95. Aukrust P, Muller F, Ueland T, et al. Enhanced levels of soluble and membrane-bound CD40 ligand in patients with unstable angina. possible reflection of T lymphocyte and platelet involvement in the pathogenesis of acute coronary syndromes. *Circulation* 1999;**100**(6):614–20.

96. Schonbeck U, Varo N, Libby P, Buring J, Ridker PM. Soluble CD.40L and cardiovascular risk in women. *Circulation* 2001;**104**(19):2266–8.

97. Heeschen C, Dimmeler S, Hamm CW, et al. Soluble CD.40 ligand in acute coronary syndromes. *N Engl J Med* 2003;**348**(12):1104–11.

98. Ludwiczek O, Kaser A, Tilg H. Plasma levels of soluble CD40 ligand are elevated in inflammatory bowel diseases. *Int J Colorectal Dis* 2003;**18**(2):142–7.

99. Seino Y, Ogawa A, Yamashita T, Fujita N, Ogata K. Multi-biomarker approach to acute coronary syndrome. *Nippon Rinsho* 2006;**64**(4):691–9.

100. Braunwald E. Unstable angina: an etiologic approach to management. *Circulation* 1998;**98**(21):2219–22.

101. Bodi V, Sanchis J, Llacer A, et al. Multimarker risk strategy for predicting 1-month and 1-year major events in non-ST-elevation acute coronary syndromes. *Am Heart J* 2005;**149**(2):268–74.

Endocrine testing in the operating room

Lakshmi V. Ramanathan and Michael S. Lewis

Overview

Improvements in medical technology have led to faster turnaround times for traditionally labor-intensive manual assays used in endocrine testing. Contributing factors include the quality of monoclonal antibodies used with more efficient platforms for immunoassays. The evolution of rapid intraoperative immunoassays provides critical information on the surgical patient in the operating room. Parathyroid hormone (PTH) and other hormones share the same characteristics –short half life, large analyte concentration gradients, rapid analysis time, and positive clinical utility.[1] This chapter focuses on rapid intraoperative immunoassay of PTH and other hormones, as well as the impact of endocrine testing in the operating room. Tests performed in the vicinity of the operating room are labeled as point-of-surgery (POS) testing.[2]

The characteristics and reference ranges[1] for analytes used in intraoperative testing and diagnosis are summarized in Table 27.1. The reference ranges indicated are for adults.

Intraoperative testing of PTH

The normal adult needs to ingest approximately 1000 mg of calcium daily to maintain calcium levels. Internal stores approximate 1 to 2 kg, with 99 percent contained in the skeleton. Deficits are compensated by slow resorption of bone. Plasma calcium is about 40 percent protein-bound to albumin and other plasma proteins. Total calcium is normally about 8.5 to 10.5 mg/dL, with ionized calcium normally 4.5 to 5 mg/dL (1.1–1.4 mmol/L).

PTH is the most important regulator of plasma calcium. It raises plasma calcium by mobilizing bone calcium and stimulating the kidneys to reabsorb more calcium and excrete more phosphorus. The concentration of free calcium in blood or extracellular fluid is the primary acute physiological regulator of PTH synthesis, metabolism, and secretion. Free calcium is detected by a calcium-sensing receptor in the plasma membrane of parathyroid cells. This receptor activates intracellular events leading to release of free calcium from intracellular stores and the opening of plasma membrane calcium channels. An increase in extracellular free calcium inhibits PTH synthesis and secretion and increases PTH metabolism, whereas a decrease has the opposite effect. An inverse sigmoidal relationship exists between PTH secretion and free calcium.

Approximately 65 percent of calcium is absorbed in the proximal tubules of the kidneys. Calcium reabsorption is closely linked to sodium and is independent of PTH. The remaining 10 percent to 20 percent of calcium is reabsorbed in the thick ascending loop of Henle, whereas PTH enhances 5 percent to 10 percent reabsorption in the distal tubule through a cyclic AMP mechanism.

PTH is one of the most important regulators of renal phosphate threshold and serum phosphate concentration. In contrast with the calcium-conserving effect of PTH in the kidneys, PTH reduces the reabsorption of phosphate from the proximal

Table 27.1. Characteristics of rapid intraoperative assays

Analyte	Half-life (min)	Reference range	Assay time (min)
PTH	5	16–87 pg/mL	15
ACTH	15	10–46 pg/mL	15
Cortisol	>90	AM: 5–25 mcg/dL	8
		PM: 2.5–12.5 mcg/dL	
Gastrin	10	0–115 pg/mL	30–60
GH	15	0.06–5.0 ng/mL	15
Insulin	9	6–27 microunits/mL	8–14
Testosterone	>60	Males: 175–781 ng/dL	18
		Females: <10–75 ng/dL	

PTH – parathyroid hormone; ACTH – adrenocorticotropic hormone; GH – growth hormone.

Table 27.2. Differential diagnosis of hypercalcemia

Related to PTH	Malignancy	Miscellaneous
Primary hyperparathyroidism	Solid tumors (breast) that produce parathyroid hormone-related protein (PTH-RP)	Granulomatous disease (sarcoid, tuberculosis), with 1,25 dihydroxy vitamin D production
Tertiary hyperparathyroidism	T-cell lymphoma that produces 1,25 dihydroxy vitamin D	Vitamin D toxicity
Multiple endocrine neoplasia	Multiple myeloma	Vitamin A toxicity
Parathyroid carcinoma	Leukemia	Hyperthyroidism
Familial hypocalciuric hypercalcemia		Adrenal insufficiency
Lithium treatment		Milk alkali syndrome
Cancer production of PTH		Aluminum toxicity
		Immobilization
		Thiazide treatment

tubule. Approximately 85 percent to 90 percent of the phosphate filtered by the kidneys is reabsorbed.

Hypercalcemia is defined as a serum calcium level less than 10.5 mg/dL. Patients are generally asymptomatic until the serum calcium levels are above 11.5 mg/dL. Treatment of hypercalcemia requires understanding the underlying disease and/or physiologic derangement. However, empirically starting with normal saline at 250 to 500 mL/hour corrects volume depletion, dilutes the ionized calcium, and inhibits calcium reabsorption by the increasing sodium excretion from the kidneys. After volume replacement is complete, a loop diuretic such as furosemide can be given to enhance excretion.[3] Calcitonin will lower calcium within two hours after injection. Pamidronate, a bisphosphate that is used for mild cases of hypercalcemia and bone resorption, is decreased because of its inhibitory effect on osteoclasts. Table 27.2 summarizes the differential diagnosis of hypercalcemia.

Hypocalcemia, on the other hand, can be caused by resistance to PTH or vitamin D calcium binding, hypomagnesemia, and other conditions. An important cause of decreased total plasma calcium is hypoalbuminemia. One way to correct for a low albumin is to add 0.8 mg/dL to the serum calcium as a correction for every 1 g/dL decrease in the albumin.

Intraoperative monitoring of PTH
Technical concepts

Immunoassays specific for various PTH fragments are available today. Antisera that have been developed for the C-terminal and N-terminal and employed in immunometric assays recognize not only the specific range, but similar fragments as well.

Recent assays for intact PTH have the necessary sensitivity for detecting circulating intact PTH in normal patients, and discriminates between normal patients and those with primary hyperparathyroidism. These assays also discriminate between primary hyperparathyroidism and hypocalcemia of malignancy when compared with previous assays, virtually without any significant overlap between these groups.

Immunometric assays have replaced radioimmunoassays for PTH. Major advances have been made in the ability to measure PTH, with amino acid sequence determination, increased

knowledge of circulating forms, secretion and metabolism, and synthesis of human PTH for antibody purification as important contributing factors. This led to the development of noncompetitive immunoassays, including the initial immunoradiometric assay (IRMA) and the immunochemiluminescent assay (ICMA).

The application of PTH assay to the operating room was realized with the availability of the chemiluminescent label that was developed by Nichols Institute Diagnostics.[1] Factors that reduce the completion time of the test include vibrating, shaking, increase in temperature to 45°C, and reducing incubation time from 22 hours to 7 minutes. EDTA plasma is the preferred sample; the complete assay, consisting of pipetting, centrifugation, incubation, washing, and reaction/reading, is accomplished in 15 minutes. The equipment required for the assay (microcentrifuge, heater/shaker apparatus, bead washer, and luminometer) fit on a cart that can be transported to the operating room. The standard curve used with each assay is stored in the luminometer and can be determined in the laboratory prior to the surgical procedure.

Subsequently, Diagnostics Products Corporation launched rapid PTH on the Immulite analyzer. The Turbo Intact PTH used in the Mount Sinai operating room is a modification of the earlier methodology on the Immulite. The assay has two incubation times, totaling 10 minutes, with overall completion time of 15 minutes, which includes sample preparation. The performance of Turbo Intact PTH on the Immulite assay was compared with the standard DPH–PTH assay.[4] Although the turbo assay was not as precise as the standard DPH–PTH assay, it had suitable intrarun precision for intraoperative declines of greater than 50 percent in PTH values.

Specimen collection and preparation

Blood is collected by venipuncture into EDTA tubes or plain tubes without anticoagulant, avoiding hemolysis. The plasma or serum is separated from the cells. It is important to keep the serum sample cold throughout the collection and separation process. Studies have shown that intact PTH is stable in whole blood when collected in EDTA tubes for up to 72 hours at room temperature (15–28°C).[5] Therefore, collection in EDTA tubes minimizes the need to keep the sample cold throughout this process.

Parameters monitored

Primary hyperparathyroidism is most commonly caused by a benign parathyroid adenoma (90% of cases) or hyperplasia (9%) and very rarely by parathyroid carcinoma. Surgical treatment includes bilateral, open-neck exploration under general anesthesia, with intraoperative frozen-section histopathological examination of the parathyroid glands.[6] Initially, urinary cyclic adenosine monophosphate was considered for intraoperative monitoring following removal of the parathyroid glands.[7] However, the testing required bladder catheterization, urine collection every 30 minutes until two hours after surgery, and was very time-consuming. Thus, the use of intraoperative testing for PTH in the operating room has increased in the past few years.

Typical baseline values for PTH in hyperparathyroid patients are about 200 pg/mL, with the trend as follows following removal of the gland:

Postisolation: 190 pg/mL
5 minutes: 160 pg/mLl
10 minutes: 90 pg/mL
20 minutes: 20 pg/mL

If there is no decline in values, this implies that the gland has not been successfully removed.

Evidence of utility

A survey conducted by the College of American Pathologists found that 39 percent of laboratories reported that rapid PTH testing was requested on all parathyroid surgeries performed.[9] The survey also found that 71 percent of the respondents performed the test within the laboratory, 6 percent within a satellite special-purpose laboratory, and 23 percent in the operating room. The cost-effectiveness of intraoperative PTH monitoring combined with preoperative imaging has resulted in simpler surgery, options of local anesthesia, and shorter hospital stays.[9] Fahy and colleagues[4] devised a computer-generated model to demonstrate that the use of rapid PTH decreases costs by $2000 per patient and the use of preoperative localization decreases costs by $3000 per patient. Other studies have shown similar savings.[10]

Many studies have demonstrated the clinical utility of intraoperative PTH monitoring. The surgeon is usually confident that complete resection of the parathyroid gland has occurred once the PTH has decreased and maintained at a level that is 50 percent below the baseline value.[10]

Practice parameters

PTH is being used as a monitor during parathyroid surgery because the production of PTH is limited to the parathyroid glands, the intact molecule has a half-life of less than five minutes, and its secretion is suppressed in normal parathyroid glands after hyperfunctioning tissue has been removed. In the typical protocol, PTH concentrations are measured at baseline before the procedure and then at 5- to 10-minute intervals following the tumor excision, with a 50 percent decrease in values observed if all hypersecreting tissue has been removed.[11]

After successful parathyroidectomy, a decrease in the serum calcium is observed within 24 hours of surgery, leading to a "hungry bone" syndrome. A decline in serum calcium usually occurs postoperatively within three to seven days. Therefore, serum calcium, magnesium, and phosphorus levels should all be monitored closely.

Testing is usually performed by licensed laboratory technologists either in the vicinity of the operating room or in the chemistry laboratory. It is essential that specimens are received by the lab as soon as possible so there is minimum delay owing to specimen transportation.

What is the future of other intraoperative testing?

Based on the success of rapid intraoperative PTH testing in terms of patient outcomes and cost savings, there is considerable interest in exploring other rapid intraoperative hormone assays. Rapid intraoperative assays take 30 minutes or less to perform. The speed of the assays has improved by modifying the sample size and temperature of the assay. Like the rapid PTH test, the other intraoperative tests are performed at 37°C or higher, which increases the rate of reaction that accelerates the rate of binding of the antibodies to the analyte. Some rapid assays use microparticle immunoassays[12] that accelerate the rate of reaction by decreasing diffusion distances and increasing the effective concentration of the capture antibodies. Although rapid intraoperative methodologies are available for insulin, growth hormone, ACTH, gastrin, and testosterone, clinical applications have been limited. More studies are needed to explore the impact of other intraoperative tests in the operating room.

References

1. Sokoll LJ, Wians FH Jr, Remaley AT. Rapid intraoperative immunoassay of parathyroid hormone and other hormones: a new paradigm for point-of-care testing. *Clin Chem* 2004;**50**:1126–1135.
2. Wians FH Jr. Intraoperative parathyroid hormone testing: a revolution in point-of-surgery testing on the horizon? *Am Clin Lab* 2000;**19**:21–22.
3. Lopez C.J. and Szolnoki J; Metabolic Derangements. In *Critical Care: The Requisites in Anesthesiology*. Philadelphia (PA) Elsevier Mosby, 2005.
4. Fahy BN, Bold RJ, Beckett L, Schneider PD. Modern Parathyroid surgery: a cost benefit analysis of localizing strategies. *Arch Surg* 2002;**137**:917–922.
5. Raff H, Shaker JL, Seifert Pe, Werner PH, Hazelrigg SR, Finding JLO. Intra operative measurement of adreno corticotrophin (ACTH) during removal of ACTH-secreting bronchial carcinoid tumors. *J Clin Endocrinol Metab* 1995;**80**:1036–1039.

6. Tamler R, Lewis MS, LiVolsi V, Genden EM. Parathyroid carcinoma: ultrasonographic and histologic features. *Thyroid* 2005;**15**:744–745.

7. Spiegel AM, Eastman ST, Attie MF, et al. Interaoperative measurement of urinary cyclic AMP to guide surgery for primary hyperthyroidism. *N Engl J Med* 1980;**303**:1457–1460.

8. Hortin GL, Carter AB. Intraoperative parathyroid hormone testing: survey of program characteristics. *Arch Pathol Lab Med* 2002;**1261**:1045–1049.

9. Johnson LR, Doherty G, Lairmore T, et al. Evaluation of the performance and clinical impart of rapid intraoperative parathyroid hormone assay in conjunction with preoperative imaging and concise parathyroidectomy. *Clin Chem* 2001;**47**:919–925.

10. Carter AB, Howanitz PJ. Intraoperative testing for parathyroid hormone: a comprehensive renewal of the use of the assay and the relevant literature. *Arch Pathol Lab Med.* 2003 127; **11**:1424–1442.

11. NIH Conference. Diagnosis and management of asymptomatic primary hyperparathyroidism: Consensus development conference statement. *Ann Intern Med* 1991;**114**:593–597.

12. Albright SV, McCant JA, Libutti SK, Bantlett DL, Alexander HR, Sampson ML, et al. Development of a rapid intraoperative immunoassay for insulin. *Ann Clin Biochem* 2002;**39**:513–515.

Temperature monitoring

David Wax and Justin Lipper

Introduction

Temperature is a measure of the average kinetic energy of a collection of particles. Body temperature is maintained in a narrow range that permits biochemical enzymatic reactions necessary for homeostasis to occur. Although normal body temperature is often considered to be 37°C, this is an oversimplification. Body temperature actually fluctuates over the course of the day (with an early morning nadir and evening peak) and also varies based on age (lower in older individuals), gender (lower in males), activity level, and site at which it is measured (Figure 28.1). Mean rectal temperatures are typically in the range of 36.7 to 37.5°C, and mean axillary temperatures are 35.5 to 37°C.[1]

Heat is a measure of the energy transferred from particles of higher temperature to those of lower temperature. Heat gain can occur as a result of physiologic (e.g. exercise, shivering), pathologic (e.g. malignant hyperthermia, infection/inflammation), or iatrogenic (e.g. overwarming) processes. Heat is also transferred within the body owing to *redistribution* from the core to the periphery and surface that occurs with the loss of regulatory mechanisms (e.g. peripheral/cutaneous vasoconstriction) during anesthesia. Heat loss from the body occurs in the typically cold operating room environment as a result of several mechanisms. Heat energy is transferred from higher to lower temperature surfaces by infrared *radiation* when there is no direct contact between the surfaces, and by *conduction* when there is direct contact between the surfaces. *Convection* contributes to heat loss when cool air currents absorb heat energy as they pass over warm body surfaces. Finally, *evaporation* of moisture from skin surfaces and surgically exposed body cavities results in loss of heat energy.

Maintenance of body temperature is the result of various physiologic sensors and effectors that appear to be integrated by the hypothalamus. These control mechanisms are impaired by anesthesia, both general and neuraxial, because of interruption of afferent, efferent, and central components of the thermoregulatory system. The resulting temperature decreases or increases can have adverse effects, may be beneficial, or may be signs of other underlying processes, making temperature monitoring an important component of perioperative care.

Thermometers

Early methods of measuring oral or rectal temperature using mercury- or alcohol-filled glass thermometers have fallen out of favor because of the risks of glass breakage and toxic spillage, as well as difficulty reading results and slow response time. Instead, newer technologies have emerged to measure temperature safely, quickly, easily, and inexpensively (Figure 28.2).

Thermocouples and thermistors

A prevalent method of measuring body temperature is using thermocouples and thermistors. A thermocouple takes advantage of the phenomenon that a conductor subjected to a temperature gradient between its ends will generate a voltage that

Figure 28.1. Diurnal variation in body temperature. Adapted from ref. 1. Thorne Research, Inc., copyright 2006. All rights reserved.

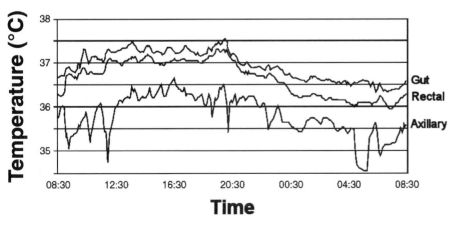

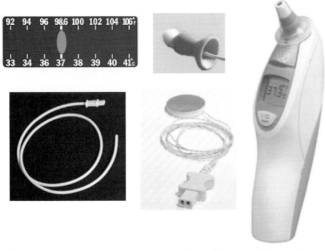

Figure 28.2. Temperature monitoring probes and devices. Clockwise from top left: liquid crystal skin temperature probe; continuous tympanic temperature probe; infrared tympanic membrane thermometer; skin temperature probe; general purpose temperature probe.

can be measured. Completing the circuit with a dissimilar metal allows measurement of the temperature difference. If the temperature of one end (the reference) is known or controlled, the temperature of the measuring (probe) end can be determined. Alternatively, a thermistor uses a semiconductor that varies in resistance based on its temperature. This resistance can be measured, and from that, the temperature can be calculated.[2]

Infrared sensors

Infrared thermometers measure the amount of infrared heat energy emitted by an object. Because they detect heat energy being given off from an object by radiation, they do not need to be in direct contact with the object. Infrared thermometers for measuring body temperature are usually designed to measure from either the forehead or the tympanic membrane. The accuracy of forehead infrared thermometers, however, has been shown to be poor in both adult and pediatric populations.[3] Similarly, many infrared ear thermometers in clinical use do not accurately pick up infrared energy from the tympanic membrane and extrapolate from areas of the outer ear.[4] Newer models, however, have shown increased accuracy and report temperatures close to that of pulmonary artery catheters.[5]

Therefore, use of infrared technology may become more prevalent.

Liquid crystal devices

Thermotropic liquid crystals have been integrated into disposable plastic strips that are used to measure temperature for nonmedical applications for which precision is not strictly required. They typically have a useful range of 34 to 40°C. Although they may not be as precise as electronic thermometers, they may be sufficient in some medical applications when other measurement methods may be problematic. The strips may be applied to the forehead when being used to measure core temperature, to the extremities during nerve blocks to monitor the temperature rise associated with a successful block, or to sites of vascular flaps to monitor blood flow indirectly. Some studies have shown that liquid crystal thermometry can vary from esophageal monitoring by up to 1°C, whereas other studies have reported that liquid crystal monitoring can accurately follow temperature trends and detect rapidly elevating temperatures.[6,7] Furthermore, it has been shown that liquid crystal monitoring is only minimally affected by redistribution of heat on induction of anesthesia, vasomotor temperature regulation (e.g. sweating and shivering), and typical ambient temperature changes.[8]

Deep tissue monitors

The concept of a deep tissue monitor is to be able to measure deep (core) body temperature with a less-invasive skin surface probe. The method uses two thermistors separated by an insulator, and a heating element integrated into the probe. The heating element adjusts dynamically to provide sufficient energy to oppose any heat loss from the skin surface, so the skin under the probe will equilibrate with and reflect deeper temperatures.[9,10] This technique has been shown to measure core body temperature effectively.[11] Despite its apparent usefulness, however, this technology is not widely used.

Monitoring sites

Various internal and external body sites are available for temperature monitoring. The suitability of each site depends on the procedure being performed, the equipment available, and the relative need for accuracy (Figure 28.3).

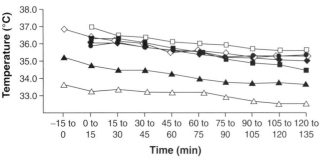

Figure 28.3. Comparison of temperature measurements at various sites during noncardiac surgery. Adapted from ref. 12. Reprinted with permission.

Legend:
□ Rectal
◇ Tympanic
◆ Esophageal
● Nasopharyngeal
■ Bladder
▲ Axillary
△ Forehead

Core/central sites

Core temperature represents the temperature of highly perfused tissues (e.g. liver, kidneys, heart). Generally, these sites (as well as the brain) are in equilibrium with one another, although regional differences may develop transiently or iatrogenically. These sites are also less influenced by vasomotor thermoregulatory mechanisms (compared with peripheral sites) and are the sites of most of the vital enzymatic reactions that require strict temperature control.

The nasopharynx can be used as an indirect but accurate measure of brain and, under equilibrium conditions, core temperature.[12] Optimal positioning requires placement of the probe past the nares and soft palate. Spontaneous breathing and gas leakage around airway devices may alter measurements at this site. Still, it is the most common site of temperature measurement during anesthesia, at least among European centers studied.[13]

The esophagus is another common location to access central temperature, although it is important to have the sensor placed in an optimal position because temperature variations of up to 6°C have been reported. The coldest temperature occurs where the heart and breath sounds are best heard (presuming the use of a combined thermometer and esophageal stethoscope) and the warmest part is 12 to 16 cm past this point.[14] Continuous gastric suctioning may also reduce measured temperatures at this site.[15] In the absence of rapid infusions of cold fluids or an open thoracic cavity, lower esophageal temperature has been shown to closely approximate brain temperature.[16]

The tympanic membrane may be a useful site for central temperature measurement because of its proximity to the internal carotid artery.[17] This location provides a measurement of brain temperature, which is particularly important because anterior hypothalamic temperature is the main regulator of thermal homeostasis.[18] Similarly, it may be useful for cases using deliberate hypothermia for brain protection. Measurements at this site may be affected by impacted cerumen, so otoscopic exam prior to measurement may help assess reliability. Improved technology for continuous monitoring at this site will help increase its utility.[19]

Central temperature can also be measured in the pulmonary artery by using a thermistor integrated into a thermodilution cardiac output pulmonary artery catheter. These measurements most accurately reflect core temperature in the absence of topical and systemic cooling during cardiopulmonary bypass. Pulmonary artery temperatures may also be lower than those measured in the nasopharynx and rectum after cardiopulmonary bypass discontinuation.[20]

Intermediate sites

Intermediate temperature monitoring sites lag behind central temperature monitors in their response to temperature change. They may be useful to supplement central measuring sites in cases using cardiopulmonary bypass when compartmental temperature changes are induced, or instead of central sites in cases in which temperature fluctuates less substantially.

Oral (i.e. sublingual) temperatures are typically slightly (0.3°C) below core temperature and may be further affected by breathing and eating or drinking. Still, oral temperature measurement is convenient in settings such as preoperative assessment and intermittent measurement in postanesthesia care units and patient wards. For rectal temperatures, discrepancies with core temperature are the result of heat-producing bacteria in the rectum, stool insulation, and cooler lower extremity venous return.[21] On the other hand, rectal sensors can be useful indicators of the temperature of poorly perfused tissues.[2] The popularity of the rectal site for perioperative use is low compared with other sites perceived to be more easily accessible, accurate, and hygienic.

Bladder temperature accuracy depends on the rate of urine flow. When urine flow is low, bladder temperature parallels rectal temperature. At high urine flow rates, bladder temperature agrees with pulmonary artery measurements.[22] In operative cases using cardiopulmonary bypass, bladder temperatures have been shown to correlate well with central temperature monitors during rewarming when compared with rectal sensors.[23]

Peripheral temperature monitoring

Peripheral temperature monitoring sites, generally on the skin surface, are subject to numerous environmental and thermoregulatory influences. Although this reduces their accuracy as a monitor of core temperature, the less-invasive nature of monitoring at such sites make it useful in many settings.

Skin surface temperatures are lower than core temperatures.[24] The most commonly used skin sites are the forehead and the axilla. With forehead sensors, the difference is consistently 2°C lower than core temperature measured, making it a reasonable estimate of core temperature after adjusting for this difference.[25] Axillary temperatures are approximately between forehead and core values, and accuracy may be improved by optimal placement of the probe over the axillary artery with the patient's arm adducted.[26]

Indications

Studies of temperature monitoring and management practice in Europe revealed that, overall, patient temperature was monitored in only 25 percent of general anesthesia cases, although 43 percent were actively warmed.[13] This suggests that many practitioners believed that actively warming patients was safe and no less effective without concomitant temperature monitoring, whereas even more practitioners seemed unconcerned about temperature management at all. For regional anesthesia cases, an even smaller percentage of cases included temperature monitoring, despite the finding that hypothermia is as common in cases using neuraxial anesthesia as in those using general anesthesia.[27]

The American Society of Anesthesiologists (ASA) standard for temperature monitoring indicates that every patient receiving anesthesia is to have temperature monitored "when clinically significant changes in body temperature are intended, anticipated, or suspected."[28] Although this wording leaves some room for interpretation, given the knowledge that both general and regional anesthesia can induce hypothermia, and that the consequences of hypothermia can be significant, it is the authors' opinion that temperature should be monitored in the vast majority of anesthetics, especially given the relative ease, safety, and low cost of such monitoring. In addition, temperature monitoring is important in preventing overheating, identifying fever, and identifying possible cases of malignant hyperthermia (even though rising temperature may be a relatively late sign of this complication). Finally, it appears that anesthesiologists are inaccurate in identifying patients who are hypothermic in the absence of a temperature monitor.[29] It is, therefore, the authors' recommendation that temperature be monitored in all patients undergoing general anesthesia for more than 30 minutes, all patients undergoing procedures longer than one hour, and all children. The 30-minute cutoff reflects the questions of interpretation and utility during this time of redistribution of body heat.[30–32]

Additional incentives to monitor temperature come from regulatory efforts toward performance improvement that have led to the establishment of quality benchmarks that clinicians are being increasingly pressured to meet.[33] One such proposal would require that colorectal surgery patients have a temperature greater than or equal to 36°C within the first 15 minutes after leaving the operating room. Achieving such goals may be aided by temperature monitoring if the data acquired are used to guide progressive interventions aimed at maintaining normothermia.

Complications

Temperature monitoring of any type is very rarely a source of significant complications. The ASA Closed Claims Project does not contain any cases directly referable to a complication of temperature monitoring. Several case reports, however, indicate the rare potential for complications from placement of temperature probes (or similar instruments): tympanic membrane perforation, epistaxis, esophageal perforation, rectal perforation, and electrical burns.[34–38]

Preexisting pathology of any potential site should prompt consideration of an alternative site. These include esophageal abnormalities (e.g. hiatal hernia, esophageal diverticulum, varices), nasopharyngeal issues (e.g. sinusitis, bleeding diatheses with increased chance of epistaxis), rectal abnormalities, and ear abnormalities (e.g. otitis, tympanostomy). Use of bladder or pulmonary artery temperature monitoring would not be advised unless bladder or pulmonary artery catheterization is required for other indications, in which case the additional use of the catheter as a temperature probe probably incurs no additional risk.

Utility

Incidental hypothermia

Rational temperature management to maintain normothermia may improve patient outcomes. As previously noted, however, many practitioners actively warm patients in the operating room without concomitant temperature monitoring. Additionally, at least one study found no independent association between use of intraoperative temperature monitoring (or warming method) and incidence of hypothermia on admission to an intensive care unit.[39] Although this may seem to suggest that monitoring of temperature is not necessarily worthwhile in preventing hypothermia and its complications, such monitoring will become increasingly important as interventions to regulate temperature become more aggressive to achieve specific clinical and regulatory goals.

There is evidence that mild perioperative hypothermia (typically defined as 34°–36°C) has deleterious effects on patient outcomes.[40] With regard to the coagulation system, mild hypothermia is thought to impair platelet aggregation and possibly other clotting mechanisms. A meta-analysis of the consequences concluded that mild hypothermia resulted in a significant increase in blood loss and transfusions.[41] Hypothermia also appears to cause hypertension and tachycardia in elderly patients; this may help explain the finding that hypothermia was an independent predictor of adverse cardiac events.[42] Mild hypothermia also appears to impair leukocytes as well as decrease tissue oxygen tension, both of which can promote wound infection and delay wound healing. Studies have indicated that mild hypothermia can significantly increase the incidence of wound infections and duration of hospitalization after colorectal surgery, and that prewarming patients before surgery can reduce surgical site infections.[43,44] In addition, hypothermia may cause patient discomfort and may delay discharge from the postanesthesia care unit.[45,46]

Therapeutic hypothermia

Hypothermia mitigates the cellular changes that lead to neuronal cell death after ischemic injury. The neuroprotective benefits of hypothermia seem clear in cases of cold-water drowning accidents and deliberate circulatory arrest during surgery. There is also evidence that early induction of moderate hypothermia in patients following cardiac arrest (but not after myocardial infarction without arrest) improves survival and neurologic outcomes.[47] Whether to warm neurologically compromised patients who spontaneously become mildly hypothermic in the course of their care also remains unsettled, because hypothermia has both potential benefits and potential risks in these patients. During cardiopulmonary bypass, there is a lack of consensus as to whether patients should be kept normothermic or have some degree of hypothermia induced, as no definite advantage of hypothermia over normothermia with regard to outcomes has been shown thus far.[48]

Hyperthermia

Temperature monitoring is also necessary to detect hyperthermia, which, similar to hypothermia, can have deleterious effects in some settings or may be an indicator of the presence of other disease processes. Hyperthermia is a relatively late sign of malignant hyperthermia, but temperature monitoring may help confirm the diagnosis and speed therapy.[49] Although mild hyperthermia may improve leukocyte function in the setting of infection, it can have adverse affects in patients whose fever is related to or in addition to actual or potential neurologic injury. For this reason, temperature monitoring is important to prevent hyperthermia during rewarming after cardiopulmonary bypass.[50] Similarly, hyperthermic patients with ischemic or hemorrhagic stroke, traumatic brain injury, subarachnoid hemorrhage, and refractory seizures may be cooled to prevent further injury.[51] However, such patients are generally cooled only to normothermic levels, as deliberate hypothermia has not been clearly proved to be beneficial in these settings.[52]

Conclusions

The likelihood that temperature monitoring can induce harm is minimal, and there is a growing body of evidence that lack of temperature control in perioperative patients is associated with complications. The authors conclude that temperature monitoring should be used in all but the briefest anesthetics (under 30 minutes' duration) and that the data should be used to guide evidence-based perioperative temperature management strategies as they evolve.

References

1. Kelly G. Body temperature variability (Part 1): a review of the history of body temperature and its variability due to site selection, biological rhythms, fitness, and aging. *Altern Med Rev* 2006;**11**(4):278–93.
2. Holdcroft A. *Body Temperature Control in Anesthesia, Surgery, and Intensive Care.* London: Balliere Tindall, 1980.
3. Suleman MI, Doufas AG, Akca O, et al. Insufficiency in a new temporal-artery thermometer for adult and pediatric patients. *Anesth Analg* 2002;**95**(1):67–71.
4. Imamura M, Matsukawa T, Ozaki M, et al. The accuracy and precision of four infrared aural canal thermometers during cardiac surgery. *Acta Anaesthsiol Scand* 1998;**42**(10):1222–6.
5. Bock M, Hohlfeld U, von Engeln K, et al. The accuracy of a new infrared ear thermometer in patients undergoing cardiac surgery. *Can J Anaesth* 2005;**52**(10):1083–7.
6. Lacoumenta S, Hall GM. Liquid crystal thermometry during anesthesia. *Anesthesia* 1984;**39**:54–56.
7. Allen GC, Horrow JC, Rosenberg H. Does forehead liquid crystal temperature accurately reflect "core" temperature? *Can J Anaesth* 1990;**37**(6):659–62.
8. Ikeda T, Sessler DI, Marder D, et al. Influence of thermoregulatory vasomotion and ambient temperature variation on the accuracy of core-temperature estimates by cutaneous liquid-crystal thermometers. *Anesthesiology* 1997;**86**(3):603–12.
9. Fox RH, Solman AJ. A new technique for monitoring the deep body temperature in man from the intact skin surface. *J Physiol* 1970;**212**:8–10.
10. Togawa T, Nemoto T, Yamazaki T, Kobayashi T. A modified internal temperature measurement device. *Med Biol Eng* 1976;**14**:361–4.
11. Matsukawa T, Sessler DI, Ozaki M, et al. Comparison of distal oesophageal temperature with "deep" and tracheal temperatures. *Can J Anaesth* 1997;**44**(4):433–8.
12. Cork RC, Vaughan RW, Humphrey LS. Precision and accuracy of intraoperative temperature monitoring. *Anesth Analg* 1983;**62**(2):211–4.
13. Torossian A; TEMMP (Thermoregulation in Europe Monitoring and Managing Patient Temperature) Study Group. Survey on intraoperative temperature management in Europe. *Eur J Anaesthesiol* 2007;**24**(8):668–75.
14. Kaufman RD. Relationship between esophageal temperature gradient and heart and lung sounds heard by esophageal stethoscope. *Anesth Analg* 1987;**66**:1046–48.
15. Nelson EJ, Grissom TE. Continuous gastric suctioning decreases measured esophageal temperature during general anesthesia. *J Clin Monit* 1996;**12**(6):429–32.
16. Whitby JD, Dunkin LJ. Cerebral, oesophageal, and nasopharyngeal temperatures. *Br J Anesth* 1971;**43**:673–6.
17. Benzinger M. Tympanic thermometry in surgery and anesthesia. *JAMA* 1969;**209**:1207–11.
18. Benzinger TH. Clinical termperature. *JAMA* 1969;**209**:1200–6.
19. Kiya T, Yamakage M, Hayase T, Satoh J, Namiki A. The usefulness of an earphone-type infrared tympanic thermometer for intraoperative core temperature monitoring. *Anesth Analg* 2007;**105**(6):1688–92.
20. Ramsay JG, Ralley FE, Whalley DG, et al. Site of temperature monitoring and prediction of afterdrop after open heart surgery. *Can Anaesth Soc J* 1985;**32**:607–12.
21. Stupfel M, Severinghaus JW. Internal body temperature gradients during anesthesia and hypothermia and effect of vagotomy. *J Appl Physiol* 1956;**9**:380–6.
22. Horrow JC, Rosenberg H. Does urinary catheter temperature reflect core temperature during cardiac surgery? *Anesthesiology* 1988;**69**:986–9.
23. Lilly JK, Boland JP, Zekan S. Urinary bladder temperature monitoring: A new index of body core temperature. *Crit Care Med* 1980;**8**:742–4.
24. Burgess GE III, Cooper JR, Marino RJ, Peuler MJ. Continuous monitoring of skin temperature using a liquid-crystal thermometer during anesthesia. *South Med J* 1978;**71**:516–8.
25. Ikeda T, Sessler DI, Marder D, Xiong J. The influence of thermoregulatory vasomotion and ambient temperature variation on the accuracy of core-temperature estimates by cutaneous liquid-crystal thermometers. *Anesthesiology* 1997;**86**:603–12.
26. Lodha R, Mukerji N, Sinha N, Pandey RM, Jain Y. Is axillary termpeature an appropriate surrogate for core temperature? *Indian J Pediatr* 2000;**67**:571–4.
27. Frank SM, Nguyen JM, Garcia CM, et al. Temperature monitoring practices during regional anesthesia. *Anesth Analg* 1999;**88**:373–7.
28. American Society of Anesthesiologists. *Standards for Basic Anesthetic Monitoring.* Park Ridge, IL: ASA, 2005.
29. Arkillic CF, Akca O, Taguchi A et al. Temperature monitoring and management during neuraxial anesthesia: an observational study. *Anesth Analg* 2000;**91**:662–6.

30. Matsukawa T, Sessler DI, Sessler AM, et al. Heat flow and distribution during induction of general anesthesia. *Anesthesiology* 1987;**82**:662–73.

31. Matsukawa T, Sessler DI, Christensen R, et al. Heat flow and distribution during epidural anesthesia. *Anesthesiology* 1995;**14**:181–6.

32. Torossian A. Thermal management during anaesthesia and thermoregulation standards for the prevention of inadvertent perioperative hypothermia. *Best Pract Res Clin Anaesthesiol* 2008;**22**(4):659–68.

33. Fry DE. Surgical site infections and the Surgical Care Improvement Project (SCIP): evolution of national quality measures. *Surg Infect (Larchmt)* 2008;**9**(6):579–84.

34. Wallace CT, Marks WE Jr, Adkins WY, Mahaffey JE. Perforation of the tympanic membrane, a complication of tympanic thermometry during anesthesia. *Anesthesiology* 1974;**41**(3):290–1.

35. James RH. An unusual complication of passing a narrow bore nasogastric tube. *Anaesthesia* 1978 Sep;**33**(8):716–8.

36. Frank JD, Brown S. Thermometers and rectal perforations in the neonate. *Arch Dis Child* 1978;**53**(10):824–5.

37. Sinha PK, Kaushik S, Neema PK. Massive epistaxis after nasopharyngeal temperature probe insertion after cardiac surgery. *J Cardiothorac Vasc Anesth* 2004;**18**(1):123–4.

38. Parker EO. Electrosurgical burn at the site of an esophageal temperature probe. *Anesthesiology* 1984; **61**:93–5.

39. Abelha FJ, Castro MA, Neves AM, Landeiro NM, Santos CC. Hypothermia in a surgical intensive care unit. *BMC Anesthesiol* 2005;**5**:7.

40. Reynolds L, Beckmann J, Kurz A. Perioperative complications of hypothermia. *Best Pract Res Clin Anaesthesiol* 2008;**22**(4):645–57.

41. Rajagopalan S, Mascha E, Na J, Sessler DI. The effects of mild perioperative hypothermia on blood loss and transfusion requirement. *Anesthesiology* 2008;**108**(1):71–7

42. Frank SM, Fleisher LA, Breslow MJ, et al. Perioperative maintenance of normothermia reduces the incidence of morbid cardiac events. A randomized clinical trial. *JAMA* 1997;**277**(14):1127–34.

43. Kurz A, Sessler DI, Lenhardt R. Perioperative normothermia to reduce the incidence of surgical-wound infection and shorten hospitalization. Study of Wound Infection and Temperature Group. *N Engl J Med* 1996;**334**(19):1209–15.

44. Melling AC, Ali B, Scott EM, Leaper DJ. Effects of preoperative warming on the incidence of wound infection after clean surgery: a randomised controlled trial. *Lancet* 2001;**358**(9285): 876–80.

45. Kurz A, Sessler DI, Narzt E, et al. Postoperative hemodynamic and thermoregulatory consequences of intraoperative core hypothermia. *J Clin Anesth* 1995;**7**(5):359–66.

46. Lenhardt R, Marker E, Goll V, et al. Mild intraoperative hypothermia prolongs postanesthetic recovery. *Anesthesiology* 1997;**87**(6):1318–23.

47. Holzer M, Behringer W. Therapeutic hypothermia after cardiac arrest and myocardial infarction. *Best Pract Res Clin Anaesthesiol* 2008;**22**(4):711–28.

48. Rees K, Beranek-Stanley M, Burke M, Ebrahim S. Hypothermia to reduce neurological damage following coronary artery bypass surgery. *Cochrane Database Syst Rev* 2001;**1**:CD002138.

49. Ali SZ, Taguchi A, Rosenberg H. Malignant hyperthermia. *Best Pract Res Clin Anaesthesiol* 2003;**17**(4):519–33.

50. Campos JM, Paniagua P. Hypothermia during cardiac surgery. *Best Pract Res Clin Anaesthesiol* 2008;**22**(4):695–709.

51. Lenhardt R, Grady M, Kurz A. Hyperthermia during anaesthesia and intensive care unit stay. *Best Pract Res Clin Anaesthesiol* 2008;**22**(4):669–94.

52. Axelrod YK, Diringer MN. Temperature management in acute neurologic disorders. *Neurol Clin* 2008;**26**(2):585–603.

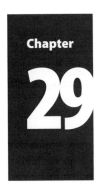

Fetal heart rate monitoring

Howard H. Bernstein

Introduction

Human birth is a normal physiologic process, with the goal of the birth of a beautiful and healthy child. Although labor usually progresses uneventfully, risks to both mother and fetus exist. Until the fourth decade of the 20th century, intrapartum maternal and fetal mortality in the United States and Europe was very common.[1,2] Fetal bradycardia with uterine contractions was first reported in 1822.[3]

Fetal monitoring, first by intermittent auscultation and later by continuous electronic monitoring, was developed with the hope of reducing the risk of fetal anoxic injury and death. It is important for the obstetric anesthesiologist to have an understanding of the physiology and terminology of fetal heart rate monitoring to communicate with our obstetrical colleagues when the assurance of fetal well-being is lost.

Oxygen delivery

The normal fetal umbilical venous and arterial partial pressures of oxygen are about 30 and 11 mmHg, respectively.[4] The fetus is adapted to maintain oxygen delivery at or above metabolic needs despite a low fetal PO_2 owing to several adaptive mechanisms. The fetus maintains a high cardiac output,

about 300 mL/kg/min, which is about four times that of the resting adult. The high cardiac output is the result, in part, of a high resting heart rate, 110 to 160 beats per minute (bpm) and to the fetal circulation. In contrast to the adult circulation, the fetal systemic and pulmonary circulations run in parallel, with a high pulmonary resistance and a low systemic resistance (Figure 29.1). This maintains right-to-left shunts, via the patent foramen ovale and the ductus arteriosus, allowing the majority of the returning systemic venous flow to bypass the pulmonary circulation. Although mixing occurs in the right atrium, the highly oxygenated blood returning through the inferior vena cava is preferentially shunted through the foramen ovale to the left ventricle, supplying the coronary and cerebral circulations. In contrast, the deoxygenated blood returning from the superior vena cava is shunted through the ductus arteriosus to the proximal descending aorta.[5]

Fetal hemoglobin also plays an important adaptive role (Figure 29.2). Normal fetal hemoglobin concentration is 20 gm%, compared with the normal 12 gm% of adult hemoglobin found in adults. In addition to the differences in hemoglobin concentrations, there are physiologic differences between adult and fetal hemoglobin. Because oxygen is more tightly bound to fetal hemoglobin than to adult hemoglobin,

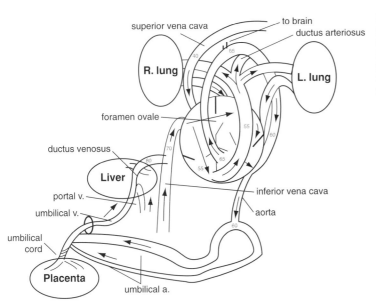

Figure 29.1. Fetal circulation with oxygen saturation. The blood with the highest oxygen saturation is shunted across the patent foramen ovale to the left ventricle, aorta, coronary, and cerebral circulations. The less oxygenated venous blood from the superior vena cava passes through the tricuspid valve to the right ventricle and pulmonary artery and shunted across the patent ductus arteriosis to the aorta, distal to the brachiocephalic vessels.

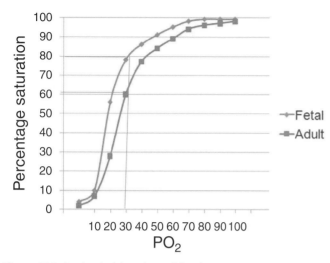

Figure 29.2. Fetal and adult oxyhemoglobin dissociation curve. At normal fetal PaO₂, 30 mmHg, oxygen saturation is 80%, whereas adult hemoglobin has a much lower saturation.

the fetal oxyhemoglobin dissociation curve is shifted to the left. At any given PaO₂, fetal hemoglobin has a higher oxygen saturation and content than adult hemoglobin. In addition, fetal hemoglobin more easily releases oxygen at the capillary bed, as fetal capillary pO₂ lies on the steep portion of the oxyhemoglobin dissociation curve.

Control of the fetal heart rate

The fetal heart rate is under autonomic control. Clinical evidence of fetal autonomic nerves is seen by 17 weeks gestational age. Rapid development of parasympathetic nerves occurs in the 18th week of gestation; sympathetic nerves begin to develop during the 20th week of gestation, increase rapidly between the 26th and 30th weeks, and slow down by the 32nd week.[6] Mean fetal heart rate slows during gestation from 175 bpm at nine weeks to about 140 bpm at the end of a normal pregnancy.[7,8] In normoxemic fetal sheep, vagal blockade with atropine results in tachycardia, and β-blockade with propranolol results in bradycardia.[9]

Fetal heart rates are not constant but rather vary over time and may be characterized by their variability and by the presence of accelerations.[10] Normal variability, also referred to as moderate variability, is defined as fluctuations in fetal heart rate of between 6 and 25 bpm. Accelerations are defined as an increase of heart rate of at least 15 bpm, acceleration duration should be between 15 seconds and 2 minutes (Figure 29.3).[10]

Normal fetal heart rate variability is caused by the influence of both parasympathetic (cardioinhibitory) and β-sympathetic (cardioacceleratory) neuronal inputs. Variability is under parasympathetic control, and accelerations are under sympathetic control.[11] Administration of atropine to fetal lambs with a normal pattern of variability results in loss of variability with the maintenance of accelerations. Subsequent administration of propranolol leads to loss of the accelerations and a slowing

of the heart rate. In addition, cortical input will affect fetal heart rate variability.[12] Cerebral ischemia may result in a loss of fetal heart rate variability. Although there is significant autonomic contribution to the control of the fetal heart rate and variability, parasympathetic and sympathetic blockade results in a 60 percent to 65 percent decrease in fetal heart variability.[13] Prostaglandins and triiodothyronine may contribute to this nonneural component of heart rate variability.[14]

The degree of fetal heart rate variability and the presence of accelerations are dependent on gestational age and fetal behavioral state, active or inactive. The active behavioral state is characterized by continuous eye movement and frequent bursts of somatic movement. Inactive or quiet sleep state is characterized by absent eye and somatic movement. Alteration between active and inactive behavioral states has been identified from 23 weeks of gestation onward.[15]

Prior to 30 weeks, the baseline fetal heart rate is similar for both active and inactive behavioral states, showing minimal variability and few accelerations with movement. After 30 weeks gestation, there is a significant reduction in baseline variability during the inactive state and increased variability during the active state (Figure 29.4).[9] In the mature fetus there is cycling between quiet and active states over 100-minute periods. Quiet states, with minimal variability and absence of accelerations, can last up to 40 minutes.[9,15] After 30 weeks, the frequency of fetal heart rate accelerations with movement increases.[9] By term, a sustained fetal tachycardia may occur when the active state is accompanied with bursts of continuous fetal movement.[15]

Fetal heart rate response to mild to moderate hypoxemia

Fetal sheep exposure to mild to moderate hypoxemia (PaO₂ 11–13 mmHg) triggers an adaptive response characterized by mild bradycardia, increased variability, increased vascular resistance, and hypertension; cardiac output is maintained but is redistributed to the brain, adrenal gland, and heart, with a decrease to peripheral organs, lung, muscle, and skin.[9,16–18] The initial fall in fetal heart rate and increase in variability is the result of an increase in cardiac vagal tone. After carotid sinus ablation, the bradycardic response to hypoxemia is lost; pretreatment with atropine abolishes the increase in variability and leads to an increase in the fetal heart rate.[19,20]

The rise in blood pressure in response to hypoxemia is under α-adrenergic control. During fetal hypoxemia, α-adrenergic blockade abolishes the rise in fetal blood pressure.[20] During mild to moderate hypoxemia, a rise in norepinephrine concentrations occurs. β-blockade of hypoxemic fetuses does not affect variability and enhanced the degree of bradycardia, implying a selective increase in sympathoadrenal tone – that is, increased adrenomedullary secretion of catecholamines. The increase in catecholamine secretion maintains fetal cardiac output and redistributes cardiac output, thus offsetting the opposing effects of increased cardiac vagal tone.[19] In chemically

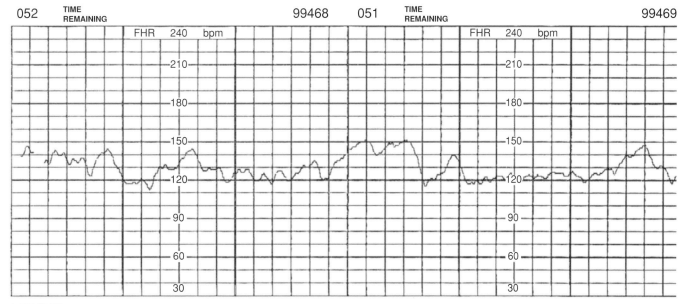

1 87 P 60

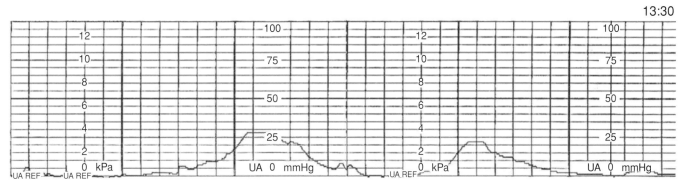

Figure 29.3. Normal fetal heart rate tracing. The top curve represents the fetal heart rate and the bottom curve represents uterine tone. Moderate variability with accelerations.

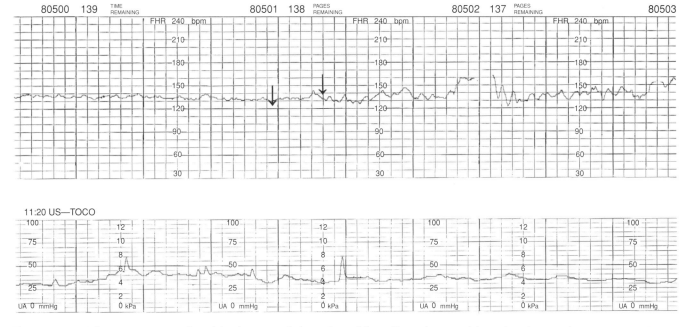

Figure 29.4. FHR demonstrating minimal variability during quiet behavioral state followed by moderate variability and accelerations during active state. Arrow marks area of change between quiet and active states.

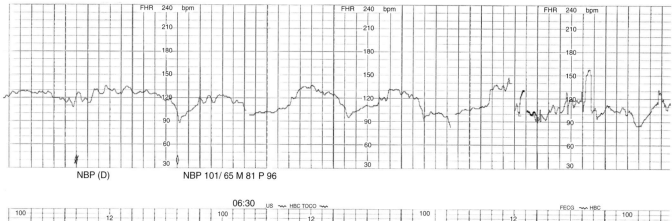

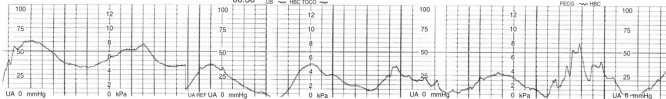

Figure 29.5. Recurrent late decelerations.

sympathectomized animals, hypoxemia led to hypotension and redistribution of the cardiac output to the muscle and intestinal organs, with decreased circulation to the brain and heart.[16]

Fetal heart rate response to phasic hypoxemia: late decelerations

The uterine vein and artery are compressed within the myometrium during a contraction, leading to a transient decrease in uterine blood flow.[21] This leads to a gradual decline in fetal PaO_2, with a gradual return to baseline after the contraction. A fall in fetal PaO_2 will result in a fetal heart rate deceleration, only when fetal PaO_2 falls below a threshold value. In experimental models employing normoxemic or chronically hypoxemic lambs, a fall below the threshold PaO_2 value resulted in a gradual delayed decline in fetal heart rate.[22,23] The decline in fetal heart rate began 20 seconds after the insult and reached its nadir after 30 seconds. This similar pattern of late decelerations is seen in humans (Figure 29.5).

Late decelerations in the normoxemic fetus are the result of a chemoreceptor-mediated reflex. Itskovitz and colleagues induced acute fetal hypoxemia in sheep by inflating a balloon in the maternal descending aorta.[23] This model produced a decline in fetal PaO_2 without the development of fetal acidemia. During hypoxemia, the fetal sheep had a delayed fall in fetal heart rate that gradually returned to baseline. There were no significant changes in fetal blood pressure. If the fetal lambs were premedicated with atropine, a delayed heart rate acceleration was observed instead of the late deceleration, implying a vagal-mediated reflex. The reflex is chemoreceptor-mediated, as it is abolished or altered after denervation of the aortic and carotid chemoreceptors.[23-25] In humans, moderate fetal heart rate variability will be maintained in the presence of late decelerations with normal fetal pH (Figure 29.6).

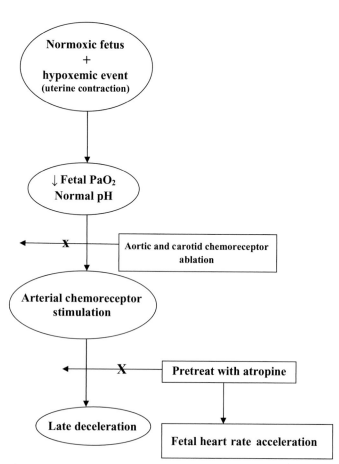

Figure 29.6. Mechanism of late decelerations: normoxic, nonacidemic fetus. Contraction leads to decreased uterine blood flow and a decline in fetal PaO_2 below threshold level, resulting in arterial chemoreceptor stimulation, increase in vagal tone, and a late deceleration. **X** = step blocked.

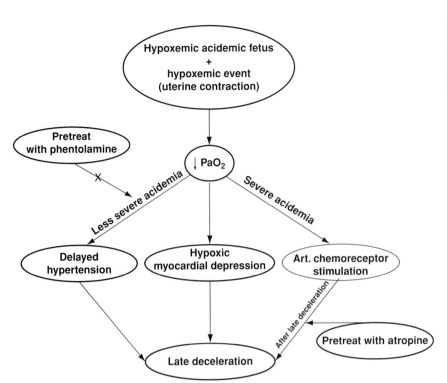

Figure 29.7. *Mechanism of late decelerations: chronically hypoxemic, acidemic fetus. Baroreceptor- and arterial chemoreceptor-mediated vagal response. Late deceleration altered but not eliminated by pretreatment with atropine and phentolamine, implying hypoxic myocardial depression.*

In an experimental model of chronically hypoxemic animals, an abrupt decrease in uterine blood flow led to a delayed fetal bradycardia and a late increase in fetal blood pressure.[23] Pretreatment with atropine altered but did not abolish the bradycardic response. Pretreatment with phentolamine abolished or reduced the hypertensive response and altered the bradycardic response; these findings implied catecholamine release as the mechanism for the fetal hypertensive response. Harris and associates[22] also noted that the deceleration was modified but not eliminated after pretreatment with atropine in the chronically hypoxemic fetus. In their study, they did not see a hypertensive response to hypoxemia, possibly because of more severe acidosis, lower pH, and base excess of their animals. They also noted a significant decline in myocardial oxygen consumption. In the presence of chronic fetal hypoxemia, an acute decrease in uterine blood flow, with resultant lowering of fetal PaO_2 and fetal pH, leads to late decelerations via an arterial chemoreceptor–vagal pathway and hypoxic myocardial depression (Figure 29.7).

Sinusoidal pattern

On rare occasions, the fetal heart rate tracing will present as repetitive sine waves, with absent variability. This may be observed with severe fetal anemia owing to Rh sensitization, feto–maternal transfusion, or in utero fetal hemorrhage, leading to fetal hypoxia with increased perinatal morbidity and mortality.[26,27] However, a sinusoidal pattern may also be seen with the administration of meperidine and butorphanol.[28,29] The etiology of the sine wave pattern is not understood (Figure 29.8).

Fetal heart rate variability

The persistent absence of fetal heart rate variability may be caused by severe fetal asphyxia and acidosis. Loss of variability is often preceded by the development of late decelerations of the fetal heart rate.[30] The presence of recurrent late decelerations in association with absent variability may be indicative of severe fetal acidosis (pH < 7.20) and a base deficit >15 mEq/L[6] There is a normal cyclic variation in fetal heart rate variability lasting 30 to 40 minutes and occurring every 1.5 to 2 hours; sufficient observation time must be allowed before deciding that fetal hypoxemia exists. In addition, fetal scalp stimulation leading to an acceleration lasting at least 15 seconds with a peak rise of at least 15 bpm over baseline is associated with a scalp pH of at least 7.20.[31,32] Causes of decreased fetal heart rate variability may include maternal narcotic and benzodiazepine administration, maternal β-blocker administration, fetal anencephaly, and fetal congenital heart block (Table 29.1).

Variable decelerations

A variable deceleration is characterized by a sudden drop in fetal heart rate, which nadirs in less than 30 seconds with no relation to the peak of the contraction (see Figure 29.9). Variable decelerations occur after umbilical cord and fetal head compressions.[33] The etiology of the decrease in heart rate is both chemo- and baroreceptor-mediated. In the exteriorized fetal goat, Barcroft demonstrated a profound rapid decrease in fetal heart rate with occlusion of the umbilical cord.[34] After vagal interruption, the bradycardic response to cord occlusion was delayed but not lost, implying a vagal efferent pathway.[35]

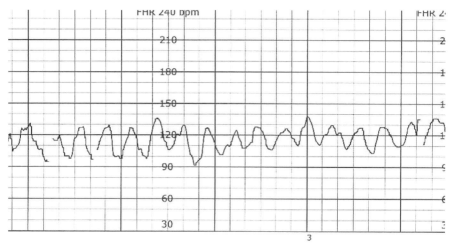

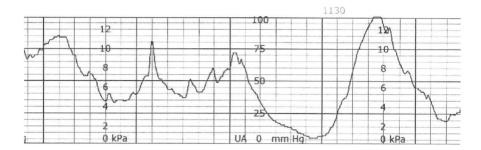

Figure 29.8. Sinusoidal fetal heart rate pattern. Notice the sine wave fetal heart pattern with absent variability. This may be the result of maternal administration of butorphanol or meperidine, but has been associated with severe fetal anemia and acidosis. This child developed severe hypoxemia and acidemia. Apgar score was 1 at one minute and 3 at five minutes. Severe hypoxic ischemic brain injury developed.

Cord occlusion has been shown to cause an acute rise in fetal blood pressure, possibly initiating a baroreceptor-mediated vagal response.[36]

Bennet and associates[37] evaluated the effect of total cord occlusion on the fetal heart rate. They studied two groups of animals, group 1 with a one-minute occlusion every five minutes and group 2 with a one-minute occlusion every 2.5 minutes. In both groups, umbilical cord occlusion was associated with an immediate rapid fall in fetal heart rate – a variable deceleration. In group 1, a sustained rise in fetal blood pressure occurred after the beginning of the deceleration, reaching its peak concomitant with the nadir of the fetal heart rate deceleration; there were minimal changes in pH. In contrast, the animals in group 2 also developed an initial hypertensive response, but with repeated cord occlusion they developed severe hypotension and metabolic acidemia. These data suggest an initial

baroreceptor-mediated reflex with a vagal efferent limb with the development of hypoxic myocardial depression as hypoxemia worsens and severe acidemia develops (Figure 29.10).

In clinical practice, mild to moderate variable decelerations are common. They are associated with the maintenance of moderate variability, normoxia, and a normal pH. In contrast, severe repetitive variable decelerations and fetal heart rate less than 90 bpm and duration of one to two minutes will lead to progressive loss of fetal heart rate variability and the development of a metabolic acidosis (Figures 29.10 and 29.11).

Early deceleration

Early decelerations are defined as a gradual decline in the fetal heart rate occurring in less than 30 seconds, with the nadir of the deceleration coinciding with the peak of the contraction. Pressure on the fetal head has been shown to result in fetal heart rate decelerations. This pressure causes an alteration in cerebral blood flow, which stimulates central nervous system vagal outflow.[38] The deceleration is blocked by atropine.[35] These early decelerations are usually not associated with fetal acidemia.[39]

Efficacy of fetal heart rate monitoring

While the goal of continuous electronic fetal monitoring was the decrease in the incidence of hypoxic brain injury and cerebral palsy (CP), this goal has not been realized. CP occurs in

---

Table 29.1. Etiology of minimal to absent fetal heart rate variability

- Cyclic changes in fetal heart rate variability: quiet cycle with decreased fetal limb and absent REM
- Fetal hypoxemia and acidemia
- Fetal congenital anomalies:
  - Anencephaly
  - Congenital heart block
- Maternal narcotic administration
- Maternal benzodiazepine administration
- Maternal β-blocker administration

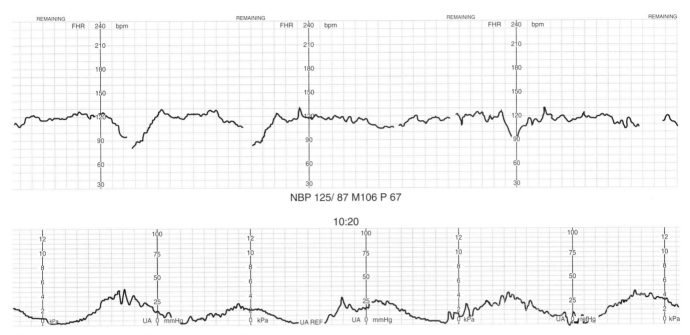

NBP 125/ 87 M106 P 67

10:20

Figure 29.9. Variable decelerations, moderate variability.

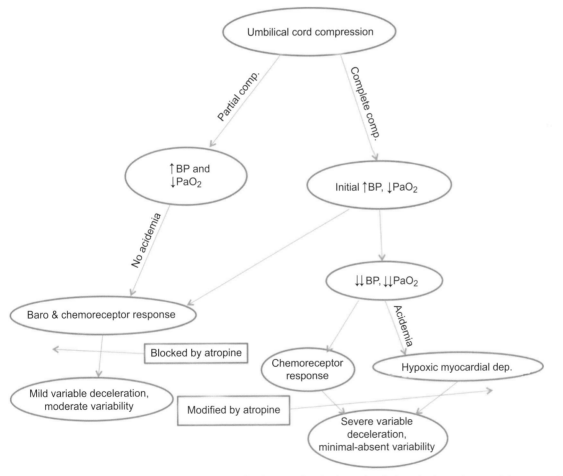

Figure 29.10. Mechanism of variable decelerations. In the absence of acidemia, cord occlusion stimulates a baro- and chemoreceptor vagal-mediated response, blocked by atropine. Frequent total cord occlusion induces severe hypoxia and acidemia. In the acidemic fetus, variable decelerations are modified but not eliminated by atropine; the deceleration is in part caused by hypoxic-induced myocardial depression.

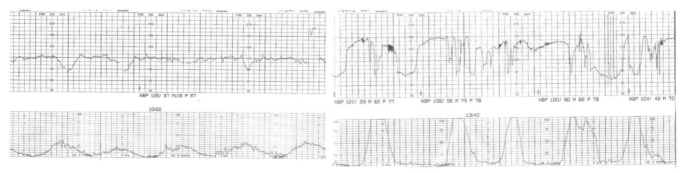

Figure 29.11. Mild and severe variable decelerations. Left panel: mild decelerations with moderate variability, normal pH. Right panel: severe variables with loss of variability and acidemia.

about 2 in 1000 live births. Multiple risk factors for the development of CP include birth asphyxia, preterm delivery, low birth weight, infection/inflammation, and multiple gestations. The proportion of CP associated with intrapartum hypoxia is only 14.5 percent.[40,41] As the majority of CP is not associated with the birth process, it is not surprising that continuous fetal monitoring has not lowered its incidence.

Despite the lack of impact on the incidence of CP, birth asphyxia, defined as a base deficit >15 mEq/L, has been associated with particular fetal heart rate patterns. Fetal tachycardia and variable and early decelerations do not distinguish between the asphyxic and the nonasphyxic fetus, as they occur at the same frequency in both groups.[42] The identification of absent fetal heart rate variability with recurrent late or prolonged decelerations during the last hour of labor may predict fetal asphyxic exposure, with a specificity of 98 percent but with a sensitivity of 17 percent; the positive predictive value was 18 percent and the negative predictive value was 98.3 percent.[42–44] Although the presence of late decelerations and decreased variability in the last hour of labor can be a useful screening test, supplementary testing is necessary to identify the large number of false-positive tests. At the present time, these tests would include either a scalp sample for pH analysis or fetal scalp stimulation. Scalp stimulation resulting in a fetal heart rate acceleration is associated with a pH of 7.19 or higher.[31,32]

Continuous versus intermittent fetal heart rate monitoring

Does continuous fetal heart rate monitoring, as opposed to intermittent monitoring, increase the probability of detecting the development of fetal hypoxia and acidemia? A study was performed randomizing women in labor with a gestational age ≥26 weeks to either continuous electronic fetal heart rate (CFHR) monitoring or intermittent auscultation (IA).[45,46] IA was performed during a contraction until 30 seconds after the end of the contraction. In the IA group, a fetal bradycardia to ≤100 bpm during and immediately after the contraction, persistent fetal heart rate baseline ≤100 bpm or persistent fetal tachycardia, or fetal heart rate ≥ 160 bpm were considered nonreassuring. In the CFHR group, late decelerations, variable decelerations, absent or minimal fetal heart rate variability, fetal tachycardia, or bradycardia were considered nonreassuring. The incidence of a nonreassuring tracing and operative delivery (cesarean section or assisted vaginal delivery) was greater in the CFHR monitored group; however, the perinatal mortality rate was higher in the IA group. The investigators concluded that the increase in perinatal morality was the result of the inability to assess variability and to detect subtle late decelerations with IA. Continuous FHR monitoring had higher sensitivity and positive and negative predictive value for detecting acidemia, compared with IA. In contrast, IA was more specific. Similar findings were found in a meta-analysis of randomized trials comparing continuous electronic fetal heart rate monitoring with IA.[47]

The American College of Obstetricians and Gynecologists (ACOG) has not come to the same conclusions. Although a higher perinatal mortality rate was detected in the IA group, this difference was based on a small number of events. If there had been one fewer perinatal death in the AI group, statistical significance would not have been met.[48] ACOG has not concluded that continuous electronic fetal monitoring has been shown to have an advantage over intermittent auscultation. In the low-risk patient, either option is deemed acceptable.[48]

Nomenclature

A large degree of inter- and intraobserver variability in the interpretation of FHR monitoring tracings has been demonstrated.[49,50] In 1997 (updated in 2008), the National Institute of Child Health and Human Development (NICHD) Research Planning Workshop published standard definitions for fetal heart rate monitoring.[10] These definitions were adopted by ACOG in 2005 and reaffirmed in 2007.[48] The definitions were developed for visual interpretation of the various fetal heart rate and contraction patterns. Definitions of the fetal heart rate patterns are summarized in Table 29.2.

A full description of the fetal heart rate tracing must include the following: (1) a quantitative description of the uterine contraction pattern; (2) baseline fetal heart rate; (3) assessment of fetal heart rate variability; (4) note on presence or absence of accelerations; (5) note on presence and type of decelerations;

Table 29.2. Definitions of FHR patterns

Baseline fetal heart rate	Mean observed FHR rounded to 5 bpm during a 10-minute window, excludes accelerations and decelerations. Normal 110 to 160 bpm at term.
Tachycardia	FHR > 160 bpm
Bradycardia	FHR < 110 bpm
Baseline FHR variability	Fluctuation in baseline FHR that is irregular in amplitude and frequency
Moderate normal variability	Amplitude range between 6 bpm and 25 bpm
Minimal variability	Amplitude range between 1 bpm and 5 bpm
Absent variability	No detectible amplitude range
FHR acceleration	Abrupt increase in heart rate, ≤30 sec to peak, peak is a rise of ≥15 bpm, with a duration of ≥15 seconds from beginning till return of baseline but <2 minutes
FHR deceleration	Decline of FHR below baseline
Late deceleration	Gradual decline in heart rate, nadir attained in ≥30 seconds, with nadir occurring after the peak of the contraction
Early deceleration	Gradual decline in heart rate, nadir attained in ≥30 seconds, with nadir coinciding with the peak of the contraction
Variable deceleration	Abrupt decline in FHR of ≥15 bpm, the nadir attained in <30 seconds
	Duration ≥15 seconds and <2 minutes
	Not necessarily related to the timing of the peak of the contraction
	Prolonged acceleration/deceleration FHR acceleration/ deceleration with a duration ≥2 minutes
Change in baseline	FHR acceleration/deceleration ≥10 minutes
Sinusoidal pattern	Smooth sine wave pattern
	Cycle frequency of 3–5/minutes
	Duration ≥20 minutes

Adapted from ref. 10.

and (6) comment on changes of the fetal heart rate tracing over time. Gestational age, fetal health, and maternal medical condition may affect the fetal heart rate tracing and must be taken into consideration when assessing fetal condition.[10] The NICHD has developed a three-tier FHR interpretive system (Table 29.3).[10]

Antepartum fetal assessment

Postdates pregnancy, intrauterine growth restriction, maternal diabetes mellitus, chronic and acute hypertension, as well as other complications of pregnancy may predispose to placental insufficiency and fetal hypoxia in the antepartum period. In the 1970s, fetal heart rate monitoring, via the oxytocin challenge test and the nonstress test, were introduced for antepartum fetal assessment. The contraction stress test, or oxytocin challenge test (OCT), consists of inducing three uterine contractions in a 20-minute window with a maternal infusion of oxytocin or via nipple stimulation.[51,52] The fetal heart rate tracing is evaluated for the presence or absence of late decelerations. The development of late decelerations in 50 percent or more of the contractions is considered a positive test, an indication for delivery. The absence of late decelerations indicates a negative test, reassuring fetal well-being. The presence of one late deceleration is nondiagnostic, and the procedure is repeated in 24 hours.[53]

The efficacy of contraction stress testing has been assessed. The false-negative rate for the OCT, defined as a fetal demise within one week, is 0.3 per 1000.[54] However, the false-positive rate is about 30 percent, with a positive predictive value of less than 35 percent, possibly leading to unnecessary induction and delivery.[55,56]

Table 29.3. FHR interpretive system

Category	Interpretation	Signs
I	Normal	• Baseline FHR 110–160 bpm • Moderate variability • No late or variable decelerations • Accelerations: present or absent • Early decelerations: present or absent
II	Indeterminate	• Unable to predict acidemia • Minimal variability • Marked variability • Absent variability: no late decelerations • No accelerations with scalp stimulation • Recurrent late decelerations with moderate variability • Prolonged deceleration ≥2 minutes and <10 minutes

III	Nonreassuring tracing	• Most predictive of acidemia
		• Absent variability in association with any of the following:
		  ○ Recurrent late deceleration
		  ○ Recurrent variable deceleration
		  ○ Bradycardia
		• Sinusoidal pattern

Adapted from ref. 10.

Table 29.4. Stillbirth rate/1000, corrected for lethal congenital anomalies and unpredictable causes of fetal demise

	NST	OCT	BPP	MBPP
Stillbirth rate	1.9 per 1000	0.3 per 1000	0.8 per 1000	0.8 per 1000

NST, nonstress test; OCT, oxytocin challenge test; BPP, full biophysical profile; MBPP, modified biophysical profile.

The nonstress test (NST) is a noninvasive method of assessing fetal well-being. The fetal heart rate is monitored by Doppler ultrasonography, and the presence of fetal heart rate accelerations is assessed. The NST is based on the association of fetal movement with acceleration in the fetal heart rate.[57] As with intrapartum FHR monitoring, an acceleration is defined as a rise above baseline of at least 15 bpm with a duration of at least 15 seconds from beginning to return to baseline. At least two accelerations in a 20-minute window is considered reassuring and is termed a reactive NST. To account for fetal quiet states, monitoring for 40 minutes may be necessary. The absence of fetal heart rate accelerations is termed a nonreactive NST, requiring further evaluation. False-positive tests are very common; 90 percent of nonreactive nonstress tests are followed by a normal OCT. The positive predictive value of a nonreactive NST is 10 percent, with a negative predictive value of 99.8 percent.[58]

The biophysical profile (BPP) consists of an NST accompanied by a fetal ultrasound evaluation assessing for fetal breathing, fetal movement, and fetal tone and determination of amniotic fluid volume. Each component is given a value of 2 if present and 0 if absent. A composite score of 10 is normal, 6 is considered equivocal, and ≤4 is abnormal. An equivocal BPP should be repeated in 24 hours. A BPP score <4 should prompt expeditious delivery; however, in the presence of severe prematurity, management should be individualized. As placental insufficiency may lead to oligohydramnios, the assessment of amniotic fluid volume, combined with a nonstress test, the modified biophysical profile (MBPP), may be used to assess fetal health. Normal amniotic fluid volume and a reactive NST are considered a reassuring, normal test. A nonreactive NST and/or decreased amniotic fluid volume are considered abnormal. As with other antepartum tests, the MBPP is associated with a high false-positive rate, 60 percent, requiring further testing with a full BPP.[59] The stillbirth rate for the normal BPP and modified BPP is 0.8/1000. The negative predictive value for the OCT, BPP, and MBPP is greater than 99.9 percent (Table 29.4).[58]

Summary

Fetal heart rate monitoring was developed with the hope of reducing the incidence of intrapartum fetal hypoxic brain injury and cerebral palsy. This goal was not accomplished, as most injuries leading to cerebral palsy occur in the antepartum period. Intrapartum monitoring is associated with a very low false-negative rate, but with a high false-positive rate. Even the most concerning pattern associated with hypoxia and acidemia,

late decelerations and loss of variability, has a positive predictive value of only 17 percent, leading to many unnecessary interventions, including forceps and cesarean delivery. Decisions regarding the management of a nonreassuring pattern must therefore also take the maternal and fetal history into consideration.

References

1. Loudon I. Maternal mortality in the past and its relevance to developing countries today. *Am J Clin Nutr* 2000;**72**(suppl): 241S–246S.
2. Woods, R. Long-term trends in fetal mortality: implications for developing countries. *Bull World Health Org, Geneva*, 2008; **86**(6):460–466.
3. De Kegaradec L. *Memoire sur l'auscultation appliqué de la grossesse*. Paris, 1822.
4. Wulf KH, Kunzel W, Lehmann V. Clinical aspects of placental gas exchange. In Longo LD, Bartels H, eds. *Respiratory Gas Exchange and Blood Flow in the Placenta*. Washington, DC: DHEW Publications, National Institute of Health, 1972.
5. Martin CB Jr. Normal fetal physiology and behavior, and adaptive responses with hypoxemia. *Semin Perinatol* 2008;**32**:239–242.
6. Ohta T, Okamura K, Kimura Y, Suzuki T, et al. Alteration in the low-frequency domain in power spectral analysis of fetal heart beat fluctuations. *Fetal Diagn Ther* 1999;**14**:92–97.
7. van Lith JM, Visser GH, Mantingh A, Beekhuis JR. Fetal heart rate in early pregnancy and chromosomal disorders. *Br J Obstet Gynaecol* 1992;**99**:741–4.
8. Pillai M, James D. The development of fetal heart rate patterns during normal pregnancy. *Am J Obstet Gynecol* 1990;**76**:812–6.
9. Yu Z, Lumbers R, Gibson KJ, Stevens AD. Effects of hypoxaemia on foetal heart rate, variability and cardiac rhythm. *Clin Exp Pharmacol Physiol* 1998;**25**:577–84.
10. Macones GA, Hankins GDV, Spong CY, Hauth J, Moore T. The 2008 National Institute of Child Health and Human Development Workshop Report on Electronic Fetal Monitoring. *Obstet Gynecol* 2008;**112**:661–66.
11. Renou P, Newman W, Wood C. Autonomic control of fetal heart rate. *Am J Obstet Gynecol* 1969;**105**:949–53.
12. Walker AM, de Preu ND, Horne RS, Berger PJ. Autonomic control of heart rate differs with electrocortical activity and chronic hypoxaemia in fetal lambs. *Dev Physiol* 1990;**14**:43–8.
13. Dalton KJ, Dawes GS, Patgrick JE. The autonomic nervous system and fetal heart rate variability. *Am J Obstet Gynecol* 1983;**146**:456–62.
14. Papp JG. Autonomic responses and neurohumoral control in the human early antenatal heart. *Basic Res Cardiol* 1988;**83**:2–9.
15. Pillai M, James D. Behavioral states in normal mature human fetuses. *Arch Dis Child* 1990;**65**:39–43.
16. Jensen A, Lang U. Foetal circulatory responses to arrest of uterine blood flow in sheep: effects of chemical sympathectomy. *J Dev Physiol* 1992;**17**:75–86.
17. Jensen A, Hohmann M, Kunzel W. Dynamic changes in organ blood flow and oxygen consumption during acute asphyxia in fetal sheep. *J Dev Physiol* 1987;**9**:543–59.
18. Jensen A, Roman C, Rudolph AM. Effects of reducing uterine blood flow on fetal blood flow distribution and oxygen delivery. *J Dev Physiol* 1991;**15**:309–23.
19. Giussani DA, McGarrigle HH, Spencer JA, et al. Effect of carotid denervation on plasma vasopressin levels during acute hypoxia in the late-gestation fetal sheep. *J Physiol* 1994;**477**:81–87.

20. Lewis AB, Donovan M, Platzker AC. Cardiovascular responses to autonomic blockade in hypoxemic fetal lambs. *Biol Neonate* 1980;**37**:233–42.

21. Greiss FC. Concepts of uterine blood flow in vivo. In *Obstetrics and Gynecology Annual*. New York: Appleton-Century-Crofts, 1973, pp. 55–83.

22. Harris JL, Krueger TR, Parer JT. Mechanisms of late decelerations of the fetal heart rate during hypoxia. *Am J Obstet Gynecol* 1982;**144**:491–96.

23. Itskovitz J, Goetzman BW, Rudolph AM. The mechanism of late deceleration of the heart rate and its relationship to oxygenation in normoxemic and chronically hypoxemic fetal lambs. *Am J Obstet Gynecol* 1982;**142**:66–73.

24. Giussani DA, Spencer JA, Moore PJ, et al. Afferent and efferent components of the cardiovascular reflex responses to acute hypoxia in term fetal sheep. *J Physiol* 1993;**461**:431–49.

25. Itskovitz J, LaGamma EF, Bristow J, Rudolph AM. Cardiovascular responses to hypoxemia in sinoaortic-denervated fetal sheep. *Pediatr Res* 1991;**30**:381–5.

26. Shenker L. Clinical experience with fetal heart rate monitoring of 1000 patients in labor. *Am J Obstet Gynecol* 1973;**115**:1111–6.

27. Rosenn B, Chetrit A, Palti Z, Hurwitz A. Sinusoidal fetal heart rate pattern due to massive feto-maternal transfusion. *Int J Gynecol Obstet* 1990;**31**:271–73.

28. Epstein H, Waxman A, Gleicher N, et al. Meperidine-induced sinusoidal fetal heart rate pattern and reversal with naloxone. *Obstet Gynecol* 1982;**59**:22S–25S.

29. Angel J, Knuppel R, Lake M. Sinusoidal fetal heart rate patterns associated with intravenous butorphanol administration. *Am J Obstet Gynecol* 1984;**149**: 465–7.

30. Paul RH, Suidan AK, Yeh SY, et al. Clinical fetal monitoring VII. The evaluation and significance of intrapartum baseline FHR variability. *Am J Obstet Gynecol* 1975;**123**:206–10.

31. Clark S, Gimovsky M, Miller FC. Fetal heart rate response to scalp blood sampling. *Am J Obstet Gynecol* **144**;706–8.

32. Clark SL, Gimovsky ML, Miller FC. The scalp stimulation test: a clinical alternative to fetal scalp blood sampling. *Am J Obstet Gynecol* 1984;**148**:274–7.

33. Ball RH, Parer JT. The physiologic mechanisms of variable decelerations. *Am J Obstet Gynecol* 1992;**166**:1683–8.

34. Barcroft J. *Researches on Prenatal Life*. Oxford: Blackwell Scientific Publications, 1946.

35. Hon EH, Bradfield AH, Hess OW. The electronic evaluation of the fetal heart rate. V. The vagal factor in fetal bradycardia. *Am J Obstet Gynecol* 1961;**82**:291–300.

36. Lee ST, Hon EH. Fetal hemodynamic response to umbilical cord compression. *Obstet Gynecol* 1964;**22**:553–62.

37. Bennet L, Westgate JA, Liu Y-C, et al. Fetal acidosis and hypotension during repeated umbilical cord occlusions are associated with enhanced chemoreflex responses in near-term sheep. *J Appl Physiol* 2005;**99**:1477–82.

38. Paul WM, Quilligan EJ, MacLachlan T. Cardiovascular phenomenon associated with fetal head compression. *Am J Obstet Gynecol* 1964;**90**: 824–6.

39. Kubli FW, Hon EH, Khazin AF, et al. Observations on heart rate and pH in the human fetus during labor. *Am J Obstet Gynecol* 1969;**104**:1190–206.

40. Graham EM, Ruis KA, Hartman AL, et al. A systematic review of the role of intrapartum hypoxia-ischemia in the causation of neonatal encephalopathy. *Am J Obstet Gynecol* 2008;**199**:587–95.

41. Clark SM, Ghulmiyyah LM, Hankins GD. Antenatal antecedents and the impact of obstetric care in the etiology of cerebral palsy. *Clin Obstet Gynecol* 2008;**51**:775–86.

42. Low JA, Victory R, Derrick EJ. Predictive value of electronic fetal monitoring for intrapartum fetal asphyxia with metabolic acidosis. *Obstet Gynecol* 1999;**93**:285–91.

43. Larma JD, Silva AM, Holcroft CJ, et al. Intrapartum electronic fetal heart rate monitoring and the identification of metabolic acidosis and hypoxic-ischemic encephalopathy. *Am J Obstet Gynecol* 2007;**197**:301.e1–301.e8.

44. Sameshima H, Ikenoue T. Predictive value of late decelerations for fetal acidemia in unselective low-risk pregnancies. *Am J Perinat* 2005;**22**:19–23.

45. Vintzileos AM, Nochimson GJ, Antsaklis A, et al. Comparison of intrapartum electronic fetal heart rate monitoring versus intermittent auscultation in detecting fetal acidemia at birth. *Am J Obstet Gynecol* 1995;**173**:1021–4.

46. Vintzileos AM, Antsaklis A, Varvarigos I, et al. A randomized trial of intrapartum electronic fetal heart rate monitoring versus intermittent auscultation. *Obstet Gynecol* 1993;**81**:899–907.

47. Vintzileos AM, Nochimson DJ, Guzman ER, et al. Intrapartum electronic fetal heart rate monitoring versus intermittent auscultation: a meta-analysis. *Obstet Gynecol* 2005;**85**: 149–55.

48. American College of Obstetricians and Gynecologists. *Intrapartum Fetal Heart Rate Monitoring*. ACOG Practice Bulletin No. 70. Washington, DC: American College of Obstetricians and Gynecologists, 2005, reconfirmed 2007.

49. Nielson PV, Stigsby B, Neckelsen C, Nim J. Intra- and inter-observer variability in the assessment of intrapartum cardiotocograms. *Acta Obstet Gynecol Scand* 1987;**66**:421–4.

50. Beaulieu MD, Fabia J, Leduc B, et al. The reproducibility of intrapartum cardiotocogram assessments. *Can Med Assoc J* 1982;**127**:214–6.

51. Capeless EL, Mann LI. Use of breast stimulation for antepartum stress testing. *Obstet Gynecol* 1984;**64**:641–5.

52. Palmer SM, Martin JN, Moreland ML, et al. Contraction stress test by nipple stimulation: efficacy and safety. *South Med J* 1986;**79**:1102–5.

53. Ray M, Freeman RK, Pine S, et al. Clinical experience with the oxytocin challenge test. *Am J Obstet Gynecol* 1972;**114**:1–9.

54. Freeman RK, Anderson G, Dorchester W. A prospective multi-institutional study of antepartum fetal heart rate monitoring. I. Risk of perinatal mortality and morbidity according to antepartum fetal heart rate test results. *Am J Obstet Gynecol* 1982;**143**:771–7.

55. Lagrew DC. The contraction stress test. *Clin Obstet Gynecol* 1995;**38**:11–25.

56. Staisch KJ, Westlake JR, Bashore RA. Blind oxytocin challenge test and perinatal outcome. *Am J Obstet Gynecol* 1980;**138**:399–403.

57. Rochard F, Schilfrin BS, Goupil F, et al. Nonstressed fetal heart rate monitoring in the antepartum period. *Am J Obstet Gynecol* 1976;**1126**:699–706.

58. American College of Obstetricians and Gynecologists. *Antepartum Fetal Surveillance*. ACOG Practice Bulletin No. 9. Washington, DC: American College of Obstetricians and Gynecologists, 1999, reconfirmed 2009.

59. Everston LR, Gauthier RJ, Schfrin BS, et al. Antepartrum fetal heart rate testing. I. Evolution of the nonstress test. *Am J Obstet Gynecol* 1979;**133**:29–33.

Pain scales

Jonathan Epstein, Diana Mungall, and Yaakov Beilin

Introduction

Pain, because of its subjective nature, is difficult for clinicians to quantify. Studies have demonstrated that when caregivers and/or family members are asked to assess patient pain, both groups tend to underestimate severe pain.[1,2] Accordingly, self-report is the gold standard for pain assessment. This quantification becomes necessary for health care providers to assess the efficacy of our interventions and to determine choices of therapy. Although numerous scales are currently employed to assess intensity and quality of pain, it is unclear which scale provides the most information in the least obtrusive manner.[3–5] Given the nature of our reliance on self-reporting, an ideal test would be both valid – measuring that which it purports to measure; and reliable – consistently performing its intended function free from errors in measurement.

The pain scales can be broken down into two distinct groups: the unidimensional group and the comprehensive group. The unidimensional group seeks to quantify the intensity of pain via a single number, or score. However, as a complex synthesis of emotional, physiologic, and behavioral factors, pain does not always lend itself to being reduced to a single digit or score. This is especially true when considering how many variables can factor into any given score at any given time. Jensen and associates pointed out that a pain scale will always be influenced by setting, fear, fatigue, and assorted motivational factors.[6] The comprehensive group seeks a more thorough evaluation of pain via sensory and behavioral components that cannot be obtained from a single number or score.

However, in an acute clinical situation, completing a protracted survey of a patient's pain is inefficient and may be cruel. Therefore, unidimensional scales are more commonly used. To date, there is little convincing data that any one of the existing unidimensional scales is preferable to another.[7] All appear to validly and reliably measure the intensity of a patient's pain. The clinician must therefore choose the scale that provides the most information with the greatest ease to the patient and the clinician. A scale useful for one particular clinical scenario may not be useful in another.

Accordingly, a thorough familiarity with the major pain scales is warranted. We consider five easily administered unidimensional scales: the Visual Analog Scale (VAS), the Verbal Rating Scale (VRS), the Numerical Rating Scale (NRS), the 11-point Box Scale (BS-11), and the face scales. These scales were chosen because they typify the verbal and visual cue-oriented pain scales. These five commonly used scales all allow for a patient's intensity of pain to be rated in a noninvasive, easily collected measure.

We also consider the McGill Pain Questionnaire (MPQ), a more comprehensive measurement designed to better assess the pain experience. By incorporating cognitive dimensions into the overall assessment of pain, sensory and affective components can be taken into account.[8,9]

The Visual Analog Scale

The VAS consists of a 10-cm-long line with each end labeled with descriptors representing extremes in pain intensity (Figure 30.1). The patient places a mark on the line that best approximates his or her level of pain. The distance from 0 to100 in millimeters or 0 to 10 in centimeters is considered the pain score. For ease of discussion, the unit of measurement, millimeters or centimeters, is usually omitted. The VAS has been tried in both horizontal and vertical orientations with similar observed validity.[7,10,11] The VAS has also been administered with and without the use of previously obtained scores as a reference point, with little observed influence. When serial scores were obtained, it did not to matter whether the patient had access to the initial pain score, the implication being that when administering the test it should be unnecessary to show the patient the initial score as a frame of reference.[12]

Given this measure's well-established validity, ease of use, and minimally invasive nature, it is frequently the instrument of choice for gauging pain intensity, especially in research studies.[2] A major strength of the VAS is that it correlates well with the other unidimensional indexes of pain, including both verbal and numeric scales.[5] Additionally, the test's relative

No pain _____ Worst Imaginable Pain

Figure 30.1. Typical 100-mm Visual Analog Scale with each end anchored with descriptors that represent extremes of pain.

0	1	2	3	4	5	6	7	8	9	10

Figure 30.2. The Box Score-11 scale.

proportionality allows the clinician to compare scores from different times in treatment.

However, there is evidence that suggests that certain groups of patients have difficulty completing or understanding how to use the VAS scale. The elderly population, in particular, may be more prone to errors with the VAS than the adult population at large.[13] It has also presented difficulty for patients with perceptual-motor problems.[14,15] In this population it may be better to use verbal scales rather than one the patient has to mark.

A study by Bodian and coworkers[12] addressed how to best interpret VAS scores in a clinically meaningful manner. Patients undergoing abdominal surgery were asked to complete a VAS the morning after abdominal surgery. At the same time patients were asked whether they needed additional pain medication. They found that grouping pain scores was more clinically meaningful than individual scores. Specifically, if patients rated their pain between 0 and 30 they were highly unlikely to require pain medication (4%), between 31 and 70 they were more likely to require pain medication (40%), and if the rating was over 70 almost all required additional pain medication (80%).

Collins and coworkers[16] also addressed how to interpret the results of the VAS. They analyzed the results from 11 studies in which patients were given a VAS to complete and were also asked to quantify their level of pain as none, mild, moderate, and severe. They found that 85 percent of patients who reported moderate pain had a VAS > 30, with a mean of 49. For those who reported severe pain, they found that 85 percent had a VAS > 54, with a mean score of 75.

Numeric Rating Scale

The Numeric Rating Scale (NRS) is an assessment tool in which patients are asked to choose a number that best corresponds with their level of pain. The scales are usually between 0 and 10 or 0 and 100. Patients are instructed to rate their pain, with 0 representing no pain and 10 (or 100) representing the worst imaginable pain. The NRS has also been shown to be both reliable and valid and to strongly correlate with the VAS.[5] An advantage of the NRS is that it can be administered in either the written or verbal form, avoiding the potential confounding variable of observer measurements. Also, with 101 possible responses on the NRS-101, this measure addresses the concerns of clinicians who feel that the responses possible on the VRS or BS-11 are too limited (see following discussion). The NRSs are probably the easiest to use, as they require no materials other than a verbally expressive patient.

Beilin and colleagues[17] assessed how best to analyze the results of the NRS and found that, as with the VAS, the NRS lends itself to grouping scores into clinically relevant quanta. This enables clinicians to stratify patients into those who need analgesia and those who would not require further intervention. In their study, women in labor with epidural analgesia were asked to rate their pain on a scale of 0 to 10, with 0 representing no pain and 10 signifying the worst possible pain. They determined that of patients who rated their pain 0 to 1, only 2 percent were likely to ask for additional pain relief. However, of those who reported their pain as 2 to 3, 51 percent requested more analgesia. Anyone rating their pain score higher than 3 almost universally (91%) requested more pain medication. With its well-documented validity, a clinician has at his or her disposal a means of adequately quantifying pain in a manner that lends itself to evaluating efficacy of treatment. This fact, combined with the NRS's ease of administration and absence of reliance on perceptual-motor skills, make this test a highly useful clinical tool.

Box Scale

The 11-digit Box Scale (BS-11) consist of numbers 0 through 10 surrounded by boxes (Figure 30.2). The patient places a mark on the box that best represents the level of pain. It essentially incorporates visual cues into the NRS. It is theorized that the boxes will allow for more discrete separation of the numbers in a patient's mind.[3] It too correlates well with the other unidimensional scores.[2,3] A drawback is the need to have a physical diagram of the scale to administer it.

Verbal Rating Scale

The VRS consists of a list of adjectives that describe pain. The descriptors range from "none" to "extremely severe." Each descriptor is then assigned a number, with 0 being assigned to the least-intense adjective. The number associated with the adjective is considered the patient's pain score. The scales usually come with four, five, or six descriptors. A representative list of adjectives is listed in Table 30.1. A shortcoming of this scale is that, unlike the VAS or the NRS, which theoretically contain infinite possibilities, the VRS forces the patient to assign

Table 30.1. Typical descriptors with the Verbal Rating Scale (VRS)

Pain score	Descriptor
0	No pain
1	Mild discomfort
2	Moderate pain
3	Excruciating pain

Pain score	Descriptor
0	No pain
1	Mild pain
2	Moderate pain
3	Severe pain
4	Very severe pain
5	Worst possible pain

The first part of the table represents the VRS 4 and the second part of the table the VRS 6.

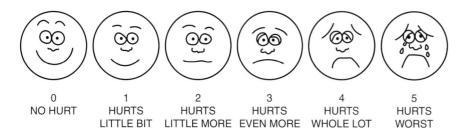

0
NO HURT

1
HURTS
LITTLE BIT

2
HURTS
LITTLE MORE

3
HURTS
EVEN MORE

4
HURTS
WHOLE LOT

5
HURTS
WORST

Figure 30.3. Wong-Baker Faces Pain Rating Scale. From Hockenberry MJ, Wilson D: *Wong's Essentials of Pediatric Nursing*, ed. 8, St. Louis, 2009 Mosby. Used with permission. Copyright © Mosby; used with permission.

the pain to just four, five, or six descriptive words. Despite this apparent shortcoming, the VRS correlates well with the VAS and the other unidimensional indexes.[2,6]

Face scales

The face scales (FSs) are composed of drawings of facial expressions representing levels of pain intensity. The simple drawings range from a smiling face connoting no pain to a frown with tears suggesting the worst imaginable pain. The faces have a letter or number assigned to each face, which then represents the patient's pain score. One of the more commonly used face scales is one developed by Wong and Baker[18] (Figure 30.3). The face scales usually have six or seven possible choices. The FS-6 and FS-7 have been shown to be both valid and reliable in children and older adults.[19,20]

Although the face scales seem particularly useful for children and older adults, they may not be as useful in the nonelderly adult population. There exists some evidence to suggest that men, in particular, may be reluctant to have their pain

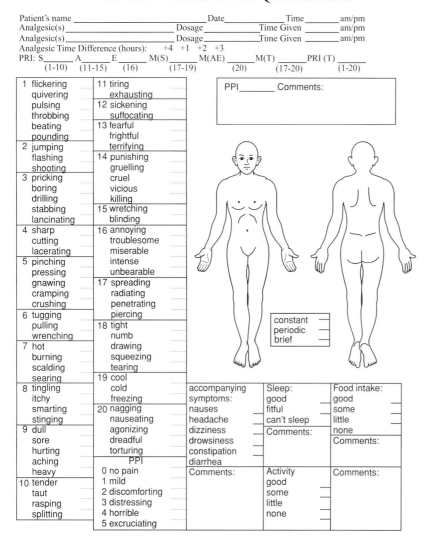

Figure 30.4. The McGill-Melzack Pain Questionnaire. The adjectives are separated into four categories: sensory (1–10), affective (11–15), evaluative (16), and miscellaneous (17–20). Each adjective is assigned a rank value, and the sum of the rank values equals the pain rating index. Additionally, the patient is asked for their current level of pain on a 0–5 scale called the present pain intensity (PPI) scale. From ref. 25.

Table 30.2. The short-form McGill Pain Questionnaire

	None	Mild	Moderate	Severe
Throbbing	0	1	2	3
Shooting	0	1	2	3
Stabbing	0	1	2	3
Sharp	0	1	2	3
Cramping	0	1	2	3
Gnawing	0	1	2	3
Hot – burning	0	1	2	3
Aching	0	1	2	3
Heavy	0	1	2	3
Tender	0	1	2	3
Splitting	0	1	2	3
Tiring – exhausting	0	1	2	3
Sickening	0	1	2	3
Fearful	0	1	2	3
Punishing – cruel	0	1	2	3

Source: See Ref. 25.

associated with a descriptive face that has tears. As tears are typically seen in the pictures correlating to the most severe level of pain, there may be a tendency to underreport the most severe pains in nonelderly adult males.[21] More research needs to be done to determine whether this test is reliable in the adult male.

The McGill Pain Questionnaire

The original McGill Pain Questionnaire (MPQ), developed by Melzack and Torgerson, was designed to provide a more comprehensive view of pain.[8] It has been shown to be a reliable and valid tool, particularly when information other than the intensity of pain is sought.[8,9,22,23] The 78 pain descriptors in the MPQ (Figure 30.4) break down the perception of pain into four distinct categories: sensory, affective, evaluative, and miscellaneous. The sensory component allows the patient to describe the type of pain and its manifestation. Examples of sensory descriptors include pounding, shooting, stabbing, sharp, crushing, and burning. The affective descriptors deal with the emotional toll that the pain exacts. Examples of descriptors from the affective category include tiring, suffocating, terrifying, and grueling. The evaluative category tries to assign a single word to describe the overall intensity of the pain. During development of the scale, it became apparent that there were words that, although infrequently used, were commonly used to describe specific pain syndromes, and these terms were added to the scale.

In addition to the four categories of descriptors, patients are asked to assess their current level of pain on a 0 to 5 scale, called the present pain intensity scale. This scale, in addition to having good reliability and validity,[9] was specifically designed to allow practitioners to differentiate between different types of pain and their causes. As Melzack pointed out, the MPQ allows clinicians to differentiate between the pain of a toothache and the pain of a pinprick.[9] In fact, the MPQ has been shown to so reliably measure distinct types of pain that it can be used in a diagnostic

fashion, as specific descriptors of pain are likely to be repeated in certain diseases. Although the MPQ gives significantly more information than the single-number intensity scales, there exist data that suggest that the MPQ functions more reliably as a measure of psychological distress than of pain intensity. Therefore, the MPQ may not be the ideal tool to assess acute pain.[24] Another problem with the scale is that it is cumbersome and takes an excessive amount of time to complete.

In an accommodation for clinicians and researchers who desire more information than pain intensity but are hesitant to administer the full MPQ, Melzack developed the short-form MPQ (Table 30.2).[25] The 15 descriptor words were selected based on their prevalence of usage on retrospective examination of the longer version of the MPQ. Descriptor words 1 through 11 represent sensory dimensions of pain and words 12 through 15 represent affective dimensions of pain. Both reliable and valid,[25] it may be of particular utility in the geriatric population, who have been noted to have some difficulty with other scales but were able to successfully complete the short-form MPQ at the same rate as other age groups.[21]

Summary, conclusions, and recommendations

The measurement of pain has become increasingly important for both clinicians and researchers. Numerous regulatory bodies call for the measurement of pain as the "fifth vital sign." However, within that very description lies the inherent difficulty of quantifying pain. Pain, by definition, cannot be a sign, because signs in medical terminology are objective. The term *symptom* is used to describe subjective information that cannot be quantified. Despite, or perhaps as a result of the difficulties in assessing pain, the Joint Commission (formerly the Joint Commission on the Accreditation of Healthcare Organizations [JCAHO]) has recommended that pain assessment be conducted in a manner "consistent with the scope of care, treatment and services and the patient's condition" and "as appropriate to the reason the patient is presenting for care or services."[26]

Despite the unquestionable importance of being able to assess a patient's pain, the practicalities of doing so remain somewhat ambiguous. For example, the New York State Department of Health (NYS DOH) advises patients that it is their right "As part of good medical care … to receive appropriate assessment and management of pain." However, there are no specific recommendations for how clinicians should implement their suggestion.[27] Nonetheless, the widespread advisories mandating the assessment of pain suggest that the health care field as a whole is recognizing that pain management is not only a patient satisfaction issue but also a means to improving the overall well-being of patients.

In an effort to incorporate the JCAHO and NYS DOH recommendations and because we believe that establishing the care and concern for patients' pain is of crucial importance, our institution has instituted a policy dedicated to ensuring optimal patient comfort. We believe that there should be a proactive pain control plan for each patient. The plan should be individualized and established mutually with the patient, family, significant others, and members of the health care team. The means by which this pain control plan is implemented involves assessing the presence, severity, and characteristics of pain. To ensure that adequate assessment takes place, assessments are to be done at the following intervals:

1. On admission or entry into the health care system.
2. After any known pain-producing event.
3. With each new report of pain.
4. Routinely at regular intervals (at least once every nursing shift).
5. After each pain management intervention at an appropriate time interval to assess the maximal (peak) effects of the therapy.
6. Prior to discharge, if indicated.

This process is monitored by a multidisciplinary committee consisting of anesthesiologists, nurses, pediatricians, geriatricians, palliative care specialists, pain management specialists, and surgeons. Additionally, patients' satisfaction with their pain management is also evaluated during their hospitalization via patient surveys coordinated by the Hospital Survey Center and again after discharge.

The goal of this review has been to demonstrate that numerous options exist for the measurement of pain. As pain assessment becomes a more important and commonly used tool in the arsenal of the clinician, the various scales with which we assess pain will become increasingly important. Whether a single-digit scale will suffice or a more thorough and comprehensive evaluation of a patient's experience of pain is warranted, a clinician has options to optimize patient care. As more research is completed, greater refinement of these scales will lead to better quantification of the dynamic process that is pain and lead to more predictive and accurate scales.

References

1. Pautex S, Berger A, Chatelain C, Herrmann F, Zulian GB. Symptom assessment in elderly cancer patients receiving palliative care. *Crit Rev Oncol Hematol* 2003;**47**:281–6.
2. Baños JE, Bosch F, Cañellas M, Bassols A, Ortega F, Bigorra J. Acceptability of visual analogue scales in the clinical setting: a comparison with verbal rating scales in postoperative pain. *Methods Find Exp Clin Pharmacol* 1989;**11**:123–7.
3. Jensen MP, Karoly P, Braver S. The measurement of clinical pain intensity: a comparison of six methods. *Pain* 1986;**27**:117–26.
4. Gagliese L, Weizblit N, Ellis W, Chan VW. The measurement of postoperative pain: a comparison of intensity scales in younger and older surgical patients. *Pain* 2005;**117**:412–20.
5. Jensen MP, Turner JA, Romano JM, Fisher LD. Comparative reliability and validity of chronic pain intensity measures. *Pain* 1999;**83**:157–62.
6. Jensen MP, Miller L, Fisher LD. Assessment of pain during medical procedures: a comparison of three scales. *Clin J Pain* 1998;**14**:343–9.
7. Downie WW, Leatham PA, Rhind VM, Wright V, Branco JA, Anderson JA. Studies with pain scale ratings. *Ann Rheum Dis* 1978;**37**:378–87.
8. Melzack R. The McGill Pain Questionnaire: from description to measurement. *Anesthesiology* 2005;**103**:199–202.
9. Melzack R. The McGill Pain Questionnaire: major properties and scoring methods. *Pain* 1975;**1**:277–99.
10. Sriwatanakul K, Kelvie W, Lasagna L, Calimlim JF, Weis OF, Mehta G. Studies with different types of visual analog scales for measurement of pain. *Clin Pharmacol Ther* 1983;**34**:234–9.
11. Joyce CR, Zutshi DW, Hrubes V, Mason RM. Comparison of fixed interval and visual analogue scales for rating chronic pain. *Eur J Clin Pharmacol* 1975;**8**:415–20.
12. Bodian CA, Freedman G, Hossain S, Eisenkraft JB, Beilin Y. The visual analog scale for pain: clinical significance in postoperative patients. *Anesthesiology* 2001;**95**:1356–61.
13. Bruera E, Kuehn N, Miller MJ, Selmser P, Macmillan K. The Edmonton Symptom Assessment System (ESAS): a simple method for the assessment of palliative care patients. *J Palliat Care* 1991; 7:6–9.
14. Gagliese L, Melzack R. Age differences in the quality of chronic pain: a preliminary study. *Pain Res Manag* 1997;**2**:157–62.
15. Kremer E, Atkinson JH, Ignelzi RJ. Measurement of pain: patient preference does not confound pain measurement. *Pain* 1981;**10**:241–8.
16. Collins SL, Moore RA, McQuay HJ. The visual analogue pain scale: what is moderate pain in millimeters? *Pain* 1997;**72**:95–97.
17. Beilin Y, Hossain S, Bodian CA. The numeric rating scale and labor epidural analgesia. *Anesth Analg* 2003;**96**:1794–8.
18. Wong DL, Hockenberry-Eaton M, Wilson D, Winkelstein ML, Schwartz P. *Wong's Essentials of Pediatric Nursing*, 6th ed. St. Louis: Mosby, 2001, p. 1301.
19. Herr KA, Mobily PR, Kohout FJ, Wagenaar D. Evaluation of the Faces Pain Scale for use with the elderly. *Clin J Pain* 1998;**14**:29–38.
20. Bieri D, Reeve RA, Champion GD, Addicoat L, Ziegler JB. The Faces Pain Scale for the self-assessment of the severity of pain experienced by children: development, initial validation, and preliminary investigation for ratio scale properties. *Pain* 1990;**41**:139–50.
21. Ramer L, Richardson JL, Cohen MZ, Bedney C, Danley KL, Judge EA. Multimeasure pain assessment in an ethnically diverse group of patients with cancer. *J Transcult Nurs* 1999;**10**:94–101.
22. Katz J, Melzack R. Measurement of pain. *Surg Clin North Am* 1999;**79**:231–52.
23. Love A, Leboeuf C, Crisp TC. Chiropractic chronic low back pain sufferers and self-report assessment methods. Part I. A reliability study of the Visual Analog Scale, the Pain Drawing and the McGill Pain Questionnaire. *J Manipulative Physiol Ther* 1989;**12**:21–5.
24. Ahles TA, Blanchard EB, Ruckdeschel JC. The multidimensional nature of cancer-related pain. *Pain* 1983;**17**:277–88.
25. Melzack R. The short-form McGill Pain Questionnaire. *Pain* 1987;**30**:191–97.
26. http://www.jointcommission.org/Standards/Requirements.
27. www.nyhealth.gov/nysdoh/opmc/main.htm.

Chapter 31

Neurologic clinical scales

Jennifer A. Frontera

Introduction

Scales for evaluation of the neurologic exam were initially developed for research purposes and to facilitate communication between practitioners across subspecialties. These scales are useful to standardize neurologic assessment, but a detailed description of the neurologic exam should be documented whenever possible. Although they have implications in terms of functional and cognitive outcome, the limitation of broad generalizations based on these scales should be recognized.

Admission clinical assessment scales

Glasgow Coma Scale

The Glasgow Coma Scale[1] was originally developed in 1974 for assessment of traumatic brain injury patients but has subsequently been applied across the spectrum of neurologic diagnoses. The scale ranges from 3 to 15. In intubated patients, the suffix "T" is placed after the score to indicate a limited assessment. Brain injury can be categorized as severe: GCS $\leq$ 8 (definition of coma); moderate to severe: GCS 9–12; and mild: GCS $\geq$13. The components of the GCS scale are in Table 31.1.

FOUR Score

The FOUR Score[2] was developed as an alternative to the GCS score to assess level of coma. Limitations of the GCS include that the verbal score cannot be assessed in intubated patients and brainstem reflexes and breathing patterns are not assessed as part of the GCS. Additionally, each component of the GCS has a different potential maximum score, whereas the FOUR Score assigns a maximum score of 4 to each category and is more intuitive. The FOUR Score has been found to have good intra- and interrater reliability and distinguishes among patients with the lowest GCS scores. The probability of in-hospital mortality has been shown to be higher for the lowest total FOUR score as compared with the lowest total GCS score. The FOUR score system is seen in Table 31.2:

Hunt–Hess Grade

The Hunt–Hess grade[3] was developed to assess the neurologic severity of patients with nontraumatic subarachnoid hemorrhage. The scale ranges from 1 (best) to 5 (worst). A score of 0 is sometimes used to refer to an unruptured cerebral aneurysm. Many practitioners refer to an admission and a postresuscitation Hunt–Hess score, meaning the score following ventriculostomy, fluid resuscitation, or treatment of elevated intracranial pressure. The postresuscitation Hunt–Hess grade is one of the strongest predictors of outcome after subarachnoid hemorrhage. The Hunt–Hess Scoring system and associated mortality rates is in Table 31.3.

World Federation of Neurological Surgeons Subarachnoid Grade

The World Federation of Neurological Surgeons (WFNS) Subarachnoid Grade[4] system, ranging from 1 (best) to 5 (worst), was devised for nontraumatic subarachnoid hemorrhage (SAH) patients as an alternative to the Hunt–Hess grading system (see Table 31.4). The WFNS scale combines the GCS score with the presence or absence of a major neurologic deficit. It has been shown to be similar to the Hunt–Hess scale in predicting outcome measured by the Glasgow Outcome Score (1 = dead, 2 = vegetative, 3 = severely disabled, 4 = moderately disabled 5 = good outcome) after SAH.[5]

Table 31.1. Glasgow Coma Scale

Verbal	Score
Alert, oriented, and conversant	5
Confused, disoriented, but conversant	4
Intelligible words, not conversant	3
Unintelligible sounds	2
No verbalization	1
Eye opening	
Spontaneous	4
To verbal stimuli	3
To painful stimuli	2
None	1
Motor	
Follows commands	6
Localizes	5
Withdraws from painful stimuli	4
Flexor posturing	3
Extensor posturing	2
No response to noxious stimuli	1

Table 31.2. FOUR Score

Eye opening	Score
Eyelids open or opened, tracking, or blinking to command	4
Eyelids open but not tracking	3
Eyelids closed but open to loud voice	2
Eyelids closed but open to pain	1
Eyelids remain closed with pain	0
Motor response	
Thumbs up, fist, or peace sign to command	4
Localizing to pain	3
Flexion response to pain	2
Extension response to pain	1
No response to pain or generalized myoclonus status	0
Brainstem reflexes	
Pupil and corneal reflexes present	4
One pupil wide and fixed	3
Pupil *or* corneal reflexes absent	2
Pupil *and* corneal reflexes absent	1
Absent pupil, corneal, and cough reflex	0
Respiration	
Not intubated, regular breathing pattern	4
Not intubated, Cheyne–Stokes breathing pattern	3
Not intubated, irregular breathing	2
Respiratory rate above ventilator set rate	1
Respiratory rate at ventilator set rate or apnea	0

Table 31.3. Hunt-Hess Grading

Grade	Clinical exam	Associated mortality	Mean Glasgow outcome score
1	Asymptomatic, mild headache, slight nuchal rigidity	1%	4
2	Cranial nerve palsy, moderate to severe headache, severe nuchal rigidity	5%	4
3	Mild focal deficit, lethargy, confusion	19%	3
4	Stupor, moderate to severe hemiparesis, early decerebrate rigidity	42%	2
5	Deep coma, decerebrate rigidity, moribund appearance	77%	2

Table 31.5. NIH Stroke Scale

1a	Level of consciousness	0 = alert; 1 = drowsy; 2 = stuporous; 3 = comatose
1b	Level of consciousness questions	0 = answers both correctly; 1 = answers one correctly; 2 = both incorrect
1c	Level of consciousness commands	0 = obeys both correctly; 1 = obeys one correctly; 2 = both incorrect
2	Best gaze	0 = normal; 1 = partial gaze palsy; 2 = forced deviation
3	Visual fields	0 = no visual loss; 1 = partial hemianopsia; 2 = complete hemianopsia; 3 = bilateral hemianopsia
4	Facial paresis	0 = normal movement; 1 = minor paresis; 2 = partial paresis; 3 = complete palsy
5–8	Right/left arm/leg motor	0 = no drift; 1 = drift; 2 = some effort vs gravity; 3 = no effort vs gravity; 4 = no movement
9	Limb ataxia	0 = absent; 1 = present in 1 limb; 2 = present in 2 or more limbs
10	Sensory	0 = normal; 1 = partial loss; 2 = dense loss
11	Best language	0 = no aphasia; 1 = mild-moderate aphasia; 2 = severe aphasia; 3 = mute
12	Dysarthria	0 = normal articulation; 1 = mild–moderate dysarthria; 2 = unintelligible or worse
13	Neglect/inattention	0 = no neglect; 1 = partial neglect; 2 = complete neglect

NIH Stroke Scale

The NIH Stroke Scale (NIHSS),[6] ranging from 0 (best) to 42 (worst), was initially meant to apply to ischemic strokes but has been used for hemorrhagic strokes as well (see Table 31.5). Certification in NIHSS testing is available online and is required for participation in many major neurologic studies.

ICH score

The ICH score[7] was developed to predict outcome after spontaneous intracerebral hemorrhage (ICH). Independent predictors of poor outcome were weighted based on the strength of their associations. Scores range from 0 (best) to 6 (worst; see Table 31.6).

Table 31.4. WFNS Subarachnoid Grading System

Grade	GCS Score	Major focal deficit (aphasia, hemiparesis)	Associated mortality %	Mean Glasgow outcome score
1	15	–	5	4
2	13–14	–	9	4
3	13–14	+	20	3
4	7–12	+/–	33	2
5	3–6	+/–	77	2

GCS = Glasgow Coma Scale.

Table 31.6. ICH Score

GCS score	ICH score points
3–4	2
5–12	1
13–15	0
ICH volume	
≥30 cm^3	1
<30 cm^3	0
IVH	
Yes	1
No	0
Infratentorial location	
Yes	1
No	0
Age	
≥80 yr	1
<80 yr	0
Total Score	**% Mortality**
	0 = 0; 1 = 13; 2 = 26; 3 = 72; 4 = 97; 5, 6 = 100

American Spinal Injury Association Scale

The American Spinal Injury Association Scale (ASIA) score,[8] ranging from A (worst) to E (best), is predictive of outcome after spinal cord injury. Ten percent to 15 percent of ASIA A patients will improve to some extent, although only 3 percent will improve to the level of ASIA D. Of ASIA B patients, 54 percent recover to ASIA C or D. Among ASIA C or D patients, 86 percent will regain some ambulatory function.[9,10] Table 31.7 describes the ASIA scoring system.

Outcome assessment scales

Modified Rankin Scale

Originally introduced in 1957[11] and modified in 1994,[12] the modified Rankin scale (mRS) was developed to assess functional outcome after stroke. The scale ranges from 0 (best) to 6 (dead) and is commonly measured at 3, 6, or 12 months after stroke (see Table 31.8).

Glasgow Outcome Scale

The Glasgow Outcome Scale (GOS)[13] was developed to assess outcome in patients with traumatic brain injury and is similar to the mRS. The scale ranges from 1 (worst, dead) to 5 (best).

Table 31.8. Modified Rankin scale

Modified Rankin scale

0	No symptoms
1	No significant disability, despite symptoms; able to carry out all usual duties and activities
2	Slight disability; unable to carry out all previous activities but able to look after own affairs without assistance
3	Moderate disability; requires some help but able to walk without assistance
4	Moderately severe disability; unable to walk without assistance and unable to attend to own bodily needs without assistance
5	Severe disability; bedridden, incontinent, and requires constant nursing care and attention
6	Dead

The extended GOS (E-GOS)[14] was developed to create more specificity in outcome by adding a quantification of upper and lower extremity disability (see Table 31.9).

Barthel Score

The Barthel score[15] assesses activities of daily living and ranges from 0 (worst) to 100 (best). The Barthel score identifies patients who are likely to be able to live independently (see Table 31.10).

Table 31.9. GOS and E-GOS scales

Glasgow outcome score	Function
1	Dead
2	Persistent vegetative state
3	Severe disability, conscious but limited communication skills, dependent for daily activities of living
4	Independent but with disabilities; able to work
5	Resumption of normal life despite minor physical or mental deficits

Extended Glasgow outcome score	Function
1	Dead
2	Vegetative state
3	Lower severe disability
4	Upper severe disability
5	Lower moderate disability
6	Upper moderate disability
7	Lower good recovery
8	Upper good recovery

Table 31.7. ASIA Score

A	B	C	D	E
Complete: No motor or sensory function below the neurologic level through sacral segments S4–S5.	Incomplete: Sensory, but not motor, function is preserved below the neurologic level and includes S4–S5.	Incomplete: Motor function is preserved below the neurologicl level, and more than half of key muscles below the neurologic level have a muscle grade less than 3. Voluntary sphincter contraction may be present.	Incomplete: Motor function is preserved below the neurologic level, and at least half of key muscles below the neurologic level have a muscle grade of 3 or more.	Normal: Motor and sensory functions are normal

Table 31.10. Barthel score

Transfer from wheelchair to bed (does patient need help getting out of chair or bed)
0   Dependent
5   With moderate help
10 With minimal help
15 Independently

Walk on level surface, propel wheelchair (score only if unable to walk)
0   Dependent
5   Independent with wheelchair propulsion (at least a block)
10 Walking with help (at least a block)
15 Walking independently (at least a block)

Ascending and descending stairs
0   Dependent
5   With help
10 Independently

Feeding (if food needs to be cut = help)
0   Dependent
5   With help
10 Independently

Grooming (wash face, comb hair, shave, clean teeth)
0   Dependent / with help
5   Independently

Dressing (includes tying shoes, fastening fasteners)
0   Dependent
5   With help
10 Independently

Toileting (getting on and off, handling clothes, wipe, flush)
0   Dependent
5   With help
10 Independently

Bathing
0   Dependent
5   Independently

Bowel continence
0   Incontinent
5   With help – enema, laxatives
10 Continent

Bladder continence
0   Incontinent
5   With help – medication/catheter
10 Continent

References

1. Teasdale G, Jennett B. Assessment of coma and impaired consciousness. A practical scale. *Lancet* 1974;**2**:81–84.
2. Wijdicks EF, Bamlet WR, Maramattom BV, Manno EM, McClelland RL. Validation of a new coma scale: the Four score. *Ann Neurol* 2005;**58**:585–593.
3. Hunt WE, Hess RM. Surgical risk as related to time of intervention in the repair of intracranial aneurysms. *J Neurosurg* 1968;**28**:14–20.
4. Report of World Federation of Neurological Surgeons Committee on a Universal Subarachnoid Hemorrhage Grading Scale. *J Neurosurg* 1988;**68**:985–986.
5. Oshiro EM, Walter KA, Piantadosi S, Witham TF, Tamargo RJ. A new subarachnoid hemorrhage grading system based on the Glasgow Coma Scale: A comparison with the Hunt and Hess and World Federation of Neurological Surgeons scales in a clinical series. *Neurosurgery* 1997;**41**:140–147; discussion 147–148.
6. www.NIHSS.com.
7. Hemphill JC 3rd, Bonovich DC, Besmertis L, Manley GT, Johnston SC. The ICH score: a simple, reliable grading scale for intracerebral hemorrhage. *Stroke* 2001;**32**:891–897.
8. Clinical assessment after acute cervical spinal cord injury. *Neurosurgery* 2002;**50**:S21–S29.
9. Waters RL, Adkins RH, Yakura JS, Sie I. Motor and sensory recovery following incomplete tetraplegia. *Arch Phys Med Rehabil* 1994;**75**:306–311.
10. Waters RL, Adkins RH, Yakura JS, Sie I. Motor and sensory recovery following incomplete paraplegia. *Arch Phys Med Rehabil* 1994;**75**:67–72.
11. Rankin J. Cerebral vascular accidents in patients over the age of 60. II. Prognosis. *Scott Med J* 1957;**2**:200–215.
12. Lindley RI, Waddell F, Livingstone M, et al. Can simple questions assess outcome after stroke? *Cerebrovascular Diseases* 1994;**4**:314–324.
13. Jennett B, Bond M. Assessment of outcome after severe brain damage. *Lancet* 1975;**1**:480–484.
14. Jennett BS, Bond MR, Brooks, N. Disability after severe head injury: observations on the use of the Glasgow Outcome Scale. *J Neurol Neurosurg Psychiatry* 1981;**44**:285–293.
15. Shah S VF, Cooper B. Preditcting discharge status at the commencement of stroke rehabilitation. *Stroke* 1989;**20**:766–769.

Chapter 32

Postanesthesia care unit assessment scales

David Bronheim and Richard S. Gist

Introduction

Admission to the postanesthesia care unit (PACU) for recovery – after sedation and general or regional anesthesia as an interim step before transfer to an inpatient unit or before discharge home – has long been the standard of care in the United States. From arrival in the PACU until the time of discharge, all patients receive essentially continuous observation, monitoring, and treatment as deemed necessary.

The length of stay in a PACU varies, based on the length and complexity of the procedure, the severity of underlying comorbidities, the time to recovery from anesthesia, and the needs for stabilization of any resultant physiologic derangements that would prevent transfer to the appropriate inpatient unit or discharge to home. Just as the length of PACU stay may vary, there may also be a need to vary the intensity of monitoring and the degree of intervention. As a consequence, care in the PACU is frequency divided into two phases. The early recovery phase (i.e. the phase one recovery period), lasts from the time of admission to the PACU until the return of protective airway reflexes, near-normal motor function, and stable respiratory and hemodynamic function. The late recovery phase (i.e. the phase two recovery period) starts from readiness for phase one discharge until readiness for discharge to home or an inpatient unit.

Under the guidelines established by the American Society of Anesthesiologists,[1] medical care as well as discharge from the PACU should be overseen by a physician capable of managing the expected complications of surgery and anesthesia. Discharge from the PACU may be accomplished by direct physician order; however, more commonly, decisions on discharge are made by members of the nursing staff experienced in the care of the PACU patient based on guidelines and protocols that use specific criteria established by the supervising department of anesthesiology. To aid in ongoing PACU assessment and to help evaluate readiness for discharge, various scoring assessment systems are widely used in the postoperative period.

The use of scoring systems to assess a patient's medical status for the purpose of ongoing medical care in the operative period dates back to the 1950s, when Dr. Virginia Apgar first proposed a system to rapidly evaluate newborns, that is still used to this day.[2] Subsequently, in 1964 Carighan and colleagues[3] proposed a complex scoring system that assessed circulatory and respiratory status as well as gastrointestinal, renal, and neurologic

status of the postoperative patient over a period of time, using a scale of 0 to 5. The complexity of this system, combined with its need for continuous and extended observation, prevented its widespread acceptance.

Since that time, several scoring systems have been proposed, modified, used, and abandoned. For example, Steward[4] used a simple scoring system, later modified by Robertson and associates,[5] that evaluated consciousness on a 0-to-4-point basis, airway on a 0-to-3-point basis, and activity on a 0-to-2-point basis, but ignored hemodynamics and signs of hypoxia independent of airway management.

Other versions of PACU recovery scoring systems have been described. For example, the REACT assessment tool was developed by nursing researchers in the early 1980s. The parameters assessed by the REACT assessment tool include respiration, energy, alertness, circulation, and temperature. It is not scored but is used as a checklist, with yes and no checkmarks, rather than as a formal scoring system.[6]

This scale, as other earlier scales that predate the use of routine pulse oximetry monitoring, not surprisingly, does not include any objective criteria for assessment of hypoxemia. It also is limited in that the other assessed parameters are poorly defined, leaving them open for broad interpretation and increased interobserver variability. These previous scales are now rarely used as the means of assessing readiness for discharge from the PACU.

The Aldrete scoring system was initially proposed by Aldrete in 1970 and is the scale most widely used today. The initial version assessed respiration, oxygenation, consciousness, circulation, and activity in a manner similar to the current version of this scoring system (see Table 32.1). These multiple parameters were graded on a scale of 0 to 2 points, with a summary score of 8 or higher being viewed as acceptable for discharge from the PACU.

This scoring system was subsequently modified in the 1990s,[8] when the use of pulse oximetry became the standard of care. At that time, the somewhat subjective assessment of hypoxemia using skin, nail bed, and mucous membrane color was replaced with objective pulse oximetry readings. The initial Aldrete scale assesses the ability of the patient to follow commands and the stability of vital signs. It may indirectly assess pain control by the change in vital signs from baseline;

Table 32.1. The Aldrete scoring system

Respiration

Able to take a deep breath and cough	2
Dyspnea or shallow breathing	1
Apnea	0

Oxygen saturation

Maintains >92% on room air	2
Supplemental O_2 to maintain saturation greater than 90%	1
Oxygen saturation <90% on supplemental O_2	0

Consciousness

Fully awake	2
Arousable on calling	1
Not responsive	0

Circulation

BP +/− 20mm Hg of preop value	2
BP +/− 20–50 mmHg of preop value	1
BP +/− 50 mmHg of preop value	0

Activity

Able to move all extremities	2
Able to move two extremities	1
Unable to move any extremity	0

Source: From ref. 8.

Table 32.2. The Post-Anesthetic Discharge Scoring Scale (PADSS)

Vital signs

BP and pulse within 20% of preoperative values	2
BP and pulse within 20–40% of preoperative values	1
BP and pulse < or > 40% of preoperative values	0

Activity

Steady gait, no dizziness or return to preoperative baseline	2
Requires assistance	1
Unable to ambulate	0

Nausea and vomiting

Minimal, treated with oral medication	2
Moderate, treated with parenteral or rectal medication	1
Severe, refractory to treatment	0

Pain

Controlled with oral medication and acceptable to the patient	2 = yes 1 = no

Surgical Bleeding

Minimal – no dressing changes	2
Moderate – up to two dressing changes	1
Severe – more than three dressing changes	0

Source: From ref. 10 and 11.

however, it does not directly assess all criteria necessary for successful outpatient discharge. Therefore, the original Aldrete scoring system, even with oximeter usage included, should be characterized as a phase one assessment tool and is not suitable for final discharge criteria from phase two locations to home. A subsequent modification in 1998 added scoring for pain, ambulation, urine output, tolerance of oral intake, and surgical bleeding as assessed by evaluating the dressings. From a total of 20 points, 18 are necessary for discharge from phase two recovery to home. The use of the Aldrete scoring system has been shown to decrease the PACU length of stay when compared with the time-based criteria used in the past.[9]

In 1995, Chung and colleagues described another comprehensive scoring system, The Post-Anesthetic Discharge Scoring System (PADSS), which is summarized in Table 32.2.[10,11] Criteria that are assessed include the vital signs, pulse and blood pressure, activity including ambulation, the presence and level of treatment of nausea and vomiting, pain control, and surgical bleeding as assessed by the number of dressing changes. The author suggests using the original Aldrete scoring system to assess readiness for phase one discharge and then subsequently using the PADSS to assess home readiness.

Chung and colleagues randomized a defined population of patients to discharge by PADSS criteria or a less well-defined clinical discharge criterion that used yes/no scoring. Although neither system was superior to the other, the PADSS criteria had more interobserver reliability and reproducibility than the clinical discharge criteria.

The PADSS exists in two forms, one that assesses tolerance of oral fluids and voiding, and a modified form, in which these criteria are deleted. This scoring tool has proven most useful in the transition from phase two postanesthesia recovery to discharge. Adverse events associated with ambulatory surgery,

such as readmission, have been examined by Chung and colleagues.[12,13] They found that surgical complications were the cause of the vast majority of readmissions and thus readmission could not be predicted from discharge assessments that were designed to evaluate complications related to anesthesia.

White described a postanesthesia fast-track score that was a melding of both the PADSS and the Modified Aldrete Scoring System (see Table 32.3).[14] Fast-tracking of ambulatory surgery patients, which involves the bypassing of the traditional phase one PACU when clinically indicated and appropriate, was first popularized in the late 1990s and has now become routine.

The parameters assessed include level of consciousness, physical activity, hemodynamic stability, oxygen saturation, pain, and emetic symptoms. Each criterion is scaled on a score of 0 to 2, with a score of 12 out of 14 needed to meet criteria to bypass traditional phase one postanesthetic recovery areas. This scale differs from the previous scales in that the assessment is done not by the PACU nursing staff but rather by the anesthesia provider, who is judging the suitability for fast-tracking before leaving the operating room. Fast-tracking works well with the patient undergoing procedures requiring monitored anesthesia care or regional anesthesia as well as certain procedures requiring general anesthesia when those procedures are short and when short-acting anesthetic agents are used. Again, it is largely the responsibility of the anesthesiologist to determine the suitability for fast-tracking past the phase one PACU, although operating room nursing personnel may be called on to assess the suitability for fast-tracking in the absence of an anesthesia provider. White and colleagues compared the fast-track criteria previously described to the Aldrete score.[14] No significant differences were found except that, not surprisingly, because the Aldrete scoring system did not assess pain and nausea and vomiting, many patients who did not meet discharge

Table 32.3. Criteria for fast-tracking after ambulatory anesthesia

Level of consciousness	
Awake	2
Arousable with minimal stimulation	1
Responsive to only tactile stimulation	0
Physical activity	
Able to move all extremities on command	2
Some weakness in movement of extremities	1
Unable to voluntarily move extremities	0
Hemodynamic stability	
BP +/– 15% of baseline	2
BP +/– 30% of baseline	1
BP +/– 50% of baseline	0
Oxygen saturation	
SpO$_2$ > 90% on room air	2
Requires supplemental O$_2$ to maintain SpO$_2$ > than 90%	1
SpO$_2$ < 90% on supplemental O$_2$	0
Pain	
None/mild discomfort	2
Moderate to severe controlled with IV analgesia	1
Persistent to severe	0
Emetic symptoms	
None or mild nausea without vomiting	2
Transient vomiting controlled with IV antiemetics	1
Persistent moderate to severe nausea and vomiting	0

Source: From ref. 14.

criteria in the fast-track scoring criteria would have adequate Aldrete scores.

All three of these widely used scoring systems are well defined and easily mastered. To date, no large-scale randomized prospective studies have been published that compare them to one another or to routine clinical assessment without a scoring system. However, from extensive clinical experience, all seem to be readily reproducible with minimal interobserver variability, and all appear to effectively assess readiness for discharge.

References

1. ASA Taskforce on Postanesthesic Care. Practice guidelines for postanesthetic care. *Anesthesiology* 2002;**96**:742–52.
2. Apgar V. A proposal for a new method of evaluation of the newborn infant. *Anesth Analg* 1953;**32**:260–267.
3. Carighan G, Kerri-Szanto M, Lavelle J. Post-anesthetic scoring system. *Anesthesiology* 1964;**25**:396–397.
4. Steward DJ. A Simplified scoring system for post-operative recovery room. *Can Anaesth Soc J* 1975;**22**:111–113.
5. Robertson G, MacGregor D, Jones C. Evaluation of doxapram for arousal from general anesthesia in outpatients. *Br J Anaesth* 1977;**49**:133–139.
6. Fraulini K, Murphy P. R.E.A.C.T. – A new system for measuring post anesthesia recovery. *Nursing* 1984;**14**:12–13.
7. Aldrete AJ, Krovlik D. The postanesthetic recovery. *Anesth Analg* 1970;**49**:924–933.
8. Aldrete JA. The post-anesthetic recovery score revisited. *J Clin Anesth* 1995;**7**:89–91.
9. Truong L, Moran JL, Blum P. Post-anesthesia unit discharge: a clinical scoring system versus traditional time-based criteria. *Anaesth Intensive Care* 2004;**32**:33–42.
10. Chung F, Chan VWS, Ong D. A post-anesthetic discharge scoring system for home readiness after ambulatory surgery. *J Clin Anesth* 1995;**7**:500–506.
11. Chung F. Discharge criteria – a new trend. *Can J Anesth* 1995;**42**:1056–1058.
12. Marshall S, Chung F. Discharge criteria and complications after ambulatory surgery. *Ambulat Anesth* 1999;**88**:508–517.
13. Chung F, Mezei G, Tong D. Adverse events in ambulatory surgery: a comparison between younger and older patients. *Can J Anesth* 1999;**99**:309–321.
14. White P, Song D. New criteria for fast tracking after outpatient anesthesia: a comparison with the modified Aldrete's scoring system. *Anesth Analg* 1999;**88**:1069–1072.

Chapter 33

Delirium monitoring
Scales and assessments

Brigid Flynn and Corey Scurlock

Introduction

Delirium is a common cause of deleterious outcomes in nearly all patient populations. Although delirium was described nearly 2500 years ago,[1] recent studies have highlighted the significance of this disorder. The word delirium stems from the Latin words, *de*, meaning "away from," and, *lira*, meaning "a furrow or track in the field." Thus, delirium means to "be off track".[2]

More scientifically, the *Diagnostic and Statistical Manual of Mental Disorders* (*DSM-IV-TR*) of the American Psychiatric Association defines delirium as a "global disturbance in consciousness and cognitive function characterized by impaired attention, disorganized thinking and memory impairment."[3] The changes seen in delirium develop over a short period of time, usually hours to days, and the symptoms follow a fluctuating course.

Fluctuations in mental status vary throughout the day, with peak intensity usually at night.[4] In addition, the history, physical examination, or laboratory data should suggest that these symptoms are caused by a general medical condition and not better accounted for by a preexisting dementia. The mental status changes of delirium are essentially reversible.

Other behavioral characterizations with delirium include disturbed sleep–wake cycles and alterations in psychomotor activity and verbalization. Interestingly, behavioral manifestations such as these were required by DSM-III criteria for the diagnosis of delirium, but not by DSM-IV criteria. In the DSM-IV criteria, behavioral manifestations are considered "features" of delirium that are commonly present.

Although numerous definitions over thousands of years have attempted to define what delirium is and is not, clinicians have yet to fully understand how to prevent, assess, and treat patients with delirium.

Types of delirium

Because of its different subtypes, the detection of delirium can be challenging. It is important to first identify the three subtypes of delirium – mixed, hypoactive, and hyperactive (Table 33.1).

The most common type of delirium is *mixed delirium*. *Hypoactive delirium* is the most unrecognized type of delirium because of its subtle symptoms; it is experienced more frequently by older patients. Purely *hyperactive delirium* is

reported to be present in a a small percentage of general medical patients (15%)[6] and an even smaller percentage of ICU patients (1%–2%).[7] Hyperactive delirium is believed to carry a higher rate of full recovery.

Hypoactive and mixed types of delirium portend a worse prognosis than hyperactive delirium. One study showed that mixed delirium patients have the highest hospital lengths of stay and six-month mortality rates, whereas hypoactive delirium trailed closely in both of these outcomes but had the highest in-hospital mortality rate.[6] Perhaps the insidious course of these types of delirium, unlike that of hyperactive delirium, delays diagnosis and treatment. Because of the difficulty in diagnosing all three subtypes of delirium, much effort is devoted to creating objective and simple bedside scoring systems for detecting and monitoring delirium.

Incidence of delirium

Delirium is so common that it is likely encountered in all medical specialties; however, some patients are at more risk than others. Delirium occurs in up to 30 percent of patients admitted to general medical wards[8,9] and in 10 percent to 60 percent of surgical patients.[10,11] The incidence of delirium in elderly patients during the perioperative period has been reported to be high as 73 percent.[12]

When considering all adult patients, 14 percent will experience postoperative delirium soon after surgery, while in the PACU.[13] Surgical patients with particularly high rates are patients who sustain a hip fracture (estimated 44%–61% incidence),[14–16] or undergo bilateral knee surgery (estimated 41% incidence)[17] or cardiac surgery (3%–47% incidence).[18] The variability in incidence rates quoted in studies is likely a result of differences in assessment instrument used, patient population characteristics (e.g. age and severity of illness), and rater variability.

Unfortunately, the complication of delirium may extend beyond hospitalization. Eleven percent of delirious patients remain delirious at hospital discharge[19] and almost 20 percent of elderly patients admitted to a postacute facility were admitted with delirium.[20] One study showed that at three months following noncardiac surgery, 14 percent of elderly patients remained with cognitive dysfunction. Notably, this incidence was not influenced by the use of general versus regional anesthesia.[21]

Table 33.1. Subtypes of delirium

Subtype of delirium	Characterization	Pathophysiology	Examples
Hyperactive	Usually well recognized; includes pulling at lines and tubes, inconsolability, agitation, paranoia, hallucinations, disorientation, unintelligible language or shouting, intense agitation.	- Cholinergic deficiency - Reduced gamma-aminobutyric acid (GABA) activity - Excess dopaminergic activity - Elevated or normal cerebral activity	Withdrawal syndromes (alcohol, benzodiazepine)
Hypoactive	Patient is withdrawn and quiet. May be misdiagnosed as depression (note: disorientation is common in delirium but is not a feature of depression). Paranoia may be present.	- May be due to sedatives or hypoxia - Overstimulation of GABA systems - Decreased cerebral metabolism[5]	Encephalopathies (hepatic, metabolic, benzodiazepine intoxication)[5]
Mixed	Patient possesses characteristics of both hyperactive and hypoactive delirium		

The highest rates of delirium are reported in patients who are admitted to the ICU. The occurrence of delirium in ventilated ICU patients is 50 percent to 81 percent,[22] whereas 48 percent of nonventilated ICU patients develop delirium.[23] Patients who develop ICU delirium have a longer hospital length of stay and a higher six-month mortality.[22] Up to 50 percent of patients display hypoactive delirium. These patients may have normal or near-normal arousal and thus go undetected if not specifically assessed with a delirium detection instrument.[22]

Significance of delirium

Delirium leads to numerous deleterious outcomes. Patients who develop delirium have longer lengths of stay in the ICU,[24] longer hospital lengths of stay,[22–24] increased time on the ventilator, and a threefold increased risk of death at six months.[22] Delirium also places elderly patients at increased risk for discharge to a nursing home after hospitalization.[9]

Patients with delirium have a higher incidence of postoperative complications, such as feeding problems, decubital ulcers,[15] increased falls, incontinence leading to bladder catheterization, and an increased risk of infection.[25] The many complications, increased lengths of stays, and increased institutional placement after hospitalization cause delirium to be one of the largest diagnostic contributors to the financial burden of health care.[14,25,26] It is estimated that costs attributable to delirium range from $16,303 to $64,421 per patient, implying that the national burden of delirium on the health care system ranges from $38 billion to $152 billion each year.[27] Finally, the negative impact on life as a result of deranged cognitive function and failure to return to the prior ability to perform activities of daily living should not be forgotten, as this can persist long after discharge.[28]

Risk factors for delirium

Numerous risk factors thought to place patients at risk for the development of delirium have been identified. However, it is likely that delirium develops in susceptible patients exposed to one or more risk factors. Figure 33.1 illustrates the interrelationship between a vulnerable patient (one or more risk factors) and exposure to precipitating factors or insults.

Table 33.2 lists both evidence-based risk factors and hypothesized risk factors for delirium, many of which are not modifiable.

As alluded to earlier, postoperative delirium is not influenced by anesthetic technique. It has been shown that elderly patients with femoral neck fractures who received epidural anesthesia versus those who received general anesthesia had no difference in the incidence of postoperative confusion.[14,31] In fact, the use of anticholinergics and preoperative depression were the most significant risk factors for postoperative delirium. Similarly, treatment of postoperative pain with epidural techniques versus intravenous agents did not significantly influence postoperative cognitive dysfunction.[32]

Among modifiable risk factors, sedatives and analgesics have been found to contribute to the development of delirium. Specifically, benzodiazepines, such as lorazepam, have been found to have a logarithmic correlation of dosage and the development of delirium (Figure 33.2).[33] Conversely, dexmedetomidine is an alpha-2 agonist that has been shown to have an ICU delirium-sparing effect.[34] When used for sedation in ICU patients, it is reported to increase days alive without delirium when compared to lorazepam sedation.[35] Possible explanations for the delirium-sparing effect seen with dexmedetomidine

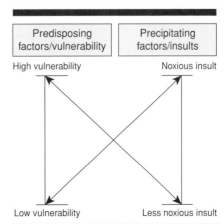

Figure 33.1. Reprinted with permission from Inouye SK, Charpentier PA. Precipitating factors for delirium in hospitalized elderly persons: predictive model and interrelationship with baseline vulnerability. *JAMA* 1996;275:852–7. Copyright © 1996 American Medical Association. All rights reserved.

Table 33.2. Modifiable and nonmodifiable risk factors for delirium

Modifiable risk factors for delirium	Nonmodifiable risk factors for delirium
Use of psychoactive drugs	Advanced age
Mechanical ventilation and ventilator dysynchrony	Preexisting cognitive impairment or dementia
Use of narcotics, benzodiazepines, dopaminergic drugs	Preexisting functional, hearing, or visual impairment
Medical comorbidities (heart failure, hypertension)	Male gender
Prolonged immobilization	Preexisting use of psychotropic agents
Abnormal blood pressure	Preexisting substance or ethanol abuse
Sleep deprivation	Stroke
Sepsis	History of mental depression
Brain ischemia/hypoxia	Prior postoperative delirium
Use of anticholinergics	Higher ASA classification
Bladder and/or central venous catheterization	Educational level (not completed high school)
Metabolic disturbances (e.g. hyponatremia)	Type of surgical procedure (e.g. hip fracture and cardiac surgeries)
Abnormal bilirubin levels[29]	Nursing home residence
Restraints	Duration of cardiopulmonary bypass
Untreated pain	
Infection (e.g. urinary tract infection)	
Malnutrition	
Blood loss; hematocrit <30%; blood transfusions[30]	

include its promotion of sedation that is similar to sleep and the absence of anticholinergic effects.

There may also be a genetic predisposition to delirium. Apolipoprotein E4 allele is the first genetic polymorphism to be implicated as a predictor of delirium duration in ICU patients.[36]

Delirium detection

Routine monitoring of patients for delirium is a standard part of patient care and is recommended by the Society of Critical Care Medicine.[37] It is believed that early detection of delirium along with a management protocol can reduce the incidence of delirium and shorten hospital length of stay.[38] Underrecognition of delirium delays proper treatment strategies; however, delirium, especially hypoactive delirium, is difficult to detect. It has been shown that critical care physicians' performance in detecting delirium remains poor, with around two-thirds of patients not being identified as delirious.[8] Lack of recognition of delirium may cause over- or undersedation of patients, both of which can lead to or increase delirium.

Although prevention of delirium is the primary goal, detection is the next step to decrease negative outcomes related to this disorder. There are numerous delirium scoring tools designed to aid the clinician in accurate and timely diagnosis. Other clinical tests, including EEG, are not as specific in the diagnosis of delirium. It is estimated that 80 percent to 90 percent of delirious patients have an abnormal EEG, with the most common finding being generalized diffuse slowing. An abnormal EEG can aid in excluding other diagnoses but is not specific for delirium.

Delirium assessment instruments
Confusion Assessment Method

Although the **Confusion Assessment Method (CAM)**[39] test was developed for nonpsychiatrists to diagnosis delirium, it does require operator training. The test is composed of nine items and has excellent validity, sensitivity, and negative predictive value. It is based on much of the criteria for delirium stated in

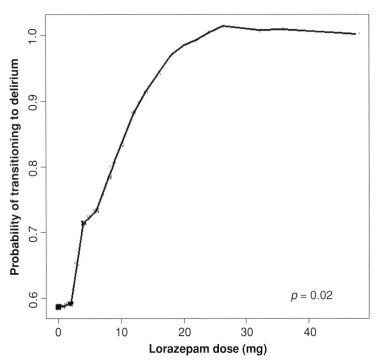

Figure 33.2. Lorazepam dose and delirium. Reprinted from ref. 33 with permission.

$p = 0.02$

the DSM-III-R, including acute onset, fluctuating course, inattention, disorganized thinking, and/or altered consciousness. Because the CAM score is based on DSM-III-R criteria, it uses behavioral manifestations as diagnostic criteria. Disadvantages of this test are that it does require some subjective clinical judgment to be used by the rater. In addition, the Mini-Mental Status Examination (MMSE) component of the test requires verbal communication, making it difficult to use in intubated patients. Finally, it does not quantify the severity of delirium but provides a yes/no dichotomous diagnosis.

Confusion Assessment Method for the Intensive Care Unit

The Confusion Assessment Method for the Intensive Care Unit (CAM-ICU)[40] is a four-feature checklist based on the CAM tool. This model was created to overcome the obstacles that inhibit cognitive evaluation in critically ill patients, namely endotracheal intubation (see Appendix A at the end of this chapter). The CAM-ICU also gives a binary result for diagnosis of delirium and is advantageous in that is allows a rapid assessment of delirium.

The test is based on DSM-IV criteria, including (a) fluctuating course, (b) inattention, (c) disorganized thinking, and (d) altered level of consciousness. It is designed to be used in conjunction with a sedation–agitation scoring system. The CAM-ICU has become the most widely accepted delirium scoring model and has been found to be sensitive, specific, and reliable in numerous patient populations, including non-ICU patients.

The CAM-ICU replaces the MMSE used in the CAM with a sedation–agitation scoring system, alleviating the need for patient verbalization. Currently, there are three validated scoring systems for monitoring sedation and agitation in ICU patients: the Sedation Agitation Scale (SAS),[41] the Richmond Agitation Sedation Scale (RASS),[42] and the Motor Activity Assessment Scale (MAAS).[43] Although sedation–agitation scoring systems are not designed to diagnose delirium, they help to identify delirious patients, because they can indicate a number of levels of agitation.[44]

Cognitive Test for Delirium

The Cognitive Test for Delirium (CTD)[45] was the first test actually created for delirium assessment in ICU patients, including those who are mechanically ventilated. It is a visual memory and attention instrument testing five domains: orientation, attention span, memory, comprehension, and vigilance. This test also incorporates the MMSE. The investigators later created an abbreviated version of the CTD using only visual attention span and recognition memory for pictures.[46]

Intensive Care Delirium Screening Checklist

The Intensive Care Delirium Screening Checklist (ICDSC)[47] is an eight-feature checklist based on DSM criteria, including fluctuating course, level of consciousness and attentiveness, orientation, disturbances in speech and/or mood, sleep/wake cycle disturbances, presence of hallucinations or delusions, and psychomotor agitation or slowing. This scoring system was developed to provide an easy and rapid delirium assessment with a dichotomous (yes/no) conclusion. It aims to incorporate information gathered during routine patient care, not requiring patient participation during the assessment. Although the sensitivity is high, it lacks specificity. Thus, this test may best be used as an effective delirium screening tool rather than for diagnostic purposes.

Delirium Detection Score

The Delirium Detection Score (DDS)[48] system also uses an eight-feature checklist giving a dichotomous evaluation of delirium. The DDS is modified from the Clinical Withdrawal Assessment for Alcohol (CIWA-Ar) score and includes signs such as tremor, myoclonus, hallucinations, and paroxysmal sweating. Although this test has been validated in ICU patients, it is not widely used because many of the features evaluated are not specific to delirium. In fact, only one of the items evaluated in the DDS, orientation assessment, corresponds to DSM-IV criteria.

NEECHAM Confusion Scale

The NEECHAM Confusion Scale[49,50] (named for the two inventors) is designed to assess for confusion but has also been validated as a delirium assessment tool. It is not based on DSM criteria. Another difference of this scoring system is that patients can be classified as "early to mild confused," "at risk," or "normal," unlike other models. It is designed to be administered by nursing staff and gives a numeric value assessment. This lengthy test assesses three categorical areas: (a) information processing, (b) behavior manifestations, and (c) physiologic variables. The measurement of physiologic parameters, such as oxygen saturation, vital function stability, and urinary continence differentiates this test from others. In ICU patients, the NEECHAM has been found to have acceptable sensitivity, specificity, and predictive value for delirium when compared with the CAM-ICU.[51]

Delirium Rating Scale

The original Delirium Rating Scale (DRS)[52,53] is a 10-item scale that allows the clinician to not only diagnose delirium, but also rate the severity of delirium. It uses DSM-III criteria as a conceptual base. Similar to the CAM, it requires some subjective clinical judgment by the rater. The DRS was later modified to address some of its limitations and was renamed the DRS-R-98. The DRS-R-98 was increased to cover 16 items and has been found to be a valid measure of delirium severity over a broad range of symptoms and is a useful diagnostic and assessment tool. It is available in French, Italian, Spanish, Dutch, Mandarin Chinese, Korean, Swedish, Japanese, German, and Indian language translations.

Memorial Delirium Assessment Scale

The 10-item Memorial Delirium Assessment Scale[54] questionnaire was first validated on hospitalized cancer and acquired immunodeficiency syndrome (AIDS) patients. As with the DRS, this test allows the clinician to rate the severity of delirium, not just diagnose it. It has been shown to have good validity and reliability when compared with other standard tests, but it is not as widely used.

Delirium Symptom Interview

The Delirium Symptom Interview (DSI)[55] detects the presence or absence of DSM-III criteria for delirium and has been validated as a useful diagnostic tool. One advantage of this model is that it requires minimal subjective clinical judgment on the part of the rater. A disadvantage of this test, when compared with other delirium assessments, is its length, which makes it more cumbersome to administer.[56] In total, there are 107 items: 63 interview questions and 44 observations.

Confusion Rating Scale

The Confusion Rating Scale (CRS)[57] was developed to detect confusion. It may have utility as a delirium screening instrument, but this is yet to be adequately tested. The CRS was designed to be administered by nurses and does not require patient participation. It is based on four items (disorientation, inappropriate communication, inappropriate behavior, and illusions/hallucinations). This tool is advantageous in that it is adaptable to a fluctuating mental status because it is a continuous assessment. Unfortunately, the CRS assesses hyperactive delirium but fails to acknowledge hypoactive delirium.

Nursing Delirium Screening Scale

The Nursing Delirium Screening Scale (Nu-DESC)[58] is an observational five-item scale, composed of the four-item CRS scale plus one additional item. The additional item incorporated is unusual psychomotor retardation, based on DSM criteria. This is thought to increase sensitivity in order to not miss hypoactive delirium. The Nu-DESC has been validated for diagnostic adequacy, and as the name implies, it is designed to be administered by nurses. A recent study in postoperative recovery room patients compared the Nu-DESC, the CAM, and the DDS scores and found the Nu-DESC to be the most sensitive test to detect delirium in this setting.[59]

Clinical Assessment of Confusion

The Clinical Assessment of Confusion-A (CAC-A)[60] is a 25-item observational scale that scores patients in areas concerning orientation, general behavior, motor response, cognitive function, and psychotic behavior. This model likely has limited clinical validity because it contains few of the DSM-IV criteria for delirium.

The Clinical Assessment of Confusion-B (CAC-B)[61] is a 58-item observational scoring system that includes all the items in the CAC-A. In addition, the CAC-B tests patients on items such as behaviors that threaten the patient's safety, speech content, and abilities concerning daily living. This model attempts to rate the severity of delirium. Although the CAC-B incorporates more of the DSM-IV delirium criteria than the CAC-A, the validity of this scoring system has not been widely studied.

Visual Analog Scale for Acute Confusion

The Visual Analog Scale for Acute Confusion (VAS-AC)[62] was adapted from the VAS-C. The "A" was added to indicate "acute," to differentiate from chronic dementia or confusion states. It uses a 100-mm analog line with 0 indicating no delirium and 100 indicating severe delirium. A hash mark is drawn by caretakers to indicate where they believe the patient falls. Despite its simplicity, the VAS-AC has actually shown good reliability and predictive validity. It may be most functional as an initial screening tool, wherein patients receiving a positive score can be further tested with a more in-depth delirium assessment.[63]

Prevention and treatment of delirium

The first and most effective therapy for delirium is prevention. Numerous nonpharmacologic interventions can be used to encourage orientation, such as frequently reminding patients of their location, situation, and the date and time.[64] Clocks, calendars, consistent nursing staff, family visitation, and pictures of family members may be helpful to lessen patient confusion about location, time, and situation.

Maintaining near-normal day and night schedules is important. Opening blinds to sunlight in the morning and minimizing noise, including television, at nighttime is likely beneficial. Some authors suggest that television may be useful in maintaining contact to the outside world; however, some patients form delusions from television programs and this can create or worsen delirium.[44] It is important to provide the patient with sensory devices such as eyeglasses and hearing aids to lessen misunderstanding and confusion. Maintaining normal physiologic function and electrolyte balance, along with prompt treatment of pain, hypoxia, and infection, are all likely to decrease the incidence of delirium. Avoiding over- and undersedation by daily interruptions of sedation will likely help prevent delirium and/or detect delirium that is present.

Avoidance of deliriogenic drugs is not always possible, but these drugs should be used cautiously. Drug classes shown to cause delirium include analgesics, antidepressants, antihistamines, antimuscarinics, steroids, dopaminergics, and benzodiazepines.[44] Obviously, the lists of drugs composing these classes are quite lengthy. Thus, each patient's medication regimen must be individualized and reassessed daily for delirium risk. Often, discontinuing the deliriogenic drug may provide cessation of delirium without further intervention.

If delirium should occur, the focus should be on treating the underlying cause or medical condition. Once this has been established, the symptoms of delirium should be treated. For rapid treatment of hyperactive delirium, the neuroleptic drug, haloperidol, is the drug of choice.[64] Haloperidol works via its potent central antidopaminergic action. It has quick onset and can be titrated to calm and sedate the patient with minimal respiratory depressing effects. There is no daily maximum dose of haloperidol; however, the ECG must be monitored for QT prolongation. Atypical antipsychotics, such as olanzapine and risperidone, have also been shown to be effective.[65] Dopamine antagonists should be used in moderation or not at all in patients with Parkinsonian symptoms. Finally, methylphenidate is a central nervous system stimulant that works by acting as a norepinephrine and dopamine reuptake inhibitor and has been suggested as a treatment for hypoactive delirium.[66]

Narcotics, benzodiazepines, and other psychotropic agents have been shown to increase delirium by 3- to 11-fold.[67] Benzodiazepines should be avoided in the treatment of delirium unless delirium is caused by alcohol or benzodiazepine withdrawal. Also, using benzodiazepines as sleep agents reduces REM sleep, which possibly predisposes patients to delirium.

Conclusions

Delirium is an extremely common and costly morbidity seen in nearly all patient populations. Although many factors can place patients at risk for delirium, not all of them are modifiable and/or avoidable. When prevention of delirium fails, clinicians must be astute in the detection of delirium to maximize treatment strategies. There are numerous validated delirium detection scoring systems, many of which are based on DSM criteria. All have advantages and disadvantages, depending on the intended use and the specific population being tested. In a surgical population, the CAM-ICU is advantageous in that it is able to be used in intubated patients and has been validated in numerous studies in the post-surgical population. Additionally, the CAM-ICU can be performed by various members of the medical care team, does not necessitate a substantial amount of time in training the examiner to proficiently perform the delirium assessment, and can be fully administered to the patient in a matter of minutes. Vigilant delirium detection must continue to be on the forefront of clinical practice as studies continue to shed more light on our understanding of this disorder.

References

1. Lipowski ZJ. *Delirium: Acute Confusional States*. New York: Oxford, 1990.
2. Smith MJ, Breitbart WS, Platt MM. A critique of instruments and methods to detect, diagnose, and rate delirium. *J Pain Symptom Manage* 1994;**10**:35–77.
3. American Psychiatric Association. *Diagnostic and Statistical Manual of Mental Disorders*. 4th ed., text revision. Washington, DC: American Psychiatric Association, 2000.
4. Chevrolet JC, Jolliet P. Clinical review: agitation and delirium in the critically ill – significance and management. *Critical Care* 2007;**11**:214.
5. Ross CA. CNS arousal systems: possible role in delirium. *Int Psychogeriatr* 1991;**3**:353–371.
6. Liptzin B, Levkoff SE. An empirical study of delirium subtypes. *Br J Psychiatry* 1992;**161**:843–845.
7. Peterson JF, Pun BT, Dittus RS, et al. Delirium and its motoric subtypes: a study of 614 critically ill patients. *J Am Geriatr Soc* 2006;**54**:479–84.
8. Francis J, Martin D, Kapoor WN. A prospective study of delirium in hospitalized elderly. *JAMA* 1990;**263**:1097–1101.
9. Levkoff SE, Evans DA, Liptzin B, et al. Delirium. The occurrence and persistence of symptoms among elderly hospitalized patients. *Arch Intern Med* 1992;**152**:334–40.
10. Parikh S, Chung C. Postoperative delirium in the elderly. *Anesth Analg* 1995;**80**:1223–1232.
11. Marcantonio ER, Goldman L, Mangione CM, et al. A clinical prediction rule for delirium after elective noncardiac surgery. *JAMA* 1994;**271**:134–139.
12. Dyer CB, Ashton CM, Teasdale TA. Postoperative delirium. A review of 80 primary data-collection studies. *Arch Intern Med* 1995;**155**:461–465.
13. Radtke FM, Francke M, Schneider M, et al. Comparison of three scores to screen for delirium in the recovery room. *Br J Anaesth* 2008;**101**:338–343.
14. Berggren D, Gustafson Y, Eriksson B, et al. Postoperative confusion after anesthesia in elderly patients with femoral neck fractures. *Anesth Analg* 1987;**66**:497–504.
15. Gustafson Y, Berggren D, Brannstrom B, et al. Acute confusional states in elderly patients treated for femoral neck fracture. *J Am Geriatr Soc* 1988;**36**:55–530.
16. Sharma PT, Sieber FE, Zakriya KJ, et al. Recovery room delirium predicts postoperative delirium after hip-fracture repair. *Anesth Analg* 2005;**101**:1215–1220.
17. Williams-Russo P, Urquhart BL, Sharrock NE, et al. Post-operative delirium: predictors and prognosis in elderly orthopedic patients. *J Am Geriatr Soc* 1992;**40**:759–767.
18. Bekker AY, Weeks EJ. Cognitive function after anaesthesia in the elderly. *Best Pract Res Clin Anaesthesiol* 2003;**17**:259–272.
19. Inouye SK, Zhang Y, Jones RN, et al. Risk factors for delirium at discharge: development and validation of a predictive model. *Arch Intern Med* 2007;**167**:1406–13.
20. Kiely DK, Bergmann MA, Zhang Y, et al. Delirium among newly admitted postacute facility patients: prevalence, symptoms, and severity. *J Gerontol Biol Sci Med Sci* 2003;**58**:M441–M445.
21. Rasmussen LS, Johnson T, Kuipers HM, et al. Does anaesthesia cause postoperative cognitive dysfunction? A randomized study of regional versus general anaesthesia in 438 elderly patients. *Acta Anaesthesiol Scand* 2003;**47**:260–266.
22. Ely EW, Shintani A, Truman B, et al. Delirium as a predictor of mortality in mechanically ventilated patients in the intensive care unit. *JAMA* 2004;**291**:1753–1762.
23. Thomason JW, Shintani A, Peterson JF, et al. Intensive care unit delirium is an independent predictor of longer hospital stay: a prospective analysis of 261 non-ventilated patients. *Crit Care* 2005;**4**:R375–R381.
24. Ely EW, Gautam S, Margolin R, et al. The impact of delirium in the intensive care unit on hospital length of stay. *Intensive Care Med* 2001;**27**:1892–1900.
25. Franco K, Litaker D, Locala J, Bronson D. The cost of delirium in the surgical patient. *Psychosomatics* 2001;**42**:68–73.
26. Milbrandt EB, Deppen S, Harrison PL, et al. Costs associated with delirium in mechanically ventilated patients. *Crit Care Med* 2004;**32**:955–962.
27. Leslie DL, Marcantonio ER, Zhang Y. One-year health care costs associated with delirium in the elderly population. *Arch Intern Med* 2008;**168**:27–32.

28. Devlin JW, Fong JJ, Fraser GL, Riker RR. Delirium assessment in the critically ill. *Intensive Care Med* 2007;**33**:929–940.

29. Dubois MJ, Bergeron N, Dumont M, et al. Delirium in an intensive care unit: a study of risk factors. *Intensive Care Med* 2001;**27**:1297–1304.

30. Marcantonio E, Goldman L, Orav E, et al. The association of intraoperative factors with the development of postoperative delirium. *Am J Med* 1998;**105**:380–384.

31. Urwin SC, Parker MJ, Griffiths R. General versus regional anaesthesia for hip fracture surgery: a meta-analysis of randomized trials. *Br J Anaesth* 2000;**84**:450–455.

32. Fong HK, Sand LP, Leung JM. The role of postoperative analgesia in delirium and cognitive decline in elderly patients: a systematic review. *Anesth Analg* 2006;**102**:1255–1266.

33. Pandharipande P, Shintani A, Peterson J, et al. Lorazepam is an independent risk factor for transitioning to delirium in intensive care unit patients. *Anesthesiology* 2006;**104**:21–26.

34. Maldonado JR, Van Der Starre PJ, Wysong A. Post-operative sedation and the incidence of ICU delirium in cardiac surgery patients. ASA Annual Meeting Abstracts. *Anesthesiology* 2003;**99**:A465.

35. Pandharipande PP, Pun BT, Herr DL, et al. Effect of sedation with dexmedetomidine vs lorazepam on acute brain dysfunction in mechanically ventilated patients: the MENDS randomized controlled trial. *JAMA* 2007;**298**:2644–2653.

36. Ely EW, Girard TD, Shintani AK, et al. Apolipoprotein E4 polymorphism as a genetic predisposition to delirium in critically ill patients. *Crit Care Med* 2007;**35**:112–7.

37. Jacobi, J, Fraser GL, Coursin DB, et al. Clinical practice guidelines for the sustained use of sedatives and analgesics in the critically ill adult. *Crit Care Med* 2002;**30**:119–141.

38. Naughton BJ, Saltzman S, Ramadan F, et al. A multifactorial intervention to reduce prevalence of delirium and shorten hospital length of stay. *J Am Geriatr Soc* 2005;**53**:18–23.

39. Inouye SK, van Dyck CH, Alessi CA, et al. Clarifying confusion: the confusion assessment method. A new method for detection of delirium. *Ann Intern Med* 1990;**113**:941–948.

40. Ely E, Margolin R, Francis J, et al. Evaluation of delirium in critically ill patients: validation of the confusion assessment method for the intensive care unit (CAM-ICU). *Crit Care Med* 2001;**29**:1370–1379.

41. Riker RR, Picard JT, Fraser GL. Prospective evaluation of the Sedation-Agitation Scale for adult critically ill patients. *Crit Care Med* 1999;**27**:1325–1329.

42. Sessler CN, Gosnell MS, Grap MJ, et al. The Richmond Agitation-Sedation Scale: validity and reliability in adult intensive care patients. *Am J Respir Crit Care Med* 2002;**166**:1338–1344.

43. Devlin JW, Boleski G, Mlynarek M, et al. Motor Activity Assessment Scale: a valid and reliable sedation scale for use with mechanically ventilated patients in an adult surgical intensive care unit. *Crit Care Med* 1999;**27**:1271–1275.

44. Borthwick M, Bourne R, Craig M, Ega A, Oxley J. Detection, prevention and treatment of delirium in critically ill patients. United Kingdom Clinical Pharmacy Association. Version 1.2, 2006.

45. Hart RP, Levenson JL, Sessler CN, et al. Validation of a cognitive test for delirium in medical ICU patients. *Psychosomatics* 1996;**37**:533–546.

46. Hart RP, Best AM, Sessler CN, Levenson JL. Abbreviated cognitive test for delirium. *J Psychosom Res* 1997;**43**:417–423.

47. Bergeron N, Dubois MJ, Dumont M, et al. Intensive Care Delirium Screening Checklist: evaluation of a new screening tool. *Intensive Care Med* 2001;**27**:859–864.

48. Otter H, Martin J, Basell K, et al. Validity and reliability of the DDS for severity of delirium in the ICU. *Neurocritical Care* 2005;**2**:150–158.

49. Neelon VJ, Champagne MT, Carlson JR, Funk SG. The NEECHAM Confusion Scale: construction, validation, and clinical testing. *Nurs Res* 1996;**45**:324–30.

50. Champagne MT, Neelon VJ, McConnell ES, Funk S. The NEECHAM confusion scale: assessing acute confusion in the hospitalized and nursing home elderly (abstr.). *Gerontologist* 1987;**27**:4A.

51. Van Rompaey B, Schuurmans MJ, Shortridge-Baggett LM, et al. A comparison of the CAM-ICU and the NEECHAM Confusion Scale in intensive care delirium assessment: an observational study in non-intubated patients. *Crit Care* 2008;**12**: R16.

52. Trzepacz PT, Baker RW, Greenhouse J. A symptom rating scale for delirium. *Psychiatry Res* 1988; **23**:89–9.

53. Trzepacz PT, Mittal D, Torres R, et al. Validation of the Delirium Rating Scale-Revised-98: comparison with the delirium rating scale and the cognitive test for delirium. *J Neuropsychiatry Clin Neurosci* 2001;**13**:229–42.

54. Breitbart W, Rosenfeld B, Roth A, et al. The Memorial Delirium Assessment Scale. *J Pain Symptom Manage* 1997;**13**:128–13.

55. Albert MS, Levkoff S, Reilly C, et al. The delirium symptom interview: an interview for the detection of delirium symptoms in hospitalized patients. *J Geriatr Psychiatry Neurol.* 1992;**5**: 14–21.

56. Smith M, Breitbart W, Platt M. A critique of instruments and methods to detect, diagnose, and rate delirium. *J Pain Symptom Manage* 1994;**10**:35–77.

57. Williams MA, Ward SE, Campbell EB. Confusion: testing versus observation. *J Gerontol Nurs* 1986;**14**:25–30.

58. Gaudreau JD, Gagnon P, Harel F, et al. Fast, systematic, and continuous delirium assessment in hospitalized patients: The Nursing Delirium Screening Scale. *J Pain Symptom Manage* 2005;**29**:368–375.

59. Radtke FM, Franck M, Schneider M, et al. Comparison of three scores to screen for delirium in the recovery room. *Br J Anaesth* 2008;**101**:338–43.

60. Vermeersch P. Development of a scale to measure confusion in hospitalized adults. Doctoral dissertation, Case Western Reserve University. *Dissertation Abstracts International.* 1986;**47**(09B):3709.

61. Vermeersch P. Clinical assessment of confusion. In Funk S, Tornquist E, Champagne M, Wiese R, eds. *Key Aspects of Elder Care: Managing Falls, Incontinence, and Cognitive Impairment.* New York: Springer, 1992;251–262.

62. Nagley S. Predicting and preventing confusion in your patients. *J Gerontol Nurs* 1986;**12**:27–31.

63. Cacchione PZ. Four acute confusion assessment instruments: reliability and validity for use in long-term care facilities. *J Gerontol Nurs* 2002;**28**:12–19.

64. Meagher DJ. Delirium: optimizing management. *BMJ* 2001;**322**:144–149.

65. Skrobik Y, Bergeron N, Dumont M, Gottfried S. Olanzapine vs haloperidol: treating delirium in a critical care setting. *Intensive Care Med* 2004;**30**:444–449.

66. Gagnon B, Low G, Schreier G. Methylphenidate hydrochloride improves cognitive function in patients with advanced cancer and hypoactive delirium: a prospective clinical study. *Rev Psychiatr Neurosci* 2005;**30**:100–107.

67. Inouye SK, Schlesinger MJ, Lyndon TJ. Delirium: a symptom of how hospital care is failing older persons and a window to improve quality of hospital care. *Am J Med* 1999;**106**:565–573.

Appendix A
RASS and CAM-ICU Worksheet

<u>Step One</u>: Sedation Assessment

The Richmond Agitation and Sedation Scale: The RASS*

Score	Term	Description	
+4	Combative	Overtly combative, violent, immediate danger to staff	
+3	Very agitated	Pulls or removes tube(s) or catheter(s); aggressive	
+2	Agitated	Frequent nonpurposeful movement, fights ventilator	
+1	Restless	Anxious but movements not aggressive vigorous	
0	Alert and calm		
−1	Drowsy	Not fully alert, but has sustained awakening (eye-opening/eye contact) to *voice* (**≥10 seconds**)	Verbal Stimulation
−2	Light sedation	Briefly awakens with eye contact to *voice* (**<10 seconds**)	Verbal Stimulation
−3	Moderate sedation	Movement or eye opening to *voice* (**but no eye contact**)	Verbal Stimulation
−4	Deep sedation	No response to voice, but movement or eye opening to *physical* stimulation	Physical Stimulation
−5	Unarousable	No response to *voice or physical* stimulation	Physical Stimulation

Procedure for RASS Assessment

1. **Observe patient**
   a. Patient is alert, restless, or agitated.   **(score 0 to +4)**
2. **If not alert, state patient's name and *say* to open eyes and look at speaker.**
   a. Patient awakens with sustained eye opening and eye contact.   **(score −1)**
   b. Patient awakens with eye opening and eye contact, but not sustained. **(score −2)**
   c. Patient has any movement in response to voice but no eye contact.   **(score −3)**
3. **When no response to verbal stimulation, physically stimulate patient by shaking shoulder and/or rubbing sternum.**
   a. Patient has any movement to physical stimulation.   **(score −4)**
   b. Patient has no response to any stimulation.   **(score −5)**

If RASS is −4 or −5, then **Stop** and **Reassess** patient at later time.
If RASS is above −4 (−3 through +4) then **Proceed to Step 2.**

*Sessler, et al. AJRCCM 2002; 166:1338–1344. Ely, et al. JAMA 2003; 289:2983–2991.

<u>Step Two</u>: Delirium Assessment

Feature 1: Acute onset of mental status changes
or a fluctuating course

and

Feature 2: Inattention

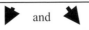 and

| **Feature 3:** Disorganized thinking | OR | **Feature 4:** Altered level of consciousness |

= DELIRIUM

CAM-ICU Worksheet

Feature 1: Acute Onset or Fluctuating Course Positive if you answer 'yes' to either 1A or 1B.	**Positive**	**Negative**
1A: Is the pt different than his/her baseline mental status? <div align="center">Or</div>**1B:** Has the pt had any fluctuation in mental status in the past 24 hours as evidenced by fluctuation on a sedation scale (e.g. RASS), GCS, or previous delirium assessment?	**Yes**	**No**
Feature 2: Inattention Positive if either score for 2A <u>or</u> 2B is less than 8. Attempt the ASE letters first. If pt is able to perform this test and the score is clear, record this score and move to Feature 3. If pt is unable to perform this test <u>or</u> the score is unclear, then perform the ASE Pictures. If you perform both tests, use the ASE Pictures' results to score the Feature.	**Positive**	**Negative**
2A: ASE Letters: record score (enter NT for not tested) <u>Directions</u>: Say to the patient, *"I am going to read you a series of 10 letters. Whenever you hear the letter 'A,' indicate by squeezing my hand."* Read letters from the following letter list in a normal tone. <div align="center">**S A V E A H A A R T**</div>Scoring: Errors are counted when patient fails to squeeze on the letter "A" and when the patient squeezes on any letter other than "A."	**Score (out of 10):** _____	
2B: ASE Pictures: record score (enter NT for not tested) Directions are included on the picture packets.	**Score (out of 10):** _____	
Feature 3: Disorganized Thinking Positive if the combined score is less than 4	**Positive**	**Negative**

3A: Yes/No Questions
(Use either Set A <u>or</u> Set B, alternate on consecutive days if necessary):
 	
     Set A   **Set B**
 1. Will a stone float on water?   1. Will a leaf float on water?
 2. Are there fish in the sea?   2. Are there elephants in the sea?
 3. Does one pound weigh more than   3. Do two pounds weigh
    two pounds?   more than one pound?
 4. Can you use a hammer to pound a nail? 4. Can you use a hammer to cut wood?
 	
Score ___(Patient earns 1 point for each correct answer out of 4)
 	
3B:Command
Say to patient: "Hold up this many fingers" (Examiner holds two fingers in front of patient) "Now do the same thing with the other hand" (Not repeating the number of fingers). *If pt is unable to move both arms, for the second part of the command ask patient "Add one more finger."
 	
Score___(Patient earns 1 point if able to successfully complete the entire command)
	Combined Score (3A + 3B):
	_____ **(out of 5)**	

Feature 4: Altered Level of Consciousness Positive if the Actual RASS score is anything other than "0" (zero)	**Positive**	**Negative**
Overall CAM-ICU (Features 1 and 2 and either Feature 3 or 4):	**Positive**	**Negative**

Intensive care unit risk scoring

Adel Bassily-Marcus and Roopa Kohli-Seth

"If something can't be quantified, its existence should be questioned."
– *Rene Descartes (1595–1650)*

Definition

Risk scoring numerically quantifies a patient's severity of illness derived from data obtained early in a hospital stay. Broadly, scores can be used to quantify severity of illness, benchmark performance, and predict mortality and other outcomes.

Background

The earliest known medical text assessing disease severity is an Egyptian papyrus that classifies 48 head injuries by severity, to define a group of patients too ill to benefit from treatment. Each case was classified by one of three different verdicts: (1) "an ailment I can treat" (favorable), (2) "an ailment I shall contend with" (uncertain), or (3) "an ailment not to be treated" (unfavorable).[1]

One of the first scoring systems widely used was the Apgar system, developed by the American anesthesiologist Virginia Apgar in 1953,[2] which assesses the vitality of newborns and is still in use worldwide.

Another scoring system that has reached maturity is the Glasgow Coma Scale (GCS),[3] developed by Teasdale and Jennings in 1974 to clinically grade consciousness after severe head injury. In fact, there is still no better clinical system to quantify the neurological exam at the bedside.

The first ICU model of disease severity, the Therapeutic Intervention Scoring System (TISS), was proposed in 1974 by Cullen and associates.[4] The basic premise was that the more seriously ill patients received more therapeutic interventions independent of a specific diagnosis, and the severity of illness could be quantified by the interventions used. However, this presumed that physicians seeing a similarly ill patient would prescribe the same therapy, which is not the case.

The introduction of the Acute Physiology and Chronic Health Evaluation (APACHE) system in 1981 by Knaus and colleagues[5] started a new era of scoring systems in critical care. Since then, many scoring systems have been developed, although only a small number are used. Several of these systems are known simply by their acronyms. These systems, or instruments, are broadly termed *general severity scores*, and aim

to stratify patients based on their severity of illness, assigning to each patient an increasing score as their severity of illness increases.

Although they were initially designed to be applicable to individual patients, it became apparent very early after their introduction that these systems could in fact be used to assess large heterogeneous groups of critically ill patients. Later, between 1985 and 1993, several groups added to this function of risk stratification the possibility of predicting a given patient's outcome probability. These improved models, now called *general outcome prediction models* or *prognostic models*, apart from their ability to stratify patients according to their severity, aim at predicting a certain outcome based on a given set of prognostic variables obtained early in the hospital stay and an associated modeling equation.

Classification of scoring systems

There is no agreed-upon classification of scoring systems that are used in critically ill patients. However, ICU scoring systems can generally be divided into four groups:

1. General risk-prognostication scores (severity of illness scores): APACHE, Simplified Acute Physiology Score (SAPS) models, Mortality Probability Model (MPM). These general outcome prediction models focus primarily on a single endpoint, survival.
2. Organ dysfunction scores (organ failure scores): Sequential Organ Failure Assessment (SOFA), Multiple-Organ Dysfunction Score (MODS), Logistic Organ Dysfunction System Score (LODS). These organ failure scores are designed to describe organ dysfunction more than to predict survival.
3. Disease-specific risk prognostication scores: GCS, Child-Pugh, Ranson, Risk-Injury-Failure-Loss-End-stage Kidney (RIFLE), Model for End-stage Liver Disease (MELD).
4. Trauma scores: Trauma Score (TS), Revised Trauma Score (RTS), Injury Severity Score (ISS), Trauma Injury Severity Score (TRISS).

Utility of scoring systems

A simple way of evaluating outcomes is to compare mortality and morbidity. Crude mortality rates cannot be used to measure

ICU performance because they do not adjust for differences in patient case mix and severity of disease. However, the standardized mortality ratio (SMR), defined as the ratio of the observed mortality rate to the expected mortality rate, does account for differences in patient case mix among ICUs, and it can therefore be used to compare the performance of individual ICUs. Thus, prognostic scoring systems permit performance-based comparisons of ICUs by adjusting for severity of disease and case mix.[6]

The scoring systems could potentially applied in five different ways:

1. Stratify patients in clinical investigations (e.g. randomized controlled trials [RCTs])
2. Quantify severity of illness for hospital and health care system administrative decisions, such as resource allocation;
3. Assess ICU performance and compare the quality of care of (a) different ICUs (e.g. it is increasingly important with proposals from the Center for Medicare and Medicaid Services to pay for superior performance, with the contemplated public release of ICU outcome data and to satisfy reporting requirements now being considered by the Joint Commission and its ORYX Core Measures program) and (b) within the same ICU over time (e.g. to assess the impact of changes in staffing rations, medical coverage);
4. Assess the prognosis of individual patients to assist families and caregivers in making decisions about ICU care;
5. Evaluate suitability of patients for novel therapy (e.g. the use of the APACHE II assessment for prescription of recombinant human-activated protein C [drotrecogin alfa]).[7]

Model creation

The ideal scoring system would have the following characteristics:

1. Variables are routinely available and easily recordable.
2. The system is well calibrated (see text that follows).
3. There is a high level of discrimination.
4. It is flexible enough to predict mortality in heterogeneous groups of patients.
5. It can be used in different countries.
6. It has the ability to predict functional status or quality of life after ICU discharge.

No scoring system currently incorporates all these features. The following outstanding issues are commonly faced when designing these systems.

Selecting target population

Most existing models are not applicable to all ICU patients. Data for patients with burns, coronary ischemia, young age,

postcardiac surgery, and very short length of stay were excluded from the development of the majority of systems.

Selecting outcome

The initial step in model creation is to determine the endpoint (typically death, organ dysfunction, resource use, duration of mechanical ventilation, ICU length of stay [LOS], or quality of life after ICU discharge or hospital discharge). Current outcome prediction models aim to predict survival status at hospital discharge. It is incorrect to use them to predict other outcomes, such as survival status at ICU discharge or at 28 days.

Variable selection

Either deductive (subjective by the use of experts consensus) or inductive (objectively using any deviation from homeostasis) selection may be used. The independent variables (e.g. age, deranged physiology, chronic health status, disease states) influence the dependent variables, such as mortality, morbidity, and length of stay. Factors thought to predict outcome (independent variables) are then evaluated against the specific outcome (dependent variable).

With the advent of large computerized databases and statistical software to accomplish techniques such as multivariate logistic regression, it has become possible to quantify the impact of multiple variables acting simultaneously on outcome.

Weight assignment

Assignment of weights to certain variables will significantly augment prognostic accuracy. For example, admission diagnosis, circumstances of ICU admission (e.g. planned or unplanned), and location and length of stay before ICU admission have important impacts on outcome.

Model performance

All predictive models developed for outcome prediction need to be validated to demonstrate their ability to predict the outcome under evaluation. This validation is especially important when the variations in case mix not accounted for by the original models may have a significant impact on its performance. The following are important aspects that should be evaluated in this context.

1. Goodness of fit (as a measure of accuracy): examine the difference between the observed frequency and the expected frequency for groups of patients. Accuracy of the scoring system measures its calibration and discrimination.

   a. Calibration: measures the degree of concordance between the expected and actual number of hospital deaths across the entire range of probabilities of death.

   b. Discrimination: the ability of the model to discriminate between survivors and nonsurvivors.

2. Uniformity of fit: The performance of the model in various subgroups of patients.

All scoring systems should also address two basic methodological issues:

1. Is the scoring system reliable? That is, will different observers (interrater reliability), or the same observer on different occasions (intrarater reliability) produce the same score given the same data?
2. Is the scoring system valid? That is, does it really measure what it is intended to measure?

System validation is tested by assessing both calibration and discrimination values. The validity of a scoring system used to predict mortality in ICU patients is generally assessed based on discrimination between survivors and nonsurvivors (discrimination) and on correspondence between observed and predicted mortality across the entire range of risk and within patient subgroups (calibration). The specific statistical method used to assess reliability is the kappa statistic. A reliability coefficient greater than 0.7, suggesting that no more than 30 percent of the score is the result of error, has been used as a statistical standard.

Calibration

Calibration describes how the instrument performs over a wide range of predicted mortalities. For example: a predictive instrument would be highly calibrated if it were accurate at mortalities of 90 percent, 50 percent, and 20 percent. Four methods have been proposed for analysis; together, these measurements have become standard practice. They are calibration curves, Z score, overall observed/expected mortality ratio (O/E ratio), and the H and the C tests proposed by Hosmer and Lemeshow (H or C depending upon whether the statistic is derived using fixed deciles of risk, H statistic, or naturally occurring deciles of sample size, C statistic). The Hosmer–Lemeshow C goodness-of-fit (HL-GOF) statistic measures how far the estimated probability for a particular case is from the probability obtained from a set of similar cases. It compares the actual and expected mortality rates across 10 defined bands of mortality risk (H^2) and 10 deciles, which include equal numbers of patients (C^2). O/E mortality ratios are calculated by dividing the observed mortality (the number of deaths) by the predicted mortality (the sum of probabilities of mortality of all patients in the sample). Ideally this ratio should be 1.00, an O/E ratio greater than 1.00 indicates a mortality that is higher than predicted, whereas an O/E ratio less than 1.00 suggests mortality that is lower than expected. A goodness-of-fit test such as Hosmer-Lemeshow statistic should have a P value greater than 0.05 (there should not be a significant difference between the model and the outcome). In general, P values of 0.2 to 0.8 are considered good.[8]

Calibration tends to decrease somewhat quickly after a model is built and is very sensitive to population changes. Improving calibration by building local models could be a partial solution to this issue, but few institutions may have enough data to develop robust local models.[9]

Discrimination

Discrimination (which is a marker of the sensitivity and specificity of a model) is the ability of the model to distinguish between patients who died and patients who survived. For example, when a scoring instrument predicts a mortality of 90 percent, discrimination is perfect if the observed mortality is 90 percent. Dicrimination is determined by calculating the area under the receiver operating characteristic curve (AUROC). The AUROC ranges from a lower limit of 0.5 for chance (i.e. coin toss) performance to 1.0 for perfect prediction. AUROC is a graphical expression of the traditional sensitivity and specificity terms. A model is considered to discriminate well when this area is greater than 0.8. The AUROC analysis is valid only if the model has first been shown to calibrate well. The calibration and discrimination components taken together have been named *goodness of fit*.[10]

Identification of subgroups of patients in which the behavior of the model is not optimal is very important and complex. The presence of such subgroups is influential in model building, and their contribution to the global error of the model can be large.[11] The most important subgroups are related to the case mix characteristics that can be related to the outcome of interest. These characteristics may include the intrahospital location before ICU admission, the surgical status, the degree of physiological reserve (age, comorbidity), and the acute diagnosis (including the presence, site, and extent of infection on ICU admission).

Large databases are often split into developmental and validation datasets. A random subset of half or more of the data is used to develop a model, and the performance is then tested on the remaining data, when discrimination and calibration of the model are determined. Determining whether a model's performance is reproducible requires external validation with completely independent data collection, which is expensive and time-consuming and has been accomplished in ICU benchmarking on only a limited basis.

In general, scoring systems need good discrimination if they are to identify nonsurvivors, and good calibration if their aim is to generate standardized mortality measures and other measures of performance based on mortality prediction. Unfortunately, general outcome scoring systems have good discrimination but poor calibration.

Customization

When the original model is not able to adequately describe the population, a recalibration is required to customize the model to counterbalance the deterioration that it may have, to improve calibration. Three different strategies could be chosen.

First-level customization (customization of the logistic equation [logit]) may be accomplished by slight modifications in the logistic equation without changing the weighs of the constituent variables. It is a mathematical translation of the original logit to get a different probability of mortality. The aim of the first-level customization is to improve the calibration of a model and not to improve discrimination. First-level customization should therefore not be considered when the improvement of discrimination is considered important.

In second-level customization, coefficients of variables in the model may also be changed. In a study on the effect of customizations, second-level customization was more effective than first-level customization in improving the calibration of the model and should probably be chosen as the preferential strategy to improve the fit of the model in a well-sized sample.

Third-level customization can be accomplished through the introduction of new prognostic variables and recomputation of all the weights and coefficients for all the variables. This technique is closer to building a new predictive model than to customizing an existing one.[12]

Commonly used scoring systems
APACHE system

APACHE is probably the best known and most widely used system. The aim of the APACHE system is to allow classification of patients on the basis of severity of illness, enable comparison between groups, provide a method to control for case mix, compare outcomes, help evaluate new therapies, and study ICU utilization.

APACHE (1981)[5]

The first physiology-based general severity-of-illness scoring system, applicable to heterogenous groups of critically ill patients, was the APACHE.

APACHE was developed in George Washington University Medical Center and published by William Knaus and associates. This model consisted of two parts: (1) the Acute Physiology Score (APS) and (2) the preadmission chronic health evaluation (CHE).

The APS was a weighted sum of each of 34 physiologic measurements obtained from the patient's clinical record within the first 32 hours of ICU admission. These variables were selected and assigned scores by a panel of expert clinicians. The 32-hour period was chosen to minimize the effect of therapeutic interventions and yet provide enough time for measurements to be available.

The second portion (CHE) was a four-category designation of preadmission health status. Determination of chronic health status was accomplished using a questionnaire that assessed the number of recent physician visits, work status, activities of daily living, and presence of cancer. The data were then subjected to logistic multiple regression, adding age, sex, operative status, and indication for admission, which yielded a mortality prediction.[13]

Strengths

APACHE was a novel system because it used a number of objective variables that were well described and commonly collected to help predict survival. It demonstrated the ability to evaluate the severity of disease in accurate reproducible form and

generate mortality predictions that were surprisingly accurate across different types of ICUs. Analysis of the study sample demonstrated good sensitivity (97%) and positive predictive value (90%), indicating that those who were predicted to survive (i.e., >50% chance) did so. Despite being the oldest system in common use, it still performs well in most validation studies. APACHE II had a slightly lower discrimination than APACHE III, SAPS II, and MPM II. Calibration was found unsatisfactory in all systems.[14]

Limitations

The model was evaluated using only 805 patients in two ICUs. There was poor specificity (49%) and negative predictive value (79%), indicating that many of those who were predicted to die actually survived. The criticisms of the APACHE centered around the large number of variables (34) required along with the 32-hour interval that made the score too complex for manual use; in addition, there was no multiinstitutional validation. In the initial publication, there was no external validation performed. Subsequently, a test of 833 patients to model the APS of APACHE using logistic regression was performed; sensitivity was found to be 60 percent and specificity to be 88 percent.[15]

APACHE II (1985)[16]

In 1985, APACHE II was introduced, with a reduced number of required variables (from 34 to 12) compared with APACHE I, and was validated in 13 large US tertiary care centers. It also introduced the concept of using the system separately for both severity scoring and mortality prediction. The selection and weighting of the variables used in the predictive equation was based on consensus opinion and the findings of previous studies (unlike the Mortality Prediction Model [MPM], which was developed using a combination of univariate and multivariate logistic regression techniques).

The model consists of 12 mandatory physiologic measurements that constitute the APS, along with age, previous health status, and ICU admission diagnosis. The 12 physiologic variables are heart rate, mean arterial blood pressure, temperature, respiratory rate, alveolar-to-arterial oxygen tension gradient, hematocrit, white blood cell count, creatinine, sodium, potassium, pH/bicarbonate, and GCS score. The collection time limit was reduced to 24 hours after ICU admission. Different weights were given for postoperative admission diagnoses, and adjustment was made for emergency surgery. APACHE II was developed from a database of medical and surgical patients that excluded patients undergoing coronary artery bypass grafting (CABG) and coronary care, burn, and pediatric patients.

Mortality probability can be calculated using the APACHE II score by assigning a patient to one of 45 diagnostic categories (29 nonoperative and 16 postoperative diagnostic categories) and using the appropriate regression equation. The mortality probability associated with a particular score is highly dependent on the disease category. Scoring is based on the most abnormal measurements during the first 24 hours in the ICU.

The total APACHE II scores range from 0 to 71 (more than 80% of patients have a score of 29 or less) and there is an increase of about 1 percent in the hospital death rate for each point increase in the score. The authors have specifically requested researchers to discontinue the use of APACHE II except in patients with severe sepsis.

Strengths

APACHE II is simpler to use and improves performance over the original model. It has remained the most widely studied and extensively used scoring system for severity of illness. It has been the method of choice for describing the severity of illness in many landmark studies.

Other claimed advantages include its applicability prospectively and retrospectively, even by nonmedical personnel, as well as reproducibility and minimal interobserver variability.

Discrimination was good (AUC = 0.863) across a wide mix of comorbidities, demographics, and geography.[8,14]

Apart from quantifying the severity of critical illness, APACHE II introduced the possibility of predicting mortality for individual patients, but it was found that mortality prediction could be used only for groups of patients and not for individual patients.

Limitations

The major limitations of the APACHE II system include the following: (1) Risk prediction was based on outcome of treatments between 1979 and 1982, and no recalibration on national databases have been done since that time. (2) The system was not designed for individual patient outcome. (3) There was selection bias – errors in prediction caused by differences in the way current patients are selected compared with criteria used in creating the database. (4) There was a failure to compensate for the lead-time bias (errors in prediction resulting from variations in timing of the ICU admission). Unless all admissions are entered at the same time in the course of their illness, the resulting predictions may not calibrate well to a new database (APACHE II underestimated mortality if it was applied to patients who were transferred from other ICUs, stepdown units, or from another hospital). (5) APACHE II does not control for pre-ICU management, which can restore a patient's physiology, leading to a lower score, thus underestimating a patient's true risk. (6) Sensitivity and specificity varied widely between comorbid conditions. (7) The derivation data set was relatively small (5813 admissions from 13 hospitals). (8) The value of this system is controversial in advanced intraabdominal sepsis and prediction of fatal multiorgan failure syndrome.[17] (9) Comparing APACHE II with physicians' prediction of outcome using AUROC suggests that the physicians impressions were significantly better than the APACHE II predictions (0.899 vs 0.796). However, APACHE II was better for less severely ill patients with mortality risk less than 30 percent.

It is known that the accuracy of APACHE II has deteriorated over time, and the lack of predictor variables of proven prognostic significance means that APACHE II mortality predictions, even when recalibrated in large contemporary databases, are likely to be inaccurate because of the absence of multiple predictor variables. The authors of APACHE II recommend that it should no longer be used to compare observed and predicted mortality, but it continues to be a useful summary measure of severity of illness.[18]

For these reasons, APACHE II should probably no longer used for mortality benchmarking, although it remains a staple for stratifying severity of illness in ICU clinical trials.

APACHE III (1991)[19]

APACHE III was introduced in 1991 and addressed the limitations of APACHE II, specifically the impact of treatment location prior to the ICU admission. There was a movement away from simplification by expanding the number of ICU diagnoses and number of variables (increased from 12 to 17, including BUN, urine output, albumin, bilirubin, and glucose), remodeling of the weights for the physiological variables, an increased number of diagnostic groups (from 45 to 78), and adjustment for location and length of stay before ICU admission, as well as inclusion of seven chronic health items: AIDS, hepatic failure, lymphoma, solid tumor with metastases, leukemia or multiple myeloma, immunocompromise, and cirrhosis.

Weighting for variables changed from group consensus in APACHE II to computer-derived weights estimated by multivariate logistic regression. New equations were added to predict LOS, duration of mechanical ventilation, risk of active therapy, and equations for daily prediction of individual outcomes (it uses daily updates of clinical information to provide a dynamic predicted mortality score similar to the MPM). Additionally, a separate predictive model was introduced to include patients who had CABG surgery.

Two updates were released after subsequent testing on patients from 1998 to 2002 (APACHE III-I, APACHE III-J). The resulting APACHE III score comprises the three subscores: age score (0–24 points) + APS (0–252 points) + chronic health evaluation (CHE; 0–23 points), and the final score ranges from 0 to 299. A five-point increase represents a significant hospital mortality risk. The single most important factor in daily risk of hospital death is the APACHE III score.

In summary, this score uses largely the same variables as APACHE II, but collects neurologic data differently. It adds two particularly important variables, the patient's origin and the lead-time bias. Although acute diagnosis is taken into account, one diagnosis must be selected.[20]

Strengths

APACHE III has superior calibration and discrimination to APACHE II. In addition to the APACHE III score (which provides an initial risk estimate), there is an APACHE III predictive equation that uses proprietary reference data on disease category and treatment location before ICU admission to provide individual risk estimates, which can be updated daily. A predicted risk of death in excess of 90 percent on any of the first seven days is associated with a 90 percent mortality rate. Data were collected on a database of 17,440 patients in 40 hospitals.

Limitations

The physiologic information must be measured over 24 hours using the worst parameter, which is challenging for data accumulation and entry. A principal ICU diagnosis must be identified; incorrect disease identification can affect the accuracy. The APACHE instrument requires precise physiologic measurement of blood pressure, whereas other systems categorizes blood pressure as high, low, or intermediate. The improvement in discrimination is modest. This system is complex, difficult to administer, and, most notably, the logistic regression coefficients and equations are proprietary information and are not freely available. These have been major barriers to its wide acceptance.

Compared with APACHE II, there is a trend for APACHE III to perform slightly better with regard to discrimination, but no consistent improvement in calibration was noted when assessing studies published in the past 10 years.[21]

APACHE IV (2006)[22]

APACHE IV was developed from data collected on 110,558 patients in 104 ICUs of 45 nonrandomly selected hospitals in the United States. The score is made up of the APS, age and admission circumstances, totaling 142 variables, of which 115 are admission diagnoses. In contrast with SAPS III, the APS was found to be the most important factor (65.6% of predictive power), followed by disease group and age. The scores range from 0 to 252. Unlike APACHE III, age, APS, and chronic health were each given a separate coefficient to calculate the probability of death in APACHE IV. The accuracy of physiologic risk adjustment was improved by adding rescaled PaO_2/FIO_2 and GCS variables and by reducing the impact of defaulting the GCS to a normal value when sedation or paralysis made direct assessment impossible. Variables are similar to those in APACHE III but new variables and different statistical modeling have been added. The number of diagnostic groups has increased from 94 to 116. A number of changes have been made for the diagnostic groups, which have been split into finer categories. For example, sepsis is separated into pulmonary sepsis, gastrointestinal sepsis, cutaneous sepsis, sepsis of unknown origin, and sepsis–other. Similarly, acute myocardial infarction is split into four groups according to the location of the infarction.[23]

APACHE IV used a different dataset for calculating the probability of death of patients admitted to the ICU following CABG. For patients admitted for acute myocardial infarction, a variable for thrombolysis therapy was added. The APACHE IV had good discrimination and calibration. Compared with APACHE III, little change was observed in discrimination, but aggregate mortality was overestimated as model age increased. The APACHE IV score is driven primarily by acute physiology (66%), age (9%), chronic health conditions (5%), admission variables (3%), ICU admission diagnosis (16%), and mechanical ventilation (1%). APACHE IV includes refined and updated models for predictions of ICU and hospital mortality during hospital days 1-7, ICU LOS, and risk of active therapy for individual patients.[14]

Strengths

APACHE IV has good discrimination (AUROC of 0.88) and good calibration. For 90 percent of the 116 ICU admission diagnoses, the ratio of observed to predicted mortality was not significantly different from 1.0.[10]

The APACHE IV model provides clinically useful ICU LOS predictions for critically ill patient groups, but its accuracy and utility are limited for individual patients. APACHE IV benchmarks for ICU stay are useful for assessing the efficiency of unit throughput and support examination of structural, managerial, and patient factors that affect ICU stay. The APACHE IV mortality equation has been placed in the public domain and is available at http://www.cerner.com/public/cerner_3.asp?id=27300.

In comparison with MPM_0-III and SAPS II, APACHE IV provides the most accurate estimate of hospital mortality for ICU patients but requires considerable resources to collect data.[24]

Limitations

APACHE IV is a complex system with 142 variables in the mortality equation, including 115 disease groups, and requires training for data entry, which is available as a web-based training manual.

The authors acknowledge the following limitations:

1. The system was developed in US ICUs; international differences in ICU structure predict that they will have an adverse impact on accuracy.

2. Data might not be nationally representative, despite the derivation from 45 different ICUs. It is a new system that has not yet been modeled and validated against a real cohort of ICU patients.

3. Although the sample was large, the results of the logistic regression analysis may have been influenced by the random assignment of patients to training or validation datasets. A large population of patients is required, and no one knows how large the dataset should be. Are data from 110,558 patients enough?

4. The prediction for an individual is only an approximate indicator of an individual's probability of mortality.

5. The use of aggregate SMR as an ICU performance benchmark is limited by factors that are not directly related to quality of care, such as frequency of treatment limitations, early discharge to skilled nursing facilities, and care before and after ICU admission.

6. As with any other system, there is an anticipation for deterioration of the system's accuracy with time, which makes it likely that the system will need to be revised and updated.[18]

Simplified Acute Physiology Score models

SAPS (1984)[25]

The Simplified Acute Physiology Score (SAPS) scoring system was developed by Le Gall in France.[26] It strived to use a simpler model than APACHE, using some of the same physiological parameters and keeping the same level of predictive ability. It was based on 679 admissions from eight French ICUs, in which 40 percent of the cases were surgical in nature. Of the 34 original APACHE variables, 14 were used (age and 13 physiologic variables: heart rate, SBP, temp, RR/mechanical ventilation, urine output, BUN, Hct, WBC, glucose, K, Na, bicarbonate, and GCS). As with APACHE, the worst values in the first 24 hours were used.

Strengths

All SAPS models share an important factor, which is the simplicity. The SAPS score is entered into a mathematical formula that can be solved on a calculator, with no commercial computer software necessary to perform the calculation. The system demonstrated the best specificity (97%) and predictive value for mortality (87.7%), whereas the APACHE system demonstrated the highest sensitivity (58%) and predictive value for surviving (90.2%).

The model became very popular in Europe, especially in France, from 1984 to 1988.

Limitations

No goodness-of-fit testing was reported. SAPS allowed only patient stratification, but not prediction of outcome.

SAPS II (1994)[27]

This was based on a European/North American database that included 13,152 patients from 137 ICUs in 12 countries.[28] Twelve physiologic variables were included in addition to age, admission type, and presence of metastatic or hematologic cancer or AIDS. Patients excluded from SAPS II were patients with age <18, burn patients, and cardiac surgery and coronary care patients. The weights for each variable were estimated using multiple logistic regression. Patients were divided between development (65%) and validation (35%) samples.

Strengths

Similar to the MPM (discussed later), SAPS II can be scored without specifying a primary diagnosis and can be fully implemented from published information. It was developed from much larger dataset than its predecessor. It has shown the ability to maintain good discrimination (ability to discriminate between patients who die or survive at hospital discharge) (AUROC 0.86) across different populations, but calibration (ability to predict mortality rate over classes risk, assessed by goodness of fit) that was initially good compared to SAPS, later deteriorated leading to the development of SAPS 3. Mortality prediction remains accurate only in patients who stay in the ICU for fewer than five days. SAPS II was found to be superior

to SAPS in general ICUs in France. It is the most commonly used scoring system in Europe.

Limitations

There is poor calibration even after two levels of customization. Data used were collected from 1991 to 1992. The accuracy of the predictive power of SAPS II was lost over time, and the mortality prediction was almost completely lost in patients who stay in the ICU for more than seven days. This system had serious case-mix bias and lead-time bias. It failed to predict mortality correctly when applied in independent samples of patients in various geographic settings.

SAPS 3(2005)[29]

SAPS 3 is based on prospective study of 19,577 patients older than 16 years of age from 307 ICUs all over the world.

SAPS 3 comprises 20 variables (17 in SAPS II) allocated in three subscores: (1) patient's characteristics before admission (5 variables); (2) circumstances of admission (5 variables); and (3) acute physiology (10 variables). The time frame of the physiologic parameters was reduced to one hour of ICU admission using worst values. Customization for specific geographical areas was developed to compute risk according to the effect of the ICU variable. Discrimination and calibration varied widely. The best predictive results were from northern Europe (SMR 0.96), and the worst were from South and Central America (SMR 1.30). A customized model (SAPS 3 PIRO) was developed for patients who were admitted with the diagnosis of infection and stayed in the ICU for more than 48 hours, with excellent calibration and discrimination.[30]

Strengths

A high-quality multinational database was built to reflect the heterogeneity of the current ICU case mix and typology all over the world. An electronic tool kit is available completely free of charge. The SAPS 3 outcome research group provides several additional resources at the project's website (www.saps3.org).

All SAPS models share the following advantages: (1) simplicity (easy and quick to compute, can be still calculated easily by hand); (2) free availability; (3) wide range of diagnoses represented; and (4) worldwide populations represented.

Limitations

In groups of surgical ICU patients, the performance of SAPS 3 was similar to that of APACHE II and SAPS II.[31]

Mortality Probability Model

MPM-I (1985)[32]

The Mortality Probability Model (MPM) was developed and validated by Teres and colleagues at Baystate Medical Center and published in 1985.[33] The original MPM (MPM-I) was based on 755 patients at a single center in 1983 and employed logistic regression to weight variables associated with hospital mortality. As in the APACHE and SAPS systems, the model excludes burn, coronary care, and cardiac surgery patients. Unlike the APACHE and SAPS systems, it does not calculate a score but computes the hospital risk of death from the presence or absence of factors in a logistic regression equation. Two models were created, one at ICU admission (MPM$_0$-I) that contained seven variables (age, systolic blood pressure, level of consciousness, type of admission, cancer, infection, and number of organ system failures), and a further prediction model (MPM$_{24}$-I) based on variables reflecting the effects of treatment at the end of the first ICU day. (MPM$_0$-I) is based on data collected within the first hour of the ICU admission, which makes the prediction treatment-independent, in contrast with APACHE, which uses the worst value within the first 24 hours. The discrimination and calibration of the model were good. MPM is not recommended for assessing prognoses for individual patients.

Strengths

MPM was developed to be a completely objective model to provide an evidence-based approach to constructing a scoring system. Very few physiologic measurements are required to simplify ICU predictions. Its utility is increased if laboratory resources are constrained, and it does not require a primary diagnosis for computation.

Limitations

All data were derived from a single institution. The system does not include a specific admission diagnosis.

MPM-II (1993)[34]

MPM-II models were developed on an international sample of 12,610 patients treated between 1989 and 1990. This was the same database used to develop SAPS-II. Prediction models for assessment at admission and at 24 hours were developed originally, but models for assessment at 48 and 72 hours were published the following year. The system allowed ongoing assessment with follow up models at 24, 48, and 72 hours. Patients under the age of 18, burn patients, coronary care patients, and cardiac surgery patients were excluded.

The admission model (MPM$_0$) contains 15 variables; the 24-hour model (MPM$_{24}$) uses five of the 15 MPM$_0$ variables plus eight additional ones. Additional variables included in MPM$_{24}$, MPM$_{48}$, and MPM$_{72}$, but not MPM$_0$, are prothrombin time, urine output, creatinine, arterial oxygenation, continuing coma or deep stupor, confirmed infection, mechanical ventilation, and intravenous vasoactive drug therapy.

MPM-II is easy to use and does not require admission diagnosis. It can be advantageous in complex ICU patients but may make an ICU performance assessment more sensitive to its case mix. The choices of variables and their weights were done by logistic regression to validate their selection. Unlike the APACHE system, which yields a score, the final result for MPM-II is expressed as a probability of death, with a range from 0 to 1.

Strengths

The strength of the MPM-II models lies in their simplicity of scoring and the possibility of sequential assessment of mortality risk throughout the ICU stay. All versions of MPM directly calculate a probability of survival from the available data, without the need to calculate a severity score first. Recent validation studies have found MPM-II to perform well. It has similar discriminatory power to SAPS II with AUROC of 0.82 and 0.84, respectively.[14] MPM$_0$-II remains the only method validated for use at the time of ICU admission.

MPM$_0$-II is an integral part of the ICU self-evaluation; external benchmarking tools are provided by Project IMPACT (Cerner Corporation, Kansas City, MO), which is widely used in North America.

Limitations

MPM-II was based on data collected from patients treated in 1989 and 1990. Recent research using Project IMPACT data suggests that MPM$_0$-II overpredicts mortality.[35]

MPM-III (2007)[36]

MPM is a component of Project IMPACT used by ICUs in the United States, Canada, and Brazil. Data collected from 125,610 patients age >18 and eligible for MPM scoring were analyzed in Project IMPACT from 2001 to 2004, when the model was updated to MPM$_0$-III. Patients were randomly split into development (60%) and validation (40%) samples and analyzed using logistic regression. New variables were added to improve calibration: patient location and lead time prior to ICU admission, code status, and a "zero-factor" term for patients with no risk factors other than age.

Strengths

The discrimination of MPM$_0$-III was very good (AUROC = 0.823) with good calibration.

This model involves the least amount of data collection and does not require a diagnosis when calculating a predicted probability of mortality. In comparison with APACHE IV and SAPS II, MPM$_0$-III is a viable alternative and can be collected at lower cost and in about one-third the amount of time as APACHE IV, without substantial loss in accuracy (MPM$_0$-III, 11.1 min; SAPS II, 19.6 min; and APACHE IV, 37.3 min).

Limitations

The utility of this model is more limited for individual care decisions. Only the admission model (MPM$_0$-III) is available. Serial evaluation is not yet possible (awaiting future work to generate MPM$_{24}$-III, MPM$_{48}$-III, and MPM$_{72}$-III). It is less accurate than APACHE IV and SAPS II in estimating hospital mortality for ICU patients.[24]

Organ dysfunction scores

The general severity scoring systems, with the exception of MPM$_{48-72}$, do not consider organ dysfunction that develops after the first 24 hours of ICU stay. Definitions of multiorgan failure do not take into account the fact that the development and resolution of organ failure is a continuum of alterations and severity, rather than a definitive event.

The majority of these scores include six key organ systems – cardiovascular, respiratory, hematologic, central nervous, renal, and hepatic – with other systems, such as the gastrointestinal system, less commonly included.

Sequential Organ Failure Assessment (1996)[37]

The Sequential Organ Failure Assessment (SOFA) was developed in 1994 during a consensus conference organized by the European Society of Intensive Care and Emergency Medicine. It was initially called the Sepsis-Related Organ Failure Assessment, as it was developed to quantitatively and objectively describe the degree of organ failure over time in septic patients. Then it was renamed the Sequential Organ Failure Assessment, as it was realized that it could be applied equally to nonseptic patients. It evaluates six systems: respiratory, coagulation, hepatic, cardiovascular, renal, and central nervous system. A score is given from 0 for normal function up to 4 for most abnormal, based on the worst values on each day recorded. Individual organ function can thus be assessed and monitored over time, and an overall global score can also be calculated. A high SOFA score (SOFA max) and a high delta SOFA (total maximum SOFA minus the admission total SOFA) have been shown to be related to a worse outcome, and the total score has been shown to increase over time in nonsurvivors compared with survivors.[38] Since its introduction, the SOFA score has also been used for predicting mortality, although it was not developed for this purpose.

Strengths

Scores are objective and independent of therapy, making variable collection uncomplicated. SOFA was designed to be simple enough for clinical use. With the number of component scores limited to six, it is less complicated than many earlier severity-of-illness scores. The combination of sequential SOFA derivatives with APACHE II/III and SAPS II models clearly improved prognostic performance of either model alone.[39,40] It is used mostly to serve as a clinical tool to follow a patient's progress over time.

Limitations

Despite its attempt at simplicity, SOFA was scored appropriately in only 48 percent of cases; accuracy was improved slightly after a refresher course, as demonstrated in a study by Tallgren and associates.[41] Studies comparing SOFA with other organ failure scores do not consistently show superiority of one scoring system over another.

Multiple-Organ Dysfunction Score (1995)[42]

John Marshall and colleagues, using literature review of clinical studies of multiple organ failure from 1969 through 1993, developed the Multiple-Organ Dysfunction Score (MODS). A database of 692 surgical ICU patients was used; 336 cases were evaluated to select the variables and the remaining 356 cases were used for validation. Similar to SOFA, six organ systems were chosen, with each organ allotted a score of 0 (indicating normal function) to 4 (most severe dysfunction) with a maximum score of 24. The worst score for each organ system in each 24-hour period was taken for calculation of the aggregate score.

Strength

The simplicity of the scoring process is excellent.

Limitations

There are problems in evaluating circulatory failure. MODS uses a composite variable pressure (CVP)-adjusted heart rate (HRXMAP/CVP), requiring CVP measurement, which is not readily available in all ICU patients.

Logistic Organ Dysfunction System (1996)[43]

The Logistic Organ Dysfunction System (LODS) is the only organ dysfunction model based on logistic regression. It was developed by Jean-Roger Le Gall using multiple logistic regression applied to selected variables from a large European–North American database (13,152 patients). It is based on the patient cohort used to derive the SAPS II and MPM II systems. Twelve variables were tested and six organ failures defined. The originality of the model is to give to each dysfunction a weight of 0 to 5 points. Four severity levels were identified, assigning the scores 0, 1, 3, or 5 for each organ system according to the severity of failure. Severe neurologic, cardiovascular, and renal failures are scored 5, severe respiratory failure and coagulopathy 3, and severe hepatic failure 1. Thus, the resulting LODS score ranged from 0 to 22 points. The LODS score is designed to be used as a once-only measure of organ dysfunction in the first 24 hours of ICU admission, rather than as a repeated assessment measure.[44]

LODS demonstrated that neurologic, cardiovascular, and renal dysfunction carried the most weight for predictive purposes, followed by pulmonary and hematologic dysfunction; hepatic dysfunction carried the least weight.

Strength

The difference between the LOD scores on day 3 and day 1 is highly predictive of the hospital outcome.

Limitation

The LODS is quite complex and the scoring system is the least used.

Physiological and Operative Severity Score for the EnUmeration of Mortality and Morbidity (1991)[45]

The Physiological and Operative Severity Score for the EnUmeration of Mortality and Morbidity (POSSUM) was developed by Copeland and associates in 1991 and has since been applied to a number of surgical groups, including orthopedic, vascular surgery (e.g. abdominal aortic aneurysm, carotid endarterectomy), head and neck surgery, gastrointestinal surgery, and recent neurosurgical patients. Originally, 48 physiologic factors and 14 operative and postoperative factors for each patient were assessed. Using multivariate analysis techniques, these were reduced to the key 12 physiologic and 6 operative factors. The 12 physiologic factors are age, cardiac history, respiratory history, blood pressure, pulse rate, GCS, hemoglobin level, white cell count, urea concentration, Na^+ level, K^+ level, and ECG. The six operative factors are operative severity, multiple procedures, total blood loss, peritoneal soiling, presence of malignancy, and mode of surgery. The physiologic score ranges from 12 through 88, and the operative score from 6 through 44. Mortality is usually stratified into four risk groups: 0 to 5 percent, 5 to 15 percent, 15 to 50 percent, and 50 to 100 percent. A modification of the POSSUM system, the Portsmouth predictor equation (P-POSSUM), adjusts mortality rates for patients in low-risk groups. V-POSSUM was designed specifically for patients undergoing vascular procedures. Interestingly, V-POSSUM predicts outcome based on preoperative physiologic factors alone, raising the question of whether operative factors can largely be omitted.[46] In a comparison with APACHE II in assessing outcome prediction for surgical patients in a high-dependency unit, the POSSUM score was of greater value.[47]

Strengths

POSSUM has been accepted as the most suitable method for surgical audit. Specialty-specific modifications seem to have improved the prognostic features of P-POSSUM, and it has become widely used and accepted as a risk scoring system.

Limitations

POSSUM may exaggerate the mortality rates in minor and intermediate surgeries and may create an impression that some units are performing better than expected if their practice is dominated by low-risk groups. P-POSSUM overpredicted morbidity and mortality in a series of major gastrointestinal and hepatobiliary operations as compared with the surgeon's opinion, especially after elective surgery.[48] It is not applicable to patients who do not undergo an operation, and is not useful in trauma or pediatric patients. It does not factor in any surgeon-related variables but does give weight to blood loss, need for reoperation, and the degree of complexity of the procedure.

National Surgical Quality Improvement Program (1998)[49]

Derived from the Department of Veterans Affairs National Surgical Quality Improvement Program (NSQIP), administered by the American College of Surgeons (ACS), became available to private-sector hospitals across the United States in 2004 to provide risk-adjusted 30-day outcome data principally relating to mortality. This equation relies on six main factors: albumin, age, ASA status, emergency procedure, disseminated cancer, and

difficulty of the operation. In the original derivation, other significantly weighted factors included resuscitation status, functional status, urea, and weight loss.[50]

Each participating hospital is required to hire a dedicated surgical clinical nurse reviewer (SCNR) to collect and enter data on 133 variables, including preoperative risk factors, intraoperative variables, and 30-day postoperative mortality and morbidity outcomes for patients undergoing major surgical procedures. The data are submitted to the ACS NSQIP through a secure Internet-based system with built-in software checks and user information prompts to ensure completeness, uniformity, and validity of the data. Data automation tools are also available to lower the data entry burden on the SCNRs and to improve the quality of the data being captured. The output of the collected data is presented in semiannual reports that include the hospital's risk adjusted outcomes expressed as observed versus expected (O/E) ratios for 30-day morbidity and mortality. These reports allow each facility to compare its outcomes with the national average and the averages in its peer group of hospitals. In addition, the website offers 24/7 access to user-friendly, real-time reports that allow hospitals to view their non–risk-adjusted data, as well as compare their data with national averages. Complete information, as well as an online application to the program, can be found on the ACS NSQIP website at http://www.acsnsqip.org.

Strengths

The original report presents the results of the Veterans Affairs' NSQIP from 1991 through 1997 and includes approximately half a million operations. One of the most extensive undertakings of its kind, NSQIP has wide usage in the United States, with a large database and validated trials. In October 2002, the Institute of Medicine named the NSQIP the "best in the nation" for measuring and reporting surgical quality and outcomes. It is the first nationally validated, risk-adjusted, outcomes-based program to measure and improve the quality of surgical care.

Limitations

Application of NSQIP to other providers or other countries is limited by lack of studies, the amount of data required, and the complexity of the coefficients to tailor the data to outcomes. It is a comprehensive scoring system but is difficult to calculate and requires a dedicated trained SCNR.

Therapeutic Intervention Scoring System (1974, 1983, 1996)[4,51,52]

The Therapeutic Intervention Scoring System (TISS) primarily evaluates needs in staffing and assessing utilization of ICU facilities rather than stratifying the severity of illness. The original score included 76 selected therapeutic activities (TISS-76), but it was updated in 1983 and further simplified in 1996 to include just 28 items, appropriately weighted (TISS-28). Its development was based on the clinical judgment of a panel of experts in selecting and attributing weights to the items. The philosophy of TISS was that the type and number of therapeutic interventions in the ICUs were related to the severity of the patient's illness. TISS was designed as a descriptor of the intensity of care and was not designed specifically to predict outcome. The TISS-28 consisted of 28 therapeutic items; each item was awarded from 1 to 8 points, depending on the degree of nursing time and nursing effort required. A 0 score indicated that an activity was not present. A total TISS-28 score was calculated by summing the scores for the selected activities. The range of scores is 0 to 79.

Strengths

TISS is one of the oldest scoring systems developed for ICUs and has proven to be a reliable measure for nursing workload and for calculations of requirements in nursing staff.

Limitations

TISS has little direct relevance in the assessment of illness severity or outcome and turned out to be insufficient for mortality prediction. TISS-28 lacks validation by large international databases.

Limitations and pitfalls of prediction models

There are several issues regarding the performance of general outcome prediction models that warrant cautious interpretation and use of the results.

Lack of individual prognostic ability

General severity scores were initially designed to be applicable to individual patients, but it became apparent very early after their introduction that they could be used only in large heterogeneous groups of critically ill patients to predict group outcomes.[53]

A good severity system provides an accurate estimate of the number of patients predicted to die among a group of similar patients; however, it does not provide a prediction of which particular patients will, in fact, die. Models were not designed for this purpose and should not be used in such a context.[54] Lemeshow and colleagues provided an insightful and succinct explanation for why scoring systems cannot predict outcome in individual patients: "Using any of the models in these severity systems (APACHE, SAPS, MPM) for ICU patients, a probability of mortality of 0.46 means that approximately 46 of 100 patients with this probability would be expected to die. One cannot, however, say whether any specific, individual patient will be one of the 46 patients who may die or one of the 54 such patients who may live."[55]

Case mix

One of the primary limitations of any objective model is that it will accurately predict only cases and populations similar to the ones used in its development. For example, in surgical ICUs with high trauma population, APACHE II will perform poorly owing to the few trauma patients (364) included in the development of its dataset. Studies have demonstrated that any variations in the proportion of certain risk factors from the development database can cause degradation of the model's performance.[9]

Model variables

The choice of model variables can also be a potential source of bias. Variable selection and weighting in earlier models was done by an expert panel. Although this ensures that the variables are clinically relevant, it can cause significant performance problems in dissimilar populations. Undue weighting by physicians of overwhelming or recently experienced events has been described. Therefore, more recent models have used objective univariate statistical methods for variable selection. This has resolved the variable selection bias component of these models to some extent, but it has obvious limitations, given the univariate nature of the selection.

Effect of indirect factors

Although the statistical techniques used are robust, they cannot capture indirect influences that affect outcome. Good examples of higher-order influences are the organization and quality of care delivered in an individual ICU. There is good evidence to suggest that the presence of a specialist in intensive care and a closed ICU improve outcome. Such factors are rarely captured in regression models.[54]

Interpretation of missing data

In a study evaluating the effect of missing data on outcome utilizing APACHE III database, it was reported that at least some data were missing in 97.8 percent of patient records.[56] Additionally, the number of missing score items was independently associated with an increased hospital mortality rate when adjusted for severity of illness. The authors concluded that missing values may lead to an underestimation of severity scores, leading in turn to underestimation of predicted hospital mortality. For this reason, further standardization of data collection is necessary.

Lead-time bias

This influence of pre-ICU stabilization on mortality prediction is often referred to as *lead-time bias*. It has been known to be a factor in the calculation of risk prediction. Inclusion of variables collected before ICU admission results in increased severity of illness scores. In an attempt to correct for this, SAPS 3 takes account of both pre-ICU hospital LOS and some therapeutic actions before ICU admission.[21]

Boyd and Grounds effect

To obtain as much data as possible, it has been common to gather data over the first 24-hour period in the ICU. Poor care in the first 24 hours will result in patients with higher predicted probability of death owing to the more extreme physiologic values allowed to develop when adequate stabilization is not performed. This effect is referred to as the Boyd and Grounds effect.[57] Scoring systems such as MPM_0-II and SAPS III prevent this by collecting data at the time of admission.[21]

Benchmarking

Health care professionals and institutions are evaluated based on performance. The fourth-generation models are well positioned for use as ICU benchmarks. These models are based on data obtained three to six years ago. From the past three decades of experience with the adult ICU prognostic models, we have learned that the systems' performances deteriorate over time. For appropriate benchmarking, the performances of the models needs to be evaluated periodically and updated when needed.[58]

Newer models with less weight on deranged physiology

In recent years, the prognostic impact of acute derangements in physiology has been consistently decreasing, whereas the impact of prior health status, physiologic reserve, and circumstances of ICU admission are increasing. These facts can be explained by several factors: (1) intensivists have learned to deal better with deranged physiology to minimize their impact on patient outcome; (2) the way researchers have developed the models can have an impact on the relative importance of different variables, with more power given to the previous health status; and (3) different sampling times of different models (admission values $\pm$ 1 hour for SAPS 3 versus worst value during first 24 hours for APACHE IV) could have an influence by providing different time windows for data collection about acute physiology.[53]

Use of organ dysfunction scores

Mortality prediction scores can be used to stratify groups of patients and assess outcome in terms of mortality. Organ dysfunction scores can help evaluate the effects of new treatments on morbidity. Mortality prediction scores provide valuable information about severity of illness of patient groups but provide little information about individual patients.[55] The use of mortality as an outcome measure may hide valuable information on improved morbidity. Although many morbidity prediction scores correlate well with outcome, they should not replace prognostic systems. The two provide different information and should be used to complement each other.[44]

Errors in model application

The potential pitfalls in application of a properly developed model fall into four major categories: data collection and entry errors, misapplication of the model (especially related to case mix), use of mortality as the sole criterion of outcome, and failure to account for sample size and chance variability when reporting results.[23]

Model customization

Several clinical case-mix, as well as nonclinical, factors are not accounted for by the scoring systems. The overall fit of a score in a particular patient sample was thought to be improved by customization using logistic regression. Customization of APACHE II and III in a large patient population from a single unit led to an improvement in the overall goodness of fit of APACHE III, but the uniformity of fit remained unsatisfactory. It is not recommended to customize models routinely.[59] Model users should keep in mind that the accuracy of these models is dynamic and should be retested periodically. When accuracy deteriorates, the models must be revised or updated. Models should be used as complements, not alternatives, to the use of clinical evaluation, especially when applied to individual patients.[60]

Physician prognostication versus scoring systems

Observational studies suggest that ICU physicians discriminate between survivors and nonsurvivors more accurately than do scoring systems in the first 24 hours of ICU admission. The overall accuracy of both predictions of patient mortality was moderate, implying limited usefulness of outcome prediction in the first 24 hours for clinical decision making.[61] Several investigators have compared prognostic scoring systems with clinical judgment. In general, the comparisons are mixed – some favor the clinician, and others favor the scoring system.[62] Neither physicians nor scoring systems are sufficiently accurate to rely on their predictions in triage and end-of-life decisions. As summarized by the Society of Critical Care Medicine's Ethics Committee, "The use of scoring systems as a sole guide to making decisions about whether to initiate or continue to provide intensive care is inappropriate."[63]

Model comparison

In a retrospective cohort study of different ICU populations, calculating SMR using APACHE II, SAPS II, and MPM_0-II showed that all three scoring systems exhibited good discrimination (AUROC > 0.80), poor calibration (with p values <0.001), and fair to moderate agreement among the three scoring systems in identifying outliers; all systems overestimated mortality. Mortality overestimation was explained by the improvement of patients' quality of care since the models were first developed, and the fact that most ICUs selected in the Project IMPACT database were self-selected, nonrepresentative samples of ICUs skewed toward high performance. The finding that most ICUs in this database were judged to be high-performing units limits the usefulness of these models in their present form for benchmarking.[6]

Future models

As the science of scoring evolves, we expect that further information about our genotypes and phenotypes will be incorporated into the process of clinical decision making. This will be used to stratify patients for risk of certain diseases and will help clinicians to choose the best therapy for an individual patient. The choice of an outcome prediction model remains the result of a tradeoff among local specificity, comparability, and global applicability. Experts forecast that in the near future we will have instruments that have the ability to zoom out, allowing assessment of large groups on the basis of major characteristics, or to zoom in on small groups on the basis of relatively minor characteristics.

Conclusions

The use of these scoring systems to stratify patients into risk categories and provide an adjusted basis for comparison of units has increased significantly in the past two decades but is still somewhat limited to the research community and administration in applicability. Experts in the field continue to recommend caution when using these models to predict individual outcomes, compare quality of care, dictate admission and discharge decisions, assess futility, or attempt health care rationing.

Severity scoring systems are useful, but it is critically important to appreciate the limitations of these scores. Recently developed scoring systems promise even better performance, but validation studies are not yet available.

"In acute diseases it is not quite safe to prognosticate either death or recovery."

Hippocrates (460 BC–377 BC)

References

1. Breasted JH. *The Edwin Smith Surgical Papyrus.* Chicago, Ill.,: The University of Chicago Press; 1930.
2. Apgar V. A proposal for a new method of evaluation of the newborn infant. *Curr Res Anesth Analg.* Jul-Aug 1953;**32**(4):260–267.
3. Teasdale G, Jennett B. Assessment of coma and impaired consciousness. A practical scale. *Lancet.* Jul 13 1974;**2**(7872):81–84.
4. Cullen DJ, Civetta JM, Briggs BA, Ferrara LC. Therapeutic intervention scoring system: a method for quantitative comparison of patient care. *Crit Care Med.* Mar-Apr 1974;**2**(2):57–60.
5. Knaus WA, Zimmerman JE, Wagner DP, Draper EA, Lawrence DE. APACHE-acute physiology and chronic health evaluation: a physiologically based classification system. *Crit Care Med.* Aug 1981;**9**(8):591–597.
6. Glance LG, Osler TM, Dick A. Rating the quality of intensive care units: is it a function of the intensive care unit scoring system? *Crit Care Med.* Sep 2002;**30**(9):1976–1982.
7. Hall JB, Schmidt GA, Wood LDH, ebrary Inc. *Principles of Critical Care,* 3rd ed. New York: McGraw-Hill, Medical Pub. Division; 2005: http://navigator-lhup.passshe.edu/login?url=http://site.ebrary.com/lib/lhup/Doc?id=10130530.
8. Rosenberg AL. Recent innovations in intensive care unit risk-prediction models. *Curr Opin Crit Care.* Aug 2002;**8**(4):321–330.
9. Ohno-Machado L, Resnic FS, Matheny ME. Prognosis in critical care. *Annu Rev Biomed Eng.* 2006;**8**:567–599.
10. Parrillo JE, Dellinger RP. *Critical Care Medicine: Principles of Diagnosis and Management in the Adult,* 3rd ed. Philadelphia, PA: Mosby Elsevier; 2008.
11. Miller ME, Hui SL, Tierney WM. Validation techniques for logistic regression models. *Stat Med.* Aug 1991;**10**(8):1213–1226.
12. Moreno R, Apolone G. Impact of different customization strategies in the performance of a general severity score. *Crit Care Med.* Dec 1997;**25**(12):2001–2008.
13. Schusterschitz N, Joannidis M. Predictive capacity of severity scoring systems in the ICU. *Contrib Nephrol.* 2007;**156**:92–100.
14. Harrison DA, Brady AR, Parry GJ, Carpenter JR, Rowan K. Recalibration of risk prediction models in a large multicenter cohort of admissions to adult, general critical care units in the United Kingdom. *Crit Care Med.* May 2006;**34**(5):1378–1388.
15. Wagner DP, Knaus WA, Draper EA. Statistical validation of a severity of illness measure. *Am J Public Health.* Aug 1983;**73**(8):878–884.
16. Knaus WA, Draper EA, Wagner DP, Zimmerman JE. APACHE II: a severity of disease classification system. *Crit Care Med.* Oct 1985;**13**(10):818–829.
17. Bosscha K, Reijnders K, Hulstaert PF, Algra A, van der Werken C. Prognostic scoring systems to predict outcome in peritonitis and intra-abdominal sepsis. *Br J Surg.* Nov 1997;**84**(11):1532–1534.
18. Zimmerman JE, Kramer AA. Outcome prediction in critical care: the Acute Physiology and Chronic Health Evaluation models. *Curr Opin Crit Care.* Oct 2008;**14**(5):491–497.
19. Knaus WA, Wagner DP, Draper EA, et al. The APACHE III prognostic system. Risk prediction of hospital mortality for critically ill hospitalized adults. *Chest.* Dec 1991;**100**(6):1619–1636.
20. Le Gall JR. The use of severity scores in the intensive care unit. *Intensive Care Med.* Dec 2005;**31**(12):1618–1623.
21. Strand K, Flaatten H. Severity scoring in the ICU: a review. *Acta Anaesthesiol Scand.* Apr 2008;**52**(4):467–478.
22. Zimmerman JE, Kramer AA, McNair DS, Malila FM. Acute Physiology and Chronic Health Evaluation (APACHE) IV: hospital mortality assessment for today's critically ill patients. *Crit Care Med.* May 2006;**34**(5):1297–1310.
23. Higgins TL. Quantifying risk and benchmarking performance in the adult intensive care unit. *J Intensive Care Med.* May-Jun 2007;**22**(3):141–156.
24. Kuzniewicz MW, Vasilevskis EE, Lane R, et al. Variation in ICU risk-adjusted mortality: impact of methods of assessment and potential confounders. *Chest.* Jun 2008;**133**(6):1319–1327.
25. Le Gall JR, Loirat P, Alperovitch A, et al. A simplified acute physiology score for ICU patients. *Crit Care Med.* Nov 1984;**12**(11):975–977.
26. Le Gall JR, Loirat P, Alperovitch A, et al. A simplified acute physiology score for ICU patients. *Crit Care Med.* Nov 1984;**12**(11):975–977.
27. Le Gall JR, Lemeshow S, Saulnier F. A new Simplified Acute Physiology Score (SAPS II) based on a European/North American multicenter study. *JAMA.* Dec 22–29 1993;**270**(24):2957–2963.
28. Predicting outcome in ICU patients. 2nd European Consensus Conference in Intensive Care Medicine. *Intensive Care Med.* May 1994;**20**(5):390–397.

29. Moreno RP, Metnitz PG, Almeida E, et al. SAPS 3–From evaluation of the patient to evaluation of the intensive care unit. Part 2: Development of a prognostic model for hospital mortality at ICU admission. *Intensive Care Med.* Oct 2005;**31**(10):1345–1355.

30. Moreno RP, Metnitz B, Adler L, Hoechtl A, Bauer P, Metnitz PG. Sepsis mortality prediction based on predisposition, infection and response. *Intensive Care Med.* Mar 2008;**34**(3):496–504.

31. Sakr Y, Krauss C, Amaral AC, et al. Comparison of the performance of SAPS II, SAPS 3, APACHE II, and their customized prognostic models in a surgical intensive care unit. *Br J Anaesth.* Dec 2008;**101**(6):798–803.

32. Lemeshow S, Teres D, Pastides H, Avrunin JS, Steingrub JS. A method for predicting survival and mortality of ICU patients using objectively derived weights. *Crit Care Med.* Jul 1985;**13**(7):519–525.

33. Teres D, Lemeshow S, Avrunin JS, Pastides H. Validation of the mortality prediction model for ICU patients. *Crit Care Med.* Mar 1987;**15**(3):208–213.

34. Lemeshow S, Teres D, Klar J, Avrunin JS, Gehlbach SH, Rapoport J. Mortality Probability Models (MPM II) based on an international cohort of intensive care unit patients. *JAMA.* Nov 24 1993;**270**(20):2478–2486.

35. Glance LG, Osler TM, Dick AW. Identifying quality outliers in a large, multiple-institution database by using customized versions of the Simplified Acute Physiology Score II and the Mortality Probability Model II0. *Crit Care Med.* Sep 2002;**30**(9):1995–2002.

36. Higgins TL, Teres D, Copes WS, Nathanson BH, Stark M, Kramer AA. Assessing contemporary intensive care unit outcome: an updated Mortality Probability Admission Model (MPM0-III). *Crit Care Med.* Mar 2007;**35**(3):827–835.

37. Vincent JL, Moreno R, Takala J, et al. The SOFA (Sepsis-related Organ Failure Assessment) score to describe organ dysfunction/failure. On behalf of the Working Group on Sepsis-Related Problems of the European Society of Intensive Care Medicine. *Intensive Care Med.* Jul 1996;**22**(7):707–710.

38. Vincent JL, de Mendonca A, Cantraine F, et al. Use of the SOFA score to assess the incidence of organ dysfunction/failure in intensive care units: results of a multicenter, prospective study. Working group on "sepsis-related problems" of the European Society of Intensive Care Medicine. *Crit Care Med.* Nov 1998;**26**(11):1793–1800.

39. Ho KM. Combining sequential organ failure assessment (SOFA) score with acute physiology and chronic health evaluation (APACHE) II score to predict hospital mortality of critically ill patients. *Anaesth Intensive Care.* Aug 2007;**35**(4):515–521.

40. Minne L, Abu-Hanna A, de Jonge E. Evaluation of SOFA-based models for predicting mortality in the ICU: A systematic review. *Crit Care.* 2008;**12**(6):R161.

41. Tallgren M, Backlund M, Hynninen M. Accuracy of Sequential Organ Failure Assessment (SOFA) scoring in clinical practice. *Acta Anaesthesiol Scand.* Jan 2009;**53**(1):39–45.

42. Marshall JC, Cook DJ, Christou NV, Bernard GR, Sprung CL, Sibbald WJ. Multiple organ dysfunction score: a reliable descriptor of a complex clinical outcome. *Crit Care Med.* Oct 1995;**23**(10):1638–1652.

43. Le Gall JR, Klar J, Lemeshow S, et al. The Logistic Organ Dysfunction system. A new way to assess organ dysfunction in the intensive care unit. ICU Scoring Group. *JAMA.* Sep 11 1996;**276**(10):802–810.

44. Vincent JL, Ferreira F, Moreno R. Scoring systems for assessing organ dysfunction and survival. *Crit Care Clin.* Apr 2000;**16**(2):353–366.

45. Copeland GP, Jones D, Walters M. POSSUM: a scoring system for surgical audit. *Br J Surg.* Mar 1991;**78**(3):355–360.

46. Galland RB. Severity scores in surgery: what for and who needs them? *Langenbecks Arch Surg.* Apr 2002;**387**(1):59–62.

47. Jones HJ, de Cossart L. Risk scoring in surgical patients. *Br J Surg.* Feb 1999;**86**(2):149–157.

48. Markus PM, Martell J, Leister I, Horstmann O, Brinker J, Becker H. Predicting postoperative morbidity by clinical assessment. *Br J Surg.* Jan 2005;**92**(1):101–106.

49. Khuri SF, Daley J, Henderson W, et al. The Department of Veterans Affairs' NSQIP: the first national, validated, outcome-based, risk-adjusted, and peer-controlled program for the measurement and enhancement of the quality of surgical care. National VA Surgical Quality Improvement Program. *Ann Surg.* Oct 1998;**228**(4):491–507.

50. Chandra A, Mangam S, Marzouk D. A review of risk scoring systems utilised in patients undergoing gastrointestinal surgery. *J Gastrointest Surg.* Aug 2009;**13**(8):1529–1538.

51. Keene AR, Cullen DJ. Therapeutic Intervention Scoring System: update 1983. *Crit Care Med.* Jan 1983;**11**(1):1–3.

52. Miranda DR, de Rijk A, Schaufeli W. Simplified Therapeutic Intervention Scoring System: the TISS-28 items–results from a multicenter study. *Crit Care Med.* Jan 1996;**24**(1):64–73.

53. Moreno RP. Outcome prediction in intensive care: why we need to reinvent the wheel. *Curr Opin Crit Care.* Oct 2008;**14**(5):483–484.

54. Ridley SA. Uncertainty and scoring systems. *Anaesthesia.* Aug 2002;**57**(8):761–767.

55. Lemeshow S, Klar J, Teres D. Outcome prediction for individual intensive care patients: useful, misused, or abused? *Intensive Care Med.* Sep 1995;**21**(9):770–776.

56. Afessa B, Keegan MT, Gajic O, Hubmayr RD, Peters SG. The influence of missing components of the Acute Physiology Score of APACHE III on the measurement of ICU performance. *Intensive Care Med.* Nov 2005;**31**(11):1537–1543.

57. Boyd O, Grounds M. Can standardized mortality ratio be used to compare quality of intensive care unit performance? *Crit Care Med.* 1994;**22**(10):1706–1709.

58. Afessa B, Gajic O, Keegan MT. Severity of illness and organ failure assessment in adult intensive care units. *Crit Care Clin.* Jul 2007;**23**(3):639–658.

59. Markgraf R, Deutschinoff G, Pientka L, Scholten T, Lorenz C. Performance of the score systems Acute Physiology and Chronic Health Evaluation II and III at an interdisciplinary intensive care unit, after customization. *Crit Care.* 2001;**5**(1):31–36.

60. Booth FV, Short M, Shorr AF, et al. Application of a population-based severity scoring system to individual patients results in frequent misclassification. *Crit Care.* Oct 5 2005;**9**(5):R522–529.

61. Sinuff T, Adhikari NK, Cook DJ, et al. Mortality predictions in the intensive care unit: comparing physicians with scoring systems. *Crit Care Med.* Mar 2006;**34**(3):878–885.

62. Herridge MS. Prognostication and intensive care unit outcome: the evolving role of scoring systems. *Clin Chest Med.* Dec 2003;**24**(4):751–762.

63. Consensus statement of the Society of Critical Care Medicine's Ethics Committee regarding futile and other possibly inadvisable treatments. *Crit Care Med.* May 1997;**25**(5):887–891.

Chapter 35

Computers and monitoring
Information management systems, alarms, and drug delivery

David Wax and Matthew Levin

Information management systems

The vast array of monitoring modalities used in the practice of anesthesia and critical care provide a snapshot of a patient's condition at any given moment. Trends of physiologic parameters, however, are often more telling than any individual measurement. Many monitoring systems, therefore, include functionality that automatically stores recent data and allows clinicians to retrieve the data in tabular or graphical format to review such trends. However, the durability of these recordings is typically limited to the time of the actual patient encounter, unless deliberately saved in some form. In addition, the data are often acquired from various stand-alone monitors, making it difficult to integrate the data from the various sources. Because retrospective review of such data at some time in the future may be beneficial for patient care, clinical research, quality improvement, administrative, and medicolegal purposes, medical records have developed to memorialize these patient encounters.

Anesthesia records

The first anesthesia records have been credited to Cushing and Codman, who created their "ether charts" beginning in 1894 in an effort to improve anesthesia care, although Snow reportedly recorded details of anesthetic care as early as the 1850s. Manual (hand-kept) anesthesia records remain in use today by the majority of practitioners and are similar in form to the earlier records, although they contain data from more monitoring modalities than were available in earlier years, as well as other data now necessary for administrative, medicolegal, and quality assurance purposes. Perioperative documentation is now a standard of care, with required elements promulgated by professional organizations. It is also a significant component of the workflow of anesthesia providers, consuming an estimated 10 percent of their time.[1–3]

Manual anesthesia records suffer from numerous inaccuracies and deficiencies in recording both physiologic variables and text-based narratives and observations; this is found in records created by practitioners of all levels of experience.[4,5] Manual recordings of physiologic values may be particularly problematic for various reasons. First, standard forms for anesthesia records are typically designed to require entries only once every 5 to 15 minutes, so transient physiologic disturbances occurring between these intervals may not be captured. Second, clinicians may be engaged in other tasks and may be unable to record monitored values at the time they are displayed, and so the data charted later from memory may be inaccurate or subject to recall bias. Finally, clinicians may deliberately omit physiologic values that they feel might be perceived to indicate suboptimal care in future case reviews.[6–10] Similarly, quality reporting based on manual records and voluntary reporting is also not optimal.[11] An additional problem of handwritten records is that extraction and tabulation of specific data elements from archives of handwritten, frequently illegible, records for research, quality assurance reporting, or administrative purposes is difficult and time-consuming.

Automatic recordkeepers

As technology advanced in other aspects of anesthesia care, innovation in recordkeeping occurred as well. As early as the 1930s, devices to automatically record some anesthetic variables had been developed, as well as new formats (e.g. punchcards) in which to manually record data that would improve the accuracy and efficiency of data extraction and analysis.[12,13] As access to computer technology increased in the 1970s and 1980s, the technology was applied to the task of anesthesia recordkeeping and led to the creation of various "home-grown" systems, and later commercial systems, for this purpose.[14–19] Other technology for automating and improving recordkeeping included video recording of patient monitors, but this never gained popularity possibly because of the difficulty with reviewing and extracting discrete data from video, the large amount of data storage space required, and possible medicolegal exposure.[20]

Anesthesia information management systems

As automatic recordkeepers (ARK) developed and began to include more functionality than just intraoperative record keeping, the term *anesthesia information management system* (AIMS) came into use. The term is an improvement over ARK in that recordkeeping is never completely automatic and still requires manual entry of data into the record (although using methods other than handwriting), and that it is a multifunctional system providing more than just a transcript of anesthetic care. There is, however, no standard set of functions that a system must have to constitute an AIMS, and implemented systems vary widely in their capabilities.

System architecture

AIMS vary in their components and architecture. A simple system may consist of a single computer workstation or personal digital assistant (PDA) with ARK software installed, whereas more elaborate systems have multiple workstations, servers, interfaces, and networked connections.

Point-of-care workstations

AIMS workstations typically consist of the components seen in Figure 35.1. A central processing unit (CPU) with features and functionality similar to standard home and office personal computers is usually sufficient to serve at the AIMS point of care, as AIMS point-of-care software does not typically require extensive data processing power. Data entry to the CPU can come

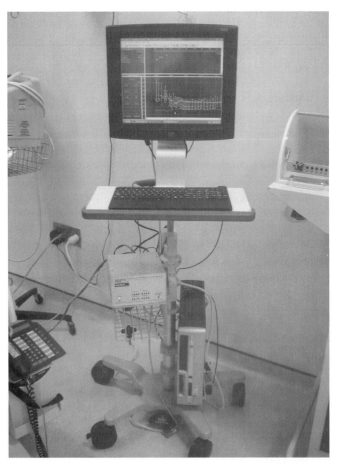

Figure 35.1. Anesthesia information management system (AIMS) point-of-care workstation consisting of computer central processing unit (CPU), sealed keyboard with integrated pointing device, touch-screen monitor, data multiplexer (to acquire data from patient monitors), and wired network connection.

from a variety of sources. A keyboard is used for text entry and ideally should be of a type that can be disinfected between cases for infection control. Voice recognition also has potential as a textual input source. A mouse, trackball, or touchpad is typically used for cursor control and must be able to be disinfected as well. A monitor is used both as the display for the AIMS software and possibly as an input device if it has touch-screen functionality for cursor control. Other input devices, such as barcode scanners, may also be integrated. A multiplexer may be required to receive data from the various patient monitors and make each source available to the CPU in sequential fashion. A local or network printer may be used for printing completed records.

The workstation may be housed on top of an anesthesia machine or drug cart or on an articulating arm attached to a wall or other stable structure, or may be on a freestanding table or frame. The location of workstations is ideally in a place that does not require that the user turn his or her back to the patient, but such positioning may be unavoidable in some settings. Mobile workstations using PDAs or tablet computers can also be used to share a workstation among low-volume locations or use on clinical rounds (e.g. remote anesthetizing locations, postoperative evaluations, pain management or critical care rounds).

Connectivity

Although a single stand-alone workstation implementation may be possible, realization of all the benefits of an AIMS requires connectivity. Each workstation, therefore, is typically connected to a server via some standard networking platform to allow each workstation to send and receive data to and from the server and shared devices. Connections can be hard-wired or wireless, and can be continuous or intermittent. (For example, operating room workstations may have wired continuous Ethernet connections, whereas a mobile workstation may have a continuous wireless 802.11 connection to an Ethernet-based WiFi router or may be used offline and only intermittently connected by wire to an Ethernet to exchange data with a server.) Network connections can be local or can connect geographically separate installations.

Data storage

The AIMS server allows centralized storage of data. This centralization provides greater storage capacity, archiving and backup efficiency, security, and availability of stored data for retrieval from any location. Various platforms are available to store data in a proprietary or open-source relational database; the choice will depend on the server operating system and AIMS software. The server also typically stores configuration data required by the workstations. Transfer of new data to the server can occur continuously as new data are acquired, or can occur in batches, between which the workstations store data locally in an offline mode. Servers may also house the AIMS software itself in configurations in which the distributed workstations function simply as minimally functional "thin-client" terminals similar to mainframe terminals. Alternatively, "thick-client" design has the complete AIMS point-of-care software on every workstation so each can run in stand-alone mode if the server fails transiently.

Software

AIMS software is available from a small number of commercial vendors or may be custom developed. Some installations use a combination of the two, using the vendor-provided software and adding functionality by integrating additional applications developed using custom programming. Basic functionality typically consists of recording intraoperative physiologic data, drug administration, fluid input and output, event timing, and narrative notes made by the clinician to document intraoperative events. Functionality also typically includes the ability to create standardized electronic forms for entering data for specific purposes (e.g. preoperative, postoperative, and critical care history and physical exam notes, procedure notes, and administrative/regulatory notes). Other functionality, such as review of old records, OR management, decision support, and the like, may be integrated. Server-level software modules may allow for extraction and reporting of data for administrative or research purposes, billing, and configuration of the entire AIMS to adapt to local practices and workflow. Security is implemented at various levels, including user management, workstation accessibility, network security, audit trails, and data backup. Various software interfaces are often necessary for the AIMS to exchange data with other systems (such as patient registration systems, OR scheduling systems, laboratory systems, monitoring devices, billing systems, and regulatory agencies).

Benefits of AIMS
Clinical documentation

Implementation of an AIMS is intended to improve clinical documentation. Several investigators have assessed the impact of an AIMS for this purpose. One study comparing AIMS-produced records to completely manual records showed that AIMS records required less practitioner time (both absolute time and percentage of case time), recorded more vital signs and clinical notes, had a similar number of artifacts, and had fewer illegible entries.[21] Another study concluded that missing or erroneous data occurred more frequently in handwritten records, especially during the first 15 minutes and last 10 minutes of a case, when greater attention to patient care is typically required and detracts from attention to documentation.[22] Vital sign data (e.g. blood pressure) were also found to be more accurate (and more variable) in AIMS records compared with manual records for aforementioned reasons.[6,23] AIMS records are still imperfect, however. Additional studies have shown that information may be incomplete even in an AIMS record owing

to dependence on free text remarks and inability to automatically present entries in logical sequences consistent with workflow, and that practitioners deliberately smooth variability and extreme values in automatically acquired physiologic data in AIMS records as well.[24,25] Overall, the improvement realized after AIMS implementation is supported by several surveys that showed that the majority of users, in both OR and obstetric settings, were satisfied with their AIMS and would not want to return to a completely manual system.[26-29]

Performance improvement and patient safety

In addition to providing better documentation of clinical care, AIMS have the potential to improve quality of care. Several studies using simple reminders in an AIMS showed that this intervention could significantly improve compliance with prophylactic antibiotic administration timing.[30-32] Another use of an AIMS is to provide decision support. In one study, an AIMS-based algorithm that alerted the clinician if a patient had multiple risk factors for postoperative nausea and vomiting nearly doubled the use of antiemetic prophylaxis for these high-risk patients.[33] Using an AIMS to screen for intraoperative markers of complications may also be helpful in identifying cases for quality assurance reviews. Studies have shown that such electronic screening yielded many more cases of interest than did voluntary reporting by clinicians.[34,35]

Technologies in common use in other industries are also beginning to be used in health care and integrated into AIMS. Use of bar codes on medication labels in conjunction with a special scanning device (Figure 35.2) may decrease medication errors and improve documentation.[36,37,38] Barcodes and radiofrequency identification tags can also be used to verify

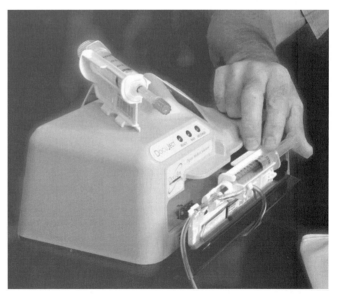

Figure 35.2. Anesthesia information management system (AIMS) medication scanning device – a device that verifies and records injections from barcoded medication syringes intended to reduce drug errors and improve documentation (DocuJect, DocuSys, Mobile, AL).

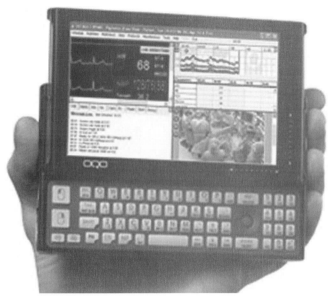

Figure 35.3. Anesthesia information management system (AIMS) remote monitoring device – handheld mobile device for monitoring real-time intraoperative physiologic data, communications, and video (Vigilance, Acuitec, Birmingham, AL).

patient identity, locate patients and vital equipment, and ensure blood product compatibility.

Other areas of improvement possible with AIMS include the ability to retrieve records of prior anesthesia encounters to identify previous problems, improvement of summary documentation for transfer of care (i.e. handoffs), guidance during emergencies (e.g. malignant hyperthermia or cardiac arrest), laboratory data interfaces that report and record pertinent lab values when they become available, alerts to worrisome trends in physiologic values beyond the simple limit alarms built into monitors, and the ability to monitor cases remotely by accessing live AIMS records from a remote workstation or PDA (Figure 35.3).

The possibility that an AIMS could actually jeopardize patient safety has been considered. With clinicians free of the need to record vital signs manually, there is potential for inattention to the vital signs that are both measured and recorded automatically. This issue was addressed in two studies that concluded that the use of an AIMS did not decrease vigilance in this regard.[39,40]

Practice and practitioner applications

Use of an AIMS creates opportunities to improve economics of practice. In addition to recording the clinical documentation that is needed to support billing, the AIMS can function as a point-of-care charge capture system as well. A complete AIMS record can contain all the necessary patient, procedure, time, and special technique information that, in combination with other patient insurance information, can be used to create a bill of service by a billing provider. Using an AIMS to drive billing can eliminate the need for paper billing vouchers and can reduce charge lag, clerical and processing costs, lost bills, days

in accounts receivable, and practitioner paperwork burden.[41] Using automatic electronic mail and PDA alerts of deficiencies in the AIMS record has also led to improved billing metrics.[42]

AIMS can also increase revenue by helping to identify potentially reimbursable items. One study showed that screening AIMS records for presence of vital signs from an invasive monitor but without supporting documentation of placement of the monitor (necessary for billing) identified a significant source of missed revenue that could be corrected.[43] Another study showed that use of an AIMS-based preoperative evaluation system by hospital coders resulted in additional abstracted diagnoses that increased hospital revenue under the diagnosis-related group (DRG) system.[44]

Not only does an AIMS allow for documenting anesthesia care, but it also has potential applications for monitoring practitioner activities. One report demonstrated a role for using an AIMS as the basis of a productivity-based compensation system for faculty and house staff in an academic anesthesia practice.[45] Another study found that an AIMS-based cost analysis was helpful in implementation of practice guidelines regarding anesthetic drug usage and could lead to significant cost savings.[46] Also reported is the use of an AIMS to help identify practitioners who may be diverting controlled substances.[47]

Research

Continued use of an AIMS leads to accumulation of large amounts of clinical data that can be used for research purposes. These data can mined (extracted) and used to test hypotheses prior to planning a prospective study, or to study things too rare, unethical, or impractical to study prospectively. (It would be too cumbersome, however, to configure an AIMS to routinely collect all conceivable data that might one day prove to be useful for research, and many outcome data of interest are typically unavailable in an AIMS because the period of post-anesthesia care is usually brief.) There is also an opportunity to combine the electronic records created by AIMS from multiple centers, allowing multicenter retrospective analyses. Such efforts are hindered, however, by the lack of standardization of structure and terminology in electronic medical records. Multiple efforts are under way to create such standards.[48] For prospective studies, an AIMS can be configured to collect necessary data elements, and an AIMS-based preoperative evaluation can be used to screen patients for inclusion in research protocols.

Barriers to AIMS

Despite the multiple benefits of AIMS, adoption of such systems has been slow, with fewer than 10 percent of academic anesthesia practices having implemented such a system by 2007. This figure was expected to increase to nearly 35% by 2009, though an actual figure has not been reported. Penetration into smaller anesthesia practices is likely much lower because of system cost and smaller volume. When asked why an AIMS had not been adopted, commonly cited reasons were related to cost, medicolegal risk, and inertia.[49]

Regarding cost, health care organizations are under budgetary pressures and are reluctant to use limited funding for projects that do not have a clear return on investment (ROI). The ROI for a hospital may be difficult to demonstrate for an AIMS, and many anesthesia groups cannot afford to purchase a system without the assistance of the hospital. In addition, much of the aforementioned functionality of an AIMS that can improve billing and regulatory compliance is not currently included in standard AIMS software but was developed by in-house development teams – a resource not available to all centers. Some things that will ameliorate the cost problem will be addition of such functionality by AIMS software vendors, creative financing options for AIMS, and overall national interest in (and government funding for) electronic health records.

The medicolegal fears of AIMS arise from concern that data that would have been omitted from a handwritten record are automatically recorded in an AIMS record, even if they are factitious/artifactual or transient. A survey addressing this issue, however, demonstrated that AIMS records had either a beneficial effect, or no effect, on outcomes of malpractice cases. No cases were hindered by the AIMS record and the majority of respondents would recommend an AIMS as part of a risk management strategy.[50] However, at least one case has been reported in which a monitoring gap in an AIMS record caused by technical failure, combined with metadata that showed that an attestation about attending anesthesiologist presence at extubation was entered prior to that event, discredited the anesthesiologist and led to a settlement. The AIMS software was later modified to show an alert when the datastream from patient monitors is unexpectedly lost, and the group created a reporting system that discouraged premature attestations (see Chapter 2).[51]

People are often resistant to change, and an AIMS is a substantial change compared with manual records. This is why one of the most important components of a successful AIMS is a local champion who is both motivated and empowered to overcome the many organizational and technical barriers to AIMS implementation. Such effort is rewarded, however, as clinicians eventually acknowledge that an AIMS improves the quality of their practice and rarely ask to switch back to manual/handwritten anesthesia records.[52]

Clinical alarm systems

Alarm systems are at the heart of modern anesthesia equipment and practice.[53,54] They can be divided broadly into two types: those that monitor equipment (technical) and those that monitor the patient (physiologic). Technical alarms tend to be immediate, indicating a fault or equipment malfunction, whereas physiologic alarms are more often anticipatory, indicating that a potential for harm exists if the alarm condition is not corrected.[55] Also, physiologic alarms are usually indirect, in that they measure derived parameters and rely on certain clinical assumptions that may not always be true.

A well-designed alarm should possess several qualities.[56,57] It should be *sensitive* (i.e. minimal false negatives) and so should reliably detect all valid triggering events. It should also be *specific* (i.e. minimal false positives) so the alarm system reliably ignores spurious or transient events that are not valid alarm triggers. Alarms should also be *distinctive*, with each alarm signal clearly indicating the nature of the alarm condition, without ambiguity. In addition, they should be *localizable*, allowing the clinician to quickly and easily identify the source of the alarm.

History

Prior to World War II, alarm systems were virtually nonexistent in anesthetic practice. Anesthesia machines were primitive, and anesthesiologists relied solely on their clinical judgment and experience to detect critical events such as equipment failure or hypoxia (e.g. by looking for cyanosis). Beginning in the 1950s, the rapid mechanization of anesthetic delivery systems both enabled and necessitated the development of monitoring systems that warned about hypoxic gas mixtures. Many of the early innovations came out of Britain. In 1956, Esplen described a low-gas warning system that consisted of an electromechanical device that sounded a bell when the pressure in a gas line fell below 5 pounds per square inch.[58] Also in 1956, Hill described an entirely different type of low gas alarm that used the relative pressure in the oxygen and nitrous oxide gas lines to control a pneumatic switch.[59] When the pressure of one gas decreased a critical amount below the other, a rubber diaphragm was unseated, causing a reed whistle to blow. The whistles had different tones, one to indicate low oxygen and the other low nitrous oxide.

By the mid-1960s, hypoxic gas mixture alarms were in common use and more sophisticated alarms began to be developed. In 1965, Lamont and Fairley reported on a ventilator alarm being used that monitored the pressure within the ventilator circuit by means of a mercury pressure switch connected to a transistor-based electronic alarm.[60] The pressure limit, as well as the length of the expiratory pause, could be adjusted via set screws or knobs. In 1970, Sawa and Ikezono described a more sophisticated ventilator alarm that could be used with both pressure- and volume-controlled ventilators.[61] Throughout the 1970s, the microprocessor revolution drove a steady improvement in the design and reliability of equipment-based alarms. In the 1980s, the refinement of capnography and the introduction and rapid adoption of pulse oximetry brought the use of physiologic alarms into the mainstream.[62] The two decades since have seen an exponential increase in both the number and complexity of alarm systems.

Standards

Several standards exist regarding alarms and their use. In agreement with the Anesthesia Patient Safety Foundation, the American Society of Anesthesiologists states that, at a minimum, alarms indicating low blood oxygenation, low oxygen concentration, low end-tidal carbon dioxide, and low pressure (i.e. breathing circuit disconnect) must be used when pulse oximetry, airway devices, or ventilators are used.[63,64]

A much more comprehensive standard has been developed by the International Electrotechnical Commission (IEC) and is intended primarily for developers and manufacturers of medical equipment.[65] This standard defines alarm categories (priorities), alarm signals, and a set of consistent control states and markings to be used by all alarm systems. The goal is a set of unified specifications that increases the usability of alarm systems by limiting the number and type of alarms and, most importantly, the frequency of false alarms.

One additional initiative that may have significant impact on alarm technology within the next few years is the Medical Device "Plug-and-Play" Interoperability Program (MD PnP). The goal of this program is to create a system of open standards that will increase interoperability among medical devices. Among other benefits, full interoperability will enable the development of intelligent alarm systems that use data from multiple devices.[66]

Auditory alarms

Auditory alarms have the advantage of being omnidirectional.[67] Although high-frequency hearing loss has the potential to interfere with alarm detection, especially in the noisy environment of an operating room, auditory alarms attract attention faster and more reliably than do visual signals, and so remain the primary alarm modality used for most anesthesia equipment.[68,69] The ideal auditory alarm should be easy to localize, easy to learn and retain, and resistant to masking by other sounds.[56] Numerous studies have shown that this is best achieved by using relatively low frequency (below about 1500 Hz), harmonic, melodic alarms, or even speech.[70,71] Speech is a particularly effective type of auditory alarm, as the meaning of the alarm is immediately obvious. In a medical setting, however, verbal warnings may be undesirable because of their relatively long transmission time and their potential to cause undue concern in patients or visitors.

Unfortunately, the current reality is that most auditory alarms are high-frequency, monotonic, and nonspecific. For example, infusion pumps use a high-decibel, high-frequency beep to indicate downstream obstruction. This alarm is both irritating and difficult to localize. Similarly, an analysis of the predicted inner ear excitation patterns of a cardiac monitor and a pulse oximeter found that the cardiac monitor completely masked the pulse oximeter, so if both alarms sounded simultaneously, the pulse oximeter would be inaudible.[71]

The drive toward standardization of alarm sounds has accelerated in recent years. The IEC defines standardized alarm sounds as well as the sequence for escalating the auditory signal. These proposed alarms are classified by system (e.g. cardiac, ventilatory) and are intended to be device- and manufacturer-independent. Controversy exists as to whether these proposed standards will achieve their desired goal, the primary concern being that the alarm sounds defined by IEC do not differ sufficiently in their acoustic dimensions (e.g. rhythm, tonality) and this may impair the ability of clinicians to differentiate the sounds quickly and easily.[72,73] Auditory alarms, unless muted, can also be distracting while the clinician tries to focus on correcting the situation that triggered the alarm. In addition, it has been shown that responses to medium-priority alarms were faster and more accurate than responses to high-priority alarms.[74] This suggests that further work needs to be done to better define the most effective audible alarm sounds.

Visual alarms

Visual alarms can convey a much greater density of information than auditory signals, with the drawback that they are more easily overlooked or ignored because they tend to be directional/localized.[69,75] Historically, because of limitations in display technology, visual alarms tended to be simple warning lights that either flashed or illuminated to indicate an alarm condition. With modern technology, such limitations have been removed and a significant amount of information can be conveyed.

By long-standing convention, the colors red and yellow are assigned to alarm states and green to normal operating conditions.[55] The IEC codifies these color conventions and goes further by defining flashing frequencies to indicate the urgency of the alarm: 0.4 Hz to 0.8 Hz for medium-priority alarms and 1.4 to 2.8 Hz for high-priority alarms.[65] The standard further specifies that the presence of a visual alarm and its priority should be perceivable at 4 meters and legible at 1 meter. Unlike audible alarms, it should not be possible to override or disable a visual alarm.[53,55] The warning should remain visible until the alarm condition has been resolved.

False alarms, limits, and artifacts

The most pervasive problem with current alarm systems is the very high percentage of false alarms (false positives). For various reasons, not the least of which is medicolegal liability, manufacturers may be overcautious when setting default alarm limits, increasing the sensitivity of their equipment at the expense of specificity.[76] One study of intraoperative alarms found that 75 percent of all alarms during a typical case were spurious, whereas only 3 percent represented actual risk to the patient.[77] The majority of false alarms were caused by patient movement or mechanical problems. A similar study in a pediatric ICU setting found that 68 percent of all alarms during the seven-day study period were false (likely related to patient movement), and only 5.5 percent were of clinical significance.[78]

Most modern anesthesia equipment allows the user to override the default alarm limits, which can improve the specificity of the alarm (i.e. reduce the number of false positives). However, if the limits are set too broadly, the alarm is effectively disabled, with potentially adverse consequences for the patient. Similarly, most audible alarms can be silenced or disabled, a practice that may be more common than realized, and potentially disastrous.[79]

A major source of false alarms is monitoring artifact.[80] Artifact can be from external sources, or it can be intrinsic to the monitoring device. Intrinsic artifact is insidious in that it is a function of the proprietary algorithms and filters used by a particular device. In general, most current monitors use simple linear filters to remove artifacts and noise. Many also do some time series averaging for parametric data (e.g. averaging heart rate over several beats). These techniques smooth out the data and remove outliers and noise but may create delay or remove valid information.

Psychology and perception

A considerable body of work exists examining the relationship between human psychology and the perception and interpretation of informational signals.[56,81,82] Evidence suggests that there are limits on the number of informational signals that can be remembered or processed simultaneously (approximately five to seven), and that the perception of urgency is highly dependent on the nature of the alarm sound. The implication is that alarms should be limited in number and should be as specific as possible. Unfortunately, this is not the case for the modern operating room environment, which can have dozens of potential alarm sources. A study of the response of attending anesthesiologists to alarms found a significant difference between the "clinical urgency" of an alarm, as determined by an independent committee of experts, and the "perceived urgency" of the alarm reported by the study subjects.[83] Furthermore, the test subjects were able to correctly identify the alarm sound (i.e. the source of the alarm) only 33 percent of the time. Similar discordance between the perceived and actual urgency of 13 commonly used OR alarms has also been reported.[84]

One solution to this problem of perceived urgency is the development of structured alarm systems. These impose a categorical/hierarchal relationship on medical equipment alarms, modeled on that used in the civilian and military aircraft industries. Alarms are divided into *warnings, cautions*, and *advisories* based on the potential harm to the patient indicated by the alarm condition.[85,86] The IEC uses *high, medium*, and *low priority* terminology to refer to the same concepts. Determination of which priority an alarm should be assigned is made by a primitive expert system that attempts to prefilter alarm data to reduce the amount of cognitive processing that needs to be done by the attending clinician.

Emerging technologies

Device manufacturers, researchers, and engineers are now focusing on the integration of the many alarms present in a modern operating room or ICU into a single unified alarm system. The goal is to minimize the distraction and inattention caused by having a multitude of alerts, as well to minimize the number of false alarms. The primary tools to accomplish this goal are expert systems that use some combination of data mining, closed-loop feedback techniques, and fuzzy logic to process alarm data from multiple sources before presenting it to the end user. *Fuzzy logic* is a term from the artificial intelligence field that refers to nonbinary decision-making algorithms.

This was demonstrated in an expert system that combined data from seven different patient monitors with fuzzy logic, based on the responses of five expert physicians to a questionnaire.[87] The result was that fewer than 1 percent of alarms reported by the expert system were false, compared with 75 percent of those that were reported by a standard monitor. The sensitivity of the expert system was 92 percent with a positive predictive value of 97 percent, versus 31 percent and 79 percent, respectively, for the standard monitor. Another group described the use of population theory and decision trees to validate conventional alarms by analogy to hypothesis testing.[88] In this model, alarms are divided into "relevant" and "nonrelevant," with the null hypothesis being "the current alarm is clinically relevant." Using a set of test data consisting of several hundred physiologic measurements, the researchers were able to demonstrate a sensitivity of 94.6 percent for clinically relevant events, with a reduction in the false alarm rate by 56.4 percent.

Expert systems depend, to some extent, on test data for developing an accurate model, making data mining techniques useful.[89] In this approach, large sets of clinical and physiologic data for various parameters are analyzed to find interrelationships that correlate with potentially hazardous conditions. The relationships that are found are then used to derive rules that are codified in the alarm system to modify the severity and priority of the various alarms.

Rapid advances in computer hardware are making new modalities, such as haptic interfaces, heads-up displays, ecological interfaces, and sonification, possible. *Haptic* refers to the use of touch as a modality for conveying information. A prototype tactile display has been developed that uses vibrating motors strapped to either the forearm or waist to alert the anesthesiologist to changes in clinical condition.[90,91] This "vibro-tactile" alarm was as easy to learn as an audible alarm but had a better identification rate for clinically significant changes in heart rate.[92]

Sonification refers to the process of converting sensed or calculated data into a continuous auditory stream. Unlike conventional auditory alarms, sonification can provide continuous background information on the state of the monitored parameter, without disrupting foreground focus. Sonification is already in widespread use in pulse oximeters that produce continual audible sounds with each pulse wave to indicate heart rate and at a pitch that conveys blood oxygen saturation information. Extension of sonification to other parameters such as respiratory rate and capnography has also been proposed.[93]

Finally, heads-up or head-mounted displays (Figure 35.4) overcome some of the limitations of current visual displays by overlaying information directly on the user's field of vision.[75] Results of experiments with such displays in anesthesia simulators have been mixed. Although they increase peripheral awareness of patient status, they were not found to improve detection of alarm conditions.[94] An alternative approach to improving visual alarms is through the use of so-called ecological interfaces or metaphor graphics.[73] These advanced techniques integrate the display of lower-level measures in a way

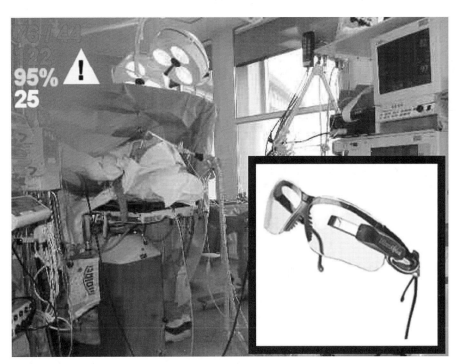

Figure 35.4. Head-mounted anesthesia display. A monocular display device mounted on safety glasses integrates physiologic data and alerts into the clinician's field of vision.

that makes higher-order physiologic functions graphically intuitive (e.g. using the area of a rectangle to represent tidal volume/respiration rate).[95] This novel presentation of data has the potential to decrease clinician response time to alarm conditions.[96,97]

Computer-assisted medication delivery

Advances in modern monitoring and anesthesia delivery have taken much of the guesswork out of anesthesia practice. However, anesthesia still remains something of an art, with some degree of trial and error and practitioner-dependent performance. To reduce the variability between practitioners and to quickly account for differences in pharmacodynamics and pharmacokinetics in different patients, computer systems have been employed to optimize anesthesia delivery.

Target-controlled infusions

Most medications are administered using weight-based dosing that is expected to achieve a certain effect in a given patient. Because most agents have limited clinical durations of action, repeat dosing is necessary to maintain effect. Intermittent bolus dosing to maintain effects may result in significant periods of time where the drug levels are more or less than desired (Figure 35.5). To maintain more stable effects and increase practitioner convenience, infusion of agents (with or without a loading dose) is used. Standard infusion devices typically allow weight-based dosing, but initial settings and subsequent adjustments depend on clinical judgment and patient response as observed by the practitioner.

With target-controlled infusion (TCI), clinicians choose a desired concentration (typically in plasma) of agent, and a

computer-driven infusion pump (Figure 35.6) calculates the dose and timing of medication based on patient parameters (e.g. weight, age) provided to it. Computer software allows complex modeling of the pharmacokinetics of the agents being delivered to predict plasma or effect-site concentrations so the target concentration is reached quickly (with minimal undershoot and overshoot) and maintained steadily over time despite accumulation, redistribution, and elimination. A commonly used model is a three-compartment model consisting of a central compartment (e.g. intravascular plasma), a rapidly equilibrating peripheral compartment (e.g. brain), and a slowly equilibrating peripheral compartment (e.g. fat).[98] Rate constants describe the movement of agent between compartments and

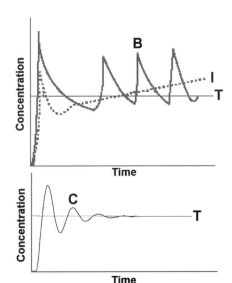

Figure 35.5. Drug concentrations by methods of delivery. Computer-controlled infusion (C) has potential to maintain target (T) concentrations more reliably than manual intermittent bolus (B) or manually controlled infusion (I) methods.

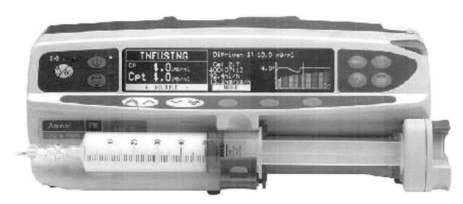

Figure 35.6. Target-controlled infusion (TCI) device – a specialized infusion pump for TCI of propofol (Diprifusor, AstraZeneca, London, UK).

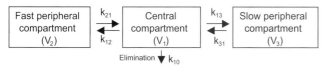

Figure 35.7. Target-controlled infusion model. A three-compartment model used for prediction of pharmacokinetics of drugs that distribute in compartments of estimated volume (V) and redistribute between compartments (and are eliminated) with rate constants (k).

elimination of active agent from the body (Figure 35.7). The rate constants are determined for different agents and are influenced by the patient parameters entered into the system.

Closed-loop medication delivery

TCI is an open-loop system because of its lack of feedback. A closed-loop system (CLS) uses feedback of the current patient state to influence subsequent agent delivery. An analagous concept is the delivery of volatile anesthetics, in which a vaporizer set to a certain concentration will add less and less volatile agent to the system per time period as the actual concentration in the expired alveolar gas that passes through it approaches the set concentration. Intravenous agents cannot be readily controlled in this manner because plasma concentrations of drugs are difficult to measure in a continuous and timely fashion. To close the loop, a source of feedback is needed. Such feedback allows for adaptive control of the infusion, whereby knowledge of the state of the set parameter is used to modify the infusion rate (Figure 35.8). Without a computer-aided CLS, such feedback is from the eyes and ears of the practitioner, who is constantly watching and listening.

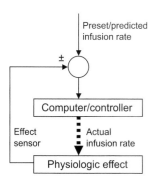

Figure 35.8. Adaptive (closed-loop) control system. A pharmacokinetic model is used to calculate an initial infusion rate, which is then continuously modified by a control function based on feedback from sensor at actual or surrogate effect site, which is compared to the target (goal) effect.

To create an automated closed-loop infusion system that does not require as much human intervention, an electronic sensor is needed to determine the current state of the variable of interest. Using these state data, proportional, integral, derivative-based, or other algorithms are used to further modify the infusion rate. But rather than using a sensor to measure the plasma concentrations of agent as predicted in TCI, the sensor is typically chosen to measure the effect of the drug rather than the concentration of the drug. This accounts for varying pharmacodynamics in individual patients as well as increasing tolerance or sensitivity to agents over time, because the effect (rather than the agent concentration) is targeted. (In this regard, even volatile agents may be better controlled by targeting the clinical effect desired rather than the agent concentration.) Examples of such sensors are heart rate and blood pressure monitors for control of vasoactive agents and analgesics, cerebral monitors (e.g. bispectral index [BIS], EEG, auditory evoked potentials) for controlling sedatives and hypnotics, myography for controlling neuromuscular blocking agents, urometry to control fluid administration, and glucometry to control insulin infusion.[99–101]

Clinical efficacy

Propofol infusion

One of the most studied applications of TCI and commercial development (Figure 35.6) has been its use for infusion of propofol.[102,103] A recent meta-analysis of 20 randomized trials comparing propofol administered by TCI for anesthesia or sedation compared with manual infusion was performed.[104] In these studies, TCI was associated with higher total doses of propofol and marginally higher drug costs, although fewer dose adjustments were required by the clinician during TCI use. No clinically significant differences were found with regard to quality of anesthesia, recovery, or adverse events. However, the reviewers did not find that the available evidence was sufficient to draw a conclusion about the value of TCI in clinical practice.

Few studies have investigated the infusion of propofol using CLS. Three studies using CLS with BIS serving as the feedback sensor in a combined 100 patients found that CLS was comparable to manual infusion in achieving target BIS values, but the CLS groups required less clinician intervention to achieve those targets.[105-107] Whether CLS can achieve enough cost savings, convenience and efficiency, or reduction in adverse events (e.g. awareness under anesthesia) to justify its own cost remains to be seen.

Volatile anesthetics

Some of the earliest reports of CLS were for controlling the delivery of volatile anesthetics using EEG, heart rate, or blood pressure feedback, but these were mostly descriptive in nature.[100] A recent study using BIS to control isoflurane delivery showed that use of CLS resulted in less overall deviation from the target BIS, less time spent outside acceptable limits, and less practitioner intervention than manual control.[108] Two recent studies showed that TCI could be used for inhalation induction with sevoflurane, although it was not necessarily superior to manual control.[109,110]

Neuromuscular blocking agents

Numerous studies of the use of TCI for administering muscle relaxants have been conducted and showed that concentrations of agent could be well-maintained by the algorithms used.[100] More recently, CLS has been applied to administering muscle relaxants. Using electromyographic feedback and various muscle relaxants, the studies suggested that CLS could control the degree of paralysis with good precision and little practitioner intervention. Also reported was the observation that infusion requirements varied at different times in the same patient to achieve the same degree of relaxation, and the CLS readily adapted to such changing pharmacodynamics.[111-113]

Analgesics

Several studies of TCI for delivery of opioids showed that, in some cases, the modeling used did not reliably produce expected target concentrations. TCI has also not been compared directly with manual infusion.[100] Use of CLS for maintenance of analgesia has mostly been in combination with a hypnotic agent. One study of CLS for alfentanil infusion using blood pressure for feedback control during balanced anesthesia found that the system provided analgesia adequate to maintain stable blood pressure.[114]

Other applications

Multiple studies of CLS have been done using blood pressure as feedback control for vasodilator (e.g. sodium nitroprusside) infusion and have shown satisfactory maintenance of target pressures.[100] Vasopressor (e.g. phenylephrine) infusion using CLS was tested in women having spinal anesthesia for elective cesarean section and kept blood pressure within target limits most of the time, although some patients still had hypotensive and/or hypertensive periods.[115]

In critical care settings, investigators have used CLS with blood pressure, left atrial pressure, and urometry to control fluid and blood product administration.[116-118] Glucose control using CLS with glucometry feedback has also been attempted but has not yet been shown to be superior to manual control strategies.[119-121]

Acknowledgment

The authors thank Felicia A. Reilly, MALS, Archivist for the Wood Library-Museum of Anesthesiology, for her help in researching historical alarms.

References

1. Fisher JA, Bromberg IL, Eisen LB. On the design of anaesthesia record forms. *Can J Anaesth* 1994;**41**:973–83.

2. Barham C. Anaesthetic records. *Anaesth Intens Care Med* 2007;**8**:12.

3. American Society of Anesthesiologists Quality Management and Departmental Administration Committee. *Statement on Documentation of Anesthesia Care*. Park Ridge, IL: ASA, 2008.

4. Rowe L, Galletly DC, Henderson RS. Accuracy of text entries within a manually compiled anaesthetic record. *Br J Anaesth* 1992;**68**:381–87.

5. Devitt JH, Rapanos T, Kurrek M, Cohen MM, Shaw M. The anesthetic record: accuracy and completeness. *Can J Anaesth* 1999;**46**(2):122–8.

6. Cook RI, McDonald JS, Nunziata E. Differences between handwritten and automatic blood pressure records. *Anesthesiology* 1989;**71**(3):385–90.

7. Lerou JG, Dirksen R, van Daele M, Nijhuis GM, Crul JF. Automated charting of physiological variables in anesthesia: a quantitative comparison of automated versus handwritten anesthesia records. *J Clin Monit* 1988;**4**(1):37–47.

8. Reich DL, Wood RK Jr, Mattar R, et al. Arterial blood pressure and heart rate discrepancies between handwritten and computerized anesthesia records. *Anesth Analg* 2000;**91**(3): 612–6.

9. Galletly DC, Rowe WL, Henderson RS. The anaesthetic record: a confidential survey on data omission or modification. *Anaesth Intensive Care* 1991;**19**(1):74–8.

10. Block FE. Normal fluctuation of physiologic cardiovascular variables during anesthesia and the phenomenon of "smoothing." *J Clin Monit* 1991;**7**(2):141–5.

11. Benson M, Junger A, Fuchs C, et al. Using an anesthesia information management system to prove a deficit in voluntary reporting of adverse events in a quality assurance program. *J Clin Monit Comput* 2000;**16**:211–7.

12. McKesson EI. The technique of recording the effects of gas-oxygen mixtures, pressures, rebreathing and carbon dioxide, with a summary of the effects. *Curr Res Anesth Anal* 1934;**13**:1–7.

13. Saklad M. A method for the collection and tabulation of of anesthesia data. *Anesth Analg* 1940;**19**:184.

14. Block FE Jr, Burton LW, Rafal MD, et al. The computer-based anesthetic monitors: the Duke Automatic Monitoring Equipment (DAME) system and the microDAME. *J Clin Monit* 1985;**1**:30–51.

15. Klocke H, Trispel S, Rau G, Hatzky U, Daub D. An anesthesia information system for monitoring and record keeping during surgical anesthesia. *J Clin Monit* 1986;**2**(4):246–61.

16. Karliczek GF, de Geus AF, Wiersma G, Oosterhaven S, Jenkins I. Carola, a computer system for automatic documentation in anesthesia. *Int J Clin Monit Comput* 1987;**4**(4):211–21.

17. Dirksen R, Lerou JG, van Daele M, Nijhuis GM, Crul JF. The clinical use of the Ohmeda Automated Anesthesia Record Keeper integrated in the Modulus II Anesthesia System. A preliminary report. *Int J Clin Monit Comput* 1987;**4**(3):135–9.

18. Gage JS, Subramanian S, Dydro JF, Poppers PJ. Automated anesthesia surgery medical record system. *Int J Clin Monit Comput* 1990;**7**(4):259–63.

19. Block FE Jr, Reynolds KM, McDonald JS. The Diatek Arkive "Organizer" patient information management system: experience at a university hospital. *J Clin Monit Comput* 1998;**14**(2):89–94.

20. Piepenbrink JC, Cullen JI Jr, Stafford TJ. A real-time anesthesia record keeping system using video. *J Clin Eng* 1990;**15**(5):391–3.

21. Edsall DW, Deshane P, Giles C, Dick D, Sloan B, Farrow J. Computerized patient anesthesia records: less time and better quality than manually produced anesthesia records. *J Clin Anesth* 1993;**5**(4):275–83.

22. Lerou JG, Dirksen R, van Daele M, Nijhuis GM, Crul JF. Automated charting of physiological variables in anesthesia: a quantitative comparison of automated versus handwritten anesthesia records. *J Clin Monit* 1988;**4**(1):37–47.

23. Reich DL, Wood RK Jr, Mattar R, et al. Arterial blood pressure and heart rate discrepancies between handwritten and computerized anesthesia records. *Anesth Analg* 2000;**91**(3):612–6.

24. Driscoll WD, Columbia MA, Peterfreund RA. An observational study of anesthesia record completeness using an anesthesia information management system. *Anesth Analg* 2007;**104**(6):1454–61.

25. Wax DB, Beilin Y, Hossain S, Lin HM, Reich DL. Manual editing of automatically recorded data in an anesthesia information management system. *Anesthesiology* 2008;**109**(5):811–5.

26. Eden A, Grach M, Goldik Z, et al. The implementation of an anesthesia information management system. *Eur J Anaesthesiol* 2006;**23**(10):882–9.

27. Coleman RL, Stanley T 3rd, Gilbert WC, et al. The implementation and acceptance of an intra-operative anesthesia information management system. *J Clin Monit* 1997;**13**(2):121–8.

28. Quinzio L, Junger A, Gottwald B, et al. User acceptance of an anaesthesia information management system. *Eur J Anaesthesiol* 2003;**20**(12):967–72.

29. Beilin Y, Wax D, Torrillo T, et al. A survey of anesthesiologists' and nurses' attitudes toward the implementation of an anesthesia information management system on a labor and delivery floor. *Int J Obstet Anesth* 2009;**18**(1):22–7.

30. O'Reilly M, Talsma A, Van Riper S, Kheterpal S, Burney R. An anesthesia information system designed to provide physician-specific feedback improves timely administration of prophylactic antibiotics. *Anesth Analg* 2006;**103**(4):908–12.

31. Wax DB, Beilin Y, Levin M, Chadha N, Krol M, Reich DL. The effect of an interactive visual reminder in an anesthesia information management system on timeliness of prophylactic antibiotic administration. *Anesth Analg* 2007;**104**(6):1462–6.

32. St. Jacques P, Sanders N, Patel N, Talbot TR, Deshpande JK, Higgins M. Improving timely surgical antibiotic prophylaxis redosing administration using computerized record prompts. *Surg Infect (Larchmt)* 2005;**6**(2):215–21.

33. Kooij FO, Klok T, Hollmann MW, Kal JE. Decision support increases guideline adherence for prescribing postoperative nausea and vomiting prophylaxis. *Anesth Analg* 2008;**106**(3):893–8.

34. Sanborn KV, Castro J, Kuroda M, Thys DM. Detection of intraoperative incidents by electronic scanning of computerized anesthesia records. Comparison with voluntary reporting. *Anesthesiology* 1996;**85**(5):977–87.

35. Benson M, Junger A, Fuchs C, et al. Using an anesthesia information management system to prove a deficit in voluntary reporting of adverse events in a quality assurance program. *J Clin Monit Comput* 2000;**16**(3):211–7.

36. Merry AF, Webster CS, Mathew DJ. A new, safety-oriented, integrated drug administration and automated anesthesia record system. *Anesth Analg* 2001;**93**(2):385–90.

37. Webster CS, Merry AF, Gander PH, Mann NK. A prospective, randomised clinical evaluation of a new safety-orientated injectable drug administration system in comparison with conventional methods. *Anaesthesia* 2004;**59**(1):80–7.

38. Nolen AL, Rodes WD 2nd. Bar-code medication administration system for anesthetics: effects on documentation and billing. *Am J Health Syst Pharm* 2008;**65**(7):655–9.

39. Allard J, Dzwonczyk R, Yablok D, Block FE Jr, McDonald JS. Effect of automatic record keeping on vigilance and record keeping time. *Br J Anaesth* 1995;**74**(5):619–26.

40. Loeb RG. Manual record keeping is not necessary for anesthesia vigilance. *J Clin Monit* 1995;**11**(1):5–8.

41. Reich DL, Kahn RA, Wax D, Palvia T, Galati M, Krol M. Development of a module for point-of-care charge capture and submission using an anesthesia information management system. *Anesthesiology* 2006;**105**(1):179–86.

42. Spring SF, Sandberg WS, Anupama S, Walsh JL, Driscoll WD, Raines DE. Automated documentation error detection and notification improves anesthesia billing performance. *Anesthesiology* 2007;**106**(1):157–63.

43. Kheterpal S, Gupta R, Blum JM, Tremper KK, O'Reilly M, Kazanjian PE. Electronic reminders improve procedure documentation compliance and professional fee reimbursement. *Anesth Analg* 2007;**104**(3):592–7.

44. Gibby GL, Paulus DA, Sirota DJ, et al. Computerized pre-anesthetic evaluation results in additional abstracted comorbidity diagnoses. *J Clin Monit* 1997;**13**(1):35–41.

45. Reich DL, Galati M, Krol M, Bodian CA, Kahn RA. A mission-based productivity compensation model for an academic anesthesiology department. *Anesth Analg* 2008;**107**(6):1981–8.

46. Lubarsky DA, Sanderson IC, Gilbert WC, et al. Using an anesthesia information management system as a cost containment tool. Description and validation. *Anesthesiology* 1997;**86**(5):1161–9.

47. Epstein RH, Gratch DM, Grunwald Z. Development of a scheduled drug diversion surveillance system based on an analysis of atypical drug transactions. *Anesth Analg* 2007;**105**(4):1053–60.

48. Warner MA, Monk TG. The impact of lack of standardized definitions on the specialty. *Anesthesiology* 2007;**107**(2):198–9.

49. Egger Halbeis CB, Epstein RH, Macario A, Pearl RG, Grunwald Z. Adoption of anesthesia information management systems by academic departments in the United States. *Anesth Analg* 2008;**107**(4):1323–9.

50. Feldman JM. Do anesthesia information systems increase malpractice exposure? Results of a survey. *Anesth Analg* 2004;**99**(3):840–3.

51. Vigoda MM, Lubarsky DA. Failure to recognize loss of incoming data in an anesthesia record-keeping system may have increased medical liability. *Anesth Analg* 2006;**102**(6):1798–802.

52. Muravchick S, Caldwell JE, Epstein RH, et al. Anesthesia information management system implementation: a practical guide. *Anesth Analg* 2008;**107**(5):1598–608.

53. Dorsch JA, Dorsch SE. *Alarm Devices. Understanding Anesthesia Equipment*, 5th ed. Philadelphia: Lippincott Williams & Wilkins, 2008, pp. 828–35.

54. Hagenouw RR. Should we be alarmed by our alarms? *Curr Opin Anaesthesiol* 2007;**20**(6):590–4.

55. Kerr JH. Symposium on anaesthetic equipment. Warning devices. *Br J Anaesth* 1985;**57**(7):696–708.

56. Edworthy J, Hellier E. Alarms and human behaviour: implications for medical alarms. *Br J Anaesth* 2006;**97**(1):12–7.

57. Edworthy J, Hellier E. Fewer but better auditory alarms will improve patient safety. *Qual Saf Health Care* 2005;**14**(3):212–5.

58. Esplen JR. A device giving warning of impending failure of the nitrous oxide or oxygen supply. *Br J Anaesth* 1956;**28**(5):226–7.

59. Hill EF. Another warning device. *Br J Anaesth* 1956;**28**(5):228–9.

60. Lamont A, Fairley HB. A pressure-sensitive ventilator alarm. *Anesthesiology* 1965;**26**:359–61.

61. Sawa T, Ikezono E. A respirator alarm for general use. *Anesthesiology* 1970;**33**(6):658–61.

62. Hedley-Whyte J. Monitoring and alarms – philosophy and practice. In Dinnick OP, Thompson PW, eds. *Baillière's Clinical Anesthesiology: International Practice and Research*. London: Baillière Tindall, 1988, pp. 379–89.

63. Olympio M. APSF workshop recommends new standards. *Anesthesia Patient Safety Foundation Newsletter*. 2004–2005;**42**:52–53.

64. American Society of Anesthesiologists. *Standards for Basic Anesthetic Monitoring*. Park Ridge, IL: ASA, 2005.

65. International Electrotechnical Commission. IEC 60601-1-8: General requirements, tests and guidance for alarm systems in medical electrical equipment and medical electrical systems, IEC 60601-1-8, 2006.

66. Goldman JM, Whitehead SF, Weininger S. Eliciting clinical requirements for the Medical Device Plug-and-Play (MD PnP) Interoperability Program. *Anesth Analg* 2006;**102**:S1–54.

67. Sanderson PM, Watson MO, Russell WJ. Advanced patient monitoring displays: tools for continuous informing. *Anesth Analg* 2005;**101**(1):161–8.

68. Wallace MS, Ashman MN, Matjasko MJ. Hearing acuity of anesthesiologists and alarm detection. *Anesthesiology* 1994;**81**(1):13–28.

69. Morris RW, Montano SR. Response times to visual and auditory alarms during anaesthesia. *Anaesth Intensive Care* 1996;**24**(6):682–4.

70. Leung YK, Smith S, Parker S, Martin R. Learning and retention of auditory warnings. International Conference on Auditory Display, Palo Alto, CA, Nov. 2–5, 1997.

71. Momtahan K, Hetu R, Tansley B. Audibility and identification of auditory alarms in the operating room and intensive care unit. *Ergonomics* 1993;**36**(10):1159–76.

72. McNeer RR, Bohorquez J, Ozdamar O, Varon AJ, Barach P. A new paradigm for the design of audible alarms that convey urgency information. *J Clin Monit Comput* 2007;**21**(6):353–63.

73. Sanderson P, Wee A, Seah E, Lacherez P, eds. Auditory alarms, medical standards, and urgency. 12th International Conference on Auditory Display, London, June 20–23, 2006.

74. Sanderson PM, Wee A, Lacherez P. Learnability and discriminability of melodic medical equipment alarms. *Anaesthesia* 2006;**61**(2):142–7.

75. Sanderson P. The multimodal world of medical monitoring displays. *Appl Ergon* 2006;**37**(4):501–12.

76. Block FE Jr, Nuutinen L, Ballast B. Optimization of alarms: a study on alarm limits, alarm sounds, and false alarms, intended to reduce annoyance. *J Clin Monit Comput* 1999;**15**(2):75–83.

77. Kestin IG, Miller BR, Lockhart CH. Auditory alarms during anesthesia monitoring. *Anesthesiology* 1988;**69**(1):106–9.

78. Lawless ST. Crying wolf: false alarms in a pediatric intensive care unit. *Crit Care Med* 1994;**22**(6):981–5.

79. Watson M, Sanderson P, Russell WJ. Tailoring reveals information requirements: the case of anesthesia alarms. *Interacting with Computers* 2004;**16**(2):271–93.

80. Takla G, Petre JH, Doyle DJ, Horibe M, Gopakumaran B. The problem of artifacts in patient monitor data during surgery: a clinical and methodological review. *Anesth Analg* 2006;**103**(5):1196–204.

81. Edworthy J. The design and implementation of non-verbal auditory warnings. *Appl Ergon* 1994;**25**(4):202–10.

82. Edworthy J, Hellier E. Auditory warnings in noisy environments. *Noise Health* 2000;**2**(6):27–40.

83. Finley GA, Cohen AJ. Perceived urgency and the anaesthetist: responses to common operating room monitor alarms. *Can J Anaesth* 1991;**38**(8):958–64.

84. Mondor TA, Finley GA. The perceived urgency of auditory warning alarms used in the hospital operating room is inappropriate. *Can J Anaesth* 2003;**50**(3):221–8.

85. Lang S. Vitalert 3200 capnometer alarm. *Can J Anaesth* 1996;**43**(9):985–6.

86. Schreiber PJ. Letters to the Editor: Anesthesia Machines(2). *Anesthesia Patient Safety Foundation Newsletter*, Summer 1996.

87. Oberli C, Urzua J, Saez C, et al. An expert system for monitor alarm integration. *J Clin Monit Comput* 1999;**15**(1):29–35.

88. Sieben W, Gather U, eds. Classifying alarms in intensive care – analogy to hypothesis testing. *Proceedings of the 11th Conference on Artificial Intelligence in Medicine*. Amsterdam: Springer-Verlag, 2007.

89. Murias G, Sales B, Blanch L. Alarms: transforming a nuisance into a reliable tool. In Vincent JL, ed. *Intensive Care Medicine Annual Update*. New York: Springer, 2007, pp. 950–7.

90. Ng G, Barralon P, Schwarz SW, Dumont G, Ansermino JM. Evaluation of a tactile display around the waist for physiological monitoring under different clinical workload conditions. *Conf Proc IEEE Eng Med Biol Soc* 2008;**2008**:1288–91.

91. Ford S, Daniels J, Lim J, et al. A novel vibrotactile display to improve the performance of anesthesiologists in a simulated critical incident. *Anesth Analg* 2008;**106**(4):1182–8.

92. Ng JY, Man JC, Fels S, Dumont G, Ansermino JM. An evaluation of a vibro-tactile display prototype for physiological monitoring. *Anesth Analg* 2005;**101**(6):1719–24.

93. Watson M, Sanderson P. Sonification supports eyes-free respiratory monitoring and task time-sharing. *Hum Factors* 2004;**46**(3):497–517.

94. Sanderson PM, Watson MO, Russell WJ, et al. Advanced auditory displays and head-mounted displays: advantages and disadvantages for monitoring by the distracted anesthesiologist. *Anesth Analg* 2008;**106**(6):1787–97.

95. Cole WG, Stewart JG. Human performance evaluation of a metaphor graphic display for respiratory data. *Methods Inf Med* 1994;**33**(4):390–6.

96. Michels P, Gravenstein D, Westenskow DR. An integrated graphic data display improves detection and identification of critical events during anesthesia. *J Clin Monit* 1997;**13**(4):249–59.

97. Blike GT, Surgenor SD, Whalen K. A graphical object display improves anesthesiologists' performance on a simulated diagnostic task. *J Clin Monit Comput* 1999;**15**(1):37–44.

98. Shafer SL, Gregg KM. Algorithms to rapidly achieve and maintain stable drug concentrations at the site of drug effect with a computer-controlled infusion pump. *J Pharmacokinet Biopharmaceut* 1992;**20**: 147–69.

99. Fields AM, Fields KM, Cannon JW. Closed-loop systems for drug delivery. *Curr Opin Anaesthesiol* 2008;**21**(4):446–51.

100. O'Hara DA, Bogen DK, Noordergraaf A. The use of computers for controlling the delivery of anesthesia. *Anesthesiology* 1992;**77**(3):563–81.

101. Kenny GN, Sutcliffe NP. Target-controlled infusions: stress free anesthesia? *J Clin Anesth* 1996;**8**(3 Suppl):15S–20S.

102. Tackley RM, Lewis GT, Prys-Roberts C, Boaden RW, Dixon J, Harvey JT. Computer controlled infusion of propofol. *Br J Anaesth* 1989;**62**(1):46–53.

103. Glen JB. The development of 'Diprifusor': a TCI system for propofol. *Anaesthesia* 1998;**53 Suppl 1**:13–21.

104. Leslie K, Clavisi O, Hargrove J. Target-controlled infusion versus manually-controlled infusion of propofol for general anaesthesia or sedation in adults. *Cochrane Database Syst Re.* 2008 Jul **16**; CD006059

105. Absalom AR, Kenny GN. Closed-loop control of propofol anaesthesia using bispectral index: performance assessment in patients receiving computer-controlled propofol and manually controlled remifentanil infusions for minor surgery. *Br J Anaesth* 2003;**90**(6):737–41.

106. Puri GD, Kumar B, Aveek J. Closed-loop anaesthesia delivery system using bispectral index: a performance assessment study. *Anaesth Intensive Care* 2007;**35**(3):357–62.

107. De Smet T, Struys MM, Neckebroek MM, Van Den Hauwe K, Bonte S, Mortier EP. The accuracy and clinical feasibility of a new Bayesian-based closed-loop control system for propofol administration using the bispectral index as a controlled variable. *Anesth Analg* 2008;**107**(4):1200–10.

108. Locher S, Stadler KS, Boehlen T, et al. A new closed-loop control system for isoflurane using bispectral index outperforms manual control. *Anesthesiology* 2004;**101**(3):591–602.

109. Nouette-Gaulain K, Lemoine P, Cros AM, Sztark F. Induction of anaesthesia with target-controlled inhalation of sevoflurane in adults with the ZEUS anaesthesia machine. *Ann Fr Anesth Reanim* 2005;**24**(7):802–6.

110. Fritsch N, Nouette-Gaulain K, Bordes M, Semjen F, Meymat Y, Cros AM. Target-controlled inhalation induction with sevoflurane in children: a prospective pilot study. *Paediatr Anaesth* 2009;**19**(2):126–32.

111. Assef SJ, Lennon RL, Jones KA, Burke MJ, Behrens TL. A versatile, computer-controlled, closed-loop system for continuous infusion of muscle relaxants. *Mayo Clin Proc* 1993;**68**(11):1074–80.

112. Schumacher PM, Stadler KS, Wirz R, Leibundgut D, Pfister CA, Zbinden AM. Model-based control of neuromuscular block using mivacurium: design and clinical verification. *Eur J Anaesthesiol* 2006;**23**(8):691–9.

113. Eleveld DJ, Proost JH, Wierda JM. Evaluation of a closed-loop muscle relaxation control system. *Anesth Analg* 2005;**101**(3):758–64.

114. Luginbühl M, Bieniok C, Leibundgut D, Wymann R, Gentilini A, Schnider TW. Closed-loop control of mean arterial blood pressure during surgery with alfentanil: clinical evaluation of a novel model-based predictive controller. *Anesthesiology* 2006;**105**(3):462–70.

115. Ngan Kee WD, Tam YH, Khaw KS, Ng FF, Critchley LA, Karmakar MK. Closed-loop feedback computer-controlled infusion of phenylephrine for maintaining blood pressure during spinal anaesthesia for caesarean section: a preliminary descriptive study. *Anaesthesia* 2007;**62**(12):1251–6.

116. Bowman RJ, Westenskow DR. A microcomputer-based fluid infusion system for the resuscitation of burn patients. *IEEE Trans Biomed Eng* 1981;**28**(6):475–9.

117. Slate JB, Sheppard LC. Automatic control of blood pressure by drug infusion. *IEEE Proc* 1982;**129**:639–45.

118. Hoskins SL, Elgjo GI, Lu J, et al. Closed-loop resuscitation of burn shock. *J Burn Care Res* 2006;**27**(3):377–85.

119. Chee F, Fernando T, van Heerden PV. Closed-loop control of blood glucose levels in critically ill patients. *Anaesth Intensive Care* 2002;**30**(3):295–307.

120. Chee F, Fernando T, van Heerden PV. Closed-loop glucose control in critically ill patients using continuous glucose monitoring system (CGMS) in real time. *IEEE Trans Inf Technol Biomed* 2003;**7**(1):43–53.

121. Chase JG, Shaw GM, Lin J, et al. Targeted glycemic reduction in critical care using closed-loop control. *Diabetes Technol Ther* 2005;**7**(2):274–82.

Appendix: Monitoring recommendations for common types of surgical procedures

Samuel DeMaria, Jr., Timothy Mooney, and Jenny Kam

(see key at bottom for interpretation of cell shading)

Procedure	ECG	NIBP Cuff	Pulse Oximeter	ETCO2 Monitor	Temperature Probe	Arterial Line	PA Catheter	TEE	EEG	SSEP/MEP/Evoked Potentials	Level of Consciousness Monitor (e.g. BIS)	Transcranial Doppler	Intracranial Pressure	Neuromuscular monitor
Standard operating room procedures														
Cystoscopy/transurethral procedures	●	●	●	●										
Prostatic surgery	●	●	●	●	●									
Lithotripsy	●	●	●	●										
Thyroid/parathyroid surgery	●	●	●	●										
Adrenal surgery	●	●	●	●		●								
Ophthalmic procedures	●	●	●	●										
Nasal surgery/sinus endoscopy	●	●	●	●										
Orthognathic and maxillofacial reconstruction	●	●	●	●	●									
Neck dissection	●	●	●	●										
Myocutaneous flap/laryngectomy/glossectomy	●	●	●	●	●	●								
Ear surgery	●	●	●	●										
Large orthopedic repairs	●	●	●	●	●									
Laparoscopic abdominal procedures	●	●	●	●	●									
Open abdominal procedures	●	●	●	●	●									
Trauma surgery	●	●	●	●	●	●	●	●						
Cardiac surgery														

Procedure	ECG	NIBP Cuff	Pulse Oximeter	ETCO2 Monitor	Temperature Probe	Arterial Line	PA Catheter	TEE	EEG	SSEP/MEP/Evoked Potentials	Level of Consciousness Monitor (e.g. BIS)	Transcranial Doppler	Intracranial Pressure	Neuromuscular monitor
Valvular repair/replacement														
CABG														
Pericardial procedures														
VAD placement														
Cryoablative procedures														
Aneurysmal/dissection repairs														
Cardiac transplantation														
Thoracic surgery														
One-lung ventilation														
Esophageal surgery														
Limited thoracotomy														
Video-assisted procedures														
Mediastinoscopy														
Bronchoscopy														
Lung transplantation														

	ECG	NIBP Cuff	Pulse Oximeter	ETCO2 Monitor	Temperature Probe	Arterial Line	PA Catheter	TEE	EEG	SSEP/MEP/Evoked Potentials	Level of Consciousness Monitor (e.g. BIS)	Transcranial Doppler	Intracranial Pressure	Neuromuscular monitor
Vascular surgery														
Endovascular repair of aorta														
Open abdominal aortic aneurysm repair														
Peripheral vascular bypass														
Carotid endarterectomy														
Vascular access creation														
Neurosurgery														
Craniotomy														
Posterior fossa surgery														
Aneurysm repairs														
Ventriculo-peritoneal shunt														
Stereotactic surgery														
Head trauma procedures														
Spine surgery														
Pituitary surgery														
Solid organ transplantation														

| | Monitor | | | | | | | | | | | | | |
Procedure	ECG	NIBP Cuff	Pulse Oximeter	ETCO2 Monitor	Temperature Probe	Arterial Line	PA Catheter	TEE	EEG	SSEP/MEP/ Evoked Potentials	Level of Consciousness Monitor (e.g. BIS)	Transcranial Doppler	Intracranial Pressure	Neuromuscular monitor
Liver transplantation	■	■	■	■	■	■	■	■						■
Renal transplantation	■	■	■	■	■	■								■
Bowel and pancreas transplantation	■	■	■	■	■	■								■
Pediatric setting		■	■	■										
Gastroschisis	■	■	■	■	■	■								
Omphalocoele	■	■	■	■	■	■								
Ductus arteriosus ligation	■	■	■	■	■	■								
Major abdominal or orthopedic case	■	■	■	■	■	■								
Congenital diaphragmatic hernia repair	■	■	■	■	■	■								
Tracheoesophageal fistula repair	■	■	■	■	■	■								
Acute epiglottitis	■	■	■	■	■									
Tonsillectomy and adenoidectomy	■	■	■	■	■									
Myringotomy and tympanostomy tube insertion	■	■	■	■	■									
Scoliosis repair	■	■	■	■	■	■								
Lumbar puncture, hepatic or renal biopsy	■	■	■	■										
Dental procedures	■	■	■	■										

Obstetrics/gynecolgy	ECG	NIBP Cuff	Pulse Oximeter	ETCO2 Monitor	Temperature Probe	Arterial Line	PA Catheter	TEE	EEG	SSEP/MEP/Evoked Potentials	Level of Consciousness Monitor (e.g. BIS)	Transcranial Doppler	Intracranial Pressure	Neuromuscular monitor
Cesarean section (nonemergent, neuraxial anesthetic)	■	■	■	■	■									■
Emergent cesarean section	■	■	■	■	■	■		■						■
Continuous labor analgesia	■	■	■											
General surgery for the parturient	■	■	■	■	■									■
Nonemergent gynecological procedures	■	■	■	■	■									■
Pelvic exenteration/tumor debulking	■	■	■	■	■	■								■
Ambulatory anesthesia	■	■	■	■										■
Hernia repair	■	■	■	■	■									■
Brief orthopedic procedures	■	■	■	■	■									■
Monitored anesthesia care	■	■	■	■	■									
Facial plastic surgery	■	■	■	■	■									■
Breast surgery and biopsy	■	■	■	■	■									■
PACU														

Monitor

	ECG	NIBP Cuff	Pulse Oximeter	ETCO2 Monitor	Temperature Probe	Arterial Line	PA Catheter	TEE	EEG	SSEP/MEP/ Evoked Potentials	Level of Consciousness Monitor (e.g. BIS)	Transcranial Doppler	Intracranial Pressure	Neuromuscular monitor
Shock patient														
Intubated patient														
Healthy ambulatory patient														
MRI suite														
Pediatric general anesthesia														
Interventional radiology and catheterization laboratory														
Neurointerventional procedures														
Vertebroplasty														
Cardiac catheterization														
Ablative procedures														

Monitor

Always
Sometimes
Rarely

Index